Geriatric Palliative Care

Geriatric Palliative Care

Edited by

R. SEAN MORRISON, MD

Hermann Merkin Professor of Palliative Care
Associate Professor
Hertzberg Palliative Care Institute
Brookdale Department of Geriatrics & Adult Development
Mount Sinai School of Medicine
New York, New York

DIANE E. MEIER, MD

Catherine Gaisman Professor of Medical Ethics
Professor
Hertzberg Palliative Care Institute
Brookdale Department of Geriatrics & Adult Development
Mount Sinai School of Medicine
New York, New York

and Deputy Editor

CAROL CAPELLO, PhD

Associate Director of Geriatric Medical Education
Division of Geriatrics and Gerontology
Weill Medical College of Cornell University
New York, New York

OXFORD
UNIVERSITY PRESS
2003

OXFORD
UNIVERSITY PRESS

Oxford   New York
Auckland   Bangkok   Buenos Aires   Cape Town   Chennai
Dar es Salaam   Delhi   Hong Kong   Istanbul   Karachi   Kolkata
Kuala Lumpur   Madrid   Melbourne   Mexico City   Mumbai
Nairobi   São Paulo   Shanghai   Taipei   Tokyo   Toronto

Published by Oxford University Press, Inc.
198 Madison Avenue, New York, New York, 10016
http://www.oup-usa.org

Library of Congress Cataloging-in-Publication Data
Geriatric palliative care / edited by R. Sean Morrison and Diane E. Meier ; deputy editor,
Carol Capello.
p. ; cm.
Includes bibliographical references and index.
ISBN 0-19-514191-1
1. Palliative treatment. 2. Terminal care. 3. Aged—Care. 4. Geriatrics. I. Morrison, R.
Sean (Rolfe Sean) II. Meier, Diane E. III. Capello, Carol.
[DNLM: 1. Geriatrics—methods. 2. Palliative Care—Aged. 3. Terminal Care—Aged.
WT 100 G366372 2003]
R726.8 .G475 2003
616′.029′0846—dc21   2002034607

2 4 6 8 9 7 5 3 1

Printed in the United States of America
on acid-free paper

To our parents,
Rolfe and Sylvia Morrison
and Paul and Louise Meier,
who taught us a love of science
and of service,

and

to our teacher Robert N. Butler
for his leadership,
his compassion,
and his commitment to
geriatrics and palliative care

Foreword

This important book represents the convergence of two radical concepts that have enormous potential to improve the quality of health care. These two concepts are geriatric medicine and palliative care. Hardly thought of by most people as radical, they represent both a reaffirmation and a rethinking of the fundamental values and approaches of medical care as it exists in the explosion of biomedical science facing us at the beginning of the twenty-first century.

Geriatric medicine emerged from the stunning observation about the increasing life expectancy of Americans and those in other developed countries. This life expectancy continues to increase at a rate that outstrips all of the predictions of demographers and economists trying to keep up with the health insurance and social security implications of increasing survival. This dramatic increase in life expectancy is an enormous success, attributable in large part to advances in civilization, standards of living, public health, and to some extent, probably increasingly, medical care intervention among the surviving elderly. Geriatric medicine recognized the fundamental physiologic processes of aging, and that physicians caring for older people needed to move beyond the single-disease, single-organ system, or single-specialty approach, to examine the interaction of multiple chronic illnesses, multiple medications, and highly variable physiologic status at the center of increasing risk. Twenty years ago, geriatricians more often than not were fending off invasive specialists, arguing that intrusive technologies were likely to be ineffective in the very old and that patients and families preferred a dignified approach to, and acceptance of, mortality. Now, however, the geriatrician's role more often than not is convincing reluctant specialists or interventionalists that a 95-year-old woman has a pretty good chance of benefiting from a surgical procedure or rehabilitation. Geriatrics, increasingly, is about survival and convincing clinicians not to be fatalistic when facing elderly patients but to seek energetically and assertively for treatable problems to improve quality of life and function. However, the base of all of this is the patient, on whose dignity and humanity all clinical interactions must be focused. At the center is a relationship. Clinicians have an enormous amount to gain from the rewarding interaction with patients, older people, and their families who are inevitably hugely grateful for someone in the healthcare profession who is willing to listen, to help navigate the complexity of the health-care system and to understand the importance of giving meaning to the outcome, whatever it is.

Palliative care, ironically, is also a "new" specialty emerging from the recognition by some clinicians that all of the wonders of modern medical technology, while they have managed to rescue many people from death, cannot ultimately eradicate mortality. The early leaders in palliative care recognized the important historical roots in medicine and nursing of caring for the dying, relieving pain and suffering, providing succor, answering questions, and abiding with the family at the bedside of a dying patient. This role in the year 2000 is as important as it was in the year 1900. In modern times, medicine is equipped with many more effective diagnostic technologies and therapeutic methods by which to relieve the suffering of the dying, thus making this set of skills even more important. Palliative care originally focused on the extremely important goal of improving the quality of care for patients at the end of life. Its focus was the quality of life for the few remaining days or weeks that a patient might have and respecting individual dignity and humanity. As this field matured over the last decade, it has recognized that predicting when death will come is difficult until the very late stages of certain illnesses. Palliative care has confronted and overturned the assumption that this model is only morally relevant when "nothing else can be done to prolong life." Modern palliative care recognizes that there is a gradual transition and balancing between the appropriateness of attempts to prolong life and vigorous palliative management of symptoms. Both can occur at the same time. Nowhere is this more true, or more important, than in the care of patients in advanced stages of illness.

More than 80% of people who die in our country die after the age of 65, and increasing numbers live well into their 80s and beyond. Thus, the vast majority of people who die each year die not in a rapid trajectory characteristic of metastatic cancer but, rather, of the accumulated insults of multiple degenerative illnesses and frailty. While this trajectory is less predictable, the ultimate prognosis remains very clear. At the center, however, is the patient and clinician, a relationship that allows a partnership into the most profound moments of life. The clinician creates relationships with patients and families, who are enormously grateful for someone who can answer perplexing questions, listen, serve as a navigator of the complex world of modern health care, and become a companion helping to give meaning to the end of life.

Thus, two radical notions converge, geriatrics and palliative care, each expanding the scope and invigorating the other. This remarkable book has been conceived, planned, and edited by two people who are experts in both fields. They have brought together the nation's most highly regarded experts in every chapter. Sean Morrison and Diane Meier are experienced researchers in geriatrics and palliative care, experienced educators, and most importantly experi-

enced clinicians who understand that at the center are the patients and the relationships. This book will become a classic the moment it is released. All of us,
as clinicians, as family members, and ultimately as patients, have been waiting
for it.

Christine K. Cassel, M.D.
Dean, School of Medicine
Oregon Health Sciences University
Portland, Oregon

Preface

Our society is facing the largest public health challenge in its history, growth of the population of older adults. Improvements in public health, antibiotics, and modern medicine have resulted in unprecedented gains in human longevity. In no prior era of human history has such a large number and proportion of the population been older adults, a leap from 5% in 1900 to over 20% by 2030. For most, the years after age 65 are a time of good health, independence, and integration of a life's work and experience. Eventually, however, most of us will develop one or more chronic illnesses with which we will live for many years before we die. Over three-quarters of deaths in the United States are due to chronic diseases of the heart, lungs, brain, and other vital organs. Even cancer, which accounts for only one-quarter of U.S. deaths, has become a chronic, multi-year illness for the majority of sufferers. It is this period of life with many years of serious illness that is the focus of this book.

Palliative care is interdisciplinary care that aims to relieve suffering and improve quality of life for patients with advanced illness and their families. It is ideally initiated at the time of diagnosis of any serious or life-threatening illness, independent of prognosis, and is delivered in concert with curative or life-prolonging efforts, provided these latter therapies are beneficial to the patient. The integrated delivery of palliative and life-prolonging efforts is not only a rational approach to the care of persons with serious and complex illness but has been shown to reduce suffering, improve satisfaction, reduce hospital costs, and ease transitions through the stages of a progressive illness. All too often, however, patients living through years of serious or advanced illness receive only repeated episodes of short-term life-prolonging efforts, followed in about one-third of cases by a few weeks of end-of-life care in the form of hospice.

In this book, the first devoted to geriatric palliative medicine, we assist physicians to reframe and broaden the medical care that they provide to older adults living with serious and chronic illness. Integrative palliative care, as defined above, allows for high-quality, long-term management of advanced illness, up to and including the period at the end of life. In this context of palliative care, the core precepts of geriatrics and palliative medicine are virtually identical: care is patient-centered, comprehensive, and holistic; patient and family together are the unit of care; high priority is given to enhancing functional independence and quality of life; regular and formal assessment is employed to ensure timely identification and treatment of problems; and an interdisciplinary team approach is required to address the spectrum of needs of patients and their families. The role of both specialties transcends the setting: care is delivered wherever the patient happens to be (home, hospital, nursing home, office), at whatever stage of illness, and for whatever diagnosis. The goal is the right care for the right patient at the right time.

This textbook would not have been possible without the invaluable contributions of many individuals. We are grateful to the staff of Oxford University Press for the encouragement, support, and assistance that they provided during the writing. At Mount Sinai, Carol Capello and Stacey Silberzweig deserve special thanks for handling the multitude of organizational details that a textbook of this magnitude entails. We thank our authors, all of whom are insanely busy individuals, for giving so generously of their time and producing such outstanding chapters. We hope that this book, the product of these collective efforts, contributes to the recognition of the unity of the missions of geriatrics and palliative medicine and in so doing improves the quality of care of our patients.

New York, New York   R.S.M.
                                                                       D.E.M.

Contents

Contributors, xvii

Introduction, xxi
R. Sean Morrison and Diane E. Meier

Part I   Overview: The Social and Cultural Context of Old Age and Frailty

1. Variability in End-of-Life Care in the United States, 3
   John E. Wennberg, Megan McAndrew Cooper, and Susan W. Tolle

2. Developmental Challenges and Opportunities for "Growth": The Inner Life at the End of Life, 17
   Robert N. Butler

3. Assessing Quality of Life and Quality of Dying in the Elderly: Implications for Clinical Practice of Palliative Medicine, 23
   J. Randall Curtis and Donald L. Patrick

4. The Place of Love in the Care of Persons with Advanced Dementia, 30
   Stephen G. Post

5. Artificial Nutrition and Hydration, 36
   Colleen Christmas and Tom Finucane

6. Age, Rationing, and Palliative Care, 46
   Daniel Callahan and Eva Topinková

7. Ethical Aspects of Geriatric Palliative Care, 55
Linda Emanuel, Madelyn A. Iris, and James R. Webster

8. Respecting Diversity, 79
Marion Danis and Risa Lavizzo-Mourey

Part II   Disease- and Syndrome-Specific Aspects of Palliative Care

9. Frailty and Its Implications for Care, 93
Jeremy D. Walston and Linda P. Fried

10. Heart Disease, 110
Julia M. Addington-Hall, Angie Rogers, Anne McCoy, and
J. Simon R. Gibbs

11. Cancer, 123
Natalie R. Sacks and Janet L. Abrahm

12. Stroke: Prognosis, Treatment, and Rehabilitation, 134
Steven R. Flanagan and Stanley Tuhrim

13. Dementia and Neurodegenerative Diseases, 160
Ellen Olson

14. Chronic Lung Disease and Lung Cancer, 173
John P. Krcmarik, Thomas J. Prendergast, E. Wesley Ely, and
James R. Runo

15. End-Stage Renal Disease and Discontinuation of Dialysis, 192
Lewis M. Cohen, Michael J. Germain, and Maura J. Brennan

Part III   Symptom Distress in Older Patients

16. Pain, 205
Bruce A. Ferrell and J. Elizabeth Whiteman

17. Dyspnea, 230
Cynthia X. Pan

18. Gastrointestinal Symptoms, 256
Nigel P. Sykes

19. Fatigue, 271
Deborah Witt Sherman and Marianne LaPorte Matzo

20. Delirium, Anxiety, and Depression, 286
Elizabeth Goy and Linda Ganzini

Part IV   Communication

21. Advance Care Planning for Frail, Older Persons, 307
Joan M. Teno

22. Doctor–Patient Communication, 314
James A. Tulsky

23. Decision Making for the Cognitively Impaired, 332
    Timothy E. Quill and Robert McCann

Part V   Structures of Care for the Chronically Ill with Palliative Care Needs

24. Can We Make the Health-Care System Work? 345
    *Janice Lynch Schuster, Sarah Myers, Susan K. Rogers, Susan C. Emmer,
    and Joanne Lynn*

25. Palliative Care in the Nursing Home, 357
    John M. Carter and Eileen Chichin

26. Family Caregivers: Burdens and Opportunities, 376
    Carol Levine

27. Home Care for Frail, Older Adults, 386
    Knight Steel and Caroline Vitale

28. Hospital-Based Palliative Care, 402
    Daniel Fischberg and Diane E. Meier

    Index, 413

Contributors

JANET L. ABRAHM, M.D.
Associate Professor, Medicine and Anesthesia
Harvard Medical School
Director, Pain and Palliative Care Program
Dana Farber Cancer Institute
Boston, Massachusetts

JULIA M. ADDINGTON-HALL, Ph.D. *hon-*
MFPHM
Professor, Palliative Care Research and Policy
Department of Palliative Care and Policy
King's College London
Weston Education Centre
London, United Kingdom

MAURA J. BRENNAN, M.D.
Director, Geriatric Consultation Program
Baystate Medical Center
Assistant Professor, Tufts University School of
Medicine
Springfield, Massachusetts

ROBERT N. BUTLER, M.D.
President and CEO, International Longevity
Center
New York, New York

DANIEL CALLAHAN, Ph.D.
Director, International Programs
The Hastings Center
Garrison, New York

JOHN M. CARTER, M.D.
Jewish Home and Hospital
New York, New York

EILEEN CHICHIN, Ph.D.
Jewish Home and Hospital
New York, New York

COLLEEN CHRISTMAS, M.D.
Assistant Professor, Medicine
Division of Geriatric Medicine and
Gerontology
Johns Hopkins University
Baltimore, Maryland

LEWIS M. COHEN, M.D.
Associate Professor, Psychiatry
Tufts University Medical Center
Director, The Renal Palliative Care Initiative
Baystate Medical Center
Springfield, Massachusetts

J. RANDALL CURTIS, M.D., M.P.H.
Associate Professor, Medicine
University of Washington
Seattle, Washington

MARION DANIS, M.D.
Head, Section on Ethics and Health Policy
Department of Clinical Bioethics
National Institutes of Health
Bethesda, Maryland

E. WESLEY ELY, M.D.
Associate Professor, Medicine
Allergy, Pulmonary and Critical Care
Health Services Research Center
Vanderbilt University School of Medicine
Nashville, Tennessee

LINDA EMANUEL, M.D., Ph.D.
Professor, Geriatric Medicine
Director, The Buehler Center on Aging
Northwestern's Feinberg School of Medicine
Chicago, Illinois

SUSAN C. EMMER, Esq.
Americans for Better Care of the Dying
Washington, D.C.

BRUCE A. FERRELL, M.D.
Associate Professor
UCLA School of Medicine
Division of Geriatrics
Los Angeles, California

TOM FINUCANE, M.D.
Professor
Johns Hopkins University School of Medicine
Baltimore, Maryland

DANIEL FISCHBERG, M.D., Ph.D.
Professor, Geriatrics and Medicine
Hertzberg Palliative Care Institute of the
Brookdale Department of Geriatric and Adult
   Development
Mount Sinai School of Medicine
New York, New York

STEVEN R. FLANAGAN, M.D.
Vice Chairman, Department of Rehabilitation
   Medicine
Mount Sinai School of Medicine
New York, New York

LINDA P. FRIED, M.D., M.P.H.
Professor and Director
Center on Aging and Health
Johns Hopkins Medical Institute
Baltimore, Maryland

LINDA GANZINI, M.D.
Professor, Psychiatry
Oregon Health and Science University
Portland, Oregon

MICHAEL J. GERMAIN, M.D., F.A.C.P.
Associate Professor, Medicine
Tufts University
Springfield, Massachusetts

J. SIMON R. GIBBS, M.D. F.R.C.P.
Senior Lecturer, Cardiology/Consultant
   Cardiologist
National Heart and Lung Institute
Faculty of Medicine, Imperial College of
   Science, Technology and Medicine
London, United Kingdom

ELIZABETH GOY, Ph.D.
Assistant Professor, Psychiatry
School of Medicine
Oregon Health and Science University
Portland, Oregon

MADELYN A. IRIS, Ph.D.
Assistant Professor, Medicine
Director, Social Sciences and Behavior Section
The Buehler Center on Aging
Northwestern's Feinberg School of Medicine
Chicago, Illinois

JOHN P. KRCMARIK, M.D.
Fellow in Pulmonary and Critical Care
   Medicine
Dartmouth-Hitchcock Medical Center
Lebanon, New Hampshire

RISA LAVIZZO-MOUREY, M.D.
Director, Institute on Aging
Chief, Division of Geriatrics
University of Pennsylvania
Philadelphia, Pennsylvania

CAROL LEVINE, M.A.
Director, Families and Health Care Project
United Hospital Fund of New York
New York, New York

JANICE LYNCH SCHUSTER
Senior Writer
Americans for Better Care of the Dying
Washington, D.C.

JOANNE LYNN, M.D.
Director, RAND Center to Improve Care for
the Dying
Arlington, Virginia

MARIANE LaPORTE MATZO, Ph.D.,
A.P.R.N., B.C., F.A.A.N.
Professor, Union Institute and University
Manchester, New Hampshire

MEGAN McANDREW COOPER, M.B.A., M.S.
Editor, the Dartmouth Atlas of Health Care
Dartmouth Medical School
Hanover, New Hampshire

ROBERT McCANN, M.D., F.A.C.P.
Associate Professor, Medicine
University of Rochester School of Medicine
and Dentistry
Chief of Medicine
Highland Hospital
Rochester, New York

ANNE McCOY, M.Sc.
Research Associate, National Heart and Lung
Institute
Faculty of Medicine, Imperial College of
Science, Technology and Medicine
London, United Kingdom

SARAH MYERS, M.P.H.
RAND Center to Improve Care of the Dying
Arlington, Virginia

ELLEN OLSON, M.D.
Bronx Veterans Hospital
Bronx, New York

CYNTHIA X. PAN, M.D.
Assistant Professor
Brookdale Department of Geriatrics and Adult
Development
Director of Education
Hertzberg Palliative Care Institute
Mount Sinai School of Medicine
New York, New York

DONALD L. PATRICK, Ph.D., M.S.P.H.
Program in Social and Behavioral Sciences
Department of Health Services
Health Sciences Center
University of Washington
Seattle, Washington

STEPHEN G. POST, Ph.D.
Professor and Associate Director, Educational
Program
School of Medicine
Case Western Reserve University
Cleveland, Ohio

THOMAS J. PRENDERGAST, M.D.
Associate Professor, Medicine and
Anesthesiology
Dartmouth-Hitchcock Medical Center
Lebanon, New Hampshire

TIMOTHY E. QUILL, M.D.
Professor, Medicine, Psychiatry, and Medical
Humanities
University of Rochester School of Medicine
and Dentistry
Rochester, New York

ANGIE ROGERS, M.Sc.
Research Fellow
Department of Palliative Care and Policy
King's College London
London, United Kingdom

SUSAN K. ROGERS, M.S., B.S.N., R.N.
Director, Education and Public Relations
Americans for Better Care of the Dying
Washington, D.C.

JAMES R. RUNO, M.D.
Fellow in Pulmonary and Critical Care
Medicine
Health Services Research Center
Vanderbilt University School of Medicine
Nashville, Tennessee

NATALIE R. SACKS, M.D.
Division of Hematology/Oncology and Cancer
Center
Hospital of the University of Pennsylvania
Philadelphia, Pennsylvania

KNIGHT STEEL, M.D.
Endowed Professor of Geriatrics
Chief, Division of Geriatrics
University of Medicine and Dentistry of New Jersey
New Jersey Medical School
Hackensack University Medical Center
Hackensack, New Jersey

NIGEL P. SYKES, M.A., B.M., B.Ch., F.R.C.G.P.
Head of Medicine and Consultation in Palliative Medicine
St. Christopher's Hospice
Honorary Senior Lecturer in Palliative Medicine
King's College
University of London
London, United Kingdom

JOAN M. TENO, M.D., M.S.
Associate Professor, Community Health and Medicine
Associate Director, Center for Gerontology and Health Care Research
Associate Medical Director, Home and Hospice Care of Rhode Island
Brown Medical School
Providence, Rhode Island

SUSAN W. TOLLE, M.D.
Director, Center for Ethics in Health Care
Oregon Health and Science University
Portland, Oregon

EVA TOPINKOVÁ, M.D., Ph.D.
Department of Geriatrics
First Medical Faculty
Charles University
Institute of Postgraduate Medical Education
Prague, Czech Republic

STANLEY TUHRIM, M.D.
Professor
Department of Neurology
Mount Sinai School of Medicine
New York, New York

JAMES A. TULSKY, M.D.
Director, Program on the Medical Encounter and Palliative Care
Durham Veterans Administration Medical Center
Associate Professor, Medicine
Associate Director, Institute on Care at the End of Life
Duke University
Durham, North Carolina

CAROLINE VITALE, M.D.
Clinical Assistant Professor, Department of Medicine
University of Medicine and Dentistry of New Jersey
New Jersey Medical School
Hackensack Medical Center
Hackensack, New Jersey

JEREMY D. WALSTON, M.D.
Associate Professor, Medicine
Johns Hopkins University School of Medicine
Baltimore, Maryland

JAMES R. WEBSTER, M.S., M.D.
Michael A. Gertz Professor of Medicine
Emeritus Director, The Buehler Center on Aging
Northwestern's Feinberg School of Medicine
Chicago, Illinois

JOHN E. WENNBERG, M.D., M.P.H.
Director, Center for the Evaluative Clinical Sciences
Peggy Y. Thomson Professor for the Evaluative Clinical Sciences
Dartmouth Medical School
Hanover, New Hampshire

J. ELIZABETH WHITEMAN, M.D.
Assistant Clinical Professor
Division of Geriatrics
UCLA School of Medicine
Los Angeles, California

DEBORAH WITT SHERMAN, Ph.D., A.P.R.N., A.N.P., B.C., F.A.A.N.
Associate Professor, Nursing
Program Coordinator of the Advanced Practice Palliative Care Master's and Post-Master's Programs
New York University
New York, New York

Introduction

In our society, the overwhelming majority of people who suffer from advanced illness are elderly. They typically die of chronic diseases, over long periods of time, with multiple coexisting problems, progressive dependence on others, and heavy care needs met mostly by family members. They spend the majority of their final months and years at home but, in most parts of the country, actually die in hospitals or nursing homes surrounded by strangers. Many of these deaths become protracted and negotiated processes, with health-care providers and family members making difficult, often wrenching, decisions about the use or discontinuation of life-prolonging technologies, such as feeding tubes, ventilators, and intravenous fluids. There is abundant evidence that the quality of life during the advanced stages of disease is often poor, characterized by inadequately treated physical distress; fragmented care systems; poor communication between doctors, patients, and families; and enormous strains on family caregiver and support systems.[1]

DEMOGRAPHY OF SERIOUS ILLNESS IN THE UNITED STATES

The median age at death in the United States is now 77 years, associated with a steady and linear decline in age-adjusted death rates since 1940. While in 1900 life expectancy at birth was less than 50 years, a girl born today may expect to live to age 79 and a boy to age 75. Those of us reaching 75 years can expect to live another 10 (men) to 12 (women) years on average. By the year 2010, life expectancy is projected to increase to 86 years for women and 79 years for men.[2,3] The result of these changes in demography has been an enormous growth in the number and health of the elderly so that by the year 2030 20% of the U.S. population will be over age 65 compared to fewer than 5% at the turn of the last century.

While death at the turn of the last century typically followed an acute infectious illness, today the leading causes of death are chronic diseases such as heart disease, cancer, and stroke. Advances in the treatment of atherosclerotic vascular disease and cancer have turned these previously rapidly fatal diseases into chronic illnesses, with which people often live for many years before death. In parallel, deaths that occurred at home in the early part of the twentieth century now occur primarily in institutions (53% in hospitals and 24% in nursing homes). The reasons for this shift in location of care prior to death are complex but related to both financial incentives[4–7] and the care burdens of chronicity and functional dependence typically accompanying life-threatening disease in the elderly. The older the patient, the higher the likelihood of death in a nursing home or hospital, with an estimated 58% of persons over age 85 spending at least some time in a nursing home in the last year of life.[7a]

These statistics, however, hide the fact that the majority of an older person's last months and years are still spent at home in the care of family members, with hospitalization and/or nursing home placement occurring primarily near the very end of life. Additionally, national figures such as these hide the substantial regional variation in location of death. In Portland, Oregon, for example, only 35% of adult deaths occur in hospitals compared to over 50% in New York City,[8] a disparity associated at least in part with differences in regional hospital bed supply and availability of adequate community supports for the seriously ill and dying. Finally, national statistics also obscure the variability in the experience of serious chronic illness that characterizes our highly diverse nation. For example, need for institutionalization or paid formal caregivers in the last months of life is significantly higher among the poor and women. Similarly, persons suffering from cognitive impairment and dementia are much more likely to spend their last years in a nursing home compared to cognitively intact elderly persons living with nondementing illnesses.

The fiscal and care system incentives promoting institutional, as opposed to home-based, care persist despite evidence that many (although not all) patients prefer to be at home and despite the existence of the Medicare Hospice Benefit. The hospice benefit was designed to provide substantial professional and material support (medications, equipment) to families caring for the dying at home for their last 6 months of life. Reasons for the low rate of utilization of the Medicare Hospice Benefit (serving about 20% of adult deaths) vary by community but include the inhibiting requirements that patients must choose to give up disease-modifying treatments in order to access hospice services, that physicians certify a prognosis of 6 months or less "if the disease follows its usual course," and that very few hours (usually 4 or less) of personal-care home attendants are covered under the benefit. In addition, the fiscal structure of the Medicare Hospice Benefit lends itself well to the relatively predictable downward trajectory of late-stage cancers or acquired immunodeficiency syndrome but not so well to the unpredictable, multiyear chronic course of other common causes of death in the elderly, like congestive heart failure, chronic lung disease, stroke, and dementing illnesses.[2]

EXPERIENCE OF ADVANCED ILLNESS IN OLDER ADULTS

Although death occurs far more commonly in the elderly than in any other age group, most research on the experience of dying has been done in younger populations and relatively little is known about how death occurs in the oldest old, those over age 75. The largest and most detailed study of adult hospital deaths in the United States, The Study to Understand Prognoses and Preferences for Outcomes and Risks of Treatments (SUPPORT),[9] focused on a relatively young population (median age 66 years) and demonstrated a high rate of untreated pain in the last few days of life, poor doctor–patient communication about the goals of medical care, and frequent use of ventilators and intensive care. There is some evidence that costly and potentially burdensome life-prolonging interventions are less frequently used among the oldest patients, independent of baseline functional measures.[10,11] Others have shown consistently high levels of untreated or undertreated pain in the elderly. In one study of elderly cancer patients in nursing homes, 26% of those with daily pain received no analgesics and 16% received only acetaminophen, a percentage that rose with increasing age and minority status.[12] Other studies comparing pain management in cognitively intact versus demented elderly with acute hip fracture found high rates of undertreatment of pain in both groups, a phenomenon that worsened with increasing age and cognitive impairment.[13,14] Similarly, a study of outpatients with cancer found that age and female sex were predictors of undertreatment, a disturbing observation given the dramatic rise in cancer prevalence and proportion of women with increasing age.[15,16] Finally, nonmalignant chronic disease is probably the most common cause of distress and disability in the elderly, affecting 42%–71% of community-dwelling older adults, and, similar to cancer pain, is consistently undertreated.[17] These data suggest that the time before death among elderly persons is often characterized by years of significant physical distress which is neither identified nor properly treated.

The dying process is also different in older adults compared to younger persons. Unlike in younger adults, for whom one disease is often the sole cause of death, death in older adults typically results from one or more major acute illnesses superimposed on multiple comorbidities (e.g., diabetes, hypertension, osteoarthritis, gait disturbances), age-related changes in organ physiology (e.g., decreased glomerular filtration rate), and progressive functional decline.

FRAILTY AS AN INDICATION FOR PALLIATIVE CARE

As discussed in Chapter 9, the frailty syndrome, independent of specific disease processes, is associated with limited life expectancy and should be considered a marker for the need for palliative care. Frailty, in fact, is the quintessential model for palliative care in older adults as optimal medical treatment for the frail patient typically includes preventive, life-prolonging, rehabilitative, and palliative measures in varying proportion and intensity based on the individual patient's needs and preferences. For example, a frail 88-year-old woman with congestive heart failure, Parkinson's disease, hypertension, diabetes, and deconditioning after hospitalization for pneumonia typically requires life-prolonging measures (treatment of heart failure, oxygen, insulin, and antibiotics), preventive measures (annual influenza vaccination), rehabilitation (home physical therapy to restore independent bed-to-chair mobility), and palliative care (advance care planning and goal setting, appointment of a health-care proxy, support for family caregivers, treatment of depression, and diuretics, oxygen, and low-dose opioids for dyspnea). Since her daughter works during the day, she also needs a 12-hour-a-day home-health aide as she is unable to care for herself independently. Thus, the model of care needed for this person with a classic geriatric frailty syndrome provides simultaneous life-prolonging, palliative, rehabilitative, and personal care (in this patient they are nearly one and the same) and, given the difficulty of prognosticating time of death in heart failure, will have to continue to do so for the remainder of the patient's life. As her condition progresses over time, increased attention to palliative measures and consideration of withdrawal of burdensome life-prolonging treatments that detract from quality of life (e.g., daily fingersticks to check blood glucose) will be necessary.

IMPACT OF SERIOUS ILLNESS ON PATIENTS AND FAMILIES

Aside from pain and other sources of physical distress, the key characteristic that distinguishes advanced illness in the elderly from that experienced by younger groups is the nearly universal occurrence of long periods of functional dependence and need for family caregivers in the last months to years of life. The SUPPORT group, focusing on a younger age cohort, found that 55% of patients had persistent and serious family caregiving needs during the course of a terminal illness,[18] a figure that rises exponentially with increasing age. Estimates based on 1996 data suggest that more than 25 million Americans deliver care to a seriously ill relative at home, on average about 18 hours per week. Assuming a conservative hourly rate of $8 for such services, this amounts to $194 billion in uncompensated care annually.[19] Although the vast majority of caregiving is done by unpaid family members (transportation, homemaker services, personal care, and more skilled nursing care), paid care supplements or provides the sole source of care in 15%–20% of patients, especially among poor elderly women living alone. Most family caregiving is provided by women (spouses and adult daughters and daughters-in-law), placing significant strains on the physical, emotional, and socioeconomic status of the caregivers.[20] Over 87% of caregivers say they need more help with transportation (62%), homemaking (55%), nursing (28%), and personal care (26%) for the patient. Caregiving in itself is a risk factor for death, major depression, and associated comorbidities.[21] Those ill and dependent patients without family caregivers or those whose caregivers can no longer provide or afford needed services are placed in nursing homes, where 20% of the over age 85 population resides.[22,23] Thus, serious illness in the oldest old is characterized by a high prevalence of untreated pain and other symptoms due to chronic conditions associated with progressive functional dependence, unpredictable disease course, and extensive family caregiver needs.

MISMATCH BETWEEN U.S. HEALTH-CARE REIMBURSEMENT AND THE NEEDS OF OLDER ADULTS

The current payment system is poorly matched to the needs of the elderly with serious and complex chronic illness. Medicare fee-for-service promotes use of procedure-based payments, hospitalization, and associated specialization and discontinuity of care. Capitated and managed-care systems attempt to avoid seriously ill or dying patients with high-intensity service needs, focusing instead on healthier, lower-cost patient populations. The Medicare Hospice Benefit was designed for patients with cancer and predictably short (under 6 month) life spans, who are willing to give up efforts to prolong life and whose families can provide for the majority of their care needs at home. None of these payment systems addresses the long-term care needs (whether at home or in a nursing home) of chronically ill and functionally dependent older adults whose prognosis is uncertain and whose medical care usually requires simultaneous efforts to prolong life, palliate symptoms, and provide support for functional dependence. Neither paid personal care services at home nor nursing home costs for the functionally dependent elderly with long-term care needs are covered by Medicare but, instead, are paid for approximately equally out-of-pocket and from Medicaid budgetary sources originally intended to provide care for the indigent. Even in nursing homes, standards of care focus on improvement of function and maintenance of weight and nutritional status, and evidence of the inevitable decline that accompanies the dying process is typically regarded as a measure of substandard care. Thus, a death in a nursing home is often viewed as evidence, particularly by state regulators, of poor care rather than an expected outcome for a frail, chronically ill older person. Similarly, quality indicators required in long-term care settings fail to either assess or reward appropriate attention to palliative measures, including relief of symptoms, support for patient- and family-centered goal setting and decision making, spiritual care, and promotion of continuity with concomitant avoidance of brink-of-death transfers to the emergency department and hospital.[24]

WHEN IS PALLIATIVE CARE APPROPRIATE IN GERIATRIC MEDICAL CARE?

Because of the nature and duration of chronic illness during old age, the timing of initiation of palliative care differs from what is usually appropriate in a younger population. The content of the palliative approach to patient care differs not in kind but in emphasis in the geriatric patient. As with younger patients, meticulous attention to symptom distress and side effect management, repeated discussions about the changing goals of medical care as the disease progresses, and support for family caregivers are all necessary in the elderly; the differences are related to the many-year duration of most geriatric chronic illnesses, the high prevalence of long-term functional and cognitive impairment in this patient population, and the associated enormous and long-term caregiver role and burden that results. Many of the characteristics of advanced old age (frailty, functional dependence, cognitive impairment, multiple comorbidities, and symptom distress) occur in a disease-independent manner or, more accurately, are multifactorial in etiology. In the frail elderly, disease-specific treatments may ameliorate or lessen the burdens of frailty, dependence, and symptom distress but are unlikely to eliminate them. Thus, markers for initiation of palliative care in the elderly are most appropriately centered on the identification and amelioration of functional and cognitive impairment, development of frailty and dependence on family caregivers, and burden of symptom distress, rather than, as is typical in advanced cancer and in traditional hospice settings, identification of a specific and advanced terminal illness or signs of poor prognosis or imminent death. Similarly, the presence of symptom distress in and of itself and whether or not it is secondary to a discrete terminal illness should prompt a comprehensive assessment and plan of treatment (Table I–1). When the time remaining is short (measured in months or years, not in decades), the quality of each of those days becomes proportionately more important and the priority accorded to the goal of improving quality of life should increase accordingly.

Similarly, while palliative care will have different goals depending on the needs and aims of each individual patient and family, the stage of a chronic illness helps to de-

Table I–1. Markers for Initiation of Palliative Care in Geriatrics

Disease-independent markers
   Frailty
   Functional dependence
   Cognitive impairment
   Symptom distress
   Family support needs

Disease-specific markers
   Symptomatic congestive heart failure
   Chronic lung disease
   Dementia
   Stroke
   Cancer
   Recurrent infection
   Degenerative joint disease causing functional
     impairment and chronic pain

termine the range and intensity of appropriate palliative care interventions (Table I–2). For example, in the early stages of a 10-year-long dementing illness, appropriate palliative interventions might include early attention to advance care planning, discussion about the preferred goals of care during later stages of illness, and health-care proxy appointment; financial planning; attention to other important tasks that need to be completed while cognition allows; disease-modifying therapies; and education, support, and counseling for family caregivers. In the middle stages of dementia, when progressive functional dependence, behavioral and physical symptoms, and increasing family burden and distress become prominent, palliative care should focus on meticulous assessment and treatment of symptom distress, practical and psychosocial support for families, and explicit planning for oncoming long-term care needs. In the advanced stages of dementia, the primary goal is the patient's physical and emotional comfort, helping families decide about the benefits and burdens of life-sustaining treatments such as tube feeding, helping families decide when and if placement in a nursing home is necessary and appropriate, attention to the family's anticipatory grief and bereavement associated with advanced-stage illness, planning for a peaceful and controlled death, and appropriate support and counseling during the bereavement process.

Table I–2. Staging of Palliative Care During the Course of a Chronic Illness

	Early	Middle	Late
Goals of care	Discuss diagnosis, prognosis, what to expect	Review understanding of diagnoses/prognosis	Communicate and assess understanding of diagnosis, disease course, prognosis
	Discuss/offer disease-modifying therapies	Review efficacy and benefit/burden of disease modifying treatment	Review appropriateness of disease-modifying treatments
	Discuss patient-centered goals, hopes, expectations from medical treatment	Reassess goals of care and expectations; prepare patient/family for shift in goals; encourage completion of important tasks, relationships, financial affairs	Review goals of care and recommend appropriate shifts in context of advanced disease; explicitly plan for a peaceful death; encourage completion of important tasks, relationships, financial affairs
Advance care planning	Advance care planning, health-care proxy appointment	Review for accuracy, current preferences, concordance of treatment with wishes, understanding of proxy role	Review for accuracy; in patient without decisional capacity, ensure relationship of treatment decisions to patient's previously stated wishes
Financial planning	Advise financial planning and consultation for estate planning, long-term care, insurance/options	Reassess adequacy of financial planning for medical, home care, prescription, long-term care, and family support needs; consider hospice referral	Review financial resources and needs; inform patient/family of financial options for personal and long-term care (hospice, Medicaid) if resources are inadequate to patient/family needs; explicitly recommend hospice, review advantages to patient and family
Symptom management	Formal symptom assessment using validated instrument management, treat identified symptoms, manage side effects, re-assess and adjust	Formal symptom assessment using validated instrument management, treat identified symptoms, manage side effects, re-assess and adjust	Formal symptom assessment using validated instrument management, treat identified symptoms, manage side effects, re-assess and adjust
Family support	Inform patient/family about support groups; ask about practical support needs (transportation, prescription drug coverage, respite care, personal care); listen	Encourage support/counseling for family caregivers; screen family caregivers for practial resource needs, stress, depression, adequacy of medical care; identify respite and practical support resources; recommend help from family/friends; raise possibility of hospice and its benefits; listen	Encourage out-of-town family to visit; refer to disease-specific support groups/counseling for family caregivers; bereavement support groups; routine inquiry about caregiver health, well-being, practical needs; offer respite care alternatives; after death, send bereavement card, call after 1–2 weeks; screen for high-risk bereavement; maintain occasional contact after patient's death; listen

(*continued*)

Table I–2. *Continued*

	Early	Middle	Late
Spiritual care	Assess desire for spiritual counseling/support	Inquire about religiosity and current engagement with religious community; refer as appropriate	Ask if referral to clergy or other spiritual support would be helpful for patient or family, especially in last days of life
Functional dependence and rehabilitation	Formally assess functional impairments, activities of daily living and instrumental activities of daily living needs; seek rehab evaluation, conditioning exercises, home safety assessment, support for instrumental activities of daily living, fall risk reduction, gait-assist devices	Review functional impairments and benefit–burden of interventions aimed at improved functional capacity	Utilize interventions to promote comfort, sense of control, ease of care for family; reassess equipment needs, safe transfers, and positioning for purposes of comfort
Comorbid disease management	Manage comorbid illness, review drug interactions; close coordination with other specialists	Review benefit–burden of comborbid disease management in terms of impact on quality and length of life	Evaluate comorbid disease management in terms of contribution to quality of life, discontinue treatments no longer of benefit

THE SIMULTANEOUS PALLIATIVE AND LIFE-PROLONGING CARE MODEL

The traditional hospice model in the United States, as codified by the Medicare Hospice Benefit, requires that patients be certified as within 6 months of death (if the disease follows its usual course) and that they choose to give up curative or life-prolonging treatments in order to access the comprehensive palliative care that hospice offers. This either–or structure for disease-modifying/curative care versus palliative care essentially forces patients to give up life-prolonging treatments in order to access palliative treatments and to reject palliative treatment in order to retain life-prolonging efforts. For the vast majority of patients living with chronic illness, both life-prolonging and palliative treatments are necessary and appropriate and the forced choice results not only in reflexive, burdensome, and costly life-prolonging treatments long after the time that they are beneficial to the patient but also in a great deal of preventable suffering during all stages of a serious or terminal illness. The model of palliative care that makes more sense, and the one promulgated in this textbook, is a simultaneous model of palliative care delivered at the same time as disease-modifying and life-prolonging treatments with the ratio and nature of these treatments varying in response to patient needs and preferences.[25–28] In the 75% of older adults living with serious illnesses other than cancer, the distinction between life-prolonging and palliative treatments is, in any case, largely illusory. In the case of congestive heart failure, where treatments with diuretics, digitalis, opiates, and oxygen are both life-prolonging and palliative, effective treatment also relieves symptom burden. A similar observation holds with chronic lung disease, end-stage renal disease, and progressive dementias. This integrated and simultaneous model of pallia-

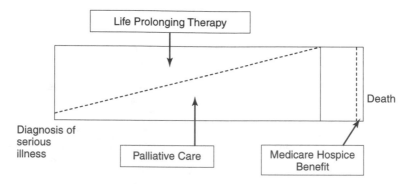

Figure I–1. Palliative care's place in the course of illness.

tive and life-prolonging care is demonstrated graphically in Figure I–1. Late in the course of any of these illnesses, when the burden of continued life-prolonging treatments outweighs their benefit, the goals of care may shift to a predominant and ultimately exclusive focus on ensuring comfort for the patient and practical and emotional support for family caregivers; a patient who has been receiving excellent palliative care along with life-prolonging measures will make the transition to hospice far more easily because the change in type of care will be gradual, rather than sudden, and driven by the patient's needs and not by the rigid and inflexible demands of the payment system.

SUMMARY AND CONCLUSION

Whereas a century ago virtually everyone died at home, surrounded by family and cared for by physicians whose primary role was the relief of suffering, today the majority of Americans die in hospitals and nursing homes, surrounded by medical technology and physicians who believe there is nothing else that they can offer. While the past 100 years have seen tremendous advances in the treatment of disease such that previously fatal illnesses (e.g., diabetes, congestive heart failure) have become chronic conditions, this progress has come at substantial cost. We have transformed the culture of the aging and illness process from an accepted part of life's experience to an unfamiliar and much feared

series of events. The majority of Americans have never witnessed a loved one die (a common experience at the turn of the century); and physicians are ill-trained, ill-equipped, and uncomfortable taking responsibility for the care of seriously ill and dying patients. The time has come to restore the balance so that "relief of suffering and cure of disease are seen as twin obligations of a medical profession that is truly dedicated to the care of the sick." [29]

Geriatric Palliative Care is a textbook devoted specifically to palliative care in the elderly. Palliative care is interdisciplinary medical care focused on the relief of suffering and achievement of the best possible quality of life for patients and their family caregivers. It involves formal symptom assessment and treatment; aid with decision making and establishing goals of care; practical and moral support for patients and their family caregivers; mobilization of community support and resources to assure a secure and safe living environment; and collaborative and seamless models of care (hospital, home, nursing home, hospice) for persons living with serious, complex, and eventually terminal illnesses.

These fundamentals bear a strong resemblance to the core precepts of geriatric medicine, and while it is true that not all older people suffer from multiple complex chronic illnesses which will ultimately lead to their death, most do and all eventually will. As a result of the successes of modern medical care, dying and death is now a geriatric phenomenon; therefore, sophisticated management for patients and families entering this stage of their lives is the province of both the geriatrician as well as all primary treating physicians. In this new textbook are chapters on practical approaches to communicating with older adults about prognosis, the likelihood of death, and patient preferences for how to use their remaining time; management of diverse sources of suffering in older adults, including distress associated with transfer from home to a nursing home, being dependent on others, and being confused; palliative approaches to caring for persons with dementia at all stages of the illness and regardless of how long the patient may have to live; and the importance of achieving a peaceful death and why physicians should care about and know how to help their patients ensure it. We hope our readers will find these useful as they accompany their patients and family caregivers through one of the most difficult and important stages of late life.

R. Sean Morrison
Diane E. Meier

REFERENCES

1. Signorielli N. Physical disabilities, impairment and safety, mental illness, and death. In: Mass Media Images and Impact on Health. Westport, CT, Greenwood Press, pp. 37–42, 1993.
2. Field MJ, Cassel CK. Approaching Death: Improving Care at the End of Life. In: Institute of Medicine, ed. Washington DC, National Academy Press, 1997.
3. Future Ift. Health and health care 2010. The forecast. The challenge. Vol. 2001, 2000.
4. Warren E, Sullivan T, Jacoby M. Medical problems and bankruptcy filings. Norton's Bankruptcy Advisor 2000.
5. Health Care Financing Administration. Highlights—National Health Expenditures, 1998. Vol. 2001, 2000.
6. Spillman B, Lubitz J. The effect of longevity on spending for acute and long term care. N Engl J Med 2000;342:1409–1415.
7. Meier DE, Morrison RS. Autonomy reconsidered. N Engl J Med 2002;346:1087–1089.
7a. National Center for Health Statistics. National Mortality Followback Survey: 1986 Summary, United States. Hyattsville, MD: Health Statistics, series 20, 1992.
8. Wennberg JE, Cooper MM, editors. The Dartmouth Atlas of Health Care 1999. American Hospital Chicago, Association Press, 1999. www.dartmouthatlas.net, accessed 10/25/02.
9. SUPPORT Principal Investigators. A controlled trial to improve care for seriously ill hospitalized patients. The Study to Understand Prognoses and Preferences for Outcomes and Risks of Treatments (SUPPORT). JAMA 1995;274:1591–1598.
10. Hamel M, Phillips R, Teno J, et al. Seriously ill hospitalized adults: do we spend less on older patients? J Am Geriatr Soc 1996;44:1043–1048.
11. Perls T, Wood E. Acute care costs of the oldest old: they cost less, their care intensity is less, and they go to nonteaching hospitals. Arch Intern Med 1996;156:754–760.
12. Bernabei R, Gambassi G, Lapane K, et al. Management of pain in elderly patients with cancer. JAMA 1998;279:1877–1882.
13. Feldt KS, Ryden MB, Miles S. Treatment of pain in cognitively impaired compared with cognitively intact older patients with hip-fracture. J Am Geriatr Soc 1998;46:1079–1085.
14. Morrison RS, Siu AL. A comparison of pain and its treatment in advanced dementia and cognitively intact patients with hip fracture. J Pain Symptom Manage 2000;19:240248.
15. Cleeland CS, Gonin R, Hatfield AK, et al. Pain and its treatment in outpatients with metastatic cancer. N Engl J Med 1994;330:592–596.
16. Stein W. Cancer pain in the elderly. In: Ferrell BR, Ferrell BA (eds.). Pain in the Elderly. Seattle, IASP Press, 1996, pp. 68–80.
17. AGS Panel on Chronic Pain in Older Persons. The management of chronic pain in older persons. J Amr Geriatr Soc 1998;46:635–651.
18. Covinsky K, Goldman L, Cook E, et al. The impact of serious illness on patients' families. JAMA 1994;272:1839–1844.
19. Arno P, Levine C, Memmott M. The economic value of informal caregiving. Health Affairs 1999;18:182–188.
20. Emanuel EJ, Fairclough DL, Slutsman J, Alpert H, Baldwin D, Emanuel L. Assistance from family members, friends, paid caregivers, and volunteers in the care of terminally ill patients. N Engl J Med 1999; 341:956–963.
21. Schulz R, Beach S. Caregiving as a risk factor for mortality: the Caregiver Health Effects Study. JAMA 1999;282:2215–2219.

22. Ferrell BA, Ferrell BR, Rivera LSO. Pain in cognitively impaired nursing home patients. J Pain Symptom Manage 1995;10:591–598.

23. Ferrell B. Overview of aging and pain. In: Ferrell BA, eds. Pain in the Elderly. Seattle: IASP Press, 1996, pp. 1–10.

24. Engle VF. Care of the living, care of the dying: reconceptualizing nursing home care. J Am Geriatr Soc 1998; 46:1172–1174.

25. Lynn J, Wilkinson AM. Quality end of life care: the case for a MediCaring demonstration. Hosp J 1998;13:151–163.

26. Lynn J. Serving patients who may die soon, and their families: the role of hospice and other services. JAMA 2001;285:925–932.

27. Lynn J. Learning to care for people with chronic illness facing the end of life. JAMA 2000;284:2508–2511.

28. Eng C, Pedulla J, Eleazer GP, McCann R, Fox N. Program of All-inclusive Care for the Elderly (PACE): an innovative model of integrated geriatric care and financing [see comments]. J Am Geriatr Soc 1997;45:223–232.

29. Cassell EJ. The nature of suffering and the goals of medicine. N Engl J Med 1982;306:639–645.

I

OVERVIEW: THE SOCIAL AND CULTURAL CONTEXT OF OLD AGE AND FRAILTY

1

Variability in End-of-Life Care in the United States

JOHN E. WENNBERG, MEGAN McANDREW COOPER, AND SUSAN W. TOLLE

The *Dartmouth Atlas of Health Care*[1] includes studies of the patterns of medical practice with regard to end-of-life care. The medical experiences of seriously ill and dying Americans vary remarkably from one community to another, as do most other aspects of health care. This chapter provides an overview of the results of these studies, discusses reasons why the variations might occur, and summarizes the current state of knowledge about the question of whether the sometimes extraordinary variation in the intensity of care among regions pays off in terms of health benefits. It also includes an interpretation of why the level of intensity of care provided to seriously ill and dying Oregonians is so much lower than it is for Americans living elsewhere, as well as examples of how the atlas data are being used to further address the quality of end-of-life care in Oregon.

The Dartmouth Atlas project is an application of the methods of small area analysis, a health-care research strategy in which the study populations to be compared are defined by place of residence. On the basis of an analysis of travel patterns for hospital care, each zip code in the United States was assigned to a hospital service area (HSA). The process resulted in 3436 geographically distinct HSAs, which were further aggregated into 306 hospital referral regions (HRRs) on the basis of referral patterns for cardiovascular surgery and neurosurgery. The end-of-life measures used in that report are summarized in Table 1–1. In our report on Oregon, data are presented for the five HRRs in Oregon and for selected HSAs in the state. For each measure, the denominator was the 18-month 1995–96 deceased Medicare population, defined as the Medicare enrollee population who died between July 1, 1995, and December 31, 1996. The methods used in the atlas (including details on how the end-of-life measures were constructed) are reported in the 1999 atlas, which is available on the Dartmouth website (http://www. dartmouthatlas.org).

Table 1–1. Measures of Intensity of Treatment in the Last 6 Months of Life

The likelihood of a hospitalized death
The likelihood of being admitted to an intensive care unit
The likelihood of spending 7 or more days in intensive care
The likelihood of being admitted to an intensive care unit during the terminal hospitalization
The number of physician visits
The number of primary-care physician visits
The number of medical-specialist physician visits
The likelihood of seeing 10 or more different physicians
Medicare reimbursements for inpatient care

Source: Dartmouth Atlas of Health Care.[1] Wennberg JE, Cooper MM, editors. The Dartmouth Atlas of Health Care 1999. Chicago, American Hospital Association Press, 1999.

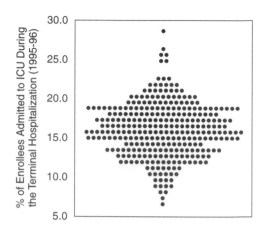

Figure 1–1. Percent of Medicare enrollees admitted to intensive care during the terminal hospitalization (1995–96). The proportion of Medicare enrollees who were admitted to intensive care at some time during the hospitalization in which they died ranged from about 6% to almost 30%. Each point represents one of the 306 hospital referral regions in the United States.

GEOGRAPHIC VARIATIONS IN THE CARE OF SERIOUSLY ILL PATIENTS: THE NATIONAL PICTURE

The quality of death Americans experience, whether relatively nonmedical (few doctor visits, low likelihood of a hospitalized death) or high-tech (many visits to different specialists, higher likelihood of dying in an intensive care unit [ICU]), is highly dependent on where they live and the health-care providers they use. This section provides an overview of the national patterns of end-of-life care, comparing the experiences of the 306 HRRs as reported in the 1999 *Dartmouth Atlas of Health Care.* Figure 1–1 shows the percent of all Medicare deaths that occurred in hospitals in which the dying person was admitted to intensive care. What this measures is not just the likelihood of a hospitalized death (there are legitimate reasons for some deaths to occur in hospitals rather than at home or in a nursing home, for example) but also the propensity of the local system to treat patients very aggressively even when death is probably imminent. Each point in the graph represents the average percent of such deaths in one of the 306 HRRs in the United States. In some parts of the country (vertical scale), only 6% or 7% of those who died had been admitted to an ICU prior to death. In other parts of the coun-

try, almost 30% of those who died had been admitted to intensive care. There was also wide variation in other measures of terminal care. For example, in 1994–95, among the Medicare population, the likelihood of a hospitalized death varied from about 20% of deaths to more than 50%.

The hospitalization of the dying is one measure of what is going on in the system, that part that has most directly "medicalized" the American experience of death. The atlas also demonstrates the extensive variation in the intensity of interventions in the seriously ill. During the last 6 months of their lives, many, if not most, Americans are seriously ill; but the amount of treatment they receive during this period varies extensively. Figure 1–2, reprinted from the 1998 edition of the *Dartmouth Atlas,* shows that the average number of days spent in hospitals during the last 6 months of life varied from fewer than 5 days to almost 23 days.

Another aspect of care that varies extensively is the frequency of physician visits. Figure 1–3 demonstrates the variation in the average number of physician visits in

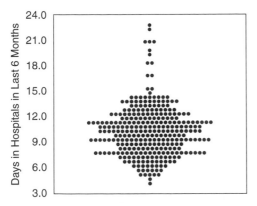

Figure 1–2. Average number of days spent in hospitals during the last 6 months of life (1994–95). The average number of days Medicare enrollees spent in acute-care hospital beds during the last 6 months of their lives varied from about 4 to almost 24. Each point on the graph represents one of the 306 hospital referral regions in the United States. (From Wennberg JE, Cooper MM, editors. The Dartmouth Atlas of Health Care 1998. AHA Publishing Chicago IL, 1998.)

the last 6 months of life among HRRs in the United States. In some regions, dying people averaged fewer than 10 encounters with physicians in their last months. In

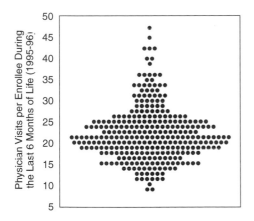

Figure 1–3. Average number of physician visits per decedent during the last 6 months of life (1995–96). The average number of physician visits per Medicare enrollee during the last 6 months of life varied from about 10 to almost 50. Each point on the graph represents one of the 306 hospital referral regions in the United States.

other regions, decedents had an average of almost 50 visits with physicians.

We looked more closely at these physician visits by dividing them between medical specialists and primary-care physicians. Together, these comprised nearly 90% of all visits. We also looked at primary-care visits according to whether they were to general internists or to family practice physicians. During the last 6 months of life, the number of visits made to medical specialists varied by a factor of more than 12, from two visits per person in the lowest-rate regions to 25 in the highest-rate region. Visits to primary-care physicians varied from 4.5 per person in the lowest-rate regions to 19.0 in the region with the highest rate.

While the number of primary-care visits and medical-specialist visits per decedent in the last 6 months of life varied substantially, we did not find that in regions where enrollees had more primary-care visits during the last 6 months of life they were less likely to have more specialist visits. In fact, there was a moderately strong positive correlation between the two ($R^2 = 0.22$), indicating that there was no substitution effect and no tendency to use primary care to reduce the use of specialty care.

Another way of measuring the intensity of the use of physician care in the last 6 months of life is to measure the number of different physicians involved in the treatment of individual enrollees, i.e., not how many times the individual saw a particular physician but how many encounters the individual had with different doctors. This "propensity to refer" was indexed by counting the number of physicians who provided one or more visits within the last 6 months of life to each patient in the 5% sample of Part B Medicare claims. According to this index, the propensity to refer varied by a factor of 27 among HRRs. Only 1.3% of enrollees in the Bloomington, Illinois, HRR and only 4.8% in the Bend, Oregon, HRR saw 10 or more physicians during their last 6 months of life. In Miami, more than one-third (34.7%) did. The propensity to refer was strongly correlated

($R^2 = 0.71$) with visit rates in the last 6 months of life.

These and other measures of the intensity of end-of-life interventions are accessible on the Dartmouth website. The site can generate a "report card" on local end-of-life measures for any selected HRR and the experience in one part of the country can be compared to that in another.

MEDICARE SPENDING AND END-OF-LIFE CARE

The Medicare program pays more than twice as much per capita for health care in some HRRs as in others. For example, in 1996, age-, sex-, and race-adjusted spending for traditional (fee-for-service) Medicare in the Miami HRR was $8414, nearly two and a half times the $3341 spent in the Minneapolis region and twice the level of the Bend region ($4231). Since all Americans pay into the Medicare Trust Fund at the same rate, regardless of residence, but some enrollees receive far more in Medicare spending than others, depending on where they live, the dollar transfers involved are enormous.

On a lifetime basis, the difference in Medicare spending between a typical 65-year-old in Miami and a typical 65-year-old in Minneapolis is more than $50,000, or equivalent to a new Lexus GS 400 with all the trimmings.[2]

The "additional" Medicare spending in high per capita reimbursement areas tends to pay for medical-specialist visits, diagnostic tests, admissions to ICU, and hospi-

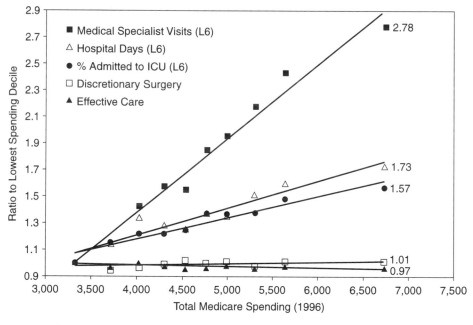

Figure 1–4. Effective care, preference-based care, and supply-sensitive care intensity among hospital referral regions grouped by enrollee spending level (1996). By grouping hospital referral regions into Medicare reimbursement deciles, we can demonstrate that the "extra" spending in high-reimbursement hospital referral regions is buying 2.78 times more specialist visits during the last 6 months of life compared to low-reimbursement areas (top line, black squares), 1.73 times more days in hospitals during the last 6 months of life (second line, white triangles), and 1.57 times more admissions to intensive care units during the last 6 months of life (third line, black circles). The dying in hospital referral regions with higher Medicare spending do not receive more discretionary surgery (fourth line, white squares) or effective care (bottom line, black triangles) than those who live in hospital referral regions with the lowest rates of Medicare reimbursement.

talizations for medical conditions. All Medicare enrollees, those who are dying and those who are not, receive more services; but the associations between overall per enrollee spending and intensity of care at the end of life are particularly strong.[3] Figure 1–4 shows the close correlation between per capita Medicare expenditures for the entire Medicare population and spending for end-of-life care.

The strong association between higher spending and greater intensity of end-of-life treatments and the lack of association between more spending and more discre-

tionary surgery or effective care can be seen in the experience of residents of four regions that represent either very high or very low levels of overall expenditure. Figure 1–5 profiles the experiences of Medicare enrollees living in four regions: Miami; Orange County, California; Portland, Oregon; and Minneapolis. Age-, sex-, and race-adjusted spending in Miami is 2.45 times higher than in Minneapolis. During the last 6 months of life, the "extra" spending purchased 6.55 times more visits to medical specialists and 2.13 times more hospital days; 2.16 times more Medicare enrollees

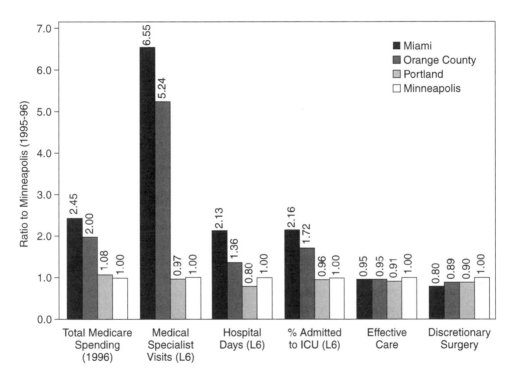

Figure 1–5. Comparison of Medicare spending, care intensity, preference-sensitive surgery, and effective care for Miami, Orange County, Minneapolis, and Portland, Oregon, hospital referral regions (1995–96). Comparing four communities provides an impression of how end-of-life treatment intensity varies depending on place of residence. Medicare enrollees in Miami were much more likely to visit multiple specialist physicians, to spend time in acute-care hospitals, and to be admitted to an intensive care unit (ICU) during their last 6 months of life than dying enrollees who lived in either Portland, Oregon, or Minneapolis. The dying in Orange County, California, had fewer such interventions than residents of Miami but were still more likely to spend time in hospitals and to visit multiple specialists than those who lived in Portland or Minneapolis. More intensity of end-of-life treatment was not associated with better access to or use of effective care (such as vaccination against pneumococcal pneumonia) or preference-sensitive care (such as surgery to relieve the symptoms of benign prostate disease); the rates of use of these services were nearly identical in all four communities. L6, care provided per decedent in the last 6 months of life.

had one or more admissions to an ICU. By contrast, rates for effective care (interventions that are of proven value, like pneumococcal pneumonia vaccinations and eye exams for diabetics) and preference-sensitive care (interventions like surgery for benign prostate disease or back pain, in which the patient's preferences and values ought to be paramount in the decision about whether or not to use the intervention) were slightly lower in Miami than in Minneapolis.

SOURCES OF VARIATION IN END-OF-LIFE CARE

What is behind the puzzling variations in end-of-life care? Differences in population rates of illness are not likely to explain the vast differences in rates of hospitalized deaths, physician visits, or other measures of end-of-life care. Why do the dying in some areas receive such aggressive and intensive treatment, while others with similar disease profiles and life expectancy who live elsewhere receive so much less intervention? Four explanations appear to be important: variations in local health-care resources, lack of guidance from current scientific evidence about the benefits of the frequency of use of supply-sensitive services, failure to accommodate patient preferences about interventions, and the propensity of physicians to deploy whatever resources are available under the assumption that more is better.

Role of Health-Care Resources

One answer to the question of why the dying in some communities are treated so much more intensively than those who are similarly ill in other communities is that the frequency of use of physician visits and hospitalizations for chronic illnesses are highly correlated with the level of resources in the local community. Most simply put, those who are dying in communities where there are more hospital beds and medical specialists per capita (Miami is a good example) are far more likely to die as hospital inpatients, see more than 10 different physi-

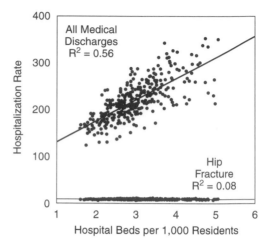

Figure 1–6. Association between hospital beds and Medicare hospitalizations for medical conditions and for hip fracture (1994–95). About half the variation in rates of hospitalizations for medical conditions can be explained by differences in the relative per capita supply of hospital beds in the region (top line, $R^2 = 0.56$). There is virtually no relationship between the rate of hospitalization for repair of hip fracture and the local per capita supply of hospital beds (bottom line, $R^2 = 0.08$). (From Wennberg and Cooper.[1])

cians, and spend time in intensive care during their last 6 months of life than are people who die in areas where there are fewer such resources (Minneapolis is an example).

Figure 1–6 demonstrates the relationship between the supply of acute care hospital beds per 1000 residents of HRRs and the rates of hospitalization for medical conditions in those regions. The relationship is strong ($R^2 = 0.56$), a phenomenon that has been referred to as *Roemer's law** or the *Field of Dreams effect*; that is, an empty hospital bed will be filled. While there is

---

*In the early 1960s, Milton Roemer, a health-services researcher interested in the use of hospitals, suggested that hospital beds, once built, will be used no matter how many there are. The relationship between the capacity of the acute hospital sector (measured in beds per 1000 residents of the local hospital referral region) and the costs of care provides an important illustration of what has become known as *Roemer's law*.

little discretion involved in the decision about whether to hospitalize people with conditions such as broken hips or those who need surgery for cancer of the colon, there is very little consensus about the indications for hospitalizing patients with such chronic conditions as congestive heart failure, diabetes, and chronic obstructive pulmonary disease. In regions where there are relatively few beds per capita, patients presenting with the latter conditions are more likely to be treated outside the hospital. In regions where the supply of beds and specialists is relatively rich, people with these conditions are more likely to be admitted to the hospital, where it is, after all, easier and more convenient for physicians to manage their care.

The phenomenon is exaggerated in hospitalizations during the last 6 months of life. Where it is relatively easy to find a hospital bed, e.g., in communities like Chicago, Philadelphia, and New Orleans, patients are more likely to have multiple hospital admissions during their last 6 months of life. In communities where hospital beds are less available, e.g., Minneapolis, San Francisco, and Denver, it is more difficult to find a bed for the seriously ill and the dying spend fewer of their last days, on average, in hospital beds.

A plausible explanation for these observations is that the threshold for hospitalization is influenced by the supply of hospital beds and other resources available for use. Faced by the challenges of managing severely ill and dying patients, even when palliation is the primary objective, the availability of resources to help manage that care seems to have a powerful influence on decision making. If the only alternative to having home care that is supervised personally by the physician is a hospital bed, many physicians and families will choose the hospital, especially if it is readily available. Clinical judgments regarding the place of final care for dying persons are made in the context of the resources, organizational structure, and culture of the local health-care system. As the Study to Understand Prognoses and Prefer-ences for Outcomes and Risks of Treatments (SUPPORT) indicates, an advance directive or other expression of personal preference will generally not be sufficient to overcome these established patterns of care.[4]

Similarly, regions where there are higher per capita supplies of specialists have higher rates of specialist visits than regions where there are fewer specialists. Figure 1–7 shows the relationship ($R^2 = 0.49$) between the supply of cardiologists per 100,000 residents of HRRs and the average number of visits to cardiologists per Medicare enrollee in those regions.[5] This stands to reason: in a region in which there are more cardiologists per capita, there are more hours of cardiologist time available in which to schedule patients, and revisit rates are higher than in regions where fewer cardiologists are available to provide services to an equal number of patients.

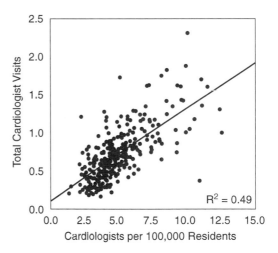

Figure 1–7. Association between the supply of cardiologists and visits to cardiologists (1992). The per capita supply of specialists is strongly correlated with the rate of visits to specialists; logically, since if there are more specialists' office hours available, more patients can visit specialists and each patient will have greater opportunity to make repeat visits. In this case, it is demonstrated that the per capita supply of cardiologists is strongly correlated ($R^2 = 0.49$) with per capita rates of visits to cardiologists.

What about Evidence-Based Medicine?

The evidence-based medicine movement has barely touched the question of the appropriate intensity of "supply-sensitive" medical care. Here, we are talking about the frequency of intervention: revisits to primary-care physicians and medical specialists, use of diagnostic tests to monitor clinical progress, and admissions of patients to acute-care and intensive-care hospital beds. The first step toward evidence-based medicine would be a well-articulated clinical theory about when and how to intervene and with what expected outcomes, which does not currently exist. For example, one searches in vain through medical texts and journal articles to find any discussion or debate about the optimal interval between revisits or when to hospitalize patients with any of the host of chronic illnesses, such as congestive heart failure, diabetes, or cancer. In the absence of medical theories, there is no opportunity to formally test efficacy, to establish the domain of evidence-based medicine. The result is that evidence-based medicine does not play much of a role in end-of-life care. What matters is the availability of supply and the cultural assumption shared by most Americans, lay and clinician alike, that more treatment is better.

What about Patient Preferences?

The SUPPORT investigators[6] reiterated the findings of two previous surveys: most Americans, when asked whether they would rather die at home or in the hospital, say that they would prefer to be at home.[7] In SUPPORT, which attempted to influence end-of-life care through intensive intervention, 391 of 479 patients expressed a wish to die at home. Only 25% of those who had expressed such a preference died in accordance with it; 55% of those who said they wanted to die at home were inpatients at the time of death. Curiously, a smaller percent of those who wanted to die in the hospital actually did so, only 46%.

Pritchard and colleagues[4] examined the factors associated with death at home.

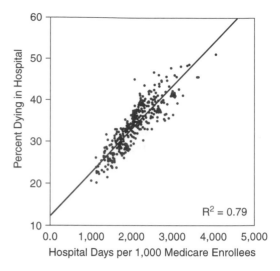

Figure 1–8. Where do Medicare enrollees die (1995–96)? In hospital referral regions where there were higher numbers of hospital days for all Medicare enrollees, those who were dying were more likely to die in a hospital bed than elsewhere (e.g., at home or in a nursing home). The relationship was very strong ($R^2 = 0.79$).

Older age, white race, being married, and diagnosis of coma or cancer were associated with a decreased risk of in-hospital death; but patients' wishes were unrelated to the place of death. Also, patient characteristics did not explain the differences in place of death. The most influential factor in the twofold difference in likelihood of a hospitalized death was the local supply of hospital beds.

Figure 1–8 demonstrates the relationship between Medicare hospital day rates and the percent of deaths that occurred in hospitals in each of the 306 HRRs (Medicare population, 1992–93). Each HRR is represented by a small dot. The HRRs assigned to the SUPPORT sites are shown in triangles. The line represents the weighted least squares regression line, in which each HRR was assigned a value weighted according to the total number of Medicare deaths in the region.[4]

The Assumption That More Is Better

In the United States, most medicine is practiced under the general assumption that more is better, i.e., that the problems facing the health-care system are those of access to care in areas where people do not have enough, rather than overexposure to interventions and their consequences. In reality, the intensity of care is governed by supply of resources and undisciplined by medical theory, medical evidence, or patient preferences. Laboring under the assumption that "more is better," our systems of care strain to deal with the burden of illness and everywhere the cry goes up that resources are scarce and that more resources and interventions are needed. However, the profession's perception of scarcity seems as strong, indeed perhaps stronger, in amply resourced, high-intensity regions such as Miami and Orange County as in low-intensity regions such as Portland and Minneapolis. Is our nation fated to an upward spiral in care intensity? Is Miami the future?

IS MORE BETTER?

There are several reasons to believe that more resources and more frequent use of resource-sensitive services are not better. A number of recent empirical studies have found no evidence that people who live in areas where the supply of resources is higher than average live longer than people who live in regions with fewer resources (e.g., doctors and hospital beds per capita). More input does not appear to result in greater longevity. Four cross-sectional studies have examined the associations between resources and mortality. Krakauer and colleagues,[8] in a national study examining associations between health-care capacity and Medicare mortality, found a small positive association between the supply of hospital beds within a region and mortality. An increase in the local bed supply of 1 bed per 1000 residents was associated with a 0.5% relative increase in mortality. McClellan and coworkers[9] also studied mortality among Medicare enrollees, using data from the 1980s and 1990s. They found a consistent and strong effect of local bed supply on mortality. Among patients with

acute myocardial infarction, residence in a region with more hospital beds per capita was associated with higher overall mortality in the year after the initial hospitalization. Using data from a 20% sample of Medicare beneficiaries and controlling for differences in age, race, sex, and socioeconomic status, Fisher et al.[10] found a similarly increased risk of death among those residing in regions with more beds per capita. Finally, Skinner and Wennberg,[11] using the statistical methods of Fisher and Welch,[12] performed a logistic regression on life expectancy for a 20% sample of the Medicare population, controlling for possible confounding factors such as level of disability, poverty rates, and underlying levels of common diseases. They found little correlation between the intensity of care near the end of life and mortality rates, whether intensity was measured by spending, days in hospitals, or ICU days near the end of life. They found a slight positive correlation between ICU days and mortality; an increase of 1.0 in the average number of ICU days in the last 6 months of life predicted a 0.8% increase in mortality.

The second reason for concern lies in the plausibility of harm from more intensive use of discretionary invasive technologies in cases where the expected benefits are least certain. Several studies have shown that the use of the ICU is dependent on availability: as the number of available ICU beds increases, the average severity of illness in admitted patients declines.[13,14] The possible mechanisms of harm from the more intensive monitoring that occurs in the ICU have been delineated.[15,16] The finding that the use of right heart catheters in the SUPPORT population was associated with increased mortality, after adjusting for extensive measures of severity of illness, is consistent with these proposed mechanisms of harm.[17] Finally, it is reasonable to assume that greater use of the hospital in high-capacity regions reflects discretionary care, i.e., hospitalization of patients who would not be treated in the hospital in regions of lower bed supply. Adverse events due to hospitalization occur in 3.7%[18] to 17.7%[18,19] of hospitalized patients. Only if the benefits of these discretionary hospitalizations exceed the risks are average outcomes likely to be better. Essentially, if hospitals have about the same incidence of infection, mismedication, or other errors among admissions, then people who live in areas where they are twice as likely to be admitted to hospitals for medical conditions have twice the exposure to these errors and twice the opportunity to be harmed by or to die from them.

If more is not better, i.e., if the marginal value of incremental investments among regions in physician visits, diagnostic tests, hospitalizations for medical conditions, and ICU use is not associated with improved health-care outcomes, then in reaching for our vision of the future, we would be advised to use Portland, Oregon, and Minneapolis as our benchmarks, rather than Orange County, California, and Miami.

PATTERNS OF PRACTICE IN OREGON

Patterns of end-of-life care can show dramatic variation among HRRs located within the same state. Indeed, the variations are often extensive among the constituent HSAs of a given HRR. The state of Oregon provides an example.

Figure 1–9 shows, by HRR of residence, the percent of Medicare decedents who were admitted one or more times to an ICU during the last 6 months of life. Four of the five regions in Oregon had rates near the bottom of the national distribution. There were variations within Oregon, however: providers treating residents of the Salem HSAs were considerably more aggressive than those serving other regions, particularly Bend.

When the Portland region was broken down into its constituent HSAs, we uncovered remarkable local variation. Figure 1–10 provides information about the Portland HSA and three contiguous areas, Hillsboro, McMinnville, and Vancouver, Washington.

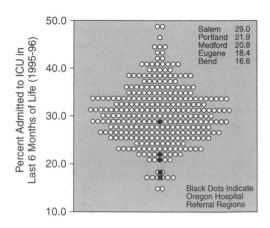

Figure 1–9. Percent of Medicare decedents admitted to intensive care during the last 6 months of life (1995–96). Nationally, the proportion of Medicare decedents admitted to an intensive care unit (ICU) one or more times during their last 6 months of life ranged from about 15% to almost 50% (white points). Rates of such admissions in Oregon's hospital referral regions ranged from 16.6% to 29.0% (black points). Each point represents one of the 306 hospital referral regions in the United States.

Figure 1–9 shows the wide variations in the likelihood of having one or more admissions to intensive care, but it does not tell us what drives particular rates of use of intensity of end-of-life care. In the final section of this chapter, we examine factors contributing to Oregon's overall conservative patterns of end-of-life care and then, acknowledging that variations still exist among Oregon communities, ask what features seem to distinguish Bend, the region with the lowest use of intensive care, from other regions.[20]

Why Is Oregon Generally So Conservative?

One reason Oregon's end-of-life statistics look different from much of the rest of the country is a statewide program of written orders. Oregon nursing homes have a higher than national average rate of do-not-resuscitate (DNR) orders for their residents. Teno and colleagues[21] in 1997 documented that 70% of nursing home residents in Portland, Oregon, had a DNR order. These

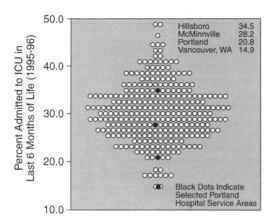

Figure 1–10. Percent of Medicare decedents admitted to intensive care during the last 6 months of life (1995–96). Nationally, the proportion of Medicare decedents admitted to an intensive care unit (ICU) one or more times during their last 6 months of life ranged from about 15% to almost 50% (white points). The variation in such admissions among decedents in hospital service areas serving residents of Oregon ranged from 14.9% to 34.5% (black points). Each point represents one of the 306 hospital referral regions in the United States.

rates continue to rise. In a 1996 study of eight Oregon nursing homes, 91% of residents had a written DNR order.[22]

However, the high rate of DNR orders cannot be the full explanation. Resuscitation efforts have such a low likelihood of being successful in some populations (e.g., those in long-term care) that whether or not cardiopulmonary resuscitation (CPR) is done is unlikely to have a measurable impact on the location of death for those who experience cardiac arrest in long-term care facilities. Something more than avoiding CPR must be having an impact on Oregon's use of ICU beds, specialty consultations, and hospitalization rates near the time of death. A critical factor might be Oregon's Physician Orders for Life-Sustaining Treatment (POLST) program, which enables physicians and nurse practitioners to write medical orders reflecting patients' wishes to set limits on life-sustaining treatments.[23] The POLST form is transportable from one care location to another. Orders can be

clearly written to focus on comfort measures, to clarify that "patient/resident is not to be hospitalized unless comfort measures fail," and to avoid transfer to an ICU in the event of hospitalization. (Of course, there remains the alternative of requesting full treatment.) A copy of the POLST form and further details about the program are available on the web (http://www.ohsu.edu/ethics).

More than 450,000 copies of the POLST form have been distributed through a voluntary statewide program. The POLST form provides clear guidance about transfer to the hospital for persons living in community settings (e.g., at home with hospice or in long-term care). Many persons with advanced illness use the form to request that the focus of their care be on maximizing comfort without transfer to a hospital. The POLST form has been particularly effective at assuring that patient wishes to limit life-sustaining treatment are followed as the patient is transferred between care settings (see Fig. 25–1).

Unlike advance directives, which have not consistently changed the impact of end-of-life care, the data suggest that the POLST program has been effective. Use of the POLST form has generally been associated with clinical care activities congruent with medical orders to limit treatment. In a prospective study of 180 nursing home residents whose POLST forms were marked "DNR" and "comfort measures only" (indicating the dying person should be transferred to the hospital only if comfort measures failed), none of the subjects received CPR, ICU care, or ventilator support during the year of the study. Thirty-eight patients died during the study period, and only two (5%) of these died in an acute-care hospital.[22]

Another factor must be the decades-long debate in Oregon over the quality of end-of-life care.[23] The changes in medical culture would not have happened without the active participation of the public. In the mid-1980s, Oregon Health Decisions conducted statewide outreach activities and distributed advance directive information through faith communities, a statewide program of "training the trainers," and town meetings. The public was bombarded with information about options in end-of-life care during intense media coverage, in 1994 and 1997, of Oregon's two public initiative votes on physician-assisted suicide. During these campaigns, extensive information about hospice care (how to enroll, how hospice works, and who benefits) was made available to the public. Specific information was disseminated about end-of-life care and choices, including how to complete an advance directive and when the POLST form is necessary to ensure that wishes and values will be understood and respected by providers.

The popular press can play a vital role in cultural change,[24] and this is certainly true in the case of Oregon. Policy change and improvements in Oregon's medical culture and end-of-life care would have been impossible without the participation of *The Oregonian*, the state's leading newspaper.[25] *The Oregonian* effectively integrated end-of-life care data with real-life stories of terminally ill Oregonians, making the statistics accessible and understandable for readers.[26,27]

Why is there still so much variation? One way to approach this question is to ask what distinguishes medical care communities with the most conservative patterns of practice from others. Deschutes County, Oregon, has the lowest rate of in-hospital deaths of the 306 HRRs in the United States. Hospice penetration in the region is high; 45% of those who died in Deschutes County in 2000 were enrolled in hospice at the time of death. Advance planning for end-of-life care has become the norm, rather than the exception, in this community; and although it is largely rural, the county provides leadership to the region in palliative care. The county has a total population of about 100,000 and only one hospital, St. Charles, which has a small designated comfort-care unit (two beds) and an effective palliative care team. The team's major focus is on hospice and palliative care and education on how to better support those who are dying at home. While

end-of-life planning is becoming the norm throughout Oregon, it is most seamless in this region. Over 90% of hospice deaths in Deschutes County occurred in a private home or homelike setting in 2000.

The Bend community uses the POLST program more extensively and in a more seamless manner than any other Oregon community. Persons in hospice, long-term care, and home health care are routinely offered the opportunity to express their wishes regarding life-sustaining treatment with the completion of a POLST form. St. Charles Hospital respects the use of the POLST form and endorses it throughout the region.

It is thus possible to identify at least the beginnings of a "system" for end-of-life care that integrates providers at various levels in the delivery system to serve the common purpose of respect for patients and their families. The emphasis on system may be key: once decisions limiting life-sustaining treatment have been made, a system is needed to assure that they are understandable, transportable, and respected in a time of crisis. Families are increasingly ready to engage in the dialogue, but the tools of traditional advance directives alone do not meet this need. Emergency medical personnel, covering physicians and nurses, find that advance directives provide insufficient information and guidance when providing end-of-life care.[28]

Can descriptive statistics regarding variation help other communities achieve systems of end-of-life care? Leaders in the Deschutes Coalition on End-of-Life Care have monitored end-of-life care in their own and other communities using the *Dartmouth Atlas* and other national, statewide, and local data (e.g., the Brown University website: www.chcr.brown.edu/dying/factsondying/htm). Descriptive statistics can focus the energy of a coalition, educate the public via the media, and provide benchmarks for evaluating care. Data can guide policy makers and health systems in developing programs to assure that patients' wishes are respected and that suffering is minimized in life's final chapter.[23,29]

In some communities, patients and their families no longer endorse the idea that more aggressive treatment is always better at the end of life. Oregon statewide studies show that most patients wish to limit life-sustaining treatments at life's end. Despite remarkably low levels of ICU days and specialty visits during the final 6 months of life, satisfaction levels with aggressiveness of treatment remain remarkably high. Family members identified from a 6% sample of 1997 Oregon death certificates were asked about the satisfaction level of treatment their family member had received during life's final months. Interviews were conducted with 475 family members. Five percent of families reported that their family member had received more life-sustaining treatment than they would have wanted, and 2% felt that they received less treatment then they had wished. The vast majority said that wishes for treatment had been respected and followed.[30]

It remains to be seen whether the experiences in Bend will help bring about change in Hillsboro; whether the documentation of variations, such as the striking differences between HSAs in the Portland area, will lead to discussions, debate, and the development of systems of care leading to patterns of end-of-life care in all parts of Oregon that reflect what patients and their families want. The Oregon experience informs the debate about which level of intervention at the end of life is right. Clearly, not every rate is right; and Oregon's efforts to establish what the dying and their families really want provide compelling evidence that much of what is being done in very high-intervention areas of the United States, as documented by the *Dartmouth Atlas*, is not only wasteful but also unwanted.

REFERENCES

1. Wennberg JE, Cooper MM (Eds.). The Quality of Medical Care in the United States: A Report on the Medicare Program. The Dartmouth Atlas of Health Care 1999. Chicago, American Hospital Assoc. Publishing, 1999.

2. Wennberg JW, Fisher ES, Skinner JS. Geography and the debate over Medicare reform. Health Aff (Millwood) 2001.

3. Skinner JS, Fisher ES, Wennberg JE. The efficiency of Medicare. National Bureau of Economic Research working paper 8395 (2001). Available at www.dartmouthatlas.org

4. Pritchard RS, Fisher ES, Teno JM, Sharp SM, Reding DJ, Knaus WA, Wennberg JE, Lynn J. Influence of patient preferences and local health system characteristics on the place of death. Study to Understand Prognoses and Preferences for Outcomes and Risks of Treatment. J Am Geriatr Soc 46:1242–1250, 1998.

5. Wennberg DE, Birkmeyer JD (Eds.). The Dartmouth Atlas of Cardiovascular Health Care. Chicago: American Hospital Associated Publishing, 2000.

6. SUPPORT Principal Investigators. A controlled trial to improve care for seriously ill hospitalized patients. The Study to Understand Prognoses and Preferences for Outcomes and Risks of Treatment (SUPPORT). JAMA 274:1591–1598, 1995.

7. Gallup Poll Organization. Knowledge and Attitudes Related to Hospice Care. Arlington, VA: National Hospice Organization, 1996.

8. Krakauer H, Baily R, et al. The systematic assessment of variations in medical practices and their outcome. Public Health Rep 110:2–12, 1995.

9. McClellan M, McNeil BJ, Newhouse JP. Does more intensive treatment of acute myocardial infarction in the elderly reduce mortality? Analysis using instrumental variables. JAMA 272:859–866, 1994.

10. Fisher ES, Wennberg JE, Stukel TA, Skinner JS, Sharp SM, Freeman JL, Gittelsohn AM. Associations among hospital capacity, utilization and mortality of US Medicare beneficiaries, controlling for sociodemographic factors. Health Serv Res 34:1351–1362, 2000.

11. Skinner JS, Wennberg JE. Regional inequality in Medicare spending: the key to Medicare reform? In: Garber A (Ed.). Frontiers in Health Policy Research, vol 3. Cambridge, MA, MIT Press, pp. 69–90, 2000.

12. Fisher ES, Welch HG. Avoiding the unintended consequences of growth in medical care: how might more be worse? JAMA 281:446–453, 1999.

13. Strauss MJ, LoGerfo JP, Yeltatzie JA, Temkin N, Hudson LD. Rationing of intensive care unit services: an everyday occurrence. JAMA 255:1143–1146, 1986.

14. Singer DE, Carr PL, Mulley AG, Thibault GE. Rationing intensive care-physician re-

sponses to a resource shortage. N Engl J Med 309:115–16, 1983.

15. Teno JM, Fisher ES, Hamel MB, Wu AW, Murphy DJ, Wenger NS, Lynn J, Harrell FE Jr. Decision-making and outcomes of prolonged ICU stays in seriously ill patients. J Am Geriatr Soc 48:70S–74S, 2000.

16. Berwick D. The SUPPORT project: lessons for action. Hastings Cent Rep 25(Suppl.): s21–s22, 1995.

17. Lynn J, Harrell F, Cohn F, Wagner D, Connors AF. Prognoses of seriously ill hospitalized patients on the days before death: implications for patient care and public policy. New Horiz 5:56–61, 1997.

18. Brennan TA, Leape LL, Laird NM, Hebert L, Localio AR, Lawthers AG, Newhouse JP, Weiler PC, Hiatt HH. Incidence of adverse events and negligence in hospitalized patients: results of the Harvard Medical Practice Study I. N Engl J Med 324:370–376, 1991.

19. Andrews LB, Stocking C, Krizek T, Gottlieb L, Krizek C, Vargish T, Siegler M. An alternative strategy for studying adverse events in medical care. Lancet 349:309–313, 1997.

20. Tolle SW. Care of the dying: clinical and financial lessons from the Oregon experience. Ann Intern Med 128:567–568, 1998.

21. Teno JM, Branco KJ, Mor V, Phillips CD, Hawes C, Morris J, et al. Changes in advance care planning in nursing homes before and after the Patient Self-Determination Act: report of a 10 state survey. J Am Geriatr Soc 45:939–944, 1997.

22. Tolle SW, Tilden VP, Nelson CA, Dunn PM. A prospective study of the efficacy of the physician order form for life-sustaining treatment. J Am Geriatr Soc 46:1097–1102, 1998.

23. Tolle SW, Tilden VP. Changing end-of-life planning: the Oregon experience. J Palliat Med 2002, in press.

24. Fein EB. Failing to discuss dying adds to pain of patient and family. New York Times 5 March 1997, sec A1, p. A14.

25. O'Keefe M. A new way of dying: public pressure has changed the way American medicine deals with end-of-life. Oregonian 29 September 1997, sec A1, pp. A18–A20.

26. Hoover-Barnett E. POLST form offers choices in care options for dying. Oregonian 2 September, 1998, see D1, p. D13.

27. Hoover-Barnett E. Doctor's orders. For 10 years, dying Oregonians have had a way to make their wishes heeded. Oregonian 24 October, 2001, sec D1, p. D4.

28. Teno JM, Licks S, Lynn J, Wenger N, Connors AF, et al. Do advance directives provide instructions that direct care? J Am Geriatr Soc 45:508–512, 1997.

29. Tolle SW, Rosenfeld AG, Tilden VP, Park BA. Oregon's low in-hospital death rates: what determines where people die and satisfaction with decisions on place of death? Ann Intern Med 130:681–685, 1999.

30. Tolle SW, Tilden VT, Rosenfield AG, Hickman SE. Family reports of barriers to optimal care of the dying. Nurs Res 49:301–317, 2000.

2

Developmental Challenges and Opportunities for "Growth": The Inner Life at the End of Life

ROBERT N. BUTLER

From the perspective of development, a dying person's thoughts, feelings, experiences, and activities during the last months, days, and moments of life may be more important than where and how that person dies or the causes of death.

This is not to say that the setting in which one dies is unimportant, nor is it meant to suggest that the cause of death, which varies in the degree of suffering it causes, is of no significance; but it is the inner life and outer conduct in the prospect of death that may be most meaningful to the individual and to the family and friends who are left behind. Coming to terms with mortality and fulfilling opportunities for "growth" even at the end of life are the last great developmental challenges, but usually there is all too little time to meet them successfully. Ambient conditions are important, specifically the availability of the best palliative care and the support of family and friends; and, of course, the absence of dementia and its destruction of the self is critical.

COMMUNICATING THE EXPERIENCE OF DYING

At death, dreams and stories of a lifetime cease in endless silence. There have been millions of deaths of *Homo sapiens* and precursors over a million years, yet we have little idea of the inner life, the thoughts, sensations, and feelings of the last moments, even days and months of life. Why is this so? We find it difficult to discuss dying and death. It is not easy to intrude on people caught up in pain and suffering, in fear and dread. Moreover, there have been no comprehensive and systematic studies of people in the process of dying, although anecdotal bedside and clinical information is available. Nonetheless, last words have been collected and accorded special power of illumination and insight, particularly prophesies and curses upon others.

Memoirs and autobiographies are also helpful. They suggest that at critical transitions in life and toward the very end, people tend to reminisce and reflect in ways

17

that are often idealized, replete with denial, and not always candid and objective. Memories are mutable, and interpretations shift. Nonetheless, as death approaches, many make efforts to come to terms with the life led. Often, this takes the form of resolving conflicts, effecting reconciliations, and atoning for deeds done or actions not taken.[1]

Many people, however, remain without a voice, some because they are not introspective and/or have limited language skills, others because they feel they have little to say; still others believe the world has little interest in them.

Socrates said, "An unexamined life is not worth living." Robert Hughes said, "An unlived life is not worth examining." Both suggest an elitist position. How do we think about the struggles for sheer survival that dominate the lives of so many? Although milestones and anniversaries dominate memories, the unplanned and unexpected turns in life are more common and have innate meaning of their own. Watching from another planet, human activities during the daily rounds of life might appear to be carried out as ritual. Some observers might divine human patterns, others randomness and even chaos.

In short, it is not possible at this time to provide truly representative as well as systematic and detailed portraits of the inner life at the end of life. Were we able to do so, we might learn both how to die better and, most of all, how to live better. There have been limited epidemiological studies of the last days of life conducted in Great Britain and at the National Institute on Aging in the United States, but they address only the external aspects. *An in-depth study is needed to help demystify the enormous fear of the unknown, death.* Examples of specific situations of particular relevance to the study of motives and feelings at the end of life include those who contemplate and carry out physician-assisted suicide, those who decide to end kidney dialysis, and those who terminate cancer treatment.

We know little about the last stage of life, other than the insights of fine writers and observers of the human condition and the few who have focused upon the stages of life, such as Carl G. Jung[2] and Erik H. Erikson.[3] The former stressed individuation with aging, and the latter the counterpoint of ego integrity versus despair.

THE TIME DIMENSION

There is a time dimension to be considered. When does end of life begin? Schopenhauer, referring to the inner psychological life, defined middle age as that point in time when people begin to count back from death instead of forward from birth.

The cheerfulness and vivacity of youth are partly due to the fact that, when we are ascending the hill of life, death is not visible: it lies down at the bottom of the other side. But once we have crossed the top of the hill, death comes in view—death, which until then, was known to us only by hearsay.[4]

What is the time frame for the imposing reality of severe chronic and/or terminal illness?

Questions arise concerning the depth of the inner life at the end of life. How profoundly is an individual coping with the end of life? Is there insight, denial, counterphobia, acceptance? How much does reality motivate a dying person to come to terms with life, reconcile strained relationships, atone for misdeeds? The wonderful play *Wit*, by Margaret Edson, about a poetry professor who is dying, informs us of the use of intellectual defenses and irony when confronted with death. Likewise, near-death experiences of a "glowing light" and something "comforting over there" may simply be defensive processes at work in our inner life, protecting us from overpowering anxiety.

Still another dimension is the age of the individual. Again, Schopenhauer said,

A complete and adequate notion of life can never be attained by anyone who does not reach old age; for it is only the old man who sees life whole and knows its natural course; it is only he who is acquainted—and this is most important—not only with its entrance, like the rest of mankind, but with its exit too; so that he alone has a full sense of its utter vanity; whilst the others never cease to labor under the false notion that everything will come right in the end.[4]

Schopenhauer considered disillusion a feature of late life.

Disillusion is the chief characteristic of old age; for by that time the fictions are gone which gave life its charm and spurred on the mind to activity; the splendors of the world have been proved null and vain; its pomp, grandeur, and magnificence are faded. A man has then found out that behind most of the things he wants, and most of the pleasures he longs for, there is very little after all; and so he comes by degrees to see that our existence is all empty and void. It is only when he is seventy years old that he quite understands the first words of the Preacher; and this again explains why it is that old men are sometimes fretful and morose.[4]

From one angle, it is difficult to imagine anything but disillusion as one moves from the hope, idealism, and aspirations of youth to the reality of human destructiveness, whether genetic or cultural. How is it possible not to become, to a degree, disillusioned and depressed? In contrast to this great pessimistic philosopher, some do leave the world with a sense of hope, offering encouragement to their survivors. Abraham Joshua Heschel said,

Old age is a major challenge to the inner life; it takes both wisdom and strength not to succumb to it. . . . Human existence cannot derive its ultimate meaning from society, because society itself is in need of meaning. . . . Old age [must] be regarded not as the age of stagnation but as the age of opportunities for inner growth.[5]

THE END OF LIFE

The courage to face death is another issue, perhaps especially for those without the supports of religion and ritual; but such support is not always necessary. Some contemporaries were disappointed that David Hume, the great English empiricist philosopher and an avowed atheist, did not repent before his death and yet died reasonably well.

As people approach the end of their lives, legacy becomes important. There is more to legacy than leaving money, real estate, and material objects. There is also the bequest of the impact of a personality, a culture, and a model of how to live and die. Some say we die as we lived, in infinite variety. Some take a last family trip together in anticipation of death. Others want only to be at home.

Probably, there are also gender differences at the end of life that have not been studied. In general, women, the kin-keepers and caregivers, live longer than men and risk the possibility of dying alone. The end-of-life inner life is influenced by the kind of end of life that was experienced by one's partner, for example, a man or woman taking care of a spouse with Alzheimer's disease. We also need to learn about racial, ethnic, and religious differences in the way people die.

Perhaps life is an end in itself, as Justice Oliver Wendell Holmes observed. Life is more than an individual physical body operating alone. Lives are part of a convoy, of linked cohorts with parents, children, friends, acquaintances, and the ambient zeitgeist. For example, the added longevity of the twentieth century did not occur in isolation. The twentieth century was marked by increasing complexity and speed of life that followed scientific discoveries and social changes. New elements of complexity further define life itself, broadening, deepening, enriching, as well as disordering the last stage of life. Indeed, a transformation of this stage is well under way, for people are living longer and better and exploring new opportunities as they age.

As an individual's life draws to a close, there is bereavement or grief over the loss of the self. Sometimes it is subtle, perhaps beyond the awareness of the individual but often obvious and acknowledged. Sometimes the dying person must emotionally support the survivors.

Accompanying the grief that a person feels, particularly in the face of a life-threatening illness, there may be self-pity as well as anxiety. An individual may experience blunt fear and anger, intensifying the sense of loss and depression, framed first by denial and last by acceptance, according to Elizabeth Kubler-Ross' valuable, if imperfect, delineation of the stages of dying. Physiological factors such as "air hunger" may complicate anxiety, fear, and dread. When depression and other emotional symptoms are present, most support treatment to bring relief. However, some would argue that such treatment might obfuscate intellectual functioning and/or diminish the suffering necessary to the normative processes of resolution and restitution. This is a sensitive professional and ethical problem.

DEATH WITH DIGNITY

Imagining one's death, of course, is not the same as experiencing it. There is only one opportunity. For some, but not all, there may be difficulty "letting go" or feeling ready to go.

There is much romanticism associated with death in general, especially the desire to die at home, when, in fact, it can be extraordinarily difficult for both the individual and the family. For the individual, there may be less security concerning the availability of pain medications, nursing, and other help. For the family, it may prove an extraordinary burden.

Part of the wish to die at home is because so much is missing in the hospital and nursing home: the ongoing presence of the family, touching and the laying on of hands, the cloak of protection offered by the familiarity of the environment, the presence of personal belongings and significant people. Theoretically, it might be possible to import some of these amenities into the hospital, just as it might be possible to import into the home some of what the hospital provides. The more than 2300 American hospices and palliative care units in hospitals constitute steps in the right direction, helping to create more appropriate environments for the dying.

In late life, older people experience loss of hearing, vision, and mobility and suffer from multiple chronic diseases that culminate in multiple system failure. We die not only biologically, but also psychologically and emotionally, and we die socially in terms of friends, relationships, and the institutions around which we organize our lives.

When people speak of "death with dignity," what is meant is a sense of autonomy, the presence of family, the status of resolution and reconciliation, a death at home. It is typically American, with its powerful libertarian streak, to stress autonomy, with the suggestion that control over dying and death are inalienable rights. The concepts of active euthanasia and physician-assisted suicide in particular depend on a belief in the reality and virtue of autonomy. Should death be totally autonomous? In considering physician-assisted suicide, there is a societal interest as well. It may be argued that the bereaved also have rights: of access, of interaction, of grief itself. Indeed, in families that have experienced suicide, the impact extends through several generations.

Twenty-seven terminally ill patients in Oregon used the physician-assisted suicide law to end their lives in 1999. In 1998, 29,383 Oregonians died of all causes. Clearly, very few individuals make use of Oregon's availability of physician-assisted suicide.

In any case, the experience of death is not just in the hands of doctors or even of the dying person. There is no genuine autonomy because dying and death are essentially pathobiological and ultimately biologically determined. While death is ultimately beyond the powers of both the physician and the patient, powerful psychological, social, and cultural factors can delay death. Data show, for example, declines in death rates before important public events, such as the Chinese New Year, and rises thereafter.

In addition to the emphasis on autonomy is the notion that one should die well, show fortitude, and at the same time experience spiritual enlightenment; but truly ideal deaths, depending on varied perspectives, are rare. For example, Sherwin Nuland, Yale University surgeon and author of *How We Die*,[6] states that many people have a difficult death. According to a report by the Department of Health and Human Services, "Management of Cancer Pain," 90% of patients with cancer can have their cancer pain managed.[7] Unfortunately, treatment itself (i.e., chemotherapy) can cause great discomfort, and physicians are frequently untrained in pain relief. A small percentage of people die in their sleep.

However, we must understand the enormous complexity of the subject, which goes beyond pain. The inner life at the end is usually embedded in physical decline, pain and suffering, grief over one's death, separation from one's surviving family and friends, and the intrusiveness of the health-care environment, including medications that may dull consciousness, so often a part of even the best palliative care.

The bottom line is that clinicians, family members, and others who are close to severely ill and terminally ill patients, whether over several years or a few months, weeks, or moments, need to be sensitive to the natural need of the dying patient to come to terms with the life that has been lived (i.e., to find meaning), effect reconciliations, resolve conflicts, atone for deeds and misdeeds. Beyond the relief of physical pain and emotional suffering, support of this process should constitute a significant component of palliative medicine. Within this context, we protest the inappropriate use of high technological interventions and suggest that their use depend only on open discussion and agreement by the patient, family, and physician. All too often there are futile and burdensome medical interventions. The patient–family–clinician interactions at this stage of life are critical to a decent death.[8] The desire for health care is not infinite or insatiable, and patients often tell us when to stop. For example, it is appropriate, even kind, to stop giving a dying patient artificial nutrition and hydration and to let the person die.

THE PHYSICIAN AND THE DYING PATIENT

Most people believe in an afterlife, but few seem in a hurry to get there. In the Judeo-Christian tradition, death was God's punishment for Eve and Adam, who had eaten of the fruit of the Tree of Knowledge, disobeying God's specific commandment.

Their behavior alone lost eternal life for all. However, in the Christian tradition, this loss is recoverable. The Book of Revelations says, "Death shall be no more, neither shall there be mourning nor crying nor pain anymore." These ideas represent the ground-level cultural framework of the Western tradition concerning death.

There are many other, often conflicting religions, concepts, and cultures. The culture of medicine offers a good example. Beginning in the twentieth century, higher expectations emerged based on solid accomplishments and the unprecedented increase in length of life. There are specific subcultures within medicine, such as the field of oncology, where the "war on cancer" had led to near feverish expectations of survival. Another mainstream subculture is critical care medicine (intensive care units). Anti-aging medicine is an aberrant movement. In these several cultures, the desires of patients and doctors reinforce each other.

An older person or any person with a terminal, serious, or life-threatening chronic illness faces many challenges and opportunities for growth near the end of life. Personal evolution continues to the very end. Clinicians must consider the importance of mental and verbal lucidity to the "examined life" when administering medications. The deathbed confession, seeking absolution and reconciliation, is an extreme expression of the life review.

Many hospital settings are religious, emphasizing the observance of religious traditions of preserving life and "the sanctity of life." Equal attention should be paid to persons of religious belief and those who do not profess a belief.

We cannot talk about a better death if there are few doctors, nurses, and other health providers well trained to provide it. We do not educate and help health-care personnel deal with death. There is little counseling and little support given to medical students when patients die. One might question how large a role in death doctors should play. It seems wasteful to create a new profession to help the individual, family, and doctor negotiate death. Better to advise the physician not to become a philosopher, a spiritual leader or clergy, but instead to remain the "attending" physician and understand what forces need to be mobilized, for example, the need for a secular death in the case of a nonbeliever and the need to call upon appropriate clergy for the religious.

If a patient does not bring up the topic of end-of-life care, the physician should do so at the beginning of their relationship and under the following circumstances: when a patient is facing imminent death, expresses the desire to die, is in the hospital with a severe progressive illness; when discussing prognosis, hopes, and fears; and when the prognosis appears poor. In truth, in a rich doctor–patient relationship, this topic should be brought up early and discussion should be ongoing.[9]

Do doctors have a pathological and excessive urge to fight death, or are they simply reflecting their culture? With the possible exception of the oncologist and the critical care physician, it is the author's impression that most physicians are reasonable in accepting death, do not undertake excessive treatment, and are mindful of the attitudes of the patient, the family, the law, the clergy, and so forth. Most people understand that many doctors have helped to negotiate the timing and circumstances of death with patients and their families. It is estimated that 70% of deaths occur after withdrawal of "death-prolonging" technologies, such as ventilators, after the request of the patient and family. If this is true, it contradicts the idea that doctors deny death and oppose it at all costs. Obviously, we need empirical studies of doctors and patients with regard to the end of life.

CONCLUSION

To summarize, it would be ideal if one could address the purpose of this chapter based on comprehensive, in-depth, empirical representative studies to delineate how people live out their last moments, days, and months of life, with particular emphasis on the nature of their inner lives, the situations in which they find themselves, and the limitations they face.

Were such information available, we would discuss, first, what we know (and what we do not) about the inner life at the end of life; second, how, ideally, people can continue to evolve emotionally at the end of life and the extent to which they can make choices and contribute to personal growth; and third, what else is intended by "development at the end of life," for example, opportunities to leave a legacy and review one's life.

The review of one's life appears to be the psychological basis for a parade of choices that necessarily underlies the development and growth of each of us. The growth of the palliative care field in the health professions and the medical academy will support the research needed to understand the lived human experience of facing death. These insights will help us to build a healthcare system that can best accompany patients and their families through this inevitable and important life stage.

REFERENCES

1. Butler RN. The life review: an interpretation of reminiscence in the aged. Psychiatry 26:65–76, 1963.
2. Jung CG. The stages of life. In: Modern Man in Search of a Soul. New York, Harcourt, Brace & World, 1933.
3. Erickson EH. The problem of ego identity. Journal Psychol Issues 1:101–164, 1959.
4. Schopenhauer A. The Ages of Life. Counsels and Maxims, trans. T. Bailey Saunders. London, Swon Sonnenschein & Co., 1990.
5. Heschel AJ. The Insecurity of Freedom. New York, Farrar, Straus, Giroux, 1966.
6. Nuland S. How We Die. New York, Knopf, 1994.
7. Agency for Health Care Policy and Research. AHCPR releases cancer pain treatment guidelines. Available at http://www.hhs.gov/news/press/pre1995pres/940302.txt
8. Lynn J., Harrold J. Handbook for Mortals. Guidance for People Facing Serious Illness. New York, Oxford University Press, 1999.
9. Block SD. Psychological considerations, growth, and transcendence at the end of life. The art of the possible. JAMA 285:2898–2905, 2001.

3

Assessing Quality of Life and Quality of Dying in the Elderly: Implications for Clinical Practice of Palliative Medicine

J. RANDALL CURTIS AND DONALD L. PATRICK

There is a growing concern that disproportionate amounts of health-care budgets are spent for end-of-life medical care, and many authors have decried the high cost of dying in our society.[1–3] A large part of the reason that this issue has received such attention is the changing age distribution of our population and the high proportion of deaths that occur in acute-care hospitals,[4] particularly in the expensive setting of the intensive care unit (ICU).[4,5] Consequently, there has been interest in finding ways to limit the aggressiveness and cost of care at the end of life. There is a widespread belief that older patients, especially older patients with a reduced quality of life due to chronic disease, do not want life-sustaining treatments at the end of life. In this chapter, we examine the empiric data surrounding this issue and challenge this assumption in the hope of providing clinicians an alternative way of viewing the role of quality of life in decisions about the use and the withholding or withdrawing of life-sustaining therapy. We also examine some new developments in the area of measuring the quality of dying.

WHAT IS QUALITY OF LIFE AND HOW IS IT MEASURED?

Quality of life is one of the commonly used patient-assessed outcomes, and use of this outcome to assess medical treatments has increased dramatically over the past three decades. A Medline search of *quality of life* in combination with *elderly* in the year 2000 identified 1665 articles, a marked increase from only 104 articles 20 years earlier. If clinicians are going to use data about of quality of life in their decision making and care recommendations for older patients, it is important that they have a basic understanding of the terminology and methodologies used in this field. Patient-assessed health outcomes can be divided into four major categories: quality of life, health status, health state preferences, and patient satisfaction with care. In this chapter, we focus on quality of life and health status measurement. Figure 3–1 shows the relationships between the terms used to describe health status and quality of life, but it is important to understand the distinctions and the overlap. This figure shows the

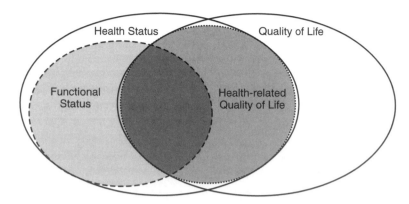

Figure 3–1. Venn diagram depicting overlapping concepts of quality of life, health status, health-related quality of life (grey circle), and functional status (light grey).

overlap in the operational definitions of these terms; several useful conceptual models have helped to advance our understanding of the interactions between these terms and clinical variables.[6,7] Quality of life and health status are important outcome measures in medicine, public health, and health policy.[8]

The term *quality of life* is widely used in clinical research and clinical care but sometimes to mean different things by different authors. In its broadest definition, the quality of an individual's life is a holistic, self-determined evaluation of satisfaction with issues important to the individual. Quality of life is influenced by many factors, including financial status, housing, employment, spirituality, social support network, and health. Consequently, many medical investigators use the more restrictive term *health-related quality of life* (HRQoL) to mean quality of life as it is affected by health. It is generally agreed that "quality of life" is considerably more comprehensive than "health status" and includes aspects of the environment that may or may not be affected by health or treatment. This distinction is not always easy to make, however, because ill health and treatment, particularly in life-threatening circumstances, can be equated with quality of life by those concerned. The term *functional status* is used to describe an individual's ability to function in such diverse realms as the phys-

ical, social, and emotional. These two terms, *HRQoL* and *functional status*, are often used interchangeably but represent different concepts. Functional status reflects the ability to perform the tasks of daily life, while HRQoL connotes the subjective experience of the impact of health status on the quality of life. Operationally, many of the instruments designed to measure HRQoL or functional status encompass both, which can make it difficult to distinguish these concepts in practical applications.

On average, functional status declines with increasing age. However, it is important to understand the confounding in this association from the burden of chronic disease. That is, if one controls for the burden of chronic diseases, the decline in functional status that occurs with increasing age becomes much less apparent.[9] Furthermore, when one examines quality of life, this confounding effect is even more apparent.[9,10] In other words, if one controls for the impact of chronic disease, one does not see a dramatic decline in overall quality of life as individuals age.

HOW DOES QUALITY OF LIFE AFFECT PATIENTS' MEDICAL DECISION MAKING?

However, elderly individuals with one or more coexisting chronic conditions often experience progressive decline in functional status and, to a lesser extent, quality of life.[11] It may seem intuitive that as patients' functional status and quality of life decrease, so will their interest in undergoing aggressive life-sustaining medical treatments. If this is true, we should be able to use quality of life as one way to understand and communicate about patients' treatment preferences for life-sustaining care at the end of life. However, as we describe below, there are several assumptions in this reasoning that are incorrect.

A number of studies have examined elderly patients' preferences for undergoing life-sustaining medical care as a function of their projected quality of life after such care. Most patients say that they would forego life-sustaining treatment if their quality of life after treatment were severely impaired.[12–15] This same finding is true for patients who know what it is like to receive intensive care because they have had a life-threatening illness treated in the ICU.[16] Most elderly patients say they would not want life-sustaining treatment if the outcome of such care were a severely reduced quality of life, such as a persistent vegetative state or dependence on others for all of the activities of daily living.

However, these data should not be extrapolated to make the assumption that patients who currently have a lower, but not severely reduced, quality of life prefer that life-sustaining treatment be withheld or withdrawn. The studies cited above use hypothetical future health states that involve a very poor quality of life, such as a persistent vegetative state or severe stroke. In fact, many of these health states involve such severe impairment that would not be possible to assess the patients' perspective while in these states because the patients cannot communicate. However, when studies measure current quality of life, there is no or very little correlation between quality of life and patients' preferences for aggressive life-sustaining medical care.[12,17–20] In a study of seriously ill, hospitalized patients over the age of 80, only a third of patients rated their current quality of life as

excellent or very good but almost 70% were willing to give up less than 1 month of 12 in exchange for excellent health.[20] Furthermore, patients were willing to trade significantly less time for a healthy life than their family members assumed they would.[20] The finding that there is little correlation between quality of life and treatment preferences is also true for patients who have received care in the ICU in the past and therefore know what this care entails.[17] One study suggested that patients with decreased HRQoL may actually prefer more aggressive medical treatment.[21]

Finally, it is important for clinicians to understand the role that the treatment itself may play in some patients' preference for life-sustaining therapy. In a study of patients' preferences for life-sustaining therapy in different health states, some patients reported that they would not want life-sustaining therapy even if the outcome were a health state that they considered to be preferable to death.[22] In these circumstances, patients seem to weigh the burdens of treatment itself in the decision to forego treatment. Nursing home residents and elderly outpatients are more likely to consider the burden of treatment than are younger, well adults. These findings suggest that clinicians should consider and discuss the burden of treatment with elderly patients and their families. However, in discussing the burden of treatment with patients, it is important to realize that many patients will find it difficult to imagine life during some treatments. For example, patients may say they want to forego short-term and long-term mechanical ventilation simply because the ventilator has a cultural image of dependence and discomfort. Others cannot picture life under dialysis treatment or chemotherapy given the lifestyle changes and fatigue involved. What patients perceive as a burden of treatment may be severely limited by a lack of relevant experience, and again, patients' hypothetical concerns are not necessarily an accurate reflection of how they would feel during or after a treatment. Complex issues like short-term mechanical ventilation may be hard to communicate and require that clinicians develop some expertise in discussing them.[23,24]

HOW DOES QUALITY OF LIFE AFFECT CLINICIANS' MEDICAL DECISION MAKING?

There is evidence that physicians make the incorrect assumption that elderly patients with lower current quality of life want less life-sustaining therapy. In a study of 258 elderly outpatients, there was no or very little significant correlation between quality of life and treatment preferences for cardiopulmonary resuscitation (CPR) or mechanical ventilation.[18] However, when these patients' primary-care physicians were asked whether they thought the patient would want CPR or mechanical ventilation, there was a significant correlation between physicians' impressions of patients' treatment preferences and the patients' quality of life. These data suggest that physicians assume that patients with lower current quality of life want less life-sustaining therapy when this is not the case. Since physicians' predictions of patients' treatment preferences may have an important effect on the treatments received,[25] these findings imply that patients with poor but measurable quality of life may receive less life-sustaining medical care than they would otherwise choose. Therefore, physicians should be careful to not make incorrect assumptions about patients' treatment preferences based on their own perspective of the patient's quality of life.

MEASURING THE QUALITY OF DYING

Improving the quality of health care for patients at the end of their lives has become a major national clinical and research objective.[4] Efforts to improve this care have included randomized, controlled trials of advance directives,[26,27] educational interventions,[5] and a comprehensive intervention that included feedback of prognostic information to patients, families, and physicians and facilitation of physician–patient communication.[5] These interventions have not demonstrated significant benefit. Part of the reason these interventions failed to improve quality of care may be due to the lack of sensitive measures of the outcomes of this care that patients and families define as important.[28] Outcome measures that accurately assess these features would allow us to identify, evaluate, and disseminate interventions that improve care at the end of life for elderly as well as younger patients. In measuring these outcomes, it may be important to differentiate the concepts of quality of life at the end of life, quality of end-of-life care, and quality of dying and death. Stewart et al.[29] developed a conceptual model that differentiates these concepts. There is a growing literature concerning quality-of-life measurement at the end of life.[29–36] To date, studies have not examined whether there are important differences between younger and elderly patients in quality of life at the end of life. There is also a growing literature on quality of end-of-life care, and researchers have investigated the important components of quality of medical care at the end of life from multiple perspectives.[37–39] There is strong interest in developing and using measures of the quality of care at the end of life to improve end-of-life care.[40,41] However, there has been little research demonstrating that these measures can be used to improve care or investigating whether elderly patients have a unique perspective on the important components of high-quality end-of-life care. If we are to identify interventions and quality-improvement efforts that improve the dying experience for patients of all ages, we will need reliable, valid, and responsive measures of these different aspects of end of life: quality of life at the end of life, quality of care at the end of life, and quality of the dying experience.

Using literature reviews and a series of qualitative studies, we have developed a measure of the *quality of dying and death* with the goal of measuring the degree to which a person's preferences for dying and the moment of death are *(1)* concordant with observations of how the person actually died as reported by others and *(2)* modified by circumstances surrounding death that may have prevented the realization of prior preferences.[42] Measuring the quality of dying and death according to this definition includes obtaining from patients their preferences about dying and death and comparing these preferences to reports from family members after death. Preliminary studies suggest that the quality of dying and death may be a valid assessment of the quality of the dying experience when used as an after-death interview with family members,[43] but further research is needed to assess its responsiveness and utility in assessing the effectiveness of interventions.

There are a number of important methodological challenges in assessing the quality of dying or the quality of end-of-life care. Because it is not possible to assess patients' experiences of the dying process or the care they received at the end of life, it is necessary to use surrogates to assess this experience. Potential surrogates include family members and health-care workers. Family members obviously have their own burdens and stressors as a loved one is dying[44,45] and their assessments may be shaped by their own experiences or by grief or other complicating factors, such as guilt.[46,47] Furthermore, different family members may have very different perspectives on the patient's experience and the assessment of the quality of death or quality of care could be affected by the time from death to the assessment.[46] Although healthcare providers are another source of information, they may spend only limited time with patients during the dying process and obviously have their own biases. Future research is needed to examine agreement across raters, the meaning of disagreements that will exist, and methods of identifying the "most accurate" rater of the quality of dying.[46]

IMPLICATIONS FOR CLINICAL PRACTICE

The belief that elderly patients with lower quality of life prefer less aggressive medical care has made it into clinical practice and bedside decision making. Unfortunately, most clinicians are not aware of the weak connection between these patients' current quality of life and their treatment preferences. Patients and doctors infrequently communicate about end-of-life care prior to life-threatening illness,[5] and family members and primary-care physicians are frequently unable to predict patients' preferences for end-of-life care.[48–50] Therefore, current medical practice runs the risk of making inaccurate assumptions about treatment preferences based on physician or surrogate interpretations of patients' quality of life. Consequently, it is important that clinicians caring for elderly patients not make assumptions about treatment preferences based on the patients' quality of life. Instead, clinicians should take the time to discuss treatment preferences and goals of therapy with patients and their families.

Quality of life at the end of life, quality of end-of-life care, and quality of dying and death will likely be important aspects of assessing interventions to improve the quality of care that we provide to elderly patients nearing the end of their lives. There are a number of such measures under development and being used in intervention studies. Further research is needed to identify those measures that provide reliable and valid assessments of these concepts and thereby assist us in identifying interventions that improve patients' experiences.

REFERENCES

1. Bayer R, Callahan D, Fletcher J, et al. The care of the terminally ill: mortality and economics. N Engl J Med 309:1490–1494, 1983.
2. Schroeder SA, Showstack JA, Schwartz J. Survival of adult high-cost patients: report of a follow-up study from nine acute-care hospitals. JAMA 245:1446–1449, 1981.

3. Turnbull AD, Carlon G, Baron R, Sichel W, Young C, Howland W. The inverse relationship between cost and survival in the critically ill cancer patient. Crit Care Med 7:20–23, 1979.

4. Field MJ, Cassel CK. Approaching Death: Improving Care at the End of Life. Institute of Medicine Report. Washington DC: National Academy Press, 1997.

5. SUPPORT Principal Investigators. A controlled trial to improve care for seriously ill hospitalized patients: the Study to Understand Prognoses and Preferences for Outcomes and Risks of Treatments (SUPPORT). JAMA 274:1591–1598, 1996.

6. Wilson IB, Cleary PD. Linking clinical variables with health-related quality of life: a conceptual model of patient outcomes. JAMA 273:59–65, 1995.

7. Patrick DL, Chiang YP. Measurement of health outcomes in treatment effectiveness evaluations: conceptual and methodological challenges. Med Care 9:II14–II27, 2000.

8. Patrick DL, Erickson P. Health Status and Health Policy: Quality of Life in Health Care Evaluation and Resource Allocation. New York: Oxford University Press, 1993.

9. Michelson H, Bolund C, Brandberg Y. Multiple chronic health problems are negatively associated with health-related quality of life irrespective of age. Qual Life Res 9:1093–1104, 2000.

10. Michalos AC, Hubley AM, Zumbo BD, Hemingway D. Health and other aspects of the quality of life of older people. Soc Indicators Res 54:239–274, 2001.

11. Patrick DL, Kinne S, Engelberg RA, Pearlman RA. Functional status and perceived quality of life in adults with and without chronic conditions. J Clin Epidemiol 53:779–785, 2000.

12. Gerety MB, Chiodo LK, Kanten DB, Tuley MR, Cornell JE. Medical treatment preferences of nursing home residents: relationship to function and concordance with surrogate decision-makers. J Am Geriatr Soc 1993:953–960, 1993.

13. Murphy DJ, Burrows D, Santilli S, et al. The influence of the probability of survival on patients' preferences regarding cardiopulmonary resuscitation. N Engl J Med 330:545–549, 1994.

14. Cohen-Mansfield J, Rabinovich BA, Lipson S, et al. The decision to execute a durable power of attorney for health care and preferences regarding the utilization of life-sustaining treatments in nursing home residents. Arch Intern Med 151:289–294, 1991.

15. Schneiderman LJ, Pearlman RA, Kaplan RM, Anderson JP, Rosenberg EM. Relationship of general advance directive instructions to specific life-sustaining treatment preferences in patients with serious illness. Arch Intern Med 152:2114–2122, 1992.

16. Elpern EH, Patterson PA, Gloskey D, Bone RC. Patients' preferences for intensive care. Crit Care Med 20:43–47, 1992.

17. Danis ML, Patrick DL, Southerland LI, Green ML. Patients' and families' preferences for medical intensive care. JAMA 260:797–802, 1988.

18. Uhlmann RF, Pearlman RA. Perceived quality of life and preferences for life-sustaining treatment in older adults. Arch Intern Med 151:495–497, 1991.

19. Starr TJ, Pearlman RA, Uhlmann RF. Quality of life and resuscitation decisions in elderly patients. J Gen Intern Med 1:373–379, 1986.

20. Tsevat J, Dawson NV, Wu AW, et al. Health values of hospitalized patients 80 years or older. JAMA 279:371–375, 1998.

21. Garrett J, Harris R, Norburn J, Patrick D. Life-sustaining treatments during terminal illness: who wants what? J Gen Intern Med 1993:361–368, 1993.

22. Patrick DL, Pearlman RA, Starks HE, Cain KC, Cole WG, Uhlmann RF. Validation of preferences for life-sustaining treatment: implications for advance care planning. Ann Intern Med 127:509–517, 1997.

23. Wenrich MD, Curtis JR, Shannon SE, Carline JD, Ambrozy DM, Ramsey PG. Communicating with dying patients within the spectrum of medical care from terminal diagnosis to death. Arch Intern Med 161:868–874, 2001.

24. Lo B, Quill T, Tulsky JA, for the ACP-ASIM End-of-Life Care Consensus Panel. Discussing palliative care with patients. Ann Intern Med 130:744–749, 1999.

25. Orentlicher D. The illusion of patient choice in end-of-life decisions. JAMA 267:2101–2104, 1992.

26. Schneiderman LJ, Kronick R, Kaplan RM, Anderson JP, Langer RD. Effects of offering advance directives on medical treatments and costs. Ann Intern Med 117:599–606, 1992.

27. Danis M, Southerland LI, Garrett JM, et al. A prospective study of advance directives for life-sustaining care. N Engl J Med 324:882–888, 1991.

28. Lo B. Improving care near the end of life: why is it so hard? JAMA 274:1634–1636, 1995.

29. Stewart AL, Teno J, Patrick DL, Lynn J. The concept of quality of life of dying per-

sons in the context of health care. J Pain Symptom Manage 17:93–108, 1999.

30. Byock IR, Merriman MP. Measuring quality of life for patients with terminal illness: the Missoula-VITAS quality of life index. Palliat Med 12:231–244, 1998.

31. Cohen SR, Mount BM, Strobel MG, Bui F. The McGill Quality of Life Questionnaire: a measure of quality of life appropriate for people with advanced disease. A preliminary study of validity and acceptability. Palliat Med 9:207–219, 1995.

32. Cohen SR, Mount BM, Bruera E, Provost M, Rowe J, Tong K. Validity of the McGill Quality of Life Questionnaire in the palliative care setting: a multi-centre Canadian study demonstrating the importance of the existential domain. Palliat Med 11:3–20, 1997.

33. Morris JN, Suissa S, Sherwood S, Wright SM, Greer D. Last days: a study of the quality of life of terminally ill cancer patients. J Chronic Dis 39:47–62, 1986.

34. Ventafridda V, De Conno F, Ripamonti C, Gamba A, Tamburini M. Quality of life assessment during a palliative care programme. Ann Oncol 1:415–420, 1990.

35. Wallston KA, Burger C, Smith RA, Baugher RJ. Comparing the quality of death for hospice and non-hospice cancer patients. Med Care 26:177–182, 1988.

36. Greer DS, Mor V, Morris JN, Sherwood S, Kidder D, Birnbaum H. An alternative in terminal care: results of the National Hospice Study. J Chronic Dis 39:9–26, 1986.

37. Singer PA, Martin DK, Kelner M. Quality end-of-life care: patients' perspective. JAMA 281:163–168, 1999.

38. Curtis JR, Wenrich MD, Carline JD, Shannon SE, Ambrozy DM, Ramsey PG. Understanding physicians' skills at providing end-of-life care: perspectives of patients, families, and health care workers. J Gen Intern Med 16:41–49, 2001.

39. Monias A, Walke L, Morrison RS, Meier DE. The effect of age on medical decisions made by patients with chronic illness. J Palliat Med 2:311–317, 1999.

40. Lynn J. Measuring quality of care at the end of life: a statement of principles. J Am Geriatr Soc 45:526–527, 1997.

41. Teno JM, Byock IR, Field MJ. Research agenda for developing measures to examine quality of life of patients diagnosed with life-limiting illness. J Pain Symptom Manage 17:75–82, 1999.

42. Patrick DL, Engelberg RA, Curtis JR. Evaluating the quality of dying and death. J Pain Symptom Manage 22:717–726, 2001.

43. Curtis JR, Patrick DL, Engelberg RA, Norris KE, Asp CH, Byock IR. A measure of the quality of dying and death: initial validation. J Pain Symptom Manage 24:17–31, 2002.

44. Emanuel EJ, Fairclough DL, Slutsman J, Emanuel LL. Understanding economic and other burdens of terminal illness: the experience of patients and their caregivers. Ann Intern Med 132:451–459, 2000.

45. Covinsky KE, Goldman L, Cook EF, et al. The impact of serious illness on patients' families. JAMA 272:1839–1844, 1994.

46. Fowler JF, Coppola KM, Teno JM. Methodological challenges for measuring quality of care at the end of life. J Pain Symptom Manage 17:114–119, 1999.

47. Hinton J. How reliable are relatives' retrospective reports of terminal illness? Patients' and relatives' accounts compared. Soc Sci Med 43:1229–1236, 1996.

48. Seckler AB, Meier DE, Mulvihill M, Cammer Paris BE. Substituted judgement: how accurate are proxy predictions? Ann Intern Med 115:92–98, 1991.

49. Suhl J, Simons P, Reedy T, Garrick T. Myth of substituted judgement: surrogate decision making regarding life support is unreliable. Arch Intern Med 154:90–96, 1994.

50. Uhlmann RF, Pearlman RA, Cain KC. Physicians' and spouses' predictions of elderly patients' resuscitation preferences. J Gerontol 43:M115–M121, 1988.

4

The Place of Love in the Care of Persons with Advanced Dementia

STEPHEN G. POST

Understanding, communication, and the celebration of the other's life in a personal manner convey a liberating and empowering sense of worth. In his book *Dementia Reconsidered: The Person Comes First,* Tom Kitwood's definition of love within the context of dementia care includes comfort in the original sense of tenderness, closeness, the calming of anxiety, and bonding.[1] Love, so defined, is itself an aspect of palliative care, which is always a great deal more than the provision of needed pain medications.

Altruistic love involves both a judgment of worth and a related "affirmative affection." It is an intentional affirmation of the other, grounded in biologically given emotional capacities that are elevated by world view (including principles, symbol, and myth) and imitation into the sphere of consistency and abiding loyalty.[2] Love is manifest in care, which is love in response to the other in need; it is manifest in compassion, which is love in response to the other in suffering; it is manifest in companion-ship, which is love attentively present with the other in ordinary moments.

LOVE'S PLACE IN PALLIATIVE CARE

Respect for choice and relief of pain and physical symptoms are central parts of palliative care, but caring also involves everything from tone of voice to the small offer to provide a family with a few hours of respite. Underlying care is a form of deep affective affirmation that is the core of altruistic love.

Altruism (*altrui,* "somebody else") is a broad classification for other-regarding actions. Altruistic love is the epitome of human altruism. Such love does not eclipse care of the self (to be loosely distinguished from self-indulgence), for without this the agent would eventually become unable to perform altruistic acts. Such love does not demand self-immolation, although it can require significant self-sacrifice; it certainly makes imperative proper self-care, for otherwise the agent of love is too exhausted and debilitated to function. The core definition of altruistic love is not sacrifice but, rather, an affective and affirming participation in the being of the other. Love is first a response to the "present actuality" of another as he or she is of irrevocable worth.

Love can be identified in part because it elicits a sense of joy in the other, who feels inwardly "a home in which it is safe." The other who receives affective affirmation and all its sequelae, such as compassion and care, will sense a freedom from anxiety, that is, a certain safe haven in love where the stress of devaluation and isolation is removed. It seems plausible to hypothesize that, emotionally and physiologically, human beings need altruistic love. Attachment theory suggests that the general need for love may derive from infant experience. The human infant requires tremendous love, and this need does not disappear over the course of the life span; however, it is modified.

People tend to remember well over the years those from whom they receive warm, generous love; conversely, people also remember those who have shamed and humiliated them. The opposite of love can be observed in episodes of malignant social psychology, which include intimidation, stigmatization, invalidation, objectification, mockery, and disparagement. There are those who convey, with tone of voice and facial expression, the message that the other's very existence rests on a mistake.

In human experience, there are certain key life events that force the self to realize that it is not the only center of value. The birth of a child and the realization of the reality of eventual death are two such events that highlight the error of thinking that all others orbit around the self in its egoism. Ethics is not about enlightened self-interest and rational self-interested choice theory. It is about an affective transformation of the self toward a deep, warm, generous, other-regarding way of life. I will add to the key life events above the challenging reality of loving and caring for a person with Alzheimer's disease (AD).

In caring for the person with AD, in seeing and responding to such a person, the self must be transformed: it must experience a decentering through the presence of the other as a call to moral life. The other's expression summons me to take another center of meaning into my world. This discovery of the other as other is often the subject of novels and plays that capture the moral transformation of the cold, uncaring egoist into an empathic other-regarding presence.

Love (synonymous with *chesed*, or *agape*), a basic solicitude, can overcome the tendency to exclude the forgetful.[3] This care is usually best expressed in "being with" the forgetful, as opposed to the "doing to" of invasive medical technologies. Many invasive medical interventions, as well as the high-tech environment of a hospital, should be avoided because they are frightening to persons with AD. Love in the basic sense of the word is the better treatment.

In general terms, no caregivers should feel that their love and care require the technological extension of the morbidity and severe dysfunction of advanced AD. Care demands an attentive presence and comfort measures, not the imposition of suffering due to burdensome treatment.

LOVE AND PERSONHOOD

Persons with cognitive disabilities need the sense of safety and peace that love creates, and this universal need must be met in the context of dying. The first principle of care for such persons is to reveal to them their value by providing attention and tenderness in love. As a culture of care, we must set aside the distorted position that a person's worth, dignity, and status as a human being under the principles of nonmaleficence and beneficence depend entirely on that person's cognitive capacities. I prefer an "I–Thou" view of personhood, which takes into account the emotional, relational, symbolic, and even spiritual capacities of the person.[4] In so far as we live in a culture dominated by heightened expectations of rationalism and economic productivity, clarity of mind and productivity inevitably influence our sense of the worth of a human life. These expectations are internalized by persons with a diagnosis of dementia, contributing to depression and despair. The dictum "I think, therefore I am" must be replaced with "I feel and relate and above all, I am."

The perils of forgetfulness are especially evident in our culture of independence and economic productivity, which so values intellect, memory, and self-control. Alzheimer's disease[5] is a quantifiable neurological atrophy that objectively assaults normal human functioning;[6] however, as medical anthropologists highlight, it is also viewed within the context of socially constructed images of the human self and its fulfillment.[7] A longitudinal study carried out in urban China, for example, by Ikels,[8] indicated that dementia does not evoke the same level of dread there as it does among Americans. Thus, the stigma associated with the mental incapacitation of dementia varies according to culture.[9]

Persons who lack certain empowering cognitive capacities are not nonpersons; rather, they have become the weakest among us and, due to their needfulness, are worthy of care. The hypercognitivist value system that shapes personhood theories of ethics is merely an example of how our culture's criteria of rationality and productivity blind us to other ways of thinking about the meaning of our humanity and the nature of humane care. I remain impressed with the work of anthropologist Charlotte Ikels, who points out that in Chinese culture the cognitive domain is not taken to be the total sum of the person, nor is the self conceptualized as essentially independent and autonomous. Thus, in the eyes of the Chinese family, the person with dementia is still "there." In Japanese culture, there are some who find in the image of dementia a release from the fetters of everyday cares and occupations.[10] This image may trivialize a disease that is a sort of human development in reverse, but there is value in seeing value in those who are demented.

For love to succeed, we must struggle to overcome the problem of stigma. Around the country, people with mild AD point to this problem in the context of workshop panels. They complain that old friends do not communicate with them directly but, instead, talk around them, that a gap surfaces. One autobiographical account of living with the diagnosis and initial decline of AD is Rev. Robert Davis' *My Journey into Alzheimer's Disease*.[11] As Davis "mourned the loss of old abilities," he nevertheless could draw on his faith: "I choose to take things moment by moment, thankful for everything that I have, instead of raging wildly at the things that I have lost" (p. 57). Even as he struggled to find a degree of peace through his religious faith, he was also keenly aware of people who "simply cannot handle being around someone who is mentally and emotionally impaired" (p. 115). As can occur in time of plague, we try to put distance between ourselves and the afflicted, especially those with a dementing disease that we would just as soon place out of sight and mind. We must not separate "them" from "us." Instead, we must support the remaining capacities and enhance the relational well-being of persons with AD using data that indicate which interventions are most helpful.[12]

The arrogance of today's so-called "ethical" theories of "personhood" was evident in the ancient Stoic ethics of universal concern for all humanity possessed of the divine spark of reason. We must go beyond Stoicism and its modern variations because it included "only the intelligent" in the divine community. An aristocratic condescension, therefore, corrupts Stoic universalism. In the love and care for persons with AD, there is no room for such condescension.

QUALITY OF LIFE AS LOVE'S CREATION

Emotional, relational, aesthetic, and spiritual forms of well-being are possible to varying degrees in people with progressive dementia.

Emotional and Relational Well-Being

Tom Kitwood and Kathleen Bredin[13] developed a description of the "culture of dementia" that is useful in appreciating emotional and relational aspects of quality of life. They provide indicators of well-being in people with severe dementia: the assertion of will or desire, usually in the form of dissent despite various coaxings; the ability to express a range of emotions; initiation of social contact (e.g., a person with dementia has a small toy dog that he treasures and places it before another person with dementia to attract attention); affectional warmth (e.g., a woman wanders back and forth in the facility without much socializing, but when people say hello to her, she gives them a kiss on the cheek and continues her wandering).[13]

There is no need to add to the above description, except to state the obvious: if a man mistakes his wife for a hat, there is no need for correction. Many a person with dementia has been badgered by those who wish to impose reality long past the point when it is a serious possibility. In the mild stage of AD, there is much to be said for trying to orient a person to reality; at some point in moderate AD, however, it becomes oppressive to impose reality upon them.

Aesthetic Well-Being

The aesthetic well-being available to people with AD is obvious to anyone who has watched art or music therapy sessions. In some cases, a person with advanced AD may still draw the same valued symbol, as though through art a sense of self is retained.[14,15] The abstract expressionist de Kooning painted his way through much of his struggle with AD. Various art critics commented that his work, while not what it had been, was nevertheless impressive. As Kay Larson, former art critic for *New York Magazine* wrote,

It would be cruel to suggest that de Kooning needed his disease to free himself. Nonetheless, the erosions of Alzheimer's could not eliminate the effects of a lifetime of discipline and love of craft. When infirmity struck, the artist was prepared. If he didn't know what he was doing, maybe it didn't matter—to him. He knew what he loved best, and it sustained him.[16]

A review of de Kooning's late art, on the one hand, indicates a loss of the sweeping power and command of brush typical of his work in the 1950s; on the other hand, there is a quality to the late work that should not be diminished.

Spiritual Well-Being

Alzheimer's disease raises the postmodernist question of the dominance of rationality in our conception of the human self. The slow disintegration of components of thought and eventually feeling found in AD raises the basic question: what does it mean to be human?

Chaplains should have a significant role in the disclosure of a diagnosis as serious as AD. They should encourage hope despite the perils of forgetfulness. Hope is a multidimensional dynamic attribute of an individual that concerns dimensions of possibility and confidence in future outcome. Hope can address secular matters, such as future plans and relationships, or religious matters of ultimate destiny. Hope is an aspect of "religious" well-being. Preservation of hope can maximize a patient's psychological adjustment to a severe disability such as dementia, as well as the capacity to participate actively in support groups, to consider consenting for AD research projects, and to make known preferences for future levels of medical treatment after the dementia becomes severe. However, some clinicians still resist telling the patient about his or her diagnosis, often because they do not wish to create despair. In the effort to retain hope, the whole ethical process of looking toward future choices is undone.

People with a diagnosis of AD often pray, for they are thrown back onto whatever faith they have in the meaningful and beneficent purposes underlying the universe. The person with a diagnosis of AD will often desire to pray with family members, to pray in religious communities, and to pray alone. The word *prayer* comes from the Latin *precari*, "to entreat" or ask earnestly. It comes from the same root as the word *precarious*, and it is in the precariousness of emerging forgetfulness that often the person with dementia is driven to prayer. Prayer is one way of enhancing hope in the future despite dementia. Chaplains and clinicians can encourage this propensity to gain strength through prayer in the midst of cognitive decline.

Even in the more advanced stages of AD, the symbolic self will persist to varying degrees. One man with AD clutched his cowboy hat whenever he went to bed, as though he knew that his self-identity was somehow connected with this symbol. It turns out that he had worn country and western garb as a steel worker for many years. He continued to clutch his hat until the day he died. Pastoral caregivers, then, may be able to reach the person with AD at some deeper symbolic level of the self, although more needs to be learned about the best forms of pastoral care in the most deeply forgetful.

Caregivers often pray for loved ones with dementia. In a study of religion variables in relation to perceived caregiver rewards, African-American women caring for elderly persons with major deficits in activities of daily living perceived greater benefits through caring based on a spiritual–religious reframing of their situation. Religiosity indicators (i.e., prayer, comfort from religion, self-rated religiosity, attendence at religious services) are especially significant as coping resources in African-American female caregivers.[17] Spirituality is a clear stress deterrent and, therefore, also impacts depression rates, which are extraordinarily high in AD caregivers. Picot et al.[17] suggest that "if religiosity indicators are shown to enhance a caregiver's perceived rewards, health care professionals could encourage caregivers to use their religiosity to reduce the negative consequences and increase the rewards of caregiving." This seems self-evident.

Other studies indicate that spirituality is an important factor in coping with the sometimes ruthless stress induced by caring for someone with AD.[18] Spirituality among AD caregivers is a central means of coping.[19] In an important study by Rabins et al.,[20] 32 family caregivers of persons with AD and 30 caregivers of persons with cancer were compared cross-sectionally to determine whether the type of illness affected the emotional state of the caregiver and to identity correlates of both undesirable and desirable emotional outcomes. While no prominent differences in negative or positive states were found between the two groups, correlates of negative and positive emotional status were identified. These include caregiver personality variables, number of social supports, and the feeling that one is supported by one's religious faith. Specifically, "emotional distress was predicted by self-reported low or absent religious faith."[20] Moreover, spirituality predicted positive emotional states in caregiving. Interestingly, the study suggested that it was "belief, rather than social contact, that was important."

The pluralistic and social scientific study of the impact of patient spirituality is very different from the theological enterprise of the seminary. Growing numbers of studies demonstrate the value of spirituality as a coping mechanism for patients with major illness. The attention given to patient spirituality and religious belief in medical education is another indication of clinical relevance.

CONCLUSION: OUR UNIVERSAL VULNERABILITY

Alasdair MacIntyre, in his recent work *Dependent Rational Animals: Why Human Beings Need the Virtues* (1999),[21] a revision of his 1997 Carus lectures, has said nothing that those involved in the world of cognitive disabilities would not readily affirm: human beings are vulnerable, mutually dependent, as well as often imperiled by lifelong disability, so we need to think about the virtues in this context. It is good to see a major philosopher take these realities so forcefully into account. MacIntyre is most concerned with the virtue of "just generosity" toward those who are disabled, especially with regard to independence and practical reasoning. He asks us to reflect on the care that we received as children and are very likely to need as we become elderly. Too often the virtues associated with the Aristotelian tradition are associated with virility, power, and patriarchy. Further developing his Thomistic Aristotelianism, MacIntyre distances himself from those features in Aristotle that are closest to Nietzsche. In focusing on vulnerability and dependence, MacIntyre affirms the feminist ethics of care.

Whether we speak in terms of an ethics of care or more broadly in terms of an ethics of love, the person with AD undergoing palliative care needs love and care in the most basic sense of these words. A family member or professional caregiver must always remember that love is the key to a good dying. Love is patient, kind in tone, and the light of a good dying. Those palliative care programs that forget the centrality of love will fail internally. All treatment of pain and discomfort should be viewed as complementary to the underlying need for love.

REFERENCES

1. Kitwood T. Dementia Reconsidered: The Person Comes First. Philadelphia: Open University Press, 1997.
2. Post SG, Underwood LG, Schloss JP, Hurlbut WB (Eds.). Altruism and Altruistic Love: Science, Philosophy, and Religion in Dialogue. New York, Oxford University Press, 2002.
3. Martin RJ, Post SG. Human dignity, dementia, and the moral basis of caregiving. In: Binstock R, Post SG, Whitehouse PJ (Eds.). Dementia and Aging: Ethics, Values, and Policy Choices. Baltimore, Johns Hopkins University Press, pp. 55–68, 1992.
4. Rudman S. Concepts of the Persons and Christian Ethics. Cambridge, Cambridge University Press, 1997.
5. Gilman S. Alzheimer's disease. Perspect Biol Med 40:230–243, 1997.
6. Fox NC, Freeborough PA, Rossor MN. Visualisation and quantification of rates of atrophy in Alzheimer's disease. Lancet 348: 94–97, 1996.
7. Herskovits E. Struggling over subjectivity: debates about the "self" and Alzheimer's disease. Med Anthropol Q 9:146–164, 1995.
8. Ikels C. The experience of dementia in China. Cult Med Psychiatry 3:257–283, 1998.
9. Yeo G, Gallagher-Thompson D (Eds.). Ethnicity and the Dementias. Bristol, PA, Taylor & Francis, 1996.
10. Ariyoshi S. The Twilight Years. New York, Kodansha International, 1984.
11. Davis R. My Journey into Alzheimer's Disease: Helpful Insights for Family and Friends. Wheaton, IL, Tyndale House, 1989.
12. Sabat SR. Recognizing and working with remaining abilities: toward improving the care of Alzheimer's disease sufferers. Am J Alzheimer Care Relat Disord Res 9:8–16, 1994.
13. Kitwood T, Bredin K. Towards a theory of dementia care: personhood and well-being. Ageing Soc 12:269–297, 1992.
14. Firlik AD. Margo's logo. JAMA 265:201, 1991.
15. Clair AA. Therapeutic Uses of Music with Older Adults. Baltimore, Health Professions Press, 1996.
16. Larson K. Willem de Kooning and Alzheimer's. World I 12:297–299, 1997.
17. Picot SJ, Debanne SM, Namazi KH, Wykle ML. Religiosity and perceived rewards of black and white caregivers. Gerontologist 37:89–101, 1997.
18. Murphey C. Day to Day: Spiritual Help When Someone You Love has Alzheimer's. Philadelphia, Westminster Press, 1988.
19. Whitlatch AM, Meddaugh DI, Langhout KJ. Religiosity among Alzheimer's disease caregivers. Am J Alzheimer Dis Relat Disord Res 12:11–20, 1992.
20. Rabins PV, Fitting MD, Eastham J, Fetting J. The emotional impact of caring for the chronically ill. Psychosomatics 31:331–336, 1990.
21. MacIntyre A. Dependent Rational Animals: Why Human Beings Need the Virtues. Chicago, Open Court, 1999.

5

Artificial Nutrition and Hydration

COLLEEN CHRISTMAS AND TOM FINUCANE

The sight of an emaciated, chronically ill elderly patient unleashes a torrent of powerful emotions. The face validity of providing nutrition to such a person is near overwhelming. Concerned family members, professional caregivers, nursing home administrators, unwitting subspecialists, purveyors of nutrition-related products, nursing home surveyors, and even personal injury lawyers may provide strong impetus to initiate feeding artificially, most likely by percutaneous endoscopic gastrostomy (PEG).

In this chapter, we show that patients and caregivers may often consent to tube feeding (or "medically administered nutrition by tube") without a full understanding of the burdens and benefits of this technology. We then review evidence about the ability of tube feeding to achieve several of the goals for which it is often initiated. Evidence about whether tube feeding palliates symptoms, provides comfort, or leads to a higher quality of life for anorexic, cachectic patients is discussed in particular detail.

DECISION MAKING AND TUBE FEEDING

Anorexia and weight loss commonly occur during serious illness. Witnessing this can be particularly distressing to family members and other caregivers. Watching a loved one "waste away" may provoke a genuinely well-intentioned and desperate effort to "do something." In the United States this frequently takes the form of artificial nutrition and hydration, often by tube feeding. The decision to initiate tube feeding seems often to be viewed as non-optional; it is frequently proposed and accepted as a necessary part of treatment.

Studying decisions about tube feeding in cognitively impaired nursing home residents, Mitchell and Lawson[1] found that while nearly 85% of decision makers reported understanding the possible benefits of tube feeding, fewer than half were aware of the risks. In fact, the decision to initiate tube feeding was often made while the patient was acutely ill and hospitalized, frequently a time of extreme duress. Only one of the 46 patients in this study had previously clearly expressed an opinion about tube feeding to a substitute decision maker, and fewer than 60% of the surrogates reported feeling certain that the patient would have wanted the feeding tube.

These findings were supported by a prospective, community-based study of 100 patients and their decision makers interviewed about the decision-making process shortly after placement of a feeding tube.[2] Most decision makers described a sense of inevitability about the decision. In this study, too, the decision was usually made at the time of an acute illness. Only 2% of decision makers reported that spoon feeding was discussed as an alternative, and 45% did not recall the proposal of any alternatives.

Documentation of informed consent for placement of a gastrostomy tube was very poor in the study of Brett and Rosenberg.[3] Discussion that included benefits of, burdens of, and alternatives to gastrostomy was documented in only one of 154 medical records of consecutive hospitalized adults who had feeding tubes placed. In over 92% of cases, a surrogate provided consent, even though the researchers found evidence that patients were competent to make their own decisions in at least 21% of records. Thus, substitute decision makers who agree to tube feeding frequently do so during acute illness, believe they have not been fully informed about the alternative approaches, and are unsure of the patient's wishes. Further, documentation of the consent process is extremely poor. We believe that legitimate options are often not presented to decision makers.

The use of tube feedings in severely impaired nursing home residents ranges from 5% in Maine to 40% in Ohio.[4] This wide regional variation suggests that physicians themselves are often uncertain as to how to proceed and tend to be influenced by local practice more so than evidence of efficacy.

NUTRITION AND MALNUTRITION

Underlying the complex issue of nutrition is a deeply seated human desire to provide nurturing and nourishment. Nutrition holds a special symbolic position rooted in social, religious, and ethical values. Though medically administered nutrition by tube is often considered food, it is important to remember that it in no way resembles usual food in appearance, in the societal context in which it is administered, or in its relation (or lack of relation) to hunger, satiety, and comfort. While all hungry people should be provided palatable food and assistance with eating if needed, patients who are anorexic may not benefit when nutrition is forced on them.

The term *malnutrition* is itself misleading and laden with emotional meaning. In one sense, it could imply that markers of nutritional status are abnormal, even though these markers can be affected by illness, regardless of nutrient intake. In another sense, it implies a condition of bad nutrition, which should improve with better nutrient intake. With the former definition, improvement with increased provision of nutrients cannot be assumed. Thus, this distinction is critical.

The word *malnutrition* often conveys a sense of shame and neglect. This ambiguity of the word and its embedded negative connotations further the impulse to seek aggressive nutritional support when a dying person is diagnosed as malnourished. It is important first to examine the evidence about the purported benefits of tube feeding, then to use this information to help negotiate through the more complex and individualized views of "what is right."

TUBE FEEDING IN ADVANCED DEMENTIA

In one common and disturbing scenario, tube feeding is considered for a patient with end-stage dementia who is having difficulty eating and losing weight. The patient is often severely demented, poorly communicative, generally recumbent, and wholly dependent on others for care. Such a patient is rarely involved in the decision to institute invasive feeding techniques near the end of life.

Evidence about the effectiveness of tube feeding in this situation is extremely limited. Although no prospective randomized trials comparing the intervention to a careful program of hand feeding have been reported, other sources of information are available. Data from retrospective analyses and prospective uncontrolled cohort studies are quite useful.

The main reasons feeding tubes are placed in patients with end-stage dementia are to prevent the clinical sequelae of malnutrition, reduce aspiration, and palliate symptoms. The most important clinical sequelae of malnutrition are death, vulnerability to infections and pressure sores, and weakness or functional decline. Here, we review the evidence about whether tube feeding has a beneficial effect on these outcomes.

Survival

There is a deeply rooted belief that demented patients who eat very little will starve to death and that death can be delayed if they are provided increased nutrition by tube. Several lines of evidence undermine this common conviction, however. First, several large, prospective but not randomized studies have demonstrated that the survival of demented nursing home residents is identical whether or not a feeding tube is utilized. Second, survival of demented patients with eating difficulties can be substantial. For example, one nonrandomized prospective study of nursing home residents found similar survival rates in four groups of patients: those who ate without difficulty, those who required assistance with feeding, those who choked when they ate, and those who refused food.[5] This suggests that eating difficulty is simply a marker of advanced disease and that overcoming this difficulty itself does not alter the ultimate course of the disease process. Third, the mortality associated with tube

feeding is quite substantial. While frequently encouraged because they are technically easy to insert, the perioperative (30 day) mortality is substantial, ranging from 6% to 24%. Further, survival after placement of a feeding tube in patients with dementia is very poor. Median survival in most studies is clearly less than 1 year after the tube is placed. One recently published meta-analysis of survival in elderly patients after placement of a feeding tube for a variety of indications demonstrated a 20% 1-month mortality and median survival of just over 6 months.[6]

Aspiration

Aspiration pneumonitis and aspiration pneumonia are a challenge to distinguish and diagnose. The former occurs when gastric contents are regurgitated into the lungs, with a resultant chemical-induced inflammation that may resolve with only supportive therapy. The latter results from misdirection of contaminated oral secretions into the lungs, in high enough inoculum to overcome host defenses and establish a tissue infection. When studied, about half of healthy adults have misdirection of oral secretions into the lungs while sleeping in a single night, but probably all persons do to variable degrees. Patients with oropharyngeal dysphagia who are unable to protect their airways during mealtimes remain vulnerable to oral secretions throughout the day and night. Placement of a feeding tube does not reduce the misdirection of oral secretions, and studies have shown regurgitation of gastric contents into the lungs is not prevented either.[7,8]

A comprehensive review of this topic published in 1996[9] found very high rates of pneumonia and death in patients with feeding tubes, particularly if a prior history of aspiration was the reason for tube placement. Further, four studies examined the rates of clinical aspiration events in patients who had feeding tubes placed for other indications.[10–13] These studies found that about 10%–15% of patients who never had aspiration pneumonia began to aspirate after placement of the tube. The presence of a feeding tube was cited as a strong risk factor for aspiration in many studies. In fact, pneumonia is the most common cause of death in patients fed by tube.

A single prospective nonrandomized study showed higher rates of aspiration events in tube-fed versus hand-fed patients with oropharyngeal dysphagia.[14] Other studies have shown that jejunostomy tubes do not have lower rates of associated aspiration than gastrostomy tubes.[15,16]

Though no randomized studies comparing tube feeding to careful feeding by hand have been published, retrospective and prospective nonrandomized studies strongly suggest that feeding tubes do not reduce the risk of aspiration in patients with neurogenic oropharyngeal dysphagia.[17–21] Indeed, no published trial has ever shown a reduction in risk with tube feeding.

Pressure Sores

The link between nutritional status and pressure sores is tenuous at best. An extensive review of these relationships found very weak associations between markers of nutritional status and pressure sores and variable effects of nutritional interventions on pressure sore development and healing.[22] Examination of over 800 patients using an administrative database showed neither accelerated healing[23] nor reduction in incidence[24] of pressure sores in nursing home patients fed by tube compared to those who were not. Because patients with dementia who receive feeding tubes are usually bedfast or poorly mobile and restraints are often employed, pressure sore outcomes could be worsened by the intervention. Further, tube-fed patients may make increased amounts of urine and stool, which could also worsen outcomes. This area has not been clarified sufficiently in prospective randomized clinical trials, but there is no good evidence to support insertion of feeding tubes for the purpose of improving pressure sore outcomes.

Infections

It is generally held that persons with poor markers of nutritional status have impaired immunity and increased risk of infection, yet most studies of nutritional interventions do not evaluate infection as an outcome. In contrast, feeding tubes are known to cause infections. As discussed above, they are a serious risk factor for the development of aspiration pneumonia. Further, they are associated with about a 5% rate of infection around the PEG insertion site, which is one source of sepsis and death in these patients.[25–32] A recent report identified feeding tubes as a strong risk factor for both colonization and clinical infection with *Clostridium difficile*,[33] and other reports demonstrate that tube feeding can be associated with both infectious and noninfectious diarrhea.[29,34] Nasogastric tubes (NGTs) may increase the propensity to develop bacterial sinusitis, and there are reports of fasciitis and myositis associated with PEG.[28,35,36] No report has ever described a reduction in clinical infections in adults with use of any type of feeding tube.

Function

People who are eating poorly, losing weight, and approaching death often become increasingly weak with decreasing functional abilities. Particularly for patients with end-stage dementia, who have limited functional reserve, these further decrements can result in total dependence with increased burden on those who provide care. Because of the association between poor oral intake and functional decline, increased nutrition may be provided to mitigate the decline. No data exist to support this practice. In fact, in one retrospective review of nursing home residents with feeding tubes, no patient had functional improvement in over 18 months of follow-up.[37] Two prospective studies cast further doubt. In a prospective, randomized trial of 100 frail nursing home residents, administration of oral nutritional supplementation for 10 weeks had no independent effect on measurements of strength or function compared to placebo, while an exercise program showed significant benefits in this time period.[38] In a small, prospective cohort study with function as a primary outcome, 123 patients consented to be studied but 46 were dead by 2 months.[39] Of the 72 survivors who were evaluated at 2 months, only seven had improvement in activities of daily living. Because tube-fed patients are usually fed semirecumbent in bed, at times with restraints used, feeding tubes may worsen immobility and strength.

PALLIATION

It is difficult, perhaps impossible, to know the experience of a patient who cannot communicate. We can look for clues of discomfort in the facial expression, posture, and behaviors; but interpreting these clues may be extremely difficult even for family members and familiar caregivers. Whether our interpretation approximates the patient's feelings is unknowable. Any data about suffering in the severely demented elderly must be based on inference. We review here the symptoms associated with poor oral intake near death, derived from investigations of patients who remain able to communicate at this time, such as some patients dying from cancer and other chronic diseases.

Data about Common Symptoms near Death

A central question facing decision makers is whether or not the provision of artificially administered nutrition and hydration can relieve suffering in chronically ill patients who are approaching death. An additional question is whether anorexic individuals near death suffer from poor oral intake.

Symptoms of hunger and thirst were quite uncommon in a prospective study of mentally aware terminal patients on an inpatient comfort care unit."[40] In this study, almost two-thirds of patients reported no hunger, and the remaining third reported initial hunger that resolved despite minimal oral intake near death. Similarly, two-thirds reported little or no thirst associated with the dying process. In all cases, the symptoms of hunger, thirst, and dry mouth were alleviated with local oral care and sips of fluid; none required invasive therapies.

Older studies demonstrated that the thirst mechanism is diminished in healthy elderly volunteers compared to younger volunteers who had nearly no oral intake for 24 hours followed by rehydration.[41] A small study of patients dying from malignant disease attempted to correlate symptoms of thirst and dry mouth to serum osmolar concentration, but no relationship could be established.[42] In these patients, then, the symptoms of hunger and thirst do not necessarily depend on volume status. Thus, those who remain communicative report that symptoms of hunger and thirst are uncommon near death, thirst mechanisms are diminished with age, and thirst does not correlate with serum osmolarity; it may not be reasonable to expect invasive food or fluid administration to improve patient comfort, even in those individuals with laboratory evidence of volume contraction.

Further, feeding tubes may themselves cause discomfort. A prospective study of 70 elderly patients who received nutrition by NGT or PEG over an 11-month period found significant agitation in both groups and frequent extubation in the group employing NGT.[43] Agitation and self-extubation occurred in two-thirds of patients during the first 2 weeks after NGT placement, while the former occurred in over 40% of patients with PEG in this same interval. Self-extubation continued to be a problem over the 11 months of follow-up in about 40% of the patients fed by NGT. In another study, about one-third of patients required PEG tube replacement at least once in the year following initial placement.[39]

Tube feeding may provoke uncomfortable symptoms. In a study of patients with motor neuron disease who were cognitively intact but unable to swallow, nasogastric feeding was associated with cough, aspiration, the development or worsening of nausea, and diminished human contact.[44] In a community-based study, the majority of patients who were able to report described at least one physical symptom related to PEG.[39] In this study, approximately 20%–30% described the onset of vomiting, diarrhea, constipation, nausea, or aspiration after initiation of tube feeding. Local infections secondary to PEG are reported to occur at a rate of 4.3%–16%, but whether these or other local effects of PEGs are painful has not been investigated. Finally, physical and chemical restraints may be used in patients with feeding tubes to reduce pulling at and removing the tube. A patient's pulling at a tube may signal irritation from this tube, and it is disturbing to think that at times this discomfort may be treated by tying down the hands rather than relief of the discomfort. Restraint use is unfortunately common: an older review of the medical records of patients who had NGT during hospitalization at a single teaching hospital showed that restraints were used on over half of these patients.[45] A more recent report on patients who received PEG tubes found restraint use in 2%.[39]

No studies have demonstrated improved quality of life or function with the use of tubes, but very few have even tried. Most patients who had PEG tubes placed were unable to communicate sufficiently to evaluate these outcomes; however, the majority of those who could speak reported little or no improvement in function, subjective health status, or life satisfaction in the year following PEG placement.[39]

There is currently no evidence that artificially administered nutrition and hydration improve patient comfort, and may actually lessen comfort.

HOW TO HELP FAMILIES THINK ABOUT PROVISION OF FOOD AND FLUIDS

Helping families think about the provision of food and fluids to their loved ones remains a formidable challenge.[46] We have reviewed above some data suggesting that families do not feel fully informed when considering artificially administered nutrition and that they are often unaware of alternatives. As always, facts are the cornerstone. Providers and decision makers need a thorough understanding of the risks, benefits, and availability of alternative methods of feeding. A self-administered audio booklet has been developed to provide information about tube feeding and hand feeding, guide the decision-making process, and operationalize the steps to decision making. This aid was found to reduce decisional conflict in substitute decision makers considering long-term tube feeding for cognitively impaired elderly patients.[47]

In some clinical situations, no data are available to describe the intervention's relative risks and benefits. During acute illness, delirium may make it impossible to provide fluid and medication to a patient. Some patients may experience rapid weight loss or severe suffering when fed by hand. Early in the course of a stroke, it is difficult to predict how much swallowing and other function the patient will regain. In these cases, it may be reasonable to consider an empiric trial of tube feeding with clearly predetermined goals of therapy.

In other situations where data are available and tend to show a lack of benefit, family members may insist on tube feeding based more on its symbolic value or on a misunderstanding of data. The impetus may arise based on the offhand remark of a friend or professional. All members of the team caring for the patient must work in unison to minimize decisional conflict. All team members should be educated about the decision to be made and the reasons behind the decision to begin or forego artificial hydration and nutrition for individual patients.

After ensuring that the decision maker comprehends the situation and the implications of various choices, helping to establish reasonable expectations is the next step. Some individuals may benefit from clear instruction to focus on what the patient would want if he or she were able to voice an opinion. It is important to emphasize that the goal is to honor the wishes of the individual patient, even if they conflict with the decision maker's wishes for the patient or with how the decision maker would decide for himself or herself in the same situation. This process can be supported by searching for indications of what the patient would want from the patient's previously expressed opinions or governing views of life.

It is critical to emphasize that the alternative to tube feeding is not "no feeding." The patient will continue to be fed and will not be abandoned. Review the data suggesting that the anorexic dying patient is not suffering from diminished nutrient intake and that feeding tubes are unlikely to help the patient live longer or more comfortably. Most importantly, make clear to the decision makers that providing less invasive techniques is not equivalent to providing lesser-quality care and may represent better-quality care. A carefully designed and individualized program of hand feeding, though very labor-intensive and less glamorous, may be proposed. The common misunderstanding that if a feeding tube is not employed, it is the same as "letting the patient starve to death" must be forcefully rejected.

A more conservative and perhaps more dignified approach to cachectic patients can be offered, though there are no prospective, randomized studies comparing these approaches to invasive ones. First, all patients with eating problems should be evaluated and treated for reversible causes of poor oral intake before invasive therapies are considered. Such treatable causes of weight loss include depression, metabolic disorders, poor access to food, and poor oral hygiene. Many medications may worsen appetite and the ability to swallow. Examples of such medications include anticholinergic medicine, which may contribute to xerostomia; sedatives and narcotics, which cause inattention; nonsteroidal anti-inflammatory medications or bisphosphonates, which could contribute to anorexia and gastroesophageal irritation; and antipsychotics, which affect swallowing function. Nonessential medications that may play a role in poor oral intake should be discontinued, and any other reversible causes of poor appetite should be treated.

Next, evaluate the diet. Food that is appealing to the patient and ethnically appropriate should be provided. Often, inappropriately restrictive diets are used without evidence of benefit. Salt should be restricted only in *dire* circumstances. Restricting sweets simply cannot be justified in the circumstances we discuss here. Diets should be liberalized to include calorie-dense foods (ice cream, gravies, butter, etc.); a variety of colors, temperatures, and textures; and individualized preferred foods. Some patients will find that finger foods are easier to eat, and others with early satiety may benefit from more frequent, smaller meals. The presentation of food to the patient should be appealing.

Attention to the social aspects of eating may be helpful as well. Ascertain the patient's eating environment preference, e.g., with only a few individuals in a quiet area versus with a large, talkative group in a more stimulating area. Limit excessively noisy or odoriferous distractions, and make note of the visual stimuli in the environment as well. Encourage eating with family and friends. Many patients will benefit from enhanced personal assistance with feeding, whether this is assistance with food preparation, occasional verbal reminders to eat more, or physical assistance with getting food and fluid into the mouth. Some patients with oropharyngeal dysphagia will require verbal reminders or gentle brushing of the cheeks and neck to trigger swallow; others may need to be instructed to swallow multiple times per bolus to be sure to clear the pharynx.

Most everyone will eat more comfortably in an upright position, and this will also lessen regurgitation of gastric contents. Make certain that the patient is comfortable when positioned to eat, for pain is a major obstacle to eating.

Finally, as noted above, many patients do not feel hunger or thirst in the terminal stages of disease; and in these patients, the focus should be provision of food and fluid whenever the patient would like it and maintenance of comfort at all times. Patients who have very little oral intake often suffer from dry lips and mouth and/or a foul taste in the mouth. Small sips of cold water or other preferred beverages may alleviate some of this discomfort. These symptoms can also be readily treated by lip lubrication with topical ointments. Attention to oral hygiene with brushes, swabs, or rinses will help to keep the oral cavity moistened and free of foul-tasting bacterial overgrowth.

These techniques are very labor-intensive and require attentive care, but they do not require skilled nursing. They can afford families, loved ones, and staff an opportunity to nurture and comfort the patient at a critical time near the end of life.

If the family continues to insist on invasive techniques at this point, a dilemma arises that is familiar in the care of demented patients: when is it morally justifiable to subject a person to treatment for the benefit of another person? If the family is extremely burdened by watching the cachectic death of a loved one, is this an indication to initiate tube feeding? Powerful extra-medical forces come into play in a situation like this. The lack of conclusive data from randomized trials sharpens the dilemma. The value of limiting conflict is sometimes decisive.

CONCLUSIONS

In caring for chronically ill adults, difficult decisions often arise where one has to choose either to accept burdensome technology in return for a chance of longer life or to accept a sooner death with more comfort and dignity. Tube feeding is not such a decision, however. The alternative is time-consuming and labor-intensive. In many cases, this is what is required for optimal care of these very vulnerable patients.

REFERENCES

1. Mitchell SL, Lawson FM. Decision-making for long-term tube-feeding in cognitively impaired elderly people. CMAJ 160:1705–1709, 1999.
2. Callahan CM, Haag KM, Buchanan NN, Nisi R. Decision-making for percutaneous endoscopic gastrostomy among older adults in a community setting. J Am Geriatr Soc 47:1105–1109, 1999.
3. Brett AS, Rosenberg JC. The adequacy of informed consent for placement of gastrostomy tubes. Arch Intern Med 161:745–748, 2001.
4. Ahronheim JC, Mulvihill M, Sieger C, Park P, Fries BE. State practice variations in the use of tube feeding for nursing home residents with severe cognitive impairment. J Am Geriatr Soc 49:148–152, 2001.
5. Volicer L, Seltzer B, Rheaume Y, et al. Eating difficulties in patients with probable dementia of the Alzheimer type. J Geriatr Psychiatry Neurol 2:188–195, 1989.
6. Mitchell SL, Tetroe JM. Survival after percutaneous endoscopic gastrostomy placement in older persons. J Gerontol A Biol Sci Med Sci 55:M735–M739, 2000.
7. Grunow JE, al-Hafidh A, Tunell WP. Gastroesophageal reflux following percutaneous endoscopic gastrostomy in children. J Pediatr Surg 24:42–44; Discussion 44–45, 1989.
8. Canal DF, Vane DW, Goto S, Gardner GP, Grosfeld JL. Changes in lower esophageal sphincter pressure (LES) after Stamm gastrostomy. J Surg Res 42:570–574, 1987.
9. Finucane TE, Bynum JP. Use of tube feeding to prevent aspiration pneumonia. Lancet 349:1421–1424, 1996.
10. Jarnagin WR, Duh QY, Mulvihill SJ, Ridge JA, Schrock TR, Way LW. The efficacy and limitations of percutaneous endoscopic gastrostomy. Arch Surg 127:261–264, 1992.
11. Weltz CR, Morris JB, Mullen JL. Surgical jejunostomy in aspiration risk patients. Ann Surg 215:140–145, 1992.
12. Cogen R, Weinryb J. Aspiration pneumonia in nursing home patients fed via gastrostomy tubes. Am J Gastroenterol 84:1509–1512, 1989.
13. Hassett JM, Sunby C, Flint LM. No elimination of aspiration pneumonia in neurologically disabled patients with feeding gastrostomy. Surg Gynecol Obstet 167:383–388, 1988.
14. Feinberg MJ, Knebl J, Tully J. Prandial aspiration and pneumonia in an elderly population followed over 3 years. Dysphagia 11:104–109, 1996.
15. Lazarus BA, Murphy JB, Culpepper L. Aspiration associated with long-term gastric versus jejunal feeding: a critical analysis of the literature. Arch Phys Med Rehabil 71:46–53, 1990.
16. Fox KA, Mularski RA, Sarfati MR, et al. Aspiration pneumonia following surgically

placed feeding tubes. Am J Surg 170: 564–556; discussion 566–567, 1995.

17. Finucane TE, Bynum JP. Use of tube feeding to prevent aspiration pneumonia. Lancet 349:1421–1424, 1996.

18. Pick N, McDonald A, Bennett N, et al. Pulmonary aspiration in a long-term care setting: clinical and laboratory observations and an analysis of risk factors. J Am Geriatr Soc 44:763–768, 1996.

19. Bourdel-Marchasson I, Dumas F, Pinganaud G, Emeriau JP, Decamps A. Audit of percutaneous endoscopic gastrostomy in long-term enteral feeding in a nursing home. Int J Qual Health Care 9:297–302, 1997.

20. Langmore SE, Terpenning MS, Schork A, et al. Predictors of aspiration pneumonia: how important is dysphagia? Dysphagia 13:69–81, 1998.

21. Feinberg MJ, Knebl J, Tully J. Prandial aspiration and pneumonia in an elderly population followed over 3 years. JAMA 282: 1365–1370, 1999.

22. Finucane TE. Malnutrition, tube feeding and pressure sores: data are incomplete. J Am Geriatr Soc 43:447–451, 1995.

23. Berlowitz DR, Ash AS, Brandeis GH, Brand HK, Halpern JL, Moskowitz MA. Rating long-term care facilities on pressure ulcer development: importance of case-mix adjustment. Ann Intern Med 124:557–563, 1996.

24. Berlowitz DR, Brandeis GH, Anderson J, Brand HK. Predictors of pressure ulcer healing among long-term care residents. J Am Geriatr Soc 45:30–34, 1997.

25. Shike M, Latkany L, Gerdes H, Bloch AS. Direct percutaneous endoscopic jejunostomies for enteral feeding. Gastrointest Endosc 44:536–540, 1996.

26. Finocchiaro C, Galletti R, Royera G, et al. Percutaneous endoscopic gastrostomy: a long-term follow-up. Nutrition 13:520–523, 1997.

27. Wasiljew BK, Ujiki GT, Beal JM. Feeding gastrostomy: complications and mortality. Am J Surg 143:194–195, 1982.

28. Lockett MA, Templeton ML, Byrne TK, Norcross ED. Percutaneous endoscopic gastrostomy complications in a tertiary-care center. Am J Surg 68:117–120, 2002.

29. Hull MA, Rawlings J, Murray FE, et al. Audit of outcome of long-term enteral nutrition by percutaneous endoscopic gastrostomy. Lancet 341:869–872, 1993.

30. Kaw M, Sekas G. Long-term follow-up of consequences of percutaneous endoscopic gastrostomy (PEG) tubes in nursing home patients. Dig Dis Sci 39:738–743, 1994.

31. Fay DE, Poplausky M, Gruber M, Lance P. Long-term enteral feeding: a retrospective comparison of delivery via percutaneous endoscopic gastrostomy and nasoenteric tubes. Am J Gastroenterol 86:1604–1609, 1991.

32. Larson DE, Burton DD, Schroeder KW, DiMagno EP. Percutaneous endoscopic gastrostomy. Indications, success, complications, and mortality in 314 consecutive patients. Gastroenterology 93:48–52, 1987.

33. Bliss DZ, Johnson S, Savik K, Clabots CR, Willard K, Gerding DN. Acquisition of Clostridium difficile and Clostridium difficile-associated diarrhea in hospitalized patients receiving tube feeding. Ann Intern Med 129:1012–1019, 1998.

34. Fernandez-Crehuet Navajas M, Jurado Chacon D, Guillen Solvas JF, Galvez Vargas R. Bacterial contamination of enteral feeds as a possible risk of nosocomial infection. J Hosp Infect 21:111–120, 1992.

35. Fox VL, Abel SD, Malas S, Duggan C, Leichtner AM. Complications following percutaneous endoscopic gastrostomy and subsequent catheter replacement in children and young adults. Gastrointest Endosc 45: 64–71, 1997.

36. Martinez P, Sanchez-Vilar O, Picon MJ, et al. Necrotizing fasciitis as complication of percutaneous endoscopic gastrostomy. Nutr Hosp 14:135–137, 1999.

37. Kaw M, Sekas G. Long-term follow-up of consequences of percutaneous endoscopic gastrostomy (PEG) tubes in nursing home patients. Dig Dis Sci 39:738–743, 1994.

38. Fiatarone MA, O'Neill EF, Ryan ND, et al. Exercise training and nutritional supplementation for physical frailty in very elderly people. N Engl J Med 330:1769–1775, 1994.

39. Callahan CM, Haag KM, Weinberger M, et al. Outcomes of percutaneous endoscopic gastrostomy among older adults in a community setting. J Am Geriatr Soc 48:1048–1054, 2000.

40. McCann RM, Hall WJ, Groth-Juncker A. Comfort care for terminally ill patients. The appropriate use of nutrition and hydration. JAMA 272:1263–1266, 1994.

41. Phillips PA, Rolls BJ, Ledingham JG, et al. Reduced thirst after water deprivation in healthy elderly men. N Engl J Med 311: 753–759, 1984.

42. Ellershaw JE, Sutcliffe JM, Saunders CM. Dehydration and the dying patient. J Pain Symptom Manage 10:192–197, 1995.

43. Ciocon JO, Silverstone FA, Graver LM, Foley CJ. Tube feedings in elderly patients. Indications, benefits, and complications. Arch Intern Med 148:429–433, 1988.

44. Scott AG, Austin HE. Nasogastric feeding in the management of severe dysphagia in motor neurone disease. Palliat Med 8:45–49, 1994.

45. Quill TE. Utilization of nasogastric feeding tubes in a group of chronically ill, elderly patients in a community hospital. Arch Intern Med 149:1937–1941, 1989.

46. Karlawish JH, Quill T, Meier DE. A consensus-based approach to providing palliative care to patients who lack decision-making capacity ACP-ASIM End-of-Life Care Consensus Panel. Ann Intern Med 18:835–840, 1999.

47. Mitchell SL, Tetroe J, O'Connor AM. A decision aid for long-term tube feeding in cognitively impaired older persons. J Am Geriatr Soc 49:313–316, 2001.

6

Age, Rationing, and Palliative Care

DANIEL CALLAHAN AND EVA TOPINKOVÁ

There is nothing so ancient in medicine as the idea of palliative care, or anything that seems so new, recently revivified after decades of neglect. Yet something is different this time. Palliative care is now set within a context of limited resources, that of health-care systems facing a steady rise in cost and increasing demands upon their services. That was not true for most of the history of medicine, which until the twentieth century could provide little in the way of effective therapy. High-technology medicine, that great contribution of the past century, is a major part of the reason for the economic pressure but accompanied as well by aging populations and increased public demand for high-quality medical care. That potent combination of forces has made the provision of health care a problem for every society, one that promises to get worse in the years ahead as the number and proportion of elderly rise.

Palliative care must, then, compete for scarce resources, which may be difficult at times. Humane caring for sick patients,

once the hallmark of good medicine, does not now have the glamour of attempts to cure them, the advantage of dramatic technologies, or the full understanding of the public or legislators. Also, it is not easy to evaluate economically as a resource investment. Cure, not care, has been the predominant note. Fortunately, despite all of the much-touted medical miracles of the past century, the force of an old insight has begun to sink in: people still get sick and die, they are still afflicted with pain and suffering, they are still cured at one time but will get sick again at another time, and old age with its burdens of frailty and disability and failing bodies is still with us. The increase in chronic illness that goes with aging and the fresh sensitivities that have developed about the care of the terminally ill mean that palliative care has an important future. A good case can be made for allocating resources to it.

Yet making a good case requires taking account of the reality of rationing and the increased need to set priorities. Rationing

46

is always a feature of health-care systems, even if that term is not openly used and even if patients and sometimes their physicians do not notice it. Rationing can come in a variety of ways. The most harsh form of rationing comes when some vital, necessary form of care or therapy is denied to patients, whether because of an inability to pay for the care (in some systems) or because the health-care system simply does not have the means to provide the care at all (common in poor countries). Less harsh rationing can come about when the necessary resource is available but in short supply, and some means must be established for deciding who gets it (as in the early days of kidney dialysis or with organ transplantation in the face of limited organ availability). The least harsh method of rationing, but probably the most widespread in developed countries, comes about when the demand for a medical treatment exceeds the affordable supply, where everyone can receive some of the treatment but not necessarily as much as may be needed or desired.

Palliative care ordinarily will fall into the last category. Depending on patient needs, it can be inexpensive, a few kind words at the right moment, or expensive, ranging from costly technological interventions (e.g., palliative radiation and surgery) to relief of persistent long-term chronic pain or suffering. Because of the wide range of palliative care possibilities and their consequent costs, every health-care system can provide some palliative care. Similarly, while every physician and nurse can develop some palliative care skills, not every health-care system may be able to afford specialized training, much less the kind of training necessary for certification as a specialist in the field.

In light of this continuum of possibilities, the most common rationing problems will likely encompass two basic questions. First, what proportion of general health-care resources ought to be devoted to palliative care in a health-care system or some subunit of a system (e.g., hospital, clinic, nursing, or home-care program)? Second, what kind and extent of specific palliative care services ought to be offered within those particular contexts?

In our opening sketch of rationing above, we looked at the concept descriptively; and that is one sense of the word *rationing*, the actual way scarce goods are allocated. A no less common sense of the term is ethical in its thrust, that of attempting to achieve an equitable distribution of scarce resources. One approach, as an economist might point out, is to examine the "opportunity costs" of palliative care, i.e., how the money that might be allocated to palliative care might otherwise be spent on other forms of health care, or whether the resources proposed for one form of care might better be spent on some other form. Still another way of approaching the issue of rationing is to specify a set of priorities among the various things that can be done for patients. If resources are scarce, what priority ought to be given to palliative care? Then, once the priority for palliative care in general is decided, and assuming that resources are still less than optimal, the next step is to determine which forms of palliative care are more or less important and, if possible, to rank-order them.

THE GOALS OF MEDICINE

The best way to approach these difficult questions, we believe, is to look first at the goals of medicine and then at appropriate medical goals for the care of the aged. Palliative care was neglected for many decades in great part because no serious effort was undertaken to examine the goals of medicine. It was assumed that they were self-evident and, as the historical record indicates, that palliative care was displaced as an important goal. An international project of the Hastings Center attempted to specify appropriate medical goals, seeking whether, across different cultures, some consensus could be achieved; and then a later project sought to clarify the most important medical goals for care of the elderly in the years ahead.[1,2] We draw upon both sources in what follows.

Medicine, historically, has pursued many purposes, some of them developed from within the profession and others stemming from outside social forces. Successful efforts to save and extend life, beginning in the eighteenth century but accelerating rapidly in the twentieth century, was the source of one major shift. Improvements in rehabilitation, surgical techniques, disease prevention by medical means (e.g., screening), and refinements in palliative care techniques were sources of still others. Different cultures, moreover, have mingled local values with what has been called *cosmopolitan medicine*, or the development of international standards for scientific medicine, symbolized by international journals and worldwide communication.

With the assistance of researchers and commentators from 14 countries, developed and developing alike, a consensus was achieved that four principles reflected a valid mix of traditional and modern values:

• the prevention of disease and injury and promotion and maintenance of health
• the relief of pain and suffering
• the care and cure of those with a malady and the care of those who cannot be cured
• the avoidance of a premature death and the pursuit of a peaceful death

Is there a fixed priority among these four goals? The research group decided that there should be no fixed priority. Disease prevention makes no sense in the case of a dying patient but is of primary importance with healthy children and adults. Thus, also, it is not reasonable and may, indeed, be cruel to pursue a cure when no cure is likely. Priorities, in short, should be determined by assessment of a particular patient's circumstances and needs, and they can change over the course of treatment. Knowing when to shift to different goals is an important part of providing good medical care; context is crucial. There is one possible exception. While it is true that, on occasion, a necessary therapy may increase a patient's pain or discomfort for a time, the aim of such therapy is eventually to reduce them. The relief of pain and suffering thus comes as close as any of the goals to having a priority in most cases. It is as important in the ordinary run of medical treatment as it is in the care of the terminally ill.

The same general principles that are pertinent for individual patients are pertinent for allocations within health-care systems. Each country has to decide what its most important population health needs are and then allocate resources accordingly. For developing countries with scarce acute-care facilities, health promotion and disease prevention will make the most sense as the leading priority, and care of children and mothers will have a high place as well. For developed countries, the management of chronic disease and the choice of the appropriate goals to do so may be the highest priority. In short, whether at the individual or the societal level, determination of the most pressing and less pressing health-care needs must be made. That determination lies at the heart of any effort to set priorities.

THE PLACE OF AGE

Should age be a determinant in choosing the appropriate goals of medicine? That is a complex question to answer. In general, the answer with individual patients is that it should not. Most procedures that can be validly and valuably carried out with younger people can now be used effectively with older people. Increasingly, few surgical or other interventions are contraindicated by age alone. At the same time, aging is not a disease but a natural condition of human life, marked by a gradual decline of many important physiological capacities and an increased risk of illness, dementia, and disability. An endlessly aggressive war against death is not an appropriate goal for elderly care, even though in many cases it can and should be forestalled; and in many other cases, it is the care and comfort of the patient that should become the focus.

Palliative care, while appropriate for all age groups, will thus take on an increased importance with the elderly.[3] That is not only because of an increase in the lesser burdens of aging, those comparatively minor aches and pains and functional losses that ordinarily go with the biology of aging, even for those in good health, but also because of a gradually increased risk of more serious disabilities. At some point, the goal of a peaceful death will become the right goal, calling for an increased intensity of palliative care and a renewed emphasis on the relief of pain and suffering. Making a judgment about these different stages of aging (when to give up the goal of cure, when to accept the coming of death) will not be easy but is still necessary to make certain that the chosen goals of care are those that are right for this patient at this stage of life.

A scarcity of resources will not make that judgment any easier. It will bring with it the temptation to bias treatment toward doing less than might be technologically optimal or to allow age itself, quite apart from individual characteristics, to determine treatment choices. Nonetheless, that scarcity cannot be ignored. At the policy level, there may be appropriate debate about the extent of resources to be allocated to programs specifically aimed at the elderly and limits set; and an equitable balance will have to be struck among the needs of children, mid-life adults, and the aged. As the Hastings Center report on resource allocation to the elderly put it, "An integrated set of priorities for young and old should be pursued . . . [and] the young and old should work together to develop those priorities."[2] Whatever decision is reached, health-care providers will then have to grapple with the resources made available and, in that context, to determine where palliative care should fit. At each stage decisions will have to be made.

PRIORITY SETTING

We have written in a general way about the goals of medicine and the setting of priorities. Some greater specificity is needed about the allocation of health system resources to both palliative care and specific patients within a system. Three major obstacles remain to be overcome in many places. The first is simply the bias, in most insurance systems, toward providing coverage for specific technological interventions rather than toward what is often perceived as more amorphous kinds of care, either very low-technology care or care that requires time and a personal presence, and the relief of symptoms that might best be classified as psychological or spiritual. A skillfully titrated morphine drip, on the one hand, and simply talking with an unhappy or agitated patient, on the other, are examples of the kind of palliative benefits often thought less valuable in comparison with more aggressive curative or rehabilitative efforts.

There is no good medical reason whatever for that kind of bias. Patients need what they need, not necessarily what hospitals or clinics think is emblematic of biomedical progress, i.e., aggressive technological interventions. If a patient's greatest need at any given moment is palliative care, then that is the most important kind of care to give.[4] It may seem utterly commonsensical to say that, but it is too often forgotten in recent years, an era that saw the idea of cure elevated to the heights and care relegated to the lower basement. The persistently reported undertreatment of pain in the elderly is a perfect example of the problem.[5]

The second great obstacle might be termed *obliviousness*. By that we mean a failure on the part of health-care personnel to notice what they are doing and to understand how they come across to patients. In a trivial sense, almost all physicians and nurses think of themselves as dedicated to the relief of pain and suffering. They think of it, when they think of it at all, as something that automatically goes with their professional role, a necessary result of carrying out their professional duties. That is not so. It must be worked at and cultivated. It is hardly an uncommon phenomenon for a patient's body to be attended to but not his or her mind or feelings. An empty intravenous bag attracts professional attention but not always an unhappy face.

The third obstacle is not unrelated to the second, a failure to understand that good palliative care requires education and refined skills. It seems too commonly believed that palliative care is, even if important, not something that requires focused attention and specialized knowledge. Even if there is a strong desire, for instance, to provide proper pain relief to the elderly, that can be done well only if it is understood to demand a knowledge about the considerable research done on pain relief in recent years and about the wide range of pharmaceuticals and other modalities available to deal with the various manifestations; and the same can be said of the emotional distress of patients, which in many cases may respond better to kind talk than to a drug but with some training may be done more effectively.

We mention these obstacles not only because they will have an influence on the priority given to palliative care in patient treatment but also because a high priority alone may not be sufficient to deal with them adequately. That can only come about if attention is paid to the cultivation of physician and nurse sensibilities, suitable palliative care education, and adequate financing. Though limited to palliative care at the end of life, an important American study looked at some of the problems standing in the way of adequate financing and, by implication, some other crucial variables.[6] As the investigators explained, they were interested in determining how leaders in various health-care organizations perceived the financial and nonfinancial barriers to palliative care and to gain their judgment on some policy options to improve the situation.

Two distinct perspectives emerged from their interviews of the leaders. There was what they called a "budget" perspective, which saw palliative care "as already implicitly included in the current reimbursement system and, therefore, part of its core programs."[6] That perspective was most common in full-risk, capitated programs, where funds are allocated to program areas according to need. By contrast, there was a "reimbursement" perspective, common in fee-for-service settings, that views end-of-life palliative care as a new service that is not reimbursed under the current financial system.

Managers holding the latter perspective tend to believe that "they are not responsible for providing this care" and "services that are not reimbursed are seen as money losers."[6] Even those working within the budget perspective, though much better off, were not entirely free of budget constraints, forced to compete with other clinical programs and to cope with the (probably inaccurate) perception that palliative care programs increase the length of stay in the hospital and, therefore, costs. More generally, those working within both systems have to cope with a cultural bias in favor of aggressive, even if often futile, treatments rather than to accept death. Aggressive procedures not only are better reimbursed than palliative care treatment but also have specific reimbursement mechanisms that the latter do not.

The authors proposed three general reforms. The first would be the establishment of quality-of-care standards, to be monitored and enforced by accreditation bodies. That accreditation would establish appropriate patient care standards and describe reimbursable palliative care services. A second reform would designate a diagnosis-related group code for end-of-life palliative care, putting it in the category of reimbursable services. The third reform would be the creation of a medical specialty for end-of-life palliative care, raising its status and improving its quality. To this recommendation we would add the following: establish it for palliative care in general, not just for terminal care. That would help emphasize its important role in accompanying all medical care. At the same time, however, there should be a decent level of palliative care education for all clinicians. Specialty service, even under ideal conditions, is not likely always to be available; and in any case, it would do great harm if clinicians felt that the existence of a specialty relieved them of palliative care responsibilities.

While claims have been made that palliative care can lower cost, we believe that it is wisest not to emphasize that possibility as a way of promoting it until, and if, solid evidence is in hand to support it.[7–11] The best argument is simply that palliative care is indispensable for good patient care, and if savings can be gained, that is fine; if not, then it must still be offered. However, this kind of argument is not sustainable in the long run. It would be wise, therefore, for the field to work with economists to develop the necessary methods to judge its economic value. As Charles Normand has effectively argued,

It is no longer adequate to argue for special treatment based on some inherent worth of the services. Failure to subject interventions to evaluation of costs and benefits will lead to even weaker arguments in the context for ever scarcer resources . . . [moreover] economic evaluation can also allow serious comparisons between palliative interventions.[9]

Having said that, the basic question remains: how high a priority ought it to have in general, and under what circumstances should it have a very high priority? We suggest that a continuum be envisioned, beginning with a minimal level of care for all, up through a maximal level for the critically or terminally ill. A minimal level is required for all patients suffering a significant degree of pain and/or suffering. Following common usage, we distinguish between *pain* (a physical phenomenon) and *suffering* (a spiritual/psychological phenomenon). By using the word *significant*, we do not mean exceptional or unusual but that level of pain or suffering sufficiently strong to disturb ordinary function, cognitive focus, and emotional stability. Individuals notoriously differ on just what that level is, and it will be the task of the clinician to determine it through a careful examination of, and conversation with, the patient. When in doubt, it is better to provide palliative care than not to do so, letting the patient

determine when it can be reduced or discontinued.

If a minimal level of palliative care is to be provided for all patients, regardless of age, there will come a point when age should make a difference. It may legitimately affect both the kind and intensity of palliative care. There are three general reasons for making such a claim. The first is that aging statistically carries with it a variety of ailments, small and great. The elderly find their youthful powers declining, their aches and pains increasing, a new one already standing by to replace or add to another. "It is," as many elderly say, "one damn thing after another." The second reason is related to the first: the meaning of illness and disability as life events change, portending a future likely to be worse than the present. For young people, it is usually otherwise. They can hope to return to normal after a medical incident; that is less likely with the elderly. Those who are aged 70 with this or that ailment cannot help noticing those who are 80 with even more, perhaps much more, of the same. It is not an attractive prospect. The third reason is that the meaning of illness takes on, in addition to the prospect of still more in the future, the whispering footsteps of death, which with every passing year lies closer at hand. Of course, that is true of someone aged 50, but (barring critical illness) the portent can be ignored, too far in the future to worry much about. This is not so by the 70s and 80s, much less the 90s: what once seemed impossible comes to seem possible, what only seemed possible becomes likely, and what seemed likely is finally revealed for what it is, inevitable, any day now.

THE CLAIM OF THE ELDERLY FOR PALLIATIVE CARE

These three points are meant only to back up an assertion: the claim of the elderly for palliative care is a strong one because they are in a situation with no exit. This does not give the elderly an automatic claim of priority over the young, but it does show why the elderly have a strong claim. In the same vein, the fact that the elderly will typically die earlier from a critical illness than the young or that their suffering is likely to be of shorter duration is no reason to give them a lower priority. Of course, the chronically ill young adult with a life-long condition has the same problem, but the more common situation of the young is that they can go in and out of illness and hope for better years. With age, that possibility gradually diminishes, and that is the source of a powerful claim to good palliative care, not just minimally adequate palliative care but of a kind to make the last years as comfortable as possible. Earlier, we contended that, of all the goals of medicine, the relief of pain and suffering ordinarily has the highest claim, one that can only rarely be put aside.

However, to argue that way hardly solves the problem of rationing and priority setting. A number of difficulties remain. We might here imagine four medical circumstances that also have a powerful competing claim, each of them able to consume considerable resources: programs of health promotion and disease prevention for children, to get them off to the best possible start in life and to lay the foundation for life-long good health; life-saving and disability-avoiding acute medical care, aiming to save people from death or disabilities that could ruin the rest of their lives; rehabilitation efforts aimed at restoring the seriously injured or disabled to an independent, functioning life; and treatment of the chronic schizophrenic or depressed patient, whose every day is a misery. With the exception of the childhood situation, each of the others carries with it a serious degree of pain and suffering, which will be relieved along with the additional benefits that the associated treatment will bring.

We do not want to argue that palliative care for the elderly should always and automatically take priority over those other treatments, but we contend that the older a person is, and the closer to death, the claim for good palliative care is as strong

as any of those mentioned. There is an important consideration in coming to that judgment: those whose lives are saved, made functional through rehabilitation, or psychologically brought back to normal, will nonetheless someday have to face aging. It is a universal condition unlike any of other, and even those children set on the path to good health will discover that it runs out in old age. Everyone is likely to need palliative care when old. That cannot be said of any other medical or psychological problem associated with the earlier stages of life. Every stage can and does have its problems, but aging is the only certain and inevitable circumstance guaranteed, sooner or later, to bring us down.

Once the relative priority to be given palliative care among an array of other medical needs is established, it may then become necessary to prioritize the available palliative care resources. The highest priority, we believe, should be given to short-term acute pain and suffering, of a kind that follows a serious surgical procedure or accompanies temporarily burdensome maladies that are ordinarily time-limited. This is perhaps the one circumstance, however, where a shortage of resources might justify less than optimal palliative care but only when it is going to be for a short time. The next highest priority should go to those patients, young or old, with serious and disabling long-term pain and suffering, of a kind that accompanies chronic illness, physical or mental. The next highest should go to efforts to improve somatic and psychological well-being and to promote symptom-free survival. Now it might be argued that it would be a mistake to give a high priority, with limited resources, to those at the end of their lives, particularly the terminally ill elderly, who can by definition benefit for only a short time. We think that reasoning to be upside down. Particularly since palliative care may be all that medicine can offer them, all they can hope for, their claim should have the highest possible priority.

We have mixed here two circumstances

that are different even if they overlap: the comparative amount of money to be made available to palliative care in relationship to other forms of medical care and the allocation of funds within palliative care budgets. Rationing and priority setting will usually be needed at both levels, and the most difficult dilemma will come about when resources are made available but insufficient to meet all reasonable needs. Rationing, in the hard sense of the term, often connotes the total denial of some needed good to some individual or group. In that circumstance, what is needed has no priority at all; it is simply eliminated from consideration. But, as noted above, a milder sense and situation is when the resource is in short supply, not adequate to meet all needs in any ideal, much less perfectly equitable, way.

In the latter circumstance, the other meaning of rationing comes into play, that of the equitable distribution of scarce resources. There are no simple principles available to determine equitable distribution, and the difficulties of determining it with palliative care make clear just why. Think of the following troublesome questions. Is it more fair to give those with the worst pain and suffering most of the resources at the expense of a much larger number whose needs are just as real but not quite so pressing? What counts as the worse situation: those suffering from severely acute physical pain of short duration or those with a low degree of psychological suffering over a longer period of time? Since individuals differ enormously in their ability to bear pain and tolerate suffering, should that matter in allocating resources? Who should decide that, the physician or the patient? Should the whining patient win out over the stoic patient?

Our general answer to these questions is that those suffering the most should receive the resources first, taking care not to use all of them on such patients. Those suffering less should receive some palliative care rather than none. A minimally adequate level should be determined, to be applied to everyone but with those worse off receiving care well above that minimum if necessary. Some difficult problems may then have to be faced, particularly with the terminally ill. How much intravenous nutrition, for instance, should be provided, or artificial ventilation or palliative chemotherapy? As with many other medical situations, judgment and experience are needed. Over time, patterns of fair allocation can be developed but always subject to periodic review and change. When it is a matter of palliative care versus other forms of care, the minimal rule should apply as well: palliative care must always be provided to some degree, but the aged should have a privileged place for the reasons noted above.

In sum, rationing is inevitable in all health-care systems, and priority setting is the best way to cope with it. A good case can be made for a high priority to be given to palliative care for the elderly. That case will be stronger in the future if supported by careful economic studies as well as by an effort to press for public and professional dialogue on the priority to be given palliative care in the competition for health-care resources. The fresh emphasis on palliative care was long overdue. Now that it is once again on the health-care agenda, it deserves careful comparison with other uses of scarce resources. Failure to do that could eventually force it to the sidelines. That would be a tragedy in the face of aging populations, who will desperately need it.

REFERENCES

1. Hastings Center. The goals of medicine: setting new priorities. Hastings Cent Rep 26: 6(Suppl) 1996.
2. Hastings Center. What do we owe the elderly: allocating social and health care resources. Hastings Cent Rep 24:2(Suppl) 1994.
3. Cleary JF, Carbone PP. Palliative medicine in the elderly. Cancer 80:1335–1347, 1997.
4. Wasson K. Ethical arguments for providing palliative care to non-cancer patients. Int J Palliat Nurs 6:66–70, 2000.
5. Teno JM, Weitzen S, Wettle T, Mohr V.

Persistent pain in nursing home residents. JAMA 205:2081, 2001.

6. Cassell CK, Ludden JM, Moon GM. Perceptions of barriers to high-quality palliative care in hospitals. Health Aff (Millwood) 5:166–172, 2000.

7. Bailes JS. Cost aspects of palliative cancer care. Semin Oncol 22(Suppl 3):64–66, 1995.

8. Warde P, Murphy MH. Measuring the cost of palliative radiotherapy. Can J Oncol 61(Suppl):90–94, 1996.

9. Normand C. Economics and evaluation of palliative care. Palliat Med 54:34–37, 1996.

10. Bruera E, Suarez-Almazo M. Cost effectiveness in palliative care. Palliat Med 12:315–316, 1998.

11. Bruner DW. Cost-effectiveness and palliative care. Semin Oncol Nurs 14:164–167, 1998.

7

Ethical Aspects of Geriatric Palliative Care

LINDA EMANUEL, MADELYN A. IRIS, AND JAMES R. WEBSTER

The dictates of ethics treat the elderly and the dying very well. Much of the real world treats them poorly. The paradox is amplified by the reality that those who care for seriously ill elders can derive profound personal and professional gratification from doing so. Indeed, geriatric palliative care can be seen as a manifestation of professionalism. Sometimes ethics is presented as the difficult balancing of competing principles in rarified situations. However, ethics also has some clear guidance, and the difficulty may be less in the analysis than in the application. This chapter summarizes the guidance as well as recurring dilemmas in the field. The first section outlines an approach to professional ethics with attention to the way precepts guide care of the seriously ill elderly. The second section delineates an approach to some of the ethical dilemmas that arise in clinical aspects of geriatric palliative care. The third section discusses challenges in social policy that have a moral claim on professionals.

MEDICAL PROFESSIONALISM

Sources of Medical Ethics

Professional ethics is a subset of general ethics. It focuses on ethical questions raised by the role and practices of professionals. Professional ethics includes the ethics of any profession, whether legal, medical, or other. Medical ethics, therefore, is a subset of professional ethics.

Medical ethics has derived its precepts and teachings from different sources. As an academic discipline and area of public interest, it experienced exponential development with the biomedical revolution, starting with the advent of life-sustaining interventions such as resuscitation and respiratory support in the 1950s and continuing until the present. This era can be characterized by the dominant influence first of religious thinkers such as Jonsen and Toulmin[1] and then of philosophical thinkers such as Beauchamp and Childress[2] and Callahan.[3] Others have contributed the perspectives of narrative ethics, economics, political theory, anthropology, role morality, and more, creating a new body of multidisciplinary perspectives.[4-8] Among the works in this multidisciplinary field, the first three editions of *Principles of Biomedical Ethics* by Beauchamp and Childress[9] have most influenced the received wisdom of ethics among professionals. In these editions, the authors distilled medical ethics principles into four types; and many people think of "beneficence, non-maleficence, autonomy, and justice" as the canons of medical ethics.

More traditional professional ethics draws on ancient as well as modern codes of ethics, such as the Hippocratic Oath, Physician's Prayer, Helsinki Declaration, American Medical Association Code of Ethics, *American College of Physicians Ethics Manual*, or the Physician's Charter.[10,11] Professional ethics places less emphasis on identifying higher-order principles and more emphasis on practical rules of conduct. These two approaches of modern medical and traditional professional ethics are compatible. Professional ethics are emphasized here because of their derivation from medical traditions that have gone through more tests of time and circumstance than any other. A useful way of considering how professional ethics relates to principles of ethics is that it identifies the legitimate purposes and conditions for medicine that are compatible with, and perhaps derived from, higher-order ethical principles. Codes of professional ethics in medicine identify the following driving purposes and conditions of practice:

- to cure;
- to care;
- to be trustworthy; and
- to contribute to the well-being of society.

A primary goal for physicians and other professionals who assist the purposes of medicine is to cure conditions of illness. Medical professionals are asked to cure the ill person's primary diagnosis and any secondary diagnoses. A concurrent second goal is to palliate any symptoms of illness or therapy that cannot be treated with curative intervention alone and to care for the person as a whole. Even in the current era of sophisticated capabilities, much of what ails people cannot be cured and thus needs palliative care.

The third major point is a condition of practice: the need for practitioners and norms of practice in medicine to be trustworthy. Recent commentaries have focused on the decline in society's trust of professionals, calling attention to a perceived impending crisis.[12,13] When some prominent commentators noted that, in a sense, the professions have a contract with society to provide services in exchange for the privilege of self-regulation, some took the message that physicians enjoy self-regulation as a kind of entitlement.[14,15] Far from having an unconditional entitlement, professionals, like others in society, are accountable.[16] The nature of illness and the nature of medical intervention make direct accountability for actions difficult. Illness causes a special kind of vulnerability. Medical intervention carries potent risks and requires special care and often special knowledge. Medical professionals must adhere tightly to the obligation to be trustworthy because the ill person has restricted options and usually has to trust someone to provide care. Indeed, a trustworthy professional has a kind of therapeutic potential and ability to comfort that comes from his or her trustworthiness alone. Trustworthiness entails the following:

- accountable adherence to norms and standards of objectively evaluated practice;
- placing priority on the needs of those served, including communication with the patient and family that allows for full informed consent for all decisions;
- subjugation (not obliteration) of financial and other self-interests to the interests of those served;
- integrity in personal conduct; and
- fair provision of medical services to all who need them.

The imperative to adhere to norms and standards of practice that have been subjected to rigorous and objective evaluation is necessary because of the vulnerable state caused by illness, on the one hand, and the specialized and possibly determinative nature of the professional's actions, on the other hand. This also gives rise to a professional obligation to be accountable for norms of practice and to provide for that accountability. This includes setting up systems such as certification, quality improvement, and disciplinary procedures.[17]

Placing the needs of the ill above those of others is motivated by the same vulnerability of the ill person. Communicating with patients and families to narrow the gap in expertise and minimize the vulnerability by maximizing the ill person's control over decisions is one manifestation of this. Subjugation of self-interests to the interests of the patient is another. Although interests are varied, financial interests are most readily regulated and serve as a case in point. Professionals are not required to have no financial gain; rather, they are not allowed to put this ahead of a patient's interests. Were professionals allowed to put self-interest first, interactions would be exploitative since the restricted options and capacities due to illness would often prevent fair negotiations.

One aspect of medical professionalism that takes up much space in most codes of ethics has to do with avoiding exploitative roles with patients. Physicians are particularly adjured to avoid sexual interaction with patients. This injunction also derives from the vulnerable state in which illness places people. Patients may not be or feel able to reject sexual advances or may be transiently enamored of the professional due to the caring role that may seem personal rather than professional. Professionals must therefore avoid all such interactions.

When some groups of people have access to more or better care than others, those who are shut out or denied aspects of care cannot be expected to find the medical system or its professionals trustworthy. Professionalism is motivated by the need it serves. If it systematically fails to respond to some peoples' needs but responds to others, it is in conflict with its own moral roots. Fair access to care is therefore an indisputable part of professionalism. Recent discussions about resource allocation in no way diminish this position; rather, fairness requires that finite resources be allocated in an openly, carefully considered fashion.

Finally, medical professionals are required by their overall role to contribute to society, most especially by protecting vulnerable values (care of the ill and protection of the public from illness) and vulnerable people (those who are ill) through their actions. In this role, medical professionals make an essential contribution to civilization as a whole.[15] Other professionals are required to make essential contributions as well, e.g., the legal profession to upholding justice, the religious professions to religious practices. In fact, all professionals make a contribution that is distinct from the contributions made by government and the private sector. In the interface between the practices of medicine that focus on the individual patient and the practices that impact society, medical professionals recognize the essential importance of activities such as public health care and support of family-based caregivers. It is also in this interface that professional activities remind society of our human limitations, that help society to infuse its culture with the legacies and wisdom of those who are ill or dying, and that help its members to realize the fulfillment of care in relation to one another. Professional advocacy exists in the direct interactions between professionals and people who are affected by illness, as well as in the realm of institutional and political advocacy for actions and policies that reflect the values of cure, care, and trustworthiness.

These four principal features of professional action—to cure, to care, to be trustworthy, and to protect vulnerable values and people—run through all that medical professionals are obligated to do.

How Professionalism Guides Geriatric Palliative Care Practice

Special obligations to elders and the terminally ill

As noted, the obligations of medical action apply to professionals for anyone who has vulnerabilities due to medical health. The goal is to minimize the source of illness (to cure or prevent) and the effect of the illness on the person (to palliate), making that person as whole as possible. These precepts apply with particular urgency to the elderly with incurable illness for several reasons.

First, the elderly are a vulnerable group in most societies. They lose the former roles they held in society, which lent them legitimacy, and key family members and friends, who would have comprised their social support network. Ageism and fears of indignity and burdensomeness can become paralyzing as elders come to feel worthless to society.

Second, those with incurable illness face possible rejection by others, which can be generated by deep-seated fears of death and dying. Culture as a whole and people as individuals can be ill-adjusted to these realities and fail to realize the ways in which the aging and terminally ill need to take on a special role in which they can contribute in perhaps intangible but still important ways.

Third, the elderly with (or without) incurable illnesses are frail in the sense that small medical events or complications may cause major functional deterioration. Their resilience to challenges and adaptability is usually reduced. For example, an iatrogenic complication such as a drug reaction may cause permanent institutionalization and complete dependence in a frail elderly patient, while in a younger person it may merely extend a hospital stay by a day or two.

Fourth, a key mental feature of frailty amplifies the vulnerability of aging and terminal illness: the high prevalence of confusional states, dementia, or delirium. Mental disability can so threaten or undermine the patient's capacity to relate (and others' capacity to relate to them) that the patient's suffering may be incomprehensible and his or her isolation that much more profound. The loneliness and thanklessness of caregiving when the patient suffers from dementia and associated psychiatric conditions are also significant and may make the task for family members and professionals especially demanding. The professional obligation to contribute to civilization motivates another feature of geriatrics and palliative care. The very old and the mortally ill have to pass on the mantle, making a bridge from the past to the future complete. These are ingredients of cultural history, mores, role continuity, and personal bearing. Medical care has an obligation to contribute to civilization by fostering the conditions under which this can happen as well as possible.

These features of professionalism and sources of vulnerability for geriatric patients in need of palliative care have structured the activities of geriatrics and of palliative care nationally and internationally.[18,19]

Features of care derived from professionalism

Goals of care and whole-person care. The two key goals of the medical professional are to cure and to care. How do these purposes translate into goals for the care of specific, contextually situated people? Both geriatrics and palliative care (especially the latter) have placed the conscious balancing of these purposes, to suit the options and goals of the patient and family, at the center of their philosophy of practice. An ideal rendering of medicine would provide each patient with a blend of care that combines curative and palliative intents according to the needs of that patient. From the time of diagnosis, patients should have palliative as well as curative care. As cure becomes elusive, the proportion of care that is of palliative intent should rise. Toward the end of life, many people will receive primarily palliative care.

People with serious illness seek care that will allow them to remain a whole person whether by curative action or by palliative care. Even when care is entirely palliative, the objective remains to make the person in his or her context as whole as possible. People with illness are a great deal more than a pathological process. People in general have physical, emotional, social, and existential aspects, all of which need to be given due respect in any encounter. This is possibly most true among medical encounters with those elderly who have a life-shortening diagnosis. Even when illness has taken major physical capacities away, the patient has dementia, or after death, care involves adaptation to keep the context as whole as possible. As people lose function, the family or care team seeks to substitute the function with some creative adaptation. When the person dies, whether by honoring a personal legacy, keeping a memory alive, or invoking a religious understanding, that person's place in the social context is kept as whole as possible. Whole-person care requires three key features: a respectful therapeutic relationship with the patient as a person, involvement of the family and community, and an interdisciplinary team.

The respectful therapeutic relationship. The need for full respect for the whole person is reflected in a recent debate over terminology. People have begun to revolt against the term *patient.* Pioneered perhaps by those facing acquired immunodeficiency syndrome (AIDS) who insisted on the term *persons living with AIDS*, people with cancer and a full range of other diagnoses are also insisting on being called *people living with cancer [illness].* Some find solace and support in the emerging community that defines itself around common experiences with illness and accept an identity that includes the illness. Others seek an identity free of illness and manage the illness as an unwelcome intruder into an illness-free personal identity.

Challenges involved in making those with mental losses as whole as possible within the therapeutic relationship have taken new strides with the school of care pioneered by Kitwood.[20] In this approach, the person is made as whole and content as possible, accepting the emotional world of meaning and relating to the person on the terms that make sense for the world as that person experiences it. This concept of respect provides for a kind of wholeness that does not attempt to restore the person to his or her former self when that is impos-

sible but, rather, seeks a sense of acceptance and, hence, wholeness on terms that are meaningful to the individual that he or she has become.

Family and community. Professional obligations to cure and care extend beyond the patient to include the family and community. Since people are connected to one another, this obligation is also found in the injunction to contribute to the well-being of society. By providing care and by fostering care that includes the family, professionals promote values that might otherwise be lost. Even in today's health-care system, when most people die in institutions and many have protracted stays in long-term care institutions, much of the care of an elderly, incurably ill person falls to the family. The relationship between the patient and the family caregiver is more important than mainstream medicine has admitted. Usually, people can identify a primary caregiver within the family. The primary caregiver, often a wife or daughter, shoulders considerable burden.[21] A larger preponderance of minorities and low-income people exist among caregivers than the general population. Just under a third of families spend their life savings and two-fifths spend down to poverty level when they are caring for a terminally ill family member.[22] Family caregivers have a higher incidence of depression and other physical illnesses than matched populations. Supporting the caregiver is therefore important for at least two reasons: to maximize the care given to the patient and to minimize the burden and risk to the health and well-being of the caregiver. Approaches to understanding and supporting the caregiver are too little considered and too rarely taught. Professionalism guides us to learn to ask how caregivers are doing; to seek resources for them from their own community and from pastors, psychologists, and social workers; and to promote social policies that take their needs into account.

The interdisciplinary medical team. Careful attention to the above features of professionalism (to cure, to care, and to contribute to the well-being of society) has made both geriatrics and palliative care attentive to the central place of the interdisciplinary team.[23] The kind of whole-picture care that both disciplines espouse is virtually impossible without it.[24] In geriatric palliative care, the kind of wholeness a person can achieve can be more dependent on the nonphysical aspects of well-being than in younger people with curable conditions. Thus, although the multidisciplinary team is not new, a more integrated version of it has come to be a central feature of quality geriatric and palliative care. Given current trends and the recommendations of a number of medical professional organizations, including the American Association of Medical Colleges, it appears that team care will become a standard of practice in the next decade.[25] In geriatrics, the team is frequently made up of core groups of physicians, specialized nurses, and social workers. Care and leadership are provided by whoever can best fulfill the needs of each individual patient. Each team member brings his or her own special knowledge, attitudes, skills, and behaviors to bear where most appropriate. On many occasions, teams will confer with other professionals, such as clergy, physical and occupational therapists, mental health specialists, and so forth. While formal teams are common, *virtual* teams, where members have informal relationships and function as needed, are often quite effective. A cardinal feature of the team is its integrative nature. The exchange between the disciplines as well as the "team-tag" of multidisciplinary teams has become an index of the philosophy of and a vehicle for integrative care.

ETHICAL ISSUES IN CLINICAL PRACTICE

Making Therapeutic Decisions

Models of therapeutic relationships/ decision making

Over the cultural developments that time has wrought, medicine has shifted its models of therapeutic relationships. The patient–physician relationship has received most attention, although many other relationships (patient–nurse, patient–social worker, patient–pastor, patient–family caregiver, and so forth) are also critical. The patient–physician relationship can be characterized in four or five different paradigms that different eras have favored: paternalistic, informational, instructional, deliberative, and situational.

The *paternalistic model* pertains if the physician is seen as a parental figure and the patient as a child-like figure; the goal is the patient's best interests, and the determiner of those best interests is the physician. Information is transmitted at the discretion of the physician. The patient is quiescent and grateful; the physician is beneficent and obliging. In reaction against paternalism and in the enthusiasm of a consumerist society, an *informational model* developed. In this, the physician merely provides information and services at the determination of the patient. The patient keeps control while the physician serves as a technician. A dissatisfaction with the informational model by many people and its inadequacy for many circumstances brought about an *instructional model*. In this model, the physician, who is seen as a teacher, also provides counsel to the patient. This approach acknowledges that people may not know what they want until they have a chance to talk it through. The goal is to realize the patient's wishes by helping the patient to articulate them with a full understanding of the information. The *deliberative model* allows that even advice may not be enough and that at times the physician should persuade the patient. So, for instance, the physician may try to persuade the patient that exercise is essential, even though he or she is not inclined to it. An advantage of this model is that it allows the professional to advocate for values that have to do with health and well-being; a disadvantage is that it can slip into paternalism. A *situational model* allows that each model has its place and that part of what the professional should do is discern which model is suitable for whom and when.

In addition to this frame of thought, another can help the reflective practitioner arrive at an ethically well-considered position: role morality. People adopt roles in relation to one another, and each role comes with a specific set of obligations and privileges. Professionals adopt a curing, caring role based on the patient's need and on the professional's ability to deliver. The role obligation is usually primarily to the ill person, then the family, the health-care team, and the community since this is usually the ordering based on need. This ordering of role obligation can remain even when the ill person has dementia or is unconscious. Both the focus and the role obligation begin to shift as the ill person becomes obtunded and death occurs, with the family taking a higher priority. However, at no point is it easy to justify acting *against* the interests of the ill person to satisfy family, team, or community needs.

> Ms. W was a 76-year-old woman with an adrenal carcinoma who had presented with cushingoid features and tuberculosis. She was fully alert and capable of usual decision making when she came to the hospital; she was able to understand and engage in a deliberative relationship, first favoring immediate surgery but readily accepting medical advice to delay until she could be made well enough for surgery. However, over the next days, tuberculous meningitis caused confusion. Her physician assumed a more paternalistic relationship with her and an instructional relationship with her family. When progressive confusion caused global incapacity, her son's role as proxy was activated and an instructional relationship between the son and physician continued, there being no difference over which care approach seemed necessary. When Ms. W became unconscious despite maximal therapy, her son and physicians transitioned her to predominantly palliative care and her family received support and, after her death 2 days later, bereavement care. Later, the son wrote a letter to the physician thanking him for the friendship shown toward his mother and the mentorship and care provided to himself and his family and remarking on how the physician managed to meet each person's changing needs.

This physician adopted the situational approach, seeking a deliberative relationship when it seemed necessary, an instructional one when it seemed sufficient, and a paternalistic one when the patient could not participate at all. He included the family in his approach to care, allowing the focus to shift toward them as Ms. W's death became imminent.

Communication

Communication is critical to building a trusting relationship. Communication includes but means more than information transmittal. It implies active listening and includes understanding of the receiver of that information. This is necessary if information is to be offered in the most useable form so that the personal meaning of that information can be appreciated. It includes communicating values, especially of care and respect.

Transmitting information. Knowledge is powerful, and professionals have a duty to make use of this power appropriately. Patients and caregivers alike identify information transmittal as an important concern that affects their experience of illness and care. Sharing knowledge and information creates a partnership rather than a hierarchy. For a majority of people in the United States, partnership is appropriate and a version of the instructional or deliberative model is sought in the therapeutic alliance.

Transmitting information about diagnosis and prognosis is not simple. Technical jargon presents one barrier. Use of statistical concepts for individual cases presents another. The professional's interpersonal communication skills are important, and variation among team members regarding what information is transmitted can present further challenges. Time and access to professional team members are necessary. Avoidance by the professionals is not acceptable. On the side of the ill person, emotional barriers to hearing charged information and limitations in medical understanding present yet further challenges. Development of communication skills and strategies to overcome these and other barriers is essential.[26]

Until recently, truth telling by professionals was considered too revealing and nondisclosure was justified by the concern that information might take hope away from the patient. In retrospect, too much of the protection was for the professional rather than the patient. Western practice has largely embraced truth telling and has rallied to reduce inappropriate use of power by guarding information.[27] Nonetheless, legitimate cultural variations remain. Even within mainstream Western culture, commentators are reviving the theme of hope and the need for some degree of "healthy denial." While withholding fundamental information, such as the malignant nature of a diagnosis, is rarely justified, allowing ambiguity along with candor, for instance by explaining decisions as "preparing for the worst but hoping for the best," may be not only excusable but the best thing to do in some situations. Allowing for the different ways in which information is handled in different patient, family, and community cultures is also appropriate. A helpful guide to staying on the right side of information management is to ask patients and, if relevant, families how they would like illness information to be handled. If the requests are discordant either among one another or with the professional's best judgment, this can be sorted out before a difficult situation occurs.

Responding to illness meaning. It can be easy for professionals to forget that patients may not know the significance or source of their symptoms. Personal meanings of illness can have powerful effects on a patient and family experience. Ethical analyses of, for instance, decisions to avoid treatment should not stop at ensuring that patients are informed and autonomous. Probing the emotional logic is also important. Thus, when an elderly woman avoids intervention for a gynecological cancer not because she is ready to let her life end naturally but rather because she feels it is just punishment for youthful errors, this is important. When an elderly man avoids opioids be-

cause he would rather fear addiction and feel alive because of it than admit that his pain is too intractable and his life expectancy too short for addiction to be relevant, this too is important. In both cases, further shared insight and deliberation could yield a better decision.

Some manifestations of illness have profound personal meaning that affects more than individual decisions. For instance, when an ill person cannot eat, expressions of family care are frustrated. Bad odors can limit personal proximity, and this can exacerbate isolation. When personal body image changes so dramatically that, say, grandchildren are frightened, this can be hurtful. When incontinence shames the elder, important relationships can be challenged. Simply by noting, whether to the ill person or to the family, the reality and that it is a normal part of the disease process the professional can open up conversations that assist adjustment and coping mechanisms.

Informed consent. Ensuring good information transfer and responding well to individual understanding about illness and prognosis is not the sum total of the professional's communication tasks. Communication about testing options, therapeutic options, and sometimes research options builds on the skills noted above. Literature exists on assisted decision-making programs for specific illnesses and options. At its simplest, each decision needs to be informed about the following features: risks of the chosen therapeutic action, in particular the serious and the common adverse events; benefits of the therapeutic action; and alternatives along with their likely outcomes.[28]

Steps involved in informed consent, as derived from the deliberative model of patient–physician relationships, include the following actions by the physician or other professional:

- giving permission and orientation: invite discussion of the topic and of relevant personal and cultural norms, identify relevant issues and acceptable approaches

- information giving (on risks, benefits, and alternatives): provide it in a way that meets the patient's information-intake style or needs
- facilitating patient self-understanding for this topic: offer education and deliberation
- allowing for patient reflection: check for stable resolution or decision
- coming to agreement: commitment to the decision by relevant parties

Informed consent worksheets that foster this approach are available.[29]

Value differences. Some communication gaps present as value differences; and conversely, some value differences present as communication gaps. The profession is obliged to adhere above all to the professional values involved in care, comfort, trustworthiness, and benefit to the community. Other values are usually best left out of patient encounters in so far as they may cause interruptions to the empathic exchange and the therapeutic encounter. So, for instance, if a patient rejects chemotherapy in favor of meditation, some physicians may wish to assert their opposition to this approach. However, a more caring approach states something like the following: "There are probably some things we should think about together before considering whether chemotherapy or meditation or both are your best option; let's first talk about what is making you consider this approach."

Distinguishing between professional values and either personal values or habits of conduct is especially necessary when they become intertwined. For instance, a professional's unexamined assumptions regarding the use of life-sustaining interventions can influence decisions. While the goal of a deliberative relationship does encourage a professional to persuade the patient and family of health-related values that are in their best interests, as noted above, the risk exists of overinfluence and paternalism. In the end, it is the patient's life and values that take precedence. Only when the professional feels unable to conscientiously participate in the requested course of action should additional steps be taken. These steps should follow a careful process and have been outlined elsewhere, for instance, for cases of futility (see also Futility below).[30]

> Mr. B was a 77-year-old retired executive with late-stage vascular dementia who lived in a nursing home. After recovery from his second aspiration pneumonia, the nursing home refused to accept him back unless he had a gastrostomy tube placed. His large extended family was reluctant to give permission since he had been clear that he did not want to be kept alive by artificial means, but they were also appalled by the prospect of letting him starve. A care conference was convened, and references were provided to show that gastrostomy tubes do not promote longevity, reduce aspiration risk, improve nutrition, or improve comfort or quality of life. A dietician provided information on cued swallowing and timing and size of meals. A different nursing home was found that would accept Mr. B without a gastrostomy tube provided that his family was willing to help on a daily basis. Mr. B died 5 months later of pneumonia. His family spoke of the times when they hand-fed him as precious and meaningful events with great periods of communication.

A team follow-up meeting revealed unanimity that this was an ideal outcome. Inadequate information and communication had allowed a situation that appeared to involve value differences. The care conference cleared up the misunderstandings.

Culture

Culture is powerful and sometimes seemingly ineffable. Different cultures show distinct patterns in matters such as life-sustaining treatment choices, understanding of death, and approaches to bereavement.[31,32] Cultural competence is an ethical imperative in so far as care and trustworthiness are compromised without it and as it contributes to the good of society. Full cultural competence may not be possible for practices that provide for a range of cultural groups. Also, variability within a culture is often as great as between cultures.[33] However, each person and family provides a source of learning. The physician who approaches each person with respect and invites that person to educate him or her in relevant aspects of the culture can attain adequate cultural competence for most encounters. Starting out a therapeutic relationship, a physician may ask how the person likes to be addressed ("What name would you like me to use for you?"), how information should be shared ("Would you like me to give information to you, to someone else you trust, or both?"), and how decisions should be made ("Do you like to make decisions alone or with someone/ others?"). Later in the relationship, it may also be helpful to ask how to plan ahead ("Should we consider possible scenarios, or should we perhaps consider what others have experienced and decided?"), how emotions are handled ("If times get difficult emotionally, what is the best way to be sure you have support?"), and how family responsibilities are understood ("If you need more care, who if anyone in your family might take on some of that care?"). These questions are both pertinent and practical, and they can open a more extensive exchange about culture if both parties so desire.

Incapacity

The high prevalence of mental compromise is a prominent feature of geriatric medicine. Mental function is so integral to a person's ability to relate to others that its compromise may seem to threaten a person's wholeness more than most other deficits in function. It also may severely limit that which makes care gratifying: appreciation. The suffering among the mentally ill may be such that some find it impossible or unbearable to imagine, let alone approach and alleviate. For these reasons, cure and comfort are that much more difficult and important. Trustworthiness is essential; these patients and their families are particularly exploitable because their circumstances are difficult and little acknowledged in communities and society generally.

Frail patients with full mental capacity. For the frail patient with full mental capacity, the professional must respond with extra efforts to compensate for the frailty. This kind of compensation can take the form of including a family member to help remember and review a medical discussion or home visiting to reduce the number of mental adjustments required by office appointments. It can take the form of responding to and coping with labile emotions in an empathic and helpful fashion and can involve providing the simplest possible medical regimen or using the most understandable form of language or nonverbal communication.

Partly incapacitated patients. Partial capacity poses a special set of problems.[34] A partially incapacitated person has to make some decisions beyond his or her capacity and others within his or her capacity. The task of the professional is to evaluate the capacity to make specific decisions. Modern ethics explains this obligation in terms of maximizing the patient's autonomy; professional ethics also sees it in terms of maximizing the patient's wholeness and comfort.

Psychiatrists have grappled with a related problem, when to overrule and when to go along with the wishes of a person who is schizophrenic, manic, or otherwise suffering from a condition that pits one aspect of the self against another in a pathological fashion. A helpful rule of thumb is to consider the psychiatrist as siding with the healthy side of the patient and against the unhealthy side. In so doing, the psychiatrist seeks to make the person as whole as possible. Similarly, when working with a partially incapacitated patient, the physician seeks to maximize the suitable potential of the healthy capacities of the patient and either over-rule or substitute for ill aspects.

Criteria for decision-specific capacity have been delineated well by Applebaum and colleagues.[35] Capacity entails making a decision, understanding relevant information, appreciating potential consequences of a decision, and having a coherent thought process. Some scholars also include another criterion: consistency of the decision with the person's values. A great deal of subjective interpretation goes into making assessments of capacity. The physician is obliged to hold himself or herself to particularly stringent levels of self-awareness, to avoid the pitfalls of projection or bias.

Globally incapacitated patients. For globally incapacitated patients, the motivation remains the same: to make the person as whole and as comfortable in all aspects of his or her experience as possible. To engage in the deliberative relational process that allows a person to realize what decisions are best, it is necessary to have someone speak in the patient's role. For globally incapacitated patients, all reasonable efforts should be made to have a proxy speak for the patient.

In keeping with the dominance of the autonomy model of medical ethics, proxies have been urged to speak in place of the patient. One standard is that of best interests: that is, the proxy should speak in place of the patient in the way that most advances the interests of the patient. However, people do not always seek what seems to be in the patient's best interests. The next standard is that of substituted judgment: that is, the proxy should seek whatever most resembles what the patient would have sought. Often, this approach is closer to a patient's desire to take the family views into account.[36] While an improvement, this standard appears to be prone to projection. A modified tack is to try to gain guidance from the person's whole life, seeking decisions that seem most compatible with the life choices the person made before the onset of mental incapacity. Use of advance care planning decisions made by the patient is another approach and is discussed below.

Emergency care decisions. Emergency care decisions fall into a special category since there is by definition rarely time to explore the patient's background enough to fully evaluate capacity or what might constitute a substituted judgment or a decision consistent with the person's life or prior decisions. Emergency decisions can usually err on the side of saving life. This is especially so since the ethics of withdrawing life support have been clarified to the point that it is acceptable to withdraw nonbeneficial or unwanted life-prolongation interventions.

Ms. M was a mildly demented, happily disposed older woman who lived with her unmarried daughter and enjoyed her church activities and visiting her other children. She spoke of her desire to enjoy life and never get stuck on a machine. Appropriate papers were completed. One morning she collapsed in her bathroom; she had suffered a stroke and was hemiplegic with a mild expressive aphasia. The physician sat with Ms. M and her local daughter, explaining that the situation was serious but not at present life-threatening and reviewing the advance directives. Ms. M nodded that these were still her wishes. Over the next 36 hours, the stroke progressed so that Ms. M became aphasic and then quite obtunded. That night, her breathing became marginal. A night team that did not know her wishes had her intubated and transferred to the intensive care unit (ICU). The next day, the physician reviewed the situation with the family. One more consultation was called; this physician felt that the outlook for long-term survival was virtually nil. Ventilatory support was withdrawn according to ICU protocols, with the family and pastor in attendance. The family was offered and took counseling. Although it was a long and painful process, everyone in the family finally came to peace with these events.

Although Ms. M was partially incapacitated, the physician found her specific decision-making capacity to be intact both before and during the immediate period after her stroke. Neither her mild dementia nor her aphasia prevented this. When she became obtunded and was clearly globally incapacitated, her prior wishes were honored. During an emergency episode at night, when her prior wishes were not known, she was given life-saving intervention; but when her wishes were available through the physician and family, care was adjusted to match her stated and documented prior wishes.

Life-Support Decisions

Medical ethics can be seen in high relief with decisions that involve life-or-death consequences. This is so even though the stakes may be as high or higher earlier in a life trajectory. Nonetheless, the clarity of analysis that has been distilled regarding life-support decisions is useful and can provide a moral compass for other decisions.

Advance care planning

Advance care planning discussions are often framed in ethics presentations as a manifestation of the principle of autonomy. They are also readily understood as being motivated by the need for trustworthiness. To be trustworthy, medical care has to be synchronous with the needs of the patient and family as well as with the social context. If care is to be guided by a synthesis of all the needs in all the dimensions of suffering, a depth of understanding is necessary that is possible only with discussion and deliberation. Patients and family members do not know their wishes in a vacuum. Physicians and other professionals cannot make good decisions based on test results alone. Advance care planning should be a relational and discursive process that may include development and evolution of personal views and capacities. The physician, the patient, and the proxy all need preparation to coordinate between one another, with the rest of the health-care team, and with the rest of the family. In a real sense, advance care planning is about team building and preparedness. It is also about coming to grips with a medical condition and allowing the patient a chance to "try out" various possibilities that might constrain how his or her last legacy is played out. It is a process that allows a healthy relationship with physical and mortal limitations. Its most practical outcome, that of having clinically relevant preference statements about future possible care, is of significant assistance when difficult care decisions

arise. In this sense, it is also helpful in avoiding conflict and mistaken decisions and is a form of preventive care.

Practical advice is available elsewhere about how to conduct advance care planning. It involves raising the topic, engaging in structured deliberation, focusing on the goals of medical care and then on specific interventions to illustrate the goals, documenting preferences, updating stated preferences, and implementing preferences. It can be assisted by using a validated worksheet to maximize the chance of understanding and documenting accurate expressions that can be translated meaningfully into medical actions. A large part can and usually should occur in the patient's home with his or her family, leaving to the physician the roles of introducing the process and checking the final expression of wishes for inconsistencies and changes over time, documenting it, and applying it. Throughout the process, common pitfalls crop up, and these too are listed in a range of helpful resources.[28,37]

> C was a midcareer professional. His widowed mother had severe chronic obstructive pulmonary disease, which was progressing more rapidly than usual. She was worried that her son had not come to terms with the fact that she was not likely to survive much longer. She asked the physician to counsel him. A meeting for the three of them was remarkable since the son confided that he had been wondering how to bring up the topic and did not know how to talk about his feelings and concerns with her. The next few months for both of them were full of gratifying memories and mutual thanks and appreciation about the accomplishments and pride that they felt in each other. C commented after his mother's death that they had "the best times we ever had; we talked about and settled everything."

The hardest part of advance care planning can be raising the topic. Once done, the rest of the discussion can be remarkably harmonious and helpful.

Futility

Futility is a subjective assessment in most cases. Futility becomes a question when the chance of providing a cure for the ill person with an intervention seems to be minimal and so outweighed by its burden or harm that care seems undermined as well. It is often not helpful to take a position regarding futility and more helpful to address the etiology of the situation and the likely outcomes of medical care. A helpful differential diagnosis of situations has been provided by Goold and Arnold[38] and includes misunderstanding, personality factors, cultural differences, and value differences. Communication lapses can often be remedied with an effort to re-approach the communication process. Personality differences can often be put aside with careful behavior or by substituting for one another in a care team. Cultural differences can usually be resolved by giving primary respect to the culture of the person who is ill. Only cases involving value differences merit ethical analysis. If this analysis does not yield helpful resolutions, use of fair process is usually successful in resolving the issue as well as possible.[39] Fair process tends to involve the following: *(1)* attempt to deliberate and reach mutually satisfactory resolution involving the patient, family, and professionals as relevant; *(2)* involve consultants; *(3)* involve the institutional ethics committee; and *(4)* transfer to another physician or institution if a better values fit can be found.

> Ms. S was a 69-year-old woman with multiple medical problems, including steroid-dependent rheumatoid arthritis and severe esophageal reflux, which had led to adult respiratory distress syndrome on one occasion. When she developed aspiration pneumonia and seemed to be headed for intubation and a long stay in the ICU again, her physician pointed out that her prognosis was poor and that she might want to accept her circumstances. Ms. S corrected her physician in no uncertain terms, pointing out that her quality of life was excellent as far as she was concerned: she saw each day as a gift; she saw her children, grandchildren, and husband every day and they seemed to appreciate her advice, counseling, and guidance.
>
> Her physician was grateful when Ms. S survived the ICU visit and returned home

none the worse for having had to teach her physician such an important lesson. Fortunately, Ms. S and her physician had a good relationship, and this miscommunication about what seemed to the physician to be futile but not so to Ms. S could be cleared up before it spun out of control.

Withdrawing and withholding
When the imperative to care over-rides the realistic possibilities for cure, it may be appropriate to avoid some interventions. Similarly, it may be appropriate to withdraw interventions that are no longer helpful. Coming to these decisions, providing alternatives that enhance comfort, and withdrawing life-sustaining interventions require trained skills. Until recently, little guidance has been available in this area. Guidance is available elsewhere in this text and in other sources. A few tips are summarized here to illustrate some ethical principles that are especially pertinent. However, it seems reasonable to say that although this area started out as one in which ethics questions predominated, it has reached ethical resolution on many general questions and dissolved into technical competence and competence in applying ethical reason.

Do-not-resuscitate orders. Cardiopulmonary resuscitation was pioneered for unexpected cardiac arrests in the operating room for patients undergoing curative surgery who were otherwise well and usually young. For the elderly and terminally ill, its outcomes are so poor that it is startling that it was ever applied to this population. The fact that it was a procedure that seemed to stave off death and that it emerged in an era when death was generally a taboo topic and its inevitability was remarkably denied may explain its use. Since realizing its extreme ineffectiveness and seeing the degree of burden it can place on those who provide such care and resuscitation recipients who survive for short periods, some have advocated that resuscitation simply never be offered.[40] The rationale can be stated as follows: resuscitation runs counter to the goals of care for patients for whom comfort is the dominant concern and for whom cure is unattainable. However, it is now a widely entrenched procedure, and it may be inconsistent with the principle of trustworthiness to make assumptions based on age and illness status without talking to the individuals concerned.

Discussion in isolation from the elucidation of goals and other life-sustaining treatment decisions should be a red flag. Resuscitation decisions should be part of an overall disposition and plan. Patients' decisions regarding resuscitation tend to be unstable in comparison to other decisions, and professionals have a hard time conducting these discussions. Likely as not, both are attributable to the cruelty of making an isolated decision about declining one last hope to live a little longer. In other words, isolated do-not-resuscitate (DNR) discussions go against the principle of comfort since they can engender sufficient psychological discomfort that they often prevent settled decisions. If patients are allowed to consider resuscitation as one intervention among many that may or may not fit with their goals, it can fall into place and be quite a comfortable and lasting decision. Professionals should be familiar with the Physician Orders for Life-Sustaining Treatments (POLST) form and similar guides to creating comprehensive orders for patients for whom life-sustaining interventions may be inappropriate.[30] A patient should not have a DNR order on his or her chart with no other orders related to it (e.g., orders regarding intubation, artificial nutrition and hydration, visiting hours, symptom management, and so forth). The professional or family member who sees this should prompt a general discussion of goals and treatment decisions.

Mechanical respiration. Early attention to withdrawing ventilator support dealt with whether it constituted euthanasia or murder. Today, these questions seem almost outrageous, such is the progress of the ethical debate and case law. It is now widely accepted that people have the right to be free of unwanted interventions even

if death results, and further, that these decisions do not cause death but, rather, avoid interference with otherwise inevitable dying. The remaining ethical issues for professionals revolve around ensuring a good decision-making process, which is discussed above, and that the actions taken provide for patient comfort. This too is covered elsewhere, including in this book.[41]

Artificial nutrition and hydration. The use of artificial feeding and hydration is a similarly well-resolved ethical question. No categorical ethical obligation exists to supply either one, and their withdrawal can be justified if they are unwanted. Nonetheless, families often have difficulty with the perception that they cannot let their relative "starve to death." Physicians and nurses may also feel ambivalent about what to do. In 1995, over 125,000 gastrostomy tubes were placed in the United States; approximately one-third of these patients had advanced dementia, and a large portion of the remainder had cancer or advanced cerebrovascular disease. Scientific studies supporting their use are sparse. Theoretically, such feeding should improve nutrition; but because of problems such as diarrhea, clogging of the tubes, severity of underlying illness, and aging of the gut with reduced absorption, nutritional status usually does not improve. Gastrostomy tubes also do not prevent aspiration pneumonia and, unfortunately, have the adverse consequences of frequently requiring patient restraints and loss of the beneficial experience of being fed by hand. Survival, functional status, and reduction of pressure sores are also not demonstrably improved by the use of feeding tubes.[42] Recently, decision aids have been developed to assist families to work through the question of whether or not to approve artificial hydration and nutrition for patients.[43] There is an extensive bioethical literature which points out that the use of feeding tubes is not mandatory and, as with other forms of treatment, can be discontinued if it is deemed inappropriate.[44] Such decisions should reflect the preferences and values of the patient following a clear previous or current determination of goals of care. Sometimes, families have emotions or religiously interpreted beliefs which lead them to the conclusion that sustenance must be continued even though the formal positions of most major religions point out that interventions are warranted only as long as there is sufficient benefit to outweigh the burdens involved to the patient. All major denominations' canons reject approaches that cause needless suffering.

Antibiotics. While antibiotics may not be intuitively included among life-sustaining interventions, their use can sustain life. While antibiotic use for comfort is sometimes indicated, infection may be chosen as the most comfortable natural death by some patients. This is not unethical.

Ms. J had adenocarcinoma of the lung and had been admitted to the hospital from home with a postobstructive pneumonia. A concerned house officer noted that she was not doing well and as yet had no life-support orders written. He approached her to confirm what he assumed was a settled choice to avoid resuscitation. Ms. J was, however, alarmed at the discussion and ended up insisting that she wanted all possible intervention. The next morning, the attending physician re-approached the issue, this time asking Ms. J to go over her goals for care and then consider a range of possible types of care, from respiratory support to surgery, artificial nutrition and hydration, and use of opioids for relief of dyspnea or pain. Ms. J made decisions that seemed much more consistent with earlier discussions; she declined resuscitation, intubation, and surgery but allowed artificial nutrition and hydration in some circumstances and accepted opioids for relevant situations. Her wishes were recorded on a POLST from.

Resuscitation decisions are difficult both because the information is difficult to convey and because the emotions that are triggered by contemplating the moment of death are strong and unpredictable. Resuscitation decisions are among the least stable of end-of-life care decisions. Consideration of, first, the goals of care and, second, a range of options

for care that are consistent with that goal tends to be more acceptable and to yield decisions that are more stable and broadly relevant.

Assisted suicide or euthanasia

Among people who attempt suicide, some of the most likely to achieve it are the elderly and especially elderly men. The question of assisted suicide or euthanasia also comes up for the terminally ill who seek to cut short the suffering. Geriatric palliative care professionals need to know how to respond when such questions arise.

Requests for physician-assisted suicide and euthanasia have generated considerable debate. Ethical arguments have not resulted in a decisive victory on either side. Arguments in favor focus on cases of intractable pain and draw on autonomy and compassion for those for whom life seems worse than death. Opposing arguments point out that the suffering that motivates requests tends to be psychosocial and associated with depression.

A compelling argument from professionalism comes from the duty to avoid harm and starts by understanding that when a professional asserts a moral position on assisted suicide there is a risk that, no matter what the position is, he or she will exacerbate the suffering. The physician who agrees that assisted suicide may be the best action risks conveying that he or she agrees that the patient's life is worth little. Opposing assisted suicide risks conveying a sense of moral judgment over the person who has made the request, and this can also exacerbate any sense of worthlessness. The physician who reveals no judgment on whether the act can ever be ethical but, rather, responds by inquiring about the suffering that is motivating the request is in a better position to heal the suffering.

Most sources of suffering, whether physical, mental, social, or existential, have remedies less dire than assisted suicide. For the few individuals who have a rational intent to shorten their intractable suffering, mostly a comfortable plan can be found that avoids life prolongation and that is not as ethically controversial or emotionally traumatic as assisted suicide can be. This is especially true of elders with terminal illness, who tend to be dependent on medical intervention for survival. If withdrawal of life-sustaining intervention does not offer a suitable plan, avoidance of unwanted nutrition and hydration is a course that has been widely accepted as ethical; and it is thought to entail minimal suffering once a person is ill enough to have lost appetite and thirst, as is often the case.

> Ms. F was a breast cancer survivor. A single person, she had cared for each of her parents until they died. She was adamant that she wanted to end her life before becoming that sick and dependent. She sought a physician who would be willing to assist her in suicide when the time came. When her surprised new physician heard of her wishes and responded by initiating an advance care planning discussion, Ms. F was interested to discover how many other options for control and dignity existed. She completed a document that entailed avoidance of life support but made no mention of assisted suicide. A year later, still in good health, Ms. F had married and seemed to be flourishing. On asking her if she would be willing to talk with medical students about her wish for assisted suicide as part of a lesson on the topic, Ms. F exclaimed: 'I never wanted assisted suicide!' She further explained that she was seeking control and dignity and had found it in her advance care plans. She was embarrassed to recall that she had once thought that assisted suicide was the only option for retaining control and dignity.

Most people who seek assisted suicide do so as a response to anticipated suffering in the psychosocial aspects of life. Realization that solutions exist to the feared situations can make assisted suicide seem irrelevant.

Research

Whereas ethics used to dictate exclusion from research on people who seemed extra vulnerable, the norms have changed to include the viewpoint that unless vulnerable groups are included in research their healthcare quality will fall behind and their right to be contributing members of society will

be unfairly abrogated. The ethics of research for elders with terminal illness includes the same concerns and procedures as for other subjects. Areas of special caution include the following.

Limited options

If a person is not resolved to dying and comfort care seems like an inadequate option, clinical trials may appear to be the only option left. Since informed consent assumes that options exist, the person who is not ready to consider palliative care a more comfortable option may not be able to make a truly informed and consenting decision. Whenever possible, assistance should be offered in reaching a better personal adjustment to the reality of dying. An alternative of comfort-focused care can then be offered, and the choice to enter a trial can be noncoerced.

Forced altruism

The immediacy of impending death and the common desire to leave something behind may cause a person to feel pressure to commit acts of altruism. Reassurance by the care team and family that the person is under no obligation to participate and that he or she is just as valuable a person now as before, even without entering a trial, can help to make the person's judgment less pressured.

Incapacity

The high prevalence of mental disability among elders with serious illness can make informed consent difficult. Proxy consent can be conducted ethically but needs special care. Additional resources on this topic can be found elsewhere.[45] Incapacity per se is not a reason for exclusion from all research. Were this the case, the most important sources of suffering for elders with serious illness would be impossible to study in the clinical setting.

Human subject concerns

Research in geriatric palliative care has the same array of human subject concerns and constraints on the investigators as other clinical areas, including the following. Subjects must be chosen in a fashion that is nonexclusionary[46] and that protects them from needless risk. Subjects must be provided with effective informed consent. Investigators must abide by standards for dealing with conflicts of interest. Further, investigators who are also clinicians must distinguish their roles to patients and family members since the fiduciary obligations are quite different: the investigator's primary fiduciary responsibility is to the science, while the clinician's primary fiduciary responsibility is to the patient. Should the roles be combined, patients and family may feel betrayed unless it is quite clear in which role the clinician/investigator is acting. These issues are dealt with in greater depth elsewhere.[47]

Conflicts of Interest

The different models of and considerations in communication and decision making and models of the therapeutic relationship assume that the professional is working in the patient's interest without complications of competing interests. Since life is full of competing interests, this is an ideal more than an achievable norm. It is, however, such an essential component of the therapeutic relationship that professionals are expected to take more measures toward that ideal than is expected of non-professionals. If professionals cannot be assumed to act in the interests of the patient, trustworthiness is impossible. Standards of management should be particularly stringent and openly accountable in geriatrics and palliative care since the population is generally less able to discern or demand redress for lapsed standards.

Conflicts of interest tend to focus on financial more than any other interests. This is partly because it is more readily quantifiable than other forms of interest and partly because it is a pervasive human motivation. Other interests can, however, be just as detrimental if they are inserted into the therapeutic relationship. The professional should be as aware of and wary about many other interests that might impede the placing of the patient's needs above his or her own. Those that involve ego gratification, such as career advancement or power, need particular attention because they are powerful motivators and often incompletely recognized.

A first premise in understanding conflicts of interest requires the recognition that they are pervasive and that the operative question is not whether or not they exist but whether they are managed within reasonable bounds. Useful rules about managing conflicts of interest include the following.[47]

Routine disclosure for institutional review
All conflicts should be disclosed or at least disclosable. Health-care institutions should have policies regarding conflicts of interest, and these should require routine mandatory reporting. This follows simply from the facts that conflicts of interest are ubiquitous and that reasonable, right-thinking individuals often have difficulty recognizing their own conflicts. Some professionals practice in settings that do not have institutional regulations. For these individuals it is harder, but a helpful index for self-assessment is whether it would be embarrassing to the professional or disconcerting to the patient or a reasonable person in either role if the situation were revealed. Should it seem to the professional that revealing the arrangement would be embarrassing or disconcerting, the professional should consider the likelihood that the situation is not compatible with a professional therapeutic relationship.

Among conflicts of interest, some are small and not obstructive to the therapeutic relationship. These situations, once disclosed, should be permitted by the institution and usually need not be disclosed to the patient or proxy.

Disclosure and imposed limitations
Other conflicts of interest are too large to be left undisclosed but nevertheless may be compatible with a therapeutic relationship. For instance, if the professional has stock in a company that supplies the drug that he or she is prescribing to a patient, the pa-

tient or proxy would likely want to know this. Then, the patient or proxy can make his or her own assessment of the professional's possible bias in favor of that drug. However, having to take these considerations into account at all can be disturbing for patients, and there is merit in avoiding conflicts such as this altogether.

Impermissible conflicts

Still other conflicts are much too large. Major holdings in a particular drug company may be of such concern that even if the professional's judgment is not biased, the perception of likely bias is so high that trustworthiness is not possible. These conflicts of interest are not compatible with professional therapeutic relationships, and the individual in question must choose between his or her holdings and the practice of medicine.

Conflicts of interest are important throughout professional practice and in other activities that require trustworthiness. They are of particular concern for professionals who care for people who are chronically vulnerable, whether due to mental incapacity or such burden of illness that they are unable to focus sufficient attention on these issues. In other words, the more readily exploitable the patient is, the more important it is to maintain stringent standards. The professional who cares for the aged facing terminal illness certainly falls into the group who need to maintain more stringent standards. The types of conflict that might be acceptable if disclosed for less impaired patients may not be acceptable for professionals caring for this population. Institutional policies on conflicts of interest and individuals' assessments of themselves or their colleagues should take this into account.

Dr. C, a geriatrician, submitted his annual conflict of interest form to his institution and disclosed the following: a mutual fund that included a proportion of investments in pharmaceutical industries; participation with a pharmaceutical company to recruit, for a fee that covered the cost of his time, patients for a clinical trial of one of their new osteo-porosis drugs; and shares in a laboratory to which he referred patients, in exchange for a referral fee, for audiometric tests. His university allowed his mutual fund to continue, required that the institutional review board ensure that patients (or their proxy) whom Dr. C, recruited for the clinical trial were aware of the financial arrangements for Dr. C, and required that Dr. C divest in the laboratory.

The university is applying the standards of *permissible, disclosure required,* and *impermissible* to these three types of financial arrangement.

Social Context

Confronting ageism

Fear of aging and the natural limits of human beings to empathetically imagine the experiences of others may be at the root of *ageism*, or bias against the aged. It can be hard to value the aged. It can be all too easy to unconsciously convey or endorse a sense of worthlessness, from which many of the elderly suffer. The emphasis placed on respect for parents and the elderly that is found in many current and ancient civilizations, for instance, in the Ten Commandments or ancient Chinese culture, reflects the dual importance and difficulty of maintaining this disposition.

Disabled communities have offered insights that are relevant for the elderly and incurable. Leading commentators have asserted that the conditions in question (quadriplegia, deafness, and many more) are defined as disabilities only in relation to dominant social constructs. With a suitable environment, conditions that are defined by the majority as disabilities need be no more limiting than the physiological and anatomical conditions with which the majority also live. In the right setting, people with special limits are able to have as much fulfillment in relationships, accomplishments, contributions to society, enjoyable sensations, and their existential life as anyone else. Establishment of this reality allows disabled communities to define themselves as a minority culture with as much dignity and sense of worth as any other community. Part of the relevance of these insights is due to the common features of ageism with bias against and intolerance of the disabled. By mustering their collective self-respect, some disabled communities have managed to change the diminished social position to which they have been relegated.

However, the elderly who also have a terminal illness may have less to muster in this regard because their illnesses may become all-consuming. For this reason, the professional has that much more of an obligation to recognize his or her own internal sources of fear and reasons for recoiling from the empathic and therapeutic relationships that professionals are supposed to provide. The professional is also in a position to foster the same process among the patient's family, friends, and community of breaking free from fears into the fulfillment of caring relationships.

Another set of insights comes from a developmental approach within palliative care, most strongly put forth by Ira Byock.[48] Noting that people grow as they make the transitions through illness, Byock asserts that there is a unique set of jobs to be done despite, and because of, declining capacity and diminishing time. People pass on roles and say and do things in relation to one another that allow these transitions. Assisting patients, family members, and communities to engage in these personal journeys allows for healthy forms of coping. These kinds of personal coping allow for a sense of wholeness for the social units in which people live. The ill person reintegrates the features that have been lodged in him or her in the people who will survive. Any and all members of the interdisciplinary team can assist with these difficult transitions and with the emotional and practical aspects of taking the necessary steps.

Mr. M was a 79-year-old man with renal failure, dependent on dialysis, who was now confronted with a new diagnosis of melanoma. He was considering forgoing further dialysis, commenting that he should already 'be a portrait on the wall' and noting that his community no longer seemed to notice him and his family called him less and less frequently. He felt valueless. After meeting with a counselor, he began to consider a question she had posed to him: did he think that the elderly and the dying have a particular role or job in life? He decided that there was one last thing he wanted to accomplish. He wanted to show his friends and particularly his grandson 'how a real man dies.' He set about an active schedule of family and community gatherings in which he took delight in telling stories, each with a lesson attached, from his earlier years, told his family of his wishes for avoiding further life support and when to stop dialysis, and set about giving away his material belongings, as he put it: "before I die—so that if they quarrel, I can settle things out before I go. A real man leaves peace behind." His family and friends were delighted not only to see Mr. M so engaged again but also to have his guidance in charting the future without him.

Mr. M had been experiencing, and passively accepting, ageism, along with the isolation and sense of worthlessness that it brings. After realizing that he had a unique developmental step to take at this stage of life and a unique set of contributions to offer, he set about living with purpose again. He and his family and community appreciated his special contributions.

Adjusting perspectives

As people age, perceptions of what constitutes the "good" life may change. For many older people, the world of social experience narrows and becomes more circumscribed, in both its scope and its frequency. However, this does not mean that quality of life decreases. As internal expectations change, what constitutes a good quality of life also changes. For example, while in middle age a good quality of life may have included the need for frequent travel, in older age the occasional trip to visit family members may suffice. Perceptions of quality of life with regard to health and disability also change as people age. Very few older people expect to live a totally pain-free or illness-free life. Instead, they are willing to adjust their activities and routines to accommodate these experiences. In fact, quality of life may be assessed by how well one can adjust, rather than by the presence or absence of the problem itself. Thus, physicians, caregivers, and others must be careful to not impose their own beliefs or values about quality of life on the older patient. While no patient should be expected to endure unremitting pain, the total absence of discomfort or even pain is not necessary for still valuing the quality of one's life.

Some of the challenge has to do with the changes in role and relationships that the life cycle's progression and illness instigate. Assistance in coping as these transitions occur can start with acknowledgment of the changes and the significance that roles in life have for all people. Assistance in realizing the rewards of different roles and the infusion of dignity into the roles that elders can have, even or especially when they have a terminal illness, is likely to be beneficial to all and arguably a minimum that is due to the elderly in civilized society. Adjustment may become a goal in itself. Inadequate adjustment, in turn, disposes to other conditions, such as depression and malnutrition. Insufficient adjustment may be in the family or professional rather than in the person living with illness. A cognitive therapist or pastor can be helpful in many of these situations, as can any other professional, friend, or family member.

TJ was always considered the matriarch of her extended family, and her children, grandchildren, and great-children often sought her opinion and counsel before making major life decisions. Thus, when she was diagnosed with Alzheimer's disease at the age of 82, her family found it difficult to accept the diagnosis and to initiate a reasonable plan of shared caring. Instead, they continued to seek TJ's opinion on a variety of matters, ignored her physician's recommendation that she move either to sheltered care or into the home of a family member, and failed to provide adequate supervision of her. Over time, however, it became clear even to the most reluctant of her children that TJ could no longer live alone and could certainly not continue to make her own financial and medical decisions. In one incident, TJ left her home dressed only in her nightgown, forgetting that she had not yet dressed. When her neighbor offered to escort her back home, TJ exhibited great embarrassment and thereafter refused to leave her home. TJ's oldest daughter sought counsel from her pastor, and after some time finally accepted the fact that her mother now required assistance from her children, rather than the other way around. TJ eventually moved into this daughter's home, and the mantle of family leadership passed to the daughter.

Recognition of, and adjustment to, disability are difficult but often the key to accessing the different sources of fulfillment available to ill elders and their families.

Abandonment, abuse/neglect, eldernapping

When the burden of care becomes too great for the caregiver, the ill person is at particular risk for neglect or abuse. Many states recognize a difference between benign and malicious neglect and that various types of abuse, such as physical, emotional, and psychological, may occur when a caregiver is overwhelmed and has no support. Interventions in cases of benign neglect usually take the form of education and assistance to caregivers, including respite and in-home support services. Malicious neglect warrants attention from the designated elder abuse intervention services and may require that the patient be relocated to a safer environment. Most states mandate reporting of abuse of all types by healthcare professionals. Abandonment of the patient, often at the emergency department, may occur in extreme cases of both abuse and neglect. While family members may not necessarily be under a legal obligation to provide care to a dying elder, social mores demand that such extreme responses be addressed and professionals should help with remedies to resolve even longstanding distress within a family.

DC had lived with his older son and his family for a number of years and was eventually diagnosed with dementia. Because DC had substantial assets, including a home that was currently occupied by a younger son, the older child sought a guardianship, to protect and conserve his father's estate. Once appointed guardian, the older son requested a court order to evict his brother from his father's house and authorization to sell the property. Upon notification by the court, the younger son filed a cross-petition for guardianship, alleging that his father was being neglected and receiving inadequate care. Eventually, the case was resolved, but the older son refused to allow his brother or any other siblings to visit DC or speak with him on the phone. DC's younger son again filed a cross-petition for guardianship, this time calling the local elder abuse service and demanding an investigation. When the case worker visited the home, she found that DC was adequately cared for but very sad, lethargic, and withdrawn. A homemaker service was recommended, and eventually the homemaker reported to her supervisor that DC continually cried out for his younger son. The social worker reported this to the elder abuse case manager, and a report was filed with the court. At the subsequent hearing in response to the counterpetition, the judge ordered that DC remain with his older son but that all family members be allowed to visit at least twice a week. A community service agency was appointed to monitor DC's progress.

Elders with disability can become as vulnerable in family quarrels as children of divorcing parents. Often, health professionals are in the only position to identify and report abuse.

SOCIAL POLICY AND ADVOCACY

This book defines a range of standards of practice in geriatric palliative care. In various places, it also points out that the accepted standards are not met in much of the real world of health-service delivery. Whether it is a matter of appropriate assessment of patients, control of symptoms, or locations of care, a wealth of evidence indicates that the gaps between standards and practices are significant. Professional ethics demands of professionals that we advocate and seek change when such gaps exist.

Education

Education for professionals is still insufficient to meet the need in both geriatrics and palliative care, although the gap is closing for both. However, until there is no gap, professionals should contribute however they can to providing education for medical students, physicians in training, and physicians in practice. Train-the-trainer programs that make use of modular modifiable units have been successful in disseminating core skills in palliative care for physicians, nurses, and other professionals. Geriatrics has evolved into a recognized discipline with fellowships and training curricula. However, in both fields, there will likely never be enough specialists to care for all of the elderly and terminally ill patients. The obligation of the geriatrician and palliative care specialist is therefore to provide not only care but also consultation and core skills to colleagues in all other relevant specialties.

Service Capacity

Service capacity development is also essential. Geriatrics and palliative care specialty services must be available. However, service capacity among other practitioners is equally important and may involve development of specialized focus among staff members, fellowship, resident and medical student rotations, regular seminars relevant to the practice issues, relevant journals and texts in the offices where patient care issues are discussed, quality consultations, and mentoring and career growth structures. Professionals who work in institutions where these capacities do not exist should advocate for their development.

Continuity of care requires coordination between different types and often different locations of care. Many of the elderly and terminally ill have to make transitions between home, hospital, and long-term care facilities. The potential for duplicative care, discordant therapeutic plans, missing information, and disjointed therapeutic relationships is great. The geriatrician and palliative care professional should make a point to advocate for institutional structures and policies that allow maximal continuity for individual patients.

Research

Outcome measurements have fallen short in both geriatrics and palliative care. In geriatrics, it became painfully obvious within the last decade that quality-of-life indices were derived using internal perceptions that characterized young and middle-aged adults and did not characterize perspectives more often found among the elderly facing life-threatening illness and its complications. Studies began to report that quality-of-life estimates were better than expected among the seriously ill and disabled.[49] Acknowledgment of the importance of the patient's internal perspective has been reasonably well achieved, but there is still a paucity of outcome instruments in the field that take this into account.[50–53]

Errors occur in medicine, as in all human activities and complex institutional systems. Since trustworthiness is such an important element in medicine and medicine involves specialized knowledge, accountability has traditionally been assigned to peers. Peers and peer-assessed standards have served as a proxy for direct assessment. As the medical knowledge of the public grows and the culture embraces it, accountability has turned more toward patients and the public than ever before. In either form, accountability for error is a critical issue. For too long, physicians and other medical professionals listened to risk management advice that cautioned against admitting error or even expressing regret at a bad outcome for fear of legal action. For too long, physicians and others have resisted the realization that other service industries have excellent approaches to safety from which medicine could learn. Medical professionals should embrace approaches to accountability for error and to error reduction. It is an essential part of professionalism. Since error in geriatrics and palliative care is especially easy as patient vigilance may be particularly compromised and error is more consequential as patients are characteristically frail and lack reserve, research on systems to reduce error is especially pertinent.[54]

Norms Development

Norms of practice are necessary for any developed field. Both geriatrics and palliative care have been developing a body of knowledge and de facto norms of practice such that it is now possible to define standards for practice. These standards can then be fostered by education and enforced by accreditation requirements. Such activities are beginning, but more progress is still needed.[55]

Professional Advocacy

Professional advocacy for patient-centered social policy is an important obligation for physicians and others in medicine. Professionals have an obligation to protect the values of care for the vulnerable among other competing values in society. Policies are often proposed that are not friendly to patient care and pose particular risks to care of the elderly or dying. In democracies, this is understandable in that the elderly and the very ill may not be well represented in the political body of voices. In nondemocratic societies that have aspirations to augmenting power and standing, the ill are readily seen as a drain on resources. In either situation, professionals have a particular role to advance the needs of the ill and the values of care since the ill cannot realize full representation without advocacy and the value of care is all too readily lost. When it seems that professional advocacy structures have become ineffective, individual professions must seek change. Recently, many professional associations seem to have been distracted and undermined by conflicts of interest or conflicts of role. If professionals need to restructure their associations or to advocate in some other way, this should be done. For geriatrics and palliative care, there are obvious advocacy priorities. The country needs to prepare for the onslaught of aging baby boomers and to plan quality, affordable, and fairly distributed geriatric and palliative care. Palliative care has much to contribute to keeping the elderly as comfortable and functional in their societal context as possible. In addition to helping individuals, its assistance for societies in crisis, whether due to culture, politics, or an epidemic of disease, can be significant.[56] Professionals and professional associations must promote these practices.

ACKNOWLEDGMENTS

We thank Dr. Joshua Hauser for his many helpful comments and Ms. Martha Jacob and Ms. J'neen Wolfe for their assistance.

REFERENCES

1. Jonsen AR, Toulmin S. The Abuse of Casuistry: A History of Moral Reasoning. Berkeley, University of California Press, 1988.
2. Beauchamp TL, Childress JF. Principles of Biomedical Ethics, 4th ed. New York, NY Oxford University Press, 1994.
3. Callahan D. The Roots of Ethics: Science, Religion and Values. New York, Plenum, 1982.
4. Brody H. Stories of Sickness. New Haven, CT, Yale University Press, 1987.
5. Fein R. Medical Care, Medical Costs: The Search for a Health Insurance Policy. San Francisco, Universe, 1999.
6. Rawls J. A Theory of Justice. Cambridge, MA, Harvard University Press, 1971.
7. Kleinman A. Writing at the Margins: Discourse Between Anthropology and Medicine. University of California Press, 1995.
8. Applbaum A. Ethics for adversaries: the morality of roles in public and professional life. Princeton, NJ, Princeton University Press, 1999.
9. Beauchamp TL, Childress JF. Principles of Biomedical Ethics, 3rd ed. New York, Oxford University Press, 1989.
10. Sohl P, Bassford R. Codes of medical ethics: traditional foundations and contemporary practice. Soc Sci Med 22:1175–1179, 1980.
11. Sox H. Medical professionalism in the new millennium: a physician charter. Ann Intern Med 136:243–246, 2002.
12. Pellegrino ED. The medical profession as a moral community. Bull NY Acad Med 66:221–232, 1990.
13. Wynia M, Latham S, Kao A, Berg J, Emanuel LL. Physician professionalism in society. N Engl J Med 341:1612–1615, 1999.
14. Starr P. The Social Transformation of American Medicine. New York, Basic Books, 1982.
15. Freidson E. Professional Dominance: The Social Structure of Medical Care. Chicago, Aldine, 1970.
16. Cruess RL, Cruess SR. Teaching medicine as a profession in the service of healing. Acad Med 72:941–952, 1997.
17. Emanuel EJ, Emanuel LL. What is accountability? Ann Intern Med 124:229–239, 1996.
18. Saunders C, Kastenbaum R (Eds). Hospice Care on the International Scene. New York, Springer, 1997.
19. Merriman A. International Geriatric Medicine. PG Economy Edition. Boston, PG Publishing, 1989.
20. Kitwood T. Dementia Reconsidered: The Person Comes First. Buckingham, UK, Open University Press, 1997.
21. Emanuel EJ, Fairclough DL, Slutsman J, Emanuel LL. Understanding economic and other burdens of terminal illness: the experience of patients and their caregivers. Ann Intern Med 132:451–459, 2000.
22. Covinsky KE, Goldman L, Cook EF, Oye R, Desbiencs N, Reding D, et al. The impact of serious illness on patients' families. SUPPORT Investigators. Study to Understand Prognoses and Preferences for Outcomes and Risks of Treatment. JAMA 272:1839–1844, 1994.
23. Siegler EL, Hyer K, Fulmer T, Mezey M, eds. Geriatric Interdisciplinary Team Training. New York, Springer, 1998.
24. Emanuel LL, von Gunten CF, Ferris FD (Eds). Whole Patient Assessment. The Education for Physicians on End-of-Life Care (EPEC) Curriculum. EPEC Project. Module 3. Robert Wood Johnson Foundation. Buehler Center on Aging, Northwestern's Feinberg School of Medicine, Chicago, IL. pp. 1–20, 1999.
25. American Geriatrics Society. Care management position statement. J Am Geriatr Soc 48:1338–1339, 2000.
26. Emanuel LL, von Guten CF, Ferris FD (Eds.). Communicating Bad News. The Education for Physicians on End-of-Life Care (EPEC) Curriculum. EPEC Project. Module 2. The Robert Wood Johnson Foundation. Buehler Center on Aging, Northwestern's Feinberg School of Medicine, pp. 1–10, 1999.

27. Pellegrino ED. Is truth telling to patients a cultural artifact? JAMA 268:1734–1735, 1992.

28. Emanuel LL, von Guten CF, Ferris FD (Eds.). Advance Care Planning. The Education for Physicians on End-of-Life Care (EPEC) Curriculum. Module 1. Buehler Center on Aging, Northwestern's Feinberg School of Medicine, Chicago, IL. 1–21, 1999.

29. Botrell MM, Alpert H, Fischbach RL, Emanuel LL. Hospital informed consent for procedure forms. Arch Surg 135:26–33, 2000.

30. Center for Ethics in Health Care. Physician Orders for Life-Sustaining Treatment (POLST). Portland, OR, Health Sciences University, 1997.

31. Kiely D, Mitchell SL, Marlow A, Murphy KM, Morris JN. Racial and state differences in the designation of advance directives in nursing home residents. J Am Geriatr Soc 49:1346–1352, 2001.

32. Luborsky M, Rubinstein RL. The dynamics of ethnic identity and bereavement among older widowers. In: Sokolovsky J (Ed.). The Cultural Context of Aging. Westport, CT, Bergin and Garvey, pp. 304–315, 1997.

33. Keith J, Fry CL, Glascock AP, Ikels C, Dickerson-Putnam J, Harpendig HC, Draper P. The aging experience: diversity and commonality across cultures. Newbury Park, CA, Sage, 1994.

34. Dresser R. Advance directives, self-determination, and personal identity. In: Hacker CMR, Vawter DE (Eds.). Advance Directives in Medicine. New York, Praeger, pp. 155–170, 1989.

35. Berg J, Appelbaum PS, Lidz CW, Parker LS. Informed Consent: Legal Theory and Clinical Practice, 2nd ed. New York, Oxford University Press, 2001.

36. Meier D, Morrison S. Autonomy reconsidered. N Engl J Med 346:1087–1089, 2002.

37. Emanuel LL DM, Pearlman RA, Singer PA. Advance care planning as a process. J Am Geriatr Soc 43:440–446, 1995.

38. Goold SD, Arnold RM. Conflicts regarding decisions to limit treatment: a differential diagnosis. JAMA 283:909–914, 2000.

39. Council on Ethical and Judicial Affairs. Medical Futility in End-of-Life Care. Chicago, American Medical Association, 1996.

40. Blackhall LJ. Must we always use CPR? N Engl J Med 317:1281–1285, 1987.

41. Emanuel LL, von Guten CF, Ferris FD (Eds.). Withholding/Withdrawing Treatment. The Education for Physicians on End-of-Life Care (EPEC) Curriculum. EPEC Project. Module 11. Buehler Center on Aging, Northwestern's Feinberg School of Medicine, Chicago, IL. pp. 1–23, 1999.

42. Campion EW. The value of geriatric interventions. N Engl J Med 332:1376–1378, 1995.

43. Mitchell S, Tetroe J, O'Connor AM. A decision aid for long term tube feeding in cognitively impaired older persons. J Am Geriatr Soc 493:313–314, 2001.

44. Gillick MR. Rethinking the role of tube feeding in patients with advanced dementia. N Engl J Med 342:208–210, 2000.

45. Levine R. Ethics and Regulation of Clinical Research, 2nd ed. New Haven, CT, Yale University Press, 1986.

46. Council on Ethical and Judicial Affairs. Subject Selection for Clinical Trials. Chicago, American Medical Association, 1997.

47. Thompson DF. Understanding financial conflict of interest. N Engl J Med 329:573–576, 1993.

48. Byock IR. Conceptual models and the outcomes of caring. J Pain Symptom Manage 17:83–92, 1999.

49. Basnett I. Health care professionals and their attitudes toward and decisions affecting disabled people. In: Albrecht G, Seelman KD, Bury M (Eds.). Handbook of Disability Studies. Newbury Park, CA, Sage, pp. 450–467, 2001.

50. Teno J, Landrum K. Toolkit of Instruments to Measure End of Life Care. Center to Improve Care of the Dying, 1996.

51. Emanuel LL, Alpert H, Emanuel EJ. Concise screening questions for clinical assessments of terminal care: the Needs near the End of Life Care Screening Tool (NEST). J Palliat Med 4:465–474, 2001.

52. Miller AM, Iris M. Health promotion attitudes and strategies in older adults. Health Educ Behav 29:249–267, 2002.

53. Berman RLH, Iris M. Approaches to self-care in later life. Qual Health Res 8:224–235, 1998.

54. Meredith S, Feldman PH, Frey D, Hall K, Arnold K, Brouwn NJ, Ray WA. Possible medication errors in home healthcare patients. J Am Geriatr Soc 49:719–724, 2001.

55. Canadian Hospice Palliative Care Association. A model to guide hospice palliative care: based on national principles and norms of practice. 2002.

56. Emanuel LL. Palliative care: a weak link in the chain of civilized life. In: Weisstub DN, Thomasma DC, Gauthier S, Tomossy GF (Eds.). International Library of Ethics, Law, and the New Medicine, vol. 12. Aging: Decisions at the End of Life, Dordrecht, Kluwer, pp. 31–47, 2001.

8

Respecting Diversity

MARION DANIS AND RISA LAVIZZO-MOUREY

Aging and death are universal life events, yet differing ethnicity, religion, socioeconomic status, and historical cohort profoundly influence the way we experience them. When patients and clinicians have a common background, these influences can provide a shared understanding and framework for coping with aging and dying. When a patient and clinician come from different cultural or religious backgrounds, grappling with the differences can be baffling. The essence of good medical practice involves recognizing that differences are an ever-present reality and appreciating that *both* the clinician or caregiver and patient are bound by beliefs, customs, experiences, prejudices, rules, and responsibilities.[1] In respecting a patient who is different, the clinician must accept diversity and recognize that human dignity transcends these differences.

In this chapter, we discuss how patients, particularly older patients, of differing ethnic and socioeconomic classes *view* aging and dying, how they *wish* to be treated during severe and terminal illness, and how they are *actually* treated during such ill-

nesses. Most importantly, we review recommendations from the medical literature about how clinicians might *best* address the needs and wishes of patients whose backgrounds differ from their own.

DEFINITION OF TERMS

In any discussion involving ethnicity, the terms *race* and *culture* are often used and warrant clarification. The biological concept of race has become scientifically outmoded since it is based on inaccurate assumptions about genetic differences. Race is poorly correlated with any biological or cultural phenomena, yet the term remains commonly used. As Sheldon and Parker write:

Modern biologists and anthropologists have rejected the scientific basis of such a categorization, for, although it must be true that phenotypic variation has a genetic basis, the point is that there is no consistent categorization across characteristics. Geographical variation in gene frequency is gradual and not qualitative; populations merge into one another. The complex and polygenic determination of human pheno-

79

type ensures that there are no typical members of groups, and the amount of variation within any ethnic group is larger than that between groups. . . . Although human variation is self-evident, the existence of definable groups or races is not. However, race is still commonly used in medical research.[2]

Thus even though the concept of race may not have a sound scientific basis, a provider's perception of a patient's race may influence or bias the care that is given. In addition, a patient's perception of his or her own racial or ethnic identity may relate to a variety of attitudes about illness and death.

As the concept of race has been discredited, the term *ethnicity* has been increasingly used to refer to shared cultural characteristics and national identity.[2] *Culture* refers to the totality of socially transmitted behavior patterns, arts, beliefs, institutions, and products of human work and thought characteristic of a community or population. It is useful to avoid thinking too simplistically about culture, as Koenig writes:

It is not a simple 'trait,' an objective, unchanging variable, located within the individual. Culture does not 'determine' behavior under certain specified circumstances. Most importantly, culture is constantly recreated and negotiated within specific social and historical contexts. . . . Seemingly simple . . . calls for 'culturally competent care' ignore the dynamic nature of culture. Moreover, in a complex postmodern world, culture can no longer be simply mapped onto a geographically isolated ethnic group. One cannot assume that a patient or family from Southern China will approach decisions about death in a certain culturally-specified fashion.[3]

While it is important to appreciate the complexity of culture, a more succinct definition may be useful: (culture) "encompasses beliefs and behaviors that are learned and shared by members of a group." [4]

EMPIRICAL EVIDENCE

Role of Ethnicity in Attitudes Toward Aging and Dying

In a classic and beautifully written book, *Death and Ethnicity,* Richard Kalish and David Reynolds[5] provide invaluable insights for clinicians who provide geriatric palliative care. Careful in-depth field interviews with over 400 Anglo, African, Japanese, and Mexican Americans in southern California and comparison with previously published literature formed the basis of their impressions. They suggested that the universal features of aging, dying, and death are as important as or more important than culturally determined features. Kalish and Reynolds found that, regardless of ethnic background, as people got older they were more likely to attend funerals, thought more about death on a daily basis, and thought more positively about their deaths.[5] Respondents reported that the most powerful influences on their attitudes to death were the death of someone else and religious background. The most important reasons people gave for not wanting to die were that death would cause grief to relatives and friends, that dying might be painful, and that they could not take care of dependents. This ranking of reasons was similar for all ethnic groups.

In a survey of the National Council on Aging in which individuals were asked what was the worst thing about being over 65, the elderly were less afraid of death (6% prevalence) than respondents under age 50. However, the worst things about being over 65 were poor health (62%) and loneliness (33%).[5] The elderly were intensely concerned about maintenance of bodily function and holding back changes of aging. In this study of ethnic differences, it is striking to read about what is common among the elderly.

Older people are significantly more likely to say they will accept death peacefully than to fight against it; they are less worried about dependents than are the young (having fewer people who do need them); they are less concerned about cessation of experiences, perhaps feeling that they have had their share and that further experiences are bought at the price of physical and psychological pain. It would appear that their entire affective response pattern regarding death has been reduced. Lacking longitudinal data, we cannot ascertain whether these feelings are the continuation into the later years of attitudes held at earlier times in life or whether the awareness of being old is the major basis. Nonetheless, these people are not in a hurry to die. They are less likely than the middle-aged or the young to espouse the idea that people should be permitted to die. And they are most likely to worry about what happens to their bodies after they die. In addition, they perceive sudden (compared to slow) deaths and accidental deaths as more tragic than do their youngers.

The old have had much more experience with death and dying; they think much more about it; they appear more ready to die, yet they do not feel death should be precipitated or occur without the opportunity to deal a little more with life. As a group, they do not seem to be in despair but they do appear to be experiencing disengagement, withdrawal, and reduction of involvement with life. . . .

The social–interactional world socializes us to reduce the focus upon inner self found in infancy by rewarding and reinforcing attachments with people, objects, and events. Then, in the late years and especially in the terminal stages, pressures for reducing attachments brought about by society again returns the individual to his inner focus, aided and abetted by aches and pains and reduced futurity. As old attachments diminish in number and intensity, re-engagement with matters directly pertaining to self are permitted. Ironically, then, the elderly are frequently chastised for self-centered behavior, which is often the only kind of behavior left to them.[5]

Subsequent literature offers a quilt-like patchwork of descriptions and comparisons, and we consider here specific points that clinicians might find valuable in the course of caring for chronically or terminally ill geriatric patients.

Role of Race, Ethnicity, Religion, and Socioeconomic Status on Attitudes toward End-of-Life Care

Ethnicity, age, religion, and socioeconomic status have strong influences on how patients wish to be treated at the end of their lives.[1,5] To be fully informed of these influences would require an encyclopedic approach. Rather, clinicians should be aware of how powerfully these influences can af-

fect patient and family attitudes about death and care at the end of life as a prerequisite to providing a strategy that may be useful in helping patients and families of any background.

Ethnicity
As Koenig states:

Cultural conceptions of the self and personhood, the location of the individual within a social group such as the family, orientation to the future, openness about discussing death, and ideas about what constitutes appropriate behavior by healers, are all directly relevant to end of life decisions.[3]

In an article that provides case studies of terminally ill patients of various ethnic origins, Klesig[6] derives several themes that are useful in practicing cross-cultural medicine. These themes develop in the course of an individual's experiences and can become apparent in their beliefs, behaviors, relationships to the family and providers, and medical expectations (Table 8–1).

Several textbooks exploring the relationship of culture and bioethics demonstrate that ethical approaches, particularly the importance placed upon the values of beneficence, autonomy, and community, differ among cultures.[7,8] Studies have also explored the way different cultures approach death.[4,5,9] Cultures vary in how individualistically oriented they are, the extent to which they encourage frank discussion of illness and death, and how active a role they encourage patients and their families to take in medical decisions. In understanding the extent to which culture influences the attitudes of ethnically diverse elderly patients, it is particularly important to recognize that the age at which they immigrated from their native country, if indeed they have immigrated, is a strong determinant of the extent to which they have acculturated to their non-native country.[10] Thus, the extent to which an elderly individual identifies with the ethnic perspective of a native or adopted country is partly, albeit not entirely, a function of this feature of personal life history.

Table 8–1. Major Themes

Experiences

Life experiences

Historic events such as political upheaval, political torture, war, traumatic losses, and migration may have
profound and lasting impact on the lives of older individuals.

Experience of illness and death

Experience and expression of pain, attitudes in the face of poor prognosis, and response to grief and loss may
vary from culture to culture.

Emotions

Patients may retain long-term mental health effects from their life experiences.
Depression, apathy, and somatization may result.

Attitudes and Beliefs

Cause of illness and practice of medicine

Understanding about the causes of illness and how to heal them may vary from culture to culture.
No matter how acculturated a person appears, during stress such as illness or death, early-learned ideas resur-
face and structure responses.

Patient–family relationships

The family is pivotal and the patient may not be viewed as separate from it.

Physician–patient relationship

Disclosure of personal information is not always appropriate on first meeting a new health care practitioner.

Bioethical pluralism

There are fundamental differences in the way American medicine conceptualizes the role of the sick person
and family in medical encounters.
The assumption that the person experiencing illness is the one to make decisions is not shared by all cultures.

Medical pluralism

Patients may seek alternative cures or therapies to cure spirits, ancestors, and or behavioral impropriety. Often Western medical treatments and alternative or native therapies are not viewed as mutually exclusive.

Behavior

Emotions are often not openly expressed or talked about.
Emotional expression may vary in culturally appropriate ways.
Family business or "secrets" may be kept from the outside world. Decision-making, receiving and disclosing
news, and orchestrating of care are concerns and responsibilities of the group.
Problems can develop if roles are reversed especially within immigrant families. This can occur when children
are put in positions of authority over parents or older adults for example in translating during medical encounters or when children are more acculturated to American life.

Modified from Klesig (Klesig 1992)
Source: Klesig.[6]

Race

As noted in the definitions above, the term
race has commonly given way to *ethnic
group*. Nonetheless, the concept of race is
often used, particularly regarding African

Americans, who have had such a harsh
experience due to racism. The views of
African-American patients have been the
focus of several studies. They are generally
reported to be more inclined to use life-

sustaining treatments than non-African Americans. For instance, in a study of Medicare enrollees, African-American patients reported being more inclined to choose life-sustaining treatments than whites when terminally ill.[11] African Americans in a nursing home have been reported to be more interested in cardiopulmonary resuscitation (CPR).[12] African Americans are less likely to prepare a living will.[13] To attribute the inclination to use life-sustaining treatments to a fear of discrimination is to oversimplify the African-American experience.

Socioeconomic status
Educational background and level of income can be related to patients' attitudes toward end-of-life care. In a study of elderly Medicare recipients,[11] individuals with less education were more inclined to want life-sustaining treatments. One can only speculate that perhaps individuals with less education are less aware of the limitations of medical technology or that a life that affords fewer opportunities makes individuals more eager to try any opportunity to prolong life.

Nationality
Lynn Payer, an American journalist who studied differing views of the practice of medicine in the United States and several western European countries, describes how varied the understanding of illness is across these countries.[14] At the risk of overgeneralizing, she reports that Germans, for example, are prone to attribute illness to a weak heart, while the French are more inclined to be concerned about liver ailments. These views have tangible consequences as illustrated by the fact that the use of digitalis is 10-fold higher in Germany than in the United States. Aside from differing beliefs about the pathophysiology of illness, there are different views about the proper style of medical practice. European critical care physicians are much less likely than physicians from the United States to use a collaborative decision-making style with patients and families and more inclined to use a style that would be considered paternalistic in the United States.[15]

If perceptions of illness vary among countries as closely linked as those in western Europe and North America, it is not surprising that attitudes among more diverse nationalities are even more disparate. Blackhall et al.[16] studied attitudes toward patient autonomy, particularly the desire for medical information and participation in decision making, among individuals residing in the United States who had various national origins. Korean Americans (47%) and Mexican Americans (65%) were less likely than European Americans (87%) and African Americans (85%) to believe that a patient should be told about a diagnosis of metastatic cancer or about a terminal prognosis and that a patient should make a life-sustaining treatment decision (28% vs. 41% vs. 60% vs. 65%, respectively). Klesig[6] has reported that the inclination to use, withhold, or remove life-sustaining treatments varies among U.S. residents of different cultural or national backgrounds.

Religion and spirituality
Religious persuasion can affect not only beliefs but practices as well. Whether an individual believes in an afterlife and whether it is acceptable to tamper with the body after death, donate organs, or observe ritual practices around the time of death vary among religions.[17] Spirituality can have a profound influence on attitudes toward illness and a consequent impact on interactions with the medical team. Kaldjian et al.[18] reported that human immunodeficiency virus (HIV)–infected individuals who perceived HIV infection as a punishment were less likely than those who believed in God's forgiveness to have had discussions about resuscitation. Individuals who reported praying daily and those who reported that God helped them when thinking about death were more likely to have a living will. Those who attended church regularly or read the Bible frequently reported being less afraid of death.[18]

Aside from having diverse views on life-sustaining treatments, different ethnic groups have different attitudes and behaviors in response to pain and pain management.[19] Given the importance of pain management in palliative care, critical care providers should be aware that individuals of different cultures might not all express their experience of pain in the same way. Whether it is for this or other reasons, minority patients tend to receive less adequate pain relief than nonminority patients.[20–22]

Perhaps one of the more important differences in the preferences of elderly ethic groups is the kind and location of supportive care they want. Many elders who live in tightly knit immigrant communities are more interested in receiving supportive care from their families than from social service workers or outside agencies and would rather receive palliative care at home than in an inpatient hospice facility. In these communities, there is unusually strong intergenerational support between elders and their children. There is some suggestion that this pattern of familial care is not only a reflection of strong preferences but may also reflect other issues, including lack of health insurance and fears or mistrust of the formal health-care sector.[23]

Despite the many reported associations between ethnic identity and preferences, it is important to be cautious about assuming that an individual's background necessarily predicts attitudes or behaviors. For example, Whittle et al.[24] report that while African Americans were less likely to say that they would undergo cardiac revascularization procedures, familiarity with procedures was a much stronger predictor of differences in desire for coronary artery bypass graft than race or ethnicity. When knowledge about the procedure was taken into account, the influence of ethnicity became insignificant. Similarly, while patients of various backgrounds may differ in their desires to have their families participate in decision making on their behalf, the accuracy of surrogate decision makers (i.e., their ability to predict patient preferences) is not correlated with ethnic background.[25]

Influence of Socioeconomic Status, Nationality, and Race on the Experience and Treatment of Aging and Dying

Socioeconomic status profoundly influences when individuals die. A growing body of literature indicates that income and social class are directly related to life expectancy. Thus, within any given country, economically less advantaged individuals die at a younger age. A variety of mechanisms are thought to play a role, including reduced access to nutrition, housing, and education; and increased social stress.[26,27] While geriatricians may not perceive these disparities in their day-to-day encounters with patients, data suggest that mortality rates from various disease processes differ between poor patients and socioeconomically advantaged patients. For each $10,000 decrement in median income, the relative risk of dying of several diseases increases by 1.5, including acquired immune deficiency syndrome, diabetes, rheumatic heart disease, chronic obstructive pulmonary disease, pneumonia, and homicide.[28]

While these comparative data are from within countries, the disparity in mortality is more stark between countries. The World Bank reports the percentage of the population over age 60 years for all of its member nations. Nineteen countries, predominantly in western and eastern Europe as well as Japan, report that 20% of their population is over age 60, while 25 countries located in Africa, the Middle East, and the Pacific report that less than 5% of their population is over age 60. These statistics are the result of the interaction of life expectancy and birth rate. Life expectancy ranges from 77.5 for men and 84.7 for women in Japan to 37.0 for men and 38.8 for women in Sierra Leone.[29]

Focusing on disparities in the United States, both socioeconomic and racial differences play a role. Life expectancy for African Americans lags behind that of whites by 13.1 years for those born in 1930, by 11.1 years for those born in 1940, and by 8.3 years for those born in 1950.[30] The medical literature provides evidence that minority and socioeconomically disadvantaged individuals generally have less access to medical care.[31] The Institute of Medicine has reported racial and ethnic disparities in the delivery of a wide range of treatments resulting in worse outcomes.[32] The use of life-sustaining treatments tends to follow this overall pattern. African Americans have slightly shorter lengths of intensive care unit (ICU) stay, although this difference is not associated with any difference in risk-adjusted hospital mortality rate.[33] They also have lower rates of organ transplantation and a lower probability of being placed on a transplantation list, even after controlling for patient preference.[34] They have lower rates of survival following CPR (odds ratio = 0.31, 95% confidence interval 0.15–0.68), even after adjusting for age, sex, initial cardiac rhythm, diagnosis of pneumonia, serum creatinine level, and acute physiology and chronic health evaluation (APACHE) score.[35] Lower rates of treatment are not the result of less desire for treatment since studies indicate that African Americans are generally more inclined to utilize them. For example, African Americans have fewer do-not-resuscitate (DNR) orders in nursing homes, an indication that they are less inclined to forgo resuscitation. Thus, studies of health services utilization raise persistent concern about disparities in treatment and the underlying causes, including bias, stereotyping, and the uncertainty that is frequently inherent in the clinical encounter.[32]

Again, while the emphasis in this discussion is on diversity, these differences must be viewed against the backdrop of a very strong overall shift in health-care services with advancing age. Use of acute-care services and their attendant life-sustaining treatments diminishes markedly with age, and use of long-term care correspondingly rises.[36]

SUGGESTIONS ABOUT CARING FOR PATIENTS OF DIVERSE BACKGROUNDS

When clinicians provide palliative care to elderly patients whose background differs from their own, they do well to bear in mind that patients of varying backgrounds may differ about the care they want while chronically ill or dying. Ironically, evidence indicates that the care that patients receive does differ, yet not in the way patients might wish. It behooves practitioners both to avoid discriminatory biases that may lead to care that is contrary to patient wishes and to avoid stereotyping and presuming to know what care patients will want. Rather, clinicians can provide optimal care by being prepared to communicate and negotiate carefully with patients and families and by tailoring the care they provide to the unique needs of each patient and family.

Differences in values can exist between any two individuals but may be even more likely when the individuals differ in gender, age, religion, culture, political affiliation, or socioeconomic class. In considering suggestions here, the discussion focuses on cross-cultural differences since these pose the greatest dilemma. While differences may exist among groups within a given culture, it is generally argued that groups within the same culture can at least express their differences in terms of a common language and moral vocabulary. While even this assumption may be somewhat simplistic, it is safe to assume that individuals of different cultures have the greatest divide between their cultural repertoires. As Jecker et al.[37] write, "Thus, cross-cultural debates often seem to introduce moral anarchy because people lack shared cultural standards or vantage points from which to communicate and resolve value differences." As Ware and Kleinman[38] suggest, "Cross-cultural conflicts may be more deeply rooted, for such differences embody not just different opinions or beliefs, but different ways of everyday living and different systems of meaning."

Relationships between health-care providers and patients are generally unequal, with clinicians playing the dominant role.[39] Much of the agenda of medical ethics over the last several decades has been to accord as much respect to the patient's perspective as possible. This attention to respect for patient preferences is particularly important when providers and patients differ in their views about what is important and valuable to them.

Ironically, this valuable approach that has been developed in Western bioethics, to respect patient autonomy by asserting the right to self-determination, may prove to be complicated. Other cultures may view the focus on the patient as an individual to be contrary to their view of the individual as inseparable from the family or community. They may also prefer a less explicit communication style than is typical of North American medical practice.

A key to making health-care decisions less ethnocentric—decisions that do not presume the superiority of one's own culture—is to develop an understanding of the differences in the use of language among cultures.[40] This requires an appreciation that the way one uses language may affect one's perception of reality. Navahos, for example, prohibit the telling of bad news because they believe that the telling may lead to the occurrence of an event.[41] Thus, the truth about bad news, which might be required to make informed treatment decisions in standard U.S. medical practice, may be perceived as disrespectful or dangerous.

In light of the importance of language, the role of interpreters can be crucial. They are not merely translators. They can be a source of cultural information; facilitate care; create trust between providers, health-care institutions, patients, families, and communities; improve continuity of care; improve access to care; mediate misunderstandings and disagreements; and act as advocates and counselors.[40] Given the pivotal role of interpreters, the clinician should learn to work effectively with them. The clinician should speak directly to the patient or family even when utilizing an interpreter and should be aware of the quality of the interpreters in his or her institution. The clinician should be aware, when having family members serve as interpreters, that the

patient's privacy may be breached and that the family member is likely to filter the conversation, which may or may not be acceptable to the patient. For these reasons, using family members as interpreters is discouraged and should be reserved for extreme circumstances.

In attending to the needs of patients of different cultural backgrounds, clinicians do well to recognize that culture can influence the way that patients experience pain and how they wish others to respond to it.[19,42] Clinicians and patients of various cultures may differ in their views of the appropriate way to express and treat pain. Patients will receive the best pain management when these differences are acknowledged and addressed.

When critically ill patients die, families of differing cultural backgrounds may have different bereavement practices.[43] While the prevailing North American view of the grieving experience is as an isolated individual experience involving detachment from the dead, acceptance of other views of the grieving process may be helpful in supporting families through their bereavement.[44] When a patient dies, the family must adjust to new events in the family life cycle and learn to function in the patient's absence. To help families requires supporting them in a manner that fits their unique circumstances as well as the bereavement expectations of their community and culture.[44]

A particularly useful general approach to caring for patients whose cultural background differs from that of the provider comes from the family practice literature. The *Teaching Framework for Cross-Cultural Health Care*, developed by Berlin and Fowkes,[45] can serve as a valuable strategy for working with patients from different cultural backgrounds regardless of how ill:

LEARN

L *Listen* with sympathy and understanding to the patient's perception of the problem

E *Explain* your perception of the problem

A *Acknowledge* and discuss the differences and similarities

R *Recommend* treatment

N *Negotiate* agreement

Specific Strategies of Caring for Severely Ill and Dying Patients

A useful series of questions, prompted by the individualized approach suggested by Koenig and Gates-Williams,[46] can serve as an outline for attending to the diverse needs of severely ill and dying patients (Table 8–2). The clinician should pay attention to the patient's language, religion, social context, beliefs, decision-making style, and social support in the process of getting familiar and working with the patient. The suggested questions can serve as a reminder about what the clinician should learn about the patient in each of these domains.

Spiritual Assessment

While we have focused on cultural influences, religious concerns are likely to be closely entwined with culture as patients muster all of their resources to face serious illness. While the clinician might be inclined to inquire about a patient's religion and assume that little more needs to be asked, it is important to realize that addressing spiritual needs requires more than merely inquiring about a patient's religious affilia-tion. A variety of strategies have been developed to help the clinician learn about a patient's spiritual values and needs.[47]

A Practical Approach to Dealing with Disagreements about Informing the Patient

Freedman[48] proposes a strategy labeled "offering truth." He argues that a patient's desire for knowledge about his or her disease is not all-or-nothing; rather, it ranges along a continuum. In the spirit of respect for patient autonomy, patients are asked how much they want to know. The discussion begins by asking what they know about the situation. If they ask why they are being queried about their knowledge, they might be told that if the clinician knows their understanding of the illness, it may save time that might otherwise be wasted on telling them things they already know, that when teaching someone it is important to have an idea of what they know in order to teach them most effectively.

The important thing is to begin to generate a dynamic within which the patient is speaking and the physician responding, rather than vice versa. Only then can the pace of conversation and level of information be controlled by the patient. The structure of the discussion, as well as the content of what the physician says, must reinforce the message: We are now establishing a new opportunity to talk and to question, but

Table 8–2. Guiding Questions

1. *Language:* What language do the patient and family prefer to use to discuss illness and disease? How openly do they wish to discuss diagnosis, prognosis, and death itself?
2. *Religion:* What is their religious background, and how avid is their religious affiliation?
   What do the patient and family think about the sanctity of life, and how do they conceive of death?
   Do they believe in miracles? Do they believe in an afterlife? Do they believe the body should be handled in a certain way after death?
3. *Social, political, and historical context:* Do any of the following factors affect the attitudes of the patient and family: the patient's status in the family, country of origin, or experiences such as poverty, refugee status, past discrimination, or lack of access to care?
4. *Beliefs:* What do they believe are the causal agents in illness, and how do these relate to the dying process?
5. *Decision-making style:* Who makes decisions about matters of importance in the family? Are the patient and family fatalistic about the course of events, or do they wish to take active control of events?
6. *Social support and resources:* What resources, including community and religious leaders, family members, and language translators, are available to aid in the complex effort of interpreting cultural dimensions of a patient's illness?

Adapted from the work of Koenig and Gates-Williams.[46]

you as the patient will have to tell us how much you want to know about your illness.[48]

A Practical Ethical Approach to Dealing with Different Perspectives

Once the clinician is familiar with the patient and family's perspective and desire for information, it can be useful to have a practical ethical approach for finding a care plan in the face of different perspectives. Jecker et al.[37] have suggested that such a plan should include the following actions:

1. Identify goals
2. Identify mutually agreeable strategies
3. Meet ethical constraints

The treatment choices should be consistent with the health-care provider's beliefs and compatible with the patient's values. If there is conflict, the clinician should re-examine his or her personal values and consider reinterpreting, reordering, or changing them in light of the case. If there are persistent disagreements, these should be adjudicated through a fair process that reflects a nonjudgmental stance.

While we have focused on the attitudes and behaviors that the individual clinician should espouse, the clinician does not and cannot operate optimally in a vacuum. Several recommendations are useful for creating a supportive institutional setting.[49]

1. Bicultural providers, translators, and others who are cognizant of the culture of patients often seen in the health-care organization should be an integral part of the organization.
2. Community leaders should be involved in policy development at the organizational and community levels.

Some specific recommendations for hospice services to ethnically diverse communities can complement individual clinicians' efforts.[23]

1. Develop hospice outreach initiates to educate elderly patients and their family caregivers about available services.
2. Recruit hospice volunteers from the ethnic community of the patient's population.

3. Increase the number of bilingual volunteers.
4. Develop multilingual educational materials using various media, including audiovisual materials, so that low-literacy patients who may make use of written material can understand and access services.

CONCLUSION

This chapter has emphasized the influence of culture, religion, and socioeconomic status on patients' experiences and preferences about critical and terminal illness. It is crucial to bear in mind that individuals within any group vary widely, a given individual may identify with a number of groups, the degree of affiliation with a culture may vary from person to person, and group affiliation may have little predictive value about a given individual's views. It is therefore particularly important to avoid stereotyping individuals. While it is important to respect and understand an individual's culture, religion, nationality, or socioeconomic background, clinicians are likely to provide the best care by being respectful of the unique qualities and attentive to the particular needs of each elderly individual they serve.

ACKNOWLEDGMENTS

We appreciate the permission of Oxford University Press to use material from the book chapter entitled, 'The role of ethnicity, race, religion, and socioeconomic status in end-of-life care in the ICU' in Managing Death in the Intensive Care Unit Curtis, JR and Rubenfeld GD, eds, 2001. The opinion expressed here are exclusively those of the authors and do not reflect policy of the National Institutes of Health or the Department of Health and Human Services.

REFERENCES

1. Surbone A, Zwitter M. Learning from the world: the editors' perspective. Ann NY Acad Sci 809:1–6, 1997.

2. Sheldon T, Parker H. Race and ethnicity in health research. J Public Health Med 14: 104–110, 1992.

3. Koenig B. Cultural diversity in decision-making about care at the end of life. In: Field M, Cassel C (Eds.). Approaching Death: Improving Care at the End of Life. Washington DC, National Academy Press, pp. 363–382, 1997.

4. Galanti G-A. Caring for Patients from Different Cultures: Case Studies from American Hospitals. Philadelphia, University of Pennsylvania Press, 1993.

5. Kalish RA, Reynolds DK. Death and Ethnicity: A Psychosocial Study. New York, Baywood, 1981.

6. Klesig J. The effects of values and culture on life-support decisions. West J Med 163:316–322, 1992.

7. Veatch RM. Medical Ethics. Boston, Jones and Bartlett, 1989.

8. Pellegrino E, Mazzarella P, Corsi P. Transcultural Dimensions in Medical Ethics. Frederick, MD, University Publishing Group, 1992.

9. Irish D, Lundquist EA. Ethnic Variations in Dying, Death, and Grief. Washington DC, Tayor and Francis, 1993.

10. Gordon, M. Assimilation in American Life. New York, Oxford University Press, 1964.

11. Garrett JM, Harris R, Norburn J, Patrick DL, Danis M. Life-sustaining treatments during terminal illness: who wants what? J Gen Intern Med 8:361–368, 1993.

12. O'Brien LA, Grisso JA, Maislin G. Nursing home residents' preferences for life-sustaining treatments [see comments]. JAMA 274:1775–1779, 1995.

13. McKinley ED, Garrett JM, Evans AT, et al. Differences in end-of-life decision making among black and white ambulatory cancer patients. J Gen Intern Med 11:651–656, 1996.

14. Payer L. Medicine and Culture: Notions of Health and Sickness in Britain, the U.S., France, and West Germany. London, V. Gollancz, 1990.

15. Vincent JL. European attitudes towards ethical problems in intensive care medicine: results of an ethical questionnaire. Intensive Care Med 16:256–264, 1990.

16. Blackhall LJ, Murphy ST, Frank G, et al. Ethnicity and attitudes toward patient autonomy. JAMA 274:820–825, 1995.

17. McQuay JE. Cross-cultural customs and beliefs related to health crises, death, and organ donation/transplantation: a guide to assist health care professionals understand different responses and provide cross-cultural assistance. Crit Care Nurs Clin North Am 7:581–594, 1995.

18. Kaldjian LC, Jekel JF, Friedland G. End-of-life decisions in HIV-positive patients: the role of spiritual beliefs. AIDS 12:103–107, 1998.

19. Martinelli A. Pain and ethnicity. AORN J 46:273–281, 1998.

20. Todd KH, Samaroo N, Hoffman JR. Ethnicity as a risk factor for inadequate emergency department analgesia. JAMA 269: 1537–1539, 1993.

21. Todd KH, Lee T, Hoffman JR. The effect of ethnicity on physician estimates of pain severity in patients with isolated extremity trauma. JAMA 271:925–928, 1994.

22. Cleeland C. Pain and treatment of pain in minority patients with cancer. Ann Intern Med 127:813–816, 1997.

23. Talamantes M, Lawler W, Espino D. Hispanic American elders: caregiving norms surrounding dying and the use of hospice services. Hospice J 10:35–49, 1995.

24. Whittle J, Conigliaro J, Grood CB, et al. Do patient preferences contribute to racial differences in cardiovascular procedure use? J Gen Intern Med 12:267–273, 1997.

25. Sulmasy DP, Terry PB, Weisman CS, et al. The accuracy of substituted judgments in patients with terminal diagnoses [see comments]. Ann Intern Med 128:621–629, 1998.

26. Leon D, Walt G. Poverty, Inequality and Health: An International Perspective. Oxford, Oxford University Press, 2001.

27. Marmot M, Wilkinson R (Eds.). Social Determinants of Health. Oxford, Oxford University Press, 2002.

28. Smith G, Gunnell D, Ben-Shlomo Y. Life-course approaches to socio-economic differentials in cause-specific adult mortality. In Leon D, Walt G (Eds.). Poverty, Inequality and Health: An International Perspective. Oxford, Oxford University Press, pp. 88–124, 2001.

29. World Health Organization. The World Health Report 2001. (Retrieved July 2, 2002) Available at: http://www.who.int/whr/

30. National Center for Health Statistics, National Vital Statistics Report. Available at: http://www.cdc.gov/nchs

31. Adler N, Boyce T. Socioeconomic inequalities in health. JAMA 269:3140–3145, 1993.

32. Smedley B, Stith A, Nelson A, Committee on Understanding and Eliminating Racial and Ethnic Disparities in Health Care (Eds.). Unequal Treatment: Confronting Racial and Ethnic Disparities in Health Care. Washington DC: National Academy Press, 2002.

33. Williams JF, Zimmerman JE, Wagner DP, et al. African-American and white patients admitted to the intensive care unit: is there

a difference in therapy and outcome? Crit Care Med 23:626–636, 1995.

34. Epstein A, Ayanian J, Keogh J, Noonan S, Armistead N, Cleary P, Weissman J, David–Kadan J, Carlson D, Fuller J, et al. Racial disparities in access to renal transplantation—clinically appropriate or due to underuse or overuse? N Engl J Med 343: 1537–1544, 2000.

35. Ebell MH, Smith M, Kruse JA, et al. Effect of race on survival following in-hospital cardiopulmonary resuscitation. J Fam Pract 40:571–577, 1995.

36. Spillman BC, Lubitz J. The effect of longevity on spending for acute and long-term care. N Engl J Med 342:1409–1415, 2000.

37. Jecker NS, Carrese JA, Pearlman RA. Caring for patients in cross-cultural settings. Hastings Cent Rep 25:6–14, 1995.

38. Ware NC, Kleinman A. Culture and somatic experience: the social course of illness in neurasthenia and chronic fatigue syndrome. Psychosom Med 54:546–560, 1992.

39. Friedson ET. Professional Dominance. New York, Atheneum, 1970.

40. Kaufert JM, Putsch RW. Communication through interpreters in healthcare: ethical dilemmas arising from differences in class, culture, language, and power. J Clin Ethics 8:71–87, 1997.

41. Carrese J, Rhodes L. Western bioethics on the Navajo reservation: benefit or harm? JAMA 274:286–289, 1995.

42. Walker AC, Tan L, George S. Impact of culture on pain management: an Australian nursing perspective. Holist Nurs Pract 9: 48–57, 1995.

43. Rosenblatt P, Walsh R, et al. Grief and Mourning in Cross-Cultural Perspectives. New Haven, CT, HRAF Press, 1976.

44. Shapiro E. Family bereavement and cultural diversity: a social development perspective. Fam Process 35:313–332, 1996.

45. Berlin EA, Fowkes WC Jr. A teaching framework for cross-cultural health care. Application in family practice. West J Med 139:934–938, 1983.

46. Koenig B, Gates-Williams J. Understanding cultural differences in caring for dying patients. West J Med 163:244–249, 1995.

47. Chambers N, Curtis JR. The interface of technology and spirituality in the ICU. In: Curtis JR, Rubenfeld GD (Eds.). Managing Death in the Intensive Care Unit: The Transition from Cure to Comfort. New York, Oxford University Press, 2001.

48. Freedman B. Offering truth. One ethical approach to the uninformed cancer patient. Arch Intern Med 153:572–576, 1993.

49. Hern HE Jr, Roenig BA, Moore IJ, et al. The difference that culture can make in end-of-life decisionmaking. Camb Q Healthc Ethics 7:27–40, 1998.

II

DISEASE- AND SYNDROME-SPECIFIC ASPECTS OF PALLIATIVE CARE

9

Frailty and Its Implications for Care

JEREMY D. WALSTON AND LINDA P. FRIED

Frailty in older adults is conceptualized by clinicians as a progressive, physiologic process marked by declines in function and physiologic reserves as well as increased vulnerability to morbidity and mortality. In its more severe form, it presages death and may be irreversible. Frailty is also frequently equated with advanced age and thought to be the final common pathway for many end-stage, chronic disease states. The transition toward frailty can include a passage from independence to one of increasing dependence on family and caregivers. The increasing burden of symptoms, increasing medical and social needs, and need for important decisions about housing and health care also mark the period of life where thoughtful and targeted palliative care should begin. Given that both the age-related physiologic declines of frailty and the chronic disease states in those who are the most frail are usually progressive and irreversible, delivery of palliative care focused on relief of suffering and enhancement of quality of life is highly germane to the medical care of frail, older adults. The

etiologic complexity of frailty together with coexisting social, psychologic, and medical issues present a considerable challenge in the delivery of palliative health care. Despite this challenge, multidisciplinary, team-based palliative approaches and the application of current geriatric knowledge can provide benefit and improve quality of life for this most vulnerable subset of older adults.

To identify those in most need of palliative care and to deliver thoughtful and comprehensive palliative care to frail, older adults, it is useful for the health-care provider to have a working understanding of the evolving definitions of frailty and its biologic basis, to recognize the common signs and symptoms of frailty, to understand how coexisting disease states and pain may worsen frailty, and to recognize the spectrum of frailty and the potential reversibility of the symptoms. To accomplish this, we will *(1)* provide a conceptual overview of frailty, *(2)* describe its clinical presentation and consequences, *(3)* summarize the present understanding of its biologic basis, *(4)* discuss criteria for the identification of frailty and its spectrum of severity, and *(5)* discuss a range of potential palliative interventions and family roles that support an improved quality of life for frail, older adults.

DEFINITION AND CONCEPTUALIZATION OF FRAILTY

Frailty has frequently been defined as a state of extreme vulnerability to a range of poor outcomes. Geriatricians often identify frailty in older adults through evidence of repeated falls and injuries, disability, susceptibility to acute illnesses, and poor ability to recover from stressors. While multiple chronic diseases (*comorbidity*) and accumulated disabilities have previously been equated with frailty, evidence is mounting that frailty represents a distinct biologic process that is age-related and can exist independently of common disease states or be initiated or exacerbated by disease.[1-3] In the modal pathway illustrated in Figure 9–1, frailty is conceptualized as a clinical entity triggered by age-related molecular changes and disease states. This clinical state is manifested through a syndrome of weakness, fatigue, and weight loss. This clinical syndrome in turn contributes to a host of consequences and poor outcomes, as detailed below.

CLINICAL PRESENTATION AND CONSEQUENCES OF FRAILTY

To provide optimal clinical and palliative care for frail, older adults, it is important to first recognize the range of signs, symptoms, and negative outcomes associated with the syndrome. Over the past several years, consensus has begun to emerge on the major clinical markers of frailty: loss of strength, decline in lean body mass, weight loss, altered balance, low levels of activity, poor endurance, and fatigue.[1,4-6] A critical mass of these symptoms and signs of frailty is associated with a range of negative clinical outcomes. For example, when both inactivity and weight loss were present, Chin et al.[5] identified a 3-year increased risk of mortality (odds ratio [OR] = 4.1, 95% confidence interval [CI] 1.8–9.4) and disability (OR = 5.2, 95% CI 1.04–25.8) in the Zutphen Elderly Study. In the Cardiovascular Health Study (CHS), the presence of three or more of five criteria for frailty, including weakness, weight loss, exhaustion, slow walking speed, and low physical activity, significantly predicted onset of falls, incidence or progression of disability, hospitalization, and mortality, even after adjusting for diseases present, health habits, age, and gender (Table 9–1).[1] Both of these studies demonstrate that frail, older adults are a highly vulnerable subset of the popu-

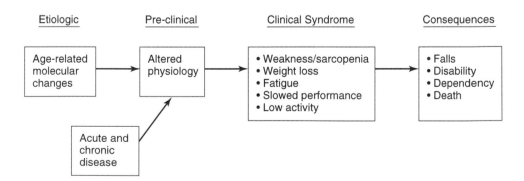

Figure 9–1. Conceptualization of frailty as a clinical syndrome with a biologic basis. In this modal pathway, disease states and age-related changes contribute to specific changes in physiology. This preclinical physiology and the resulting clinical syndrome of frailty contribute to the vulnerability and poor outcomes observed in frail, older adults.

Table 9–1. Baseline Frailty Status Independently Predicts Falls, Disability, Hospitalizations, and Death over Follow-up of 3 and 7 Years, Adjusting for Covariates*

	No frailty (reference)	3-year follow-up (95% CI)	7-year follow-up (95% CI)
Incident falls	HR = 1.0	HR = 1.29 (1.00–1.68) $p = 0.054$	HR = 1.23 (0.99–1.54) —
Worsening mobility†	HR = 1.0	HR = 1.50 (1.23–1.82) $p = 0.0001$	HR = 1.36 (1.51–1.62) $p = 0.0003$
Worsening ADL disability‡	HR = 1.0	HR = 1.98 (1.54–2.55) $p < 0.0001$	HR = 1.79 (1.47–2.17) $p < 0.0001$
First hospitalization	HR = 1.0	HR = 1.29 (1.09–1.54) $p = 0.004$	HR = 1.27 (1.11–1.46) $p = 0.0008$
Death	HR = 1.0	HR = 2.24 (1.51–3.33) $p = 0.0001$	HR = 1.63 (1.27–2.08) $p = 0.0001$

Data from the Cardiovascular Health Study, a cohort of community-dwelling men and women 65–101 years at baseline (1). Hazard Ratio (HR) and 95% confidence interval (CI) for those frail compared to nonfrail at the two follow-up time points. Adjusted for covariates including age, gender, indicator for minority cohort, income, smoking status, brachial and tibial blood pressure, fasting glucose, albumin creatinine, carotid stenosis, history of congestive heart failure, cognitive function, major electrocardiographic abnormality, use of diuretics, problems with activities of daily living (ADL), self-report health measures, Center for Epidemiologic Studies modified depression measure. HR is the ratio or risk of frailty group (frail) relative to the nonfrail group with regard to the event of interest (e.g., first fall, death).
†Defined as an increase of one unit of mobility score relative to baseline.
‡Defined as an increase of one unit of ADL score relative to baseline.

lation. This subset includes those who are most likely to need palliative interventions.

Although the physiologic processes that contribute to frailty are not thought to directly contribute to pain syndromes, frail, older adults often have multiple medical illnesses and a propensity toward falls and injuries that can make them more likely to suffer from pain.[7] A number of studies suggest that pain in older adults is, in general, under-estimated and undertreated. This occurs for a variety of reasons, including risk of adverse drug reactions, under recognition of chronic anxiety and depression, physiologic differences in the sensation of pain, and under-reporting by older patients.[8–10] New tools have been developed to identify pain in older populations, and recent developments in the understanding of the physiologic targeting of pain medications and improved treatment of chronic depression and anxiety have made the identification and treatment of pain an integral part of palliative care for frail, older adults, as described below.[7]

BIOLOGIC BASIS OF FRAILTY

To help conceptualize the complex interactions between etiologies, physiology, the clinical syndrome, and the consequences of frailty, we have previously proposed a theoretical cycle of frailty that provides a framework for understanding these relationships (Fig. 9–2). In this framework, a decline in skeletal muscle mass, usually a result of age, genetic influences, and/or environmental factors, leads to clinical declines in strength, exercise tolerance, and walking speed. These changes, in turn, predict the development of disability and dependence.[1] This cycle likely involves, ultimately, a downward spiral in function and activity, which further reinforces the loss of muscle mass; disability; and a range of poor outcomes. Also illustrated in this cycle of frailty are a number of potential physiologic entry points into the downward spiral, such as neuroendocrine dysregulation or inflammation secondary to disease states. These theoretical trigger points may

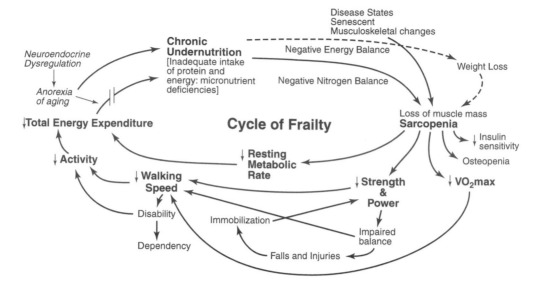

Figure 9–2. Cycle of frailty, a conceptual pathway that illustrates the initiation of frailty at multiple points of entry and a spiral of decreased mobility and activity, thus precipitating the transition from a preclinical toward a clinically apparent state. (Reprinted, with permission, from Fried et al. Frailty and failure to thrive. In: Hazzard W. (Ed.) Principles of Geriatric Medicine and Gerontology, New York, McGraw-Hill, 1998, pp. 1387–1402.

also provide guidance in the development of both preventive and palliative treatments of frailty in older adults (Fig. 9–2).

The physiology and biology of frailty are only now being elucidated with the recent use of screening criteria that help to identify frail, older adults free of confounding disease states.[1–3,5,11] The sections that follow first summarize the current understanding of the subclinical physiology that may contribute to the clinical syndrome of frailty, then describe the current knowledge of etiologic mechanisms. These mechanisms are thought to be age-related molecular changes, termed here *primary frailty*, and acute and chronic disease states, termed *secondary frailty*. Figure 9–3 illustrates the possible physiologic and etiologic components of frailty.

Subclinical Physiology of Frailty

Sarcopenia

Central to most physiologic models of frailty is *sarcopenia*, the loss of skeletal muscle mass.[4,12,13] Muscle mass and strength are usually highest between ages 20 and 30, after which they begin to decline.[14–16] These declines in muscle mass and strength accelerate after age 50, when strength falls at a rate of 10%–15% per decade of life, and even faster after age 75. This well-characterized physiologic decline has several potential etiologies, including age-related changes in type I muscle fibers, muscle atrophy, and alterations in endocrine, immune system, and central and peripheral nervous system functions with age and/or disease.[17]

Endocrine changes

Several specific hormones in the endocrine system play important roles in skeletal and muscle metabolism. Age-related or disease-influenced changes in the regulation of these hormones likely impact the development of many of the signs and symptoms of frailty. The decline in sex steroids with aging, starting with a sharp decrease in estrogen production in women at menopause and the slower but ongoing decline in testosterone production in men, leads to declines in muscle mass and muscle strength.[18–20] Other important components of the endocrine system that may contribute

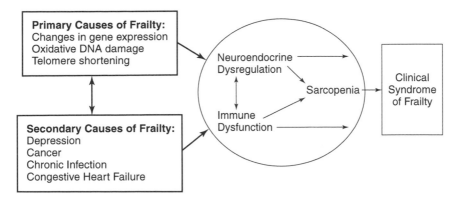

Figure 9–3. Hypothesized etiologic factors along the modal pathway to frailty. Interacting disease and age-related physiologic declines contribute, separately and together, to the development of signs and symptoms of frailty and to the range of poor outcomes observed in frailty.

to frailty include growth hormone (GH) and insulin-like growth factor-I (IGF-1). Age-related loss of normal, pulsatile production of GH and its major messenger, IGF-1 were not associated with loss of lean body mass in a longitudinal study of aging that included healthy men and women.[21] However, Cappola et al.[22] demonstrated an association between lower levels of IGF-1 and lower strength and decreased mobility in older women, both disabled and non-disabled, suggesting a potential role for this axis in the development of frailty. Finally, the loss of tight regulation of the hypothalamic–pituitary–adrenal axis has been implicated in an age-related increase in cortisol production. Several human studies have demonstrated a decrease in the ability of older adults to suppress cortisol secretion after the cessation of a stressful event; in time, prolonged cortisol elevation may contribute to decreased skeletal muscle mass and strength and onset or progression of frailty.[23–27] Each of these components of the endocrine system has well-documented age-related changes that may contribute to the syndrome of frailty. In addition, many of these changes become exaggerated in times of acute and chronic illness. For example, testosterone secretion is acutely lowered from baseline levels in patients with rheumatoid arthritis and lung cancer, two inflammatory conditions that produce muscle weakness and fatigue similar to frailty.[28–30] Both age-related changes and disease-induced alterations in these specific endocrinologic systems likely contribute to the subclinical physiology of frailty.

Inflammatory changes

Inflammation, characterized by chronic immune system activation and elevation of serum levels of the proinflammatory cytokine interleukin-6 (IL-6), appears to be increased persistently in subpopulations of older adults and in those who are frail. Interleukin-6 is a potent inflammatory cytokine that is tightly regulated by the immune system. Its increase with age appears to be due, in part, to the loss of suppression of its expression that parallels declines in estrogen and testosterone secretion.[31] Several studies have demonstrated that high levels of serum IL-6 predict the development of disability and increased mortality in older adults.[32,33] We have demonstrated a correlation between increased IL-6 and frailty in a laboratory-based study of older adults.[11] Additionally, increased serum C-reactive protein, an acute-phase reaction marker directly upregulated by IL-6, was associated with a validated frailty phenotype in the population-based cohort of the CHS.[2]

Normally IL-6 is expressed in times of infection, illness, trauma, or other stress. It is also chronically elevated in several specific disease states, including autoimmune disorders, severe congestive heart failure (CHF), some malignancies, and chronic infections. The effects of chronic IL-6 elevation in association with disease are consistent with the signs and symptoms of frailty, including loss of lean body mass, osteopenia, anemia, anorexia, and decreased hepatic protein synthesis.[31] Although other inflammatory mediators have been associated with disease-related wasting syndromes, IL-6 is most frequently shown to be predictive of poor functional and clinical outcomes in these diseases and in frailty.[32,33] Although there are presently no treatments available to ameliorate the signs and symptoms of frailty thought to be secondary to elevated IL-6, this and other inflammatory mediators are important potential targets for future interventions that target wasting symptoms and fatigue associated with frailty.

In summary, several interactive physiologic systems (skeletal muscle, endocrine, and inflammatory) appear to underlie the development of the geriatric syndrome of frailty. For each of these systems, there is good evidence that age-related changes in expression or regulation could lead to increased vulnerability to poor outcomes in a subset of older adults and that the aggregate alterations may have synergistic effects. Each of these physiologic systems can be induced into similar dysregulation by acute or chronic illness. This, in turn, supports the hypothesis of primary and secondary syndromes of frailty with similar physiology driving both primary frailty and the wasting syndromes that result from several chronic disease states, especially end-stage disease. Increased knowledge of this physiology and of potential etiologies may foster improved symptomatic care treatments targeting anorexia, exhaustion, fatigue, and weakness, symptoms that exist across the spectrum of frailty and medical illness.

Potential Etiologies of Primary Frailty: Age-Related Molecular Changes

Frailty has been postulated to stem from age-related declines in multiple physiologic systems that, in the aggregate, contribute to a syndromic presentation of weakness, fatigue, low activity, and low levels of energy. Buchner and Wagner[34] conceptualized frailty as a cumulative, age-related state of reduced physiologic reserve that is influenced by, but also exists independently of, specific diseases. They further proposed that neurologic control, mechanical performance, and alterations in energy metabolism are the major components of frailty. Others have speculated that the cumulative loss of complexity in biologic control mechanisms, especially loss of physiologic regulatory mechanisms in cardiovascular, neuroendocrine, and bone metabolism systems, contributes to the vulnerability observed in frail, older adults.[35] These conceptualizations of frailty as complex, age-related, multisystem declines have highlighted the gaps in knowledge of the molecular etiologic changes that may trigger the altered physiology described in the previous section. As suggested by theory and the evidence to date, cumulative, complex age-related changes likely contribute to the development of frailty. Although the area of molecular research is largely unexplored, several age-related molecular changes are excellent candidates as etiologic factors but require further study; (1) cumulative oxidative damage to DNA, which in turn may lead to selective loss of proteins critical to energy metabolism or other physiologic pathways; (2) telomere loss and, hence, loss of important gene transcription in older adults, which may lead to selective decline in regulatory mechanisms; (3) genetic variation that becomes more relevant with increasing age and loss or gain of transcription factors; and (4) finite cellular reproductive cycles with increased cellular senescence. More detailed study and understanding of these potential molecular etiologies of primary frailty may lead to improved interventions that target the fatigue and weakness which greatly impact the quality of life of frail, older adults.

Secondary Frailty: Disease-Induced Physiologic Changes

There are marked similarities in the wasting syndrome associated with both selected chronic disease states and primary frailty. These chronic diseases include malignancy, severe CHF, depression, rheumatoid arthritis, and chronic infections. Investigators have demonstrated a wasting syndrome like frailty in patients with advanced human immunodeficiency virus, with similar characteristics of weakness, lean body mass decline, anorexia, and high rates of morbidity and mortality.[36,37] Cardiac cachexia is a well-described wasting syndrome that develops in approximately 16% of individuals who have CHF.[38] It is characterized by high levels of inflammatory cytokines, resultant muscle loss, and neuroendocrine dysregulation.[39] In addition to these specific disease states, a recent study of frail, older adults, the CHS, has demonstrated an association of clinical and subclinical cardiovascular disease with frailty.[3] The relationship was especially strong between CHF and frailty, suggesting a related physiologic pathway for CHF and the physiologic changes that lead to frailty. All of these disease states have an end-stage syndrome consistent with frailty, an inflammatory component, and muscle mass decline. We have therefore proposed a biologic model for frailty in which age-related molecular changes (primary frailty) and disease-triggered frailty (secondary frailty) or a combination of both trigger a common, subclinical physiologic change that leads to frailty (Fig. 9–3).

IDENTIFICATION OF AT-RISK FRAIL, OLDER ADULTS FOR TARGETED TREATMENT AND PREVENTION

Over the past few years, several studies have focused on identifying characteristics of frail, older adults that are predictive of poor outcomes. Some of the most important identifying characteristics of frailty include slow walking speed, weak grip strength, weight loss, low levels of physical activity, and fatigue.[1–5] These five criteria serve as the basis for a frailty screening exam to identify the most vulnerable subset of older adults. Those who meet three of the five criteria are deemed frail, those who meet one or two are deemed intermediate, and those who meet none are deemed nonfrail. This screening method was validated in a large population of community-dwelling older adults through the demonstration that frailty so defined identified a subset at high risk of functional decline, falls, hospitalization, and increased mortality at 3 and 7 years' follow-up.[1] In the same study, about 7% of the cohort met three or more frailty criteria and 45% fell into the intermediate category; that is, they had an intermediate risk of the same outcomes and were at high risk of progressing to frailty. Although these measurements have not been widely employed in clinical practice, these screening criteria, displayed in Table 9–2, may prove useful in the identification of frail, older adults in need of palliative interventions.

Chin et al.[5] identified a subset of these clinical markers, inactivity and weight loss, as predictive of disability and mortality in the Zutphen Elderly Study cohort. They considered frailty to be inactivity combined with low energy intake, weight loss, and low body mass index and determined that inactivity plus weight loss was the combination of these factors most predictive of the development of disability.[5] This further

Table 9–2. Validated Screening Criteria Used to Identify Frail, Older Adults in the Cardiovascular Health Study Cohort*

Weight loss
   10 or more pounds lost unintentionally in prior year

Grip strength
   Lowest 20% (by gender, body mass index)

Walking speed over 15 ft
   Slowest 20% (by gender, height)

Exhaustion
   Self-report

Activity levels
   Lowest 20% by gender
     Males: <383 kcal/week
     Females: <270 kcal/week

Source: Adapted from Fried et al. Frailty in older adults: evidence for a phenotype. J Gerontol 56A:M1–M11, 2001.
*Participants who met 3–5 criteria were deemed frail, those who meet one or two criteria were deemed intermediate or prefrail, and those who met no criterion were deemed not frail.

supports inactivity and weight loss as useful clinical markers of frailty. The prior study[1] found that use of three markers, rather than two, conferred improved specificity in identifying those at risk.

Although these two studies provided useful clinical markers to identify frailty in community-dwelling populations, there has been little, if any, investigation of the full spectrum of frailty and of its end stages. Verdery[40,41] and Berkman et al.[42] conceptualized this end-of-life phase as "failure to thrive." These authors hypothesized that a late or end stage of frailty exists that is irreversible, that nutritional and other interventions have minimal impact, and that this stage of frailty presages death. Although it is not yet clear that higher numbers of clinical signs and symptoms of frailty equate with end-stage frailty or failure to thrive, it is likely that these signs and symptoms are cumulative and that higher numbers of symptoms equate with greater severity. Since this more advanced stage of frailty is likely to be found in nursing homes or assisted living residents who manifest loss of ability to perform the activities of daily living, it is important to have a range of palliative care interventions for outpatient, inpatient, and long-term care settings to cover the range of frailty.

TREATMENT OPTIONS FOR FRAIL, OLDER ADULTS

In those who are at the end of life due to end-stage disease and/or severe frailty, maximizing quality of life through palliative care is paramount. In those frail, older adults who are not clearly in a terminal condition but suffer considerably from chronic disease and/or symptoms of frailty, palliative treatment that provides comfort but not necessarily cure is also an important part of any treatment plan. Palliative approaches to care across the spectrum of frailty include decreasing the amount of time in the hospital, preventing nursing home admissions, maintaining or improving functional status, and improving overall sense of well-being through a variety of medical, psychologic and social interventions. These goals are a hallmark of the practice of palliative care as well as geriatric medicine and are especially appropriate for the frail, older population.

Because frail, older adults are found throughout the health-care continuum, it is important to have treatment approaches for ambulatory as well as hospitalized patients. For most settings, multidisciplinary approaches to frail, older adults have been demonstrated to improve outcomes, as described below. Because frail patients may present in a spectrum from mild to severe end-stage frailty, it is also important to target interventions as appropriate to stage, especially if the patient has reached the end of life and has no possibility of improved health status or function. As the patient transitions into frailty and palliative care, it is critical to include the patient in any goal setting, treatment plans, and follow-up care. The following sections outline geriatric interventions that are applicable across the spectrum of frailty as well as interventions based on specific physiology that may play an important role in the future. Figure 9–4 illustrates the spectrum of frailty and a range of phase-specific palliative interventions covered in the text below.

Ambulatory Assessment and Treatment

Comprehensive geriatric assessment
Once the vulnerable, frail, older adult has been identified using the clinical signs and symptoms described above, a comprehensive geriatric assessment with the development and implementation of a multidisciplinary treatment plan may prove beneficial to the patient by both improving quality of life and decreasing a range of poor outcomes.[4] The multidisciplinary assessment and care team usually consists of a geriatrician or other medical practitioner experienced in the care of older adults, a nurse and/or social worker, and a physical or occupational therapist, if available. These professionals assess the patient, with history taken from caregivers, followed by a detailed discussion and synthesis of the data. Goals are set and treatment plans de-

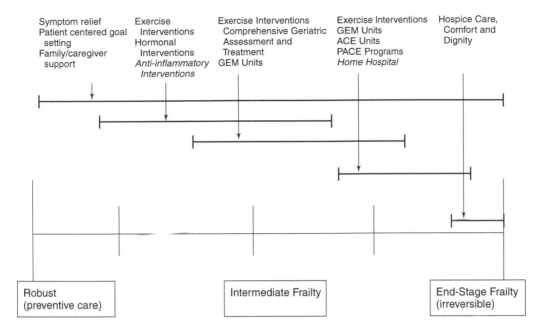

Figure 9–4. Spectrum of frailty in older adults, with suggested stage-appropriate palliative interventions. Those interventions under development are in italics. GEM, geriatric evaluation and management; ACE, acute care for elders; PACE, program of all-inclusive care for the elderly.

veloped with the patient and caregivers. Multidisiplinary geriatric assessments with ongoing follow-up care targeted at frail, older adults have been more successful than single visits.[43,44] For example, one-time multidisciplinary geriatric consultation targeted at a frail, ambulatory population coupled with the development and implementation of a treatment plan has been demonstrated to significantly reduce declines in function and quality of life.[44,45]

In any comprehensive geriatric assessment of a frail, older adult, it is of critical importance to rule out any potentially treatable causes of frailty. Because a number of treatable illnesses, including occult malignancy, chronic CHF, giant cell arteritis, rheumatoid arthritis, chronic infection, Parkinson's disease, and major depression, can present with signs and symptoms similar to frailty, the clinician must take special care to diagnose and treat these conditions when present.

After treatable medical conditions are identified and the levels of frailty and po-

tential vulnerability established, a treatment plan is developed by the participating clinicians and discussed and revised with the patient and caregiver. Most studies show that the benefit of comprehensive geriatric assessment comes only when the treatment plan is actually implemented, monitored, and revised through close follow-up.[45–47] Because of the wide variability in functional and medical conditions of frail, older adults, targeted interventions designed for a range of living situations, functional abilities, and severe frailty are necessary. Below are potential comprehensive treatment approaches that may benefit frail, older adults at many levels of severity. The overall goal of these treatment plans is palliation of symptoms and improvement in quality of life.

Comprehensive geriatric interdisciplinary treatment plans
Several studies have demonstrated the effectiveness of ongoing follow-up treatment plans and progress by nurse practitioners

with training in geriatric medicine. Stuck et al.[46] demonstrated reduction of onset of disability and of nursing home stays through annual geriatric-specialized nurse practitioner visits, including assessments, education, and recommendations, compared to usual medical care. Leveille et al.[47] demonstrated decreases in both the rate of functional decline and hospitalization using a targeted, multicomponent disability prevention and disease self-management program led by a nurse practitioner in a study of chronically ill, older adults who were deemed frail based on disability status. Other studies have demonstrated some efficacy of ongoing interventions by members of multidisciplinary teams, including physical therapists. Tinetti et al.[48] demonstrated a modest reduction in falls with a clinical intervention focused on minimizing multiple fall risk factors.

Geriatric evaluation and management units

Over the last two decades, comprehensive outpatient geriatric evaluation and management (GEM) units have proven efficacious in improving quality of life in older adults.[45,49] Although these interventions have not been targeted at frailty per se, frail, older adults are thought to be those most likely to benefit from them. For example, Boult et al.[45] identified a population of older adults at high risk for hospitalization and randomized them into either a GEM group or their usual medical care provider, who was informed of the higher hospitalization risk. After a 12- to 18-month follow-up period, those who received a comprehensive geriatric assessment followed by interdisciplinary primary care were significantly less likely than controls to lose function, to experience increased health-related restrictions in their daily activities, or to use home health services. The intervention did not affect mortality or use of health-care services and cost approximately $1350 per person above the usual medical fees.[45] Although more expensive than usual care, this approach appears to be effective at slowing functional

decline and improving quality of life, two of the most important goals of palliative care. It is, however, labor-intensive and requires intensive coordination of care, as appropriate to complex, frail, and ill older patients.

Physiologic system-targeted interventions

In addition to the effective multidisciplinary comprehensive care interventions targeted at the most frail and chronically ill older adults, substantial evidence supports the use of interventions targeted at specific components of frailty. Resistance or strengthening exercise interventions for skeletal muscle are well studied and clearly benefit the full spectrum of frail, older adults. Nutrition interventions are less clearly beneficial but probably useful in a subset of frail adults as a supplement to resistance exercise but not alone. Pain assessments and interventions are a critical component of any palliative care plan and, therefore, included in this section. Also included are discussions of inflammatory and hormonal interventions. While they are not yet clinically indicated for treatment or amelioration of frailty, those systems will very likely be future targets of intervention and are therefore included.

Exercise interventions

Numerous studies have demonstrated that exercise interventions are beneficial along the full continuum of frailty and its outcomes. In a study of very elderly, frail, nursing home subjects, progressive resistance exercise training markedly increased lean body mass, muscle strength, gait velocity, stair-climbing power, and spontaneous physical activity.[50] Another study of weight training in very elderly, frail, older adults demonstrated increased protein synthesis during a 6-month training period.[51] Other types of exercise have also been demonstrated to be beneficial in preventing falls in frail, older adults. In the Frailty and Injuries: Cooperative Studies of Intervention Techniques (FICSIT) trial, those participants who participated in a tai chi balance intervention had significantly fewer falls during and after the intervention period.[52] The same trial evaluated the effect of endurance exercise and showed minimal decrease in falls for that intervention.[52] In a recent meta-analysis of the effects of exercise on quality of life in the FICSIT cohort, investigators found that exercise produced small but significant improvements in emotional well-being and a trend toward improved social satisfaction.[53] Although exercise did not improve the perceptions of general health in this group, it did not increase bodily pain.[53] In a large review of both cross-sectional and longitudinal studies of chronically ill or frail, older adults who remain physically active, participants consistently reported feelings of increased well-being with high levels of physical activity.[54]

In summary, resistance exercise, as well as tai chi, have been studied in frail older adults. Each intervention has demonstrated some benefit in terms of function, quality of life, falls, and overall well-being across the spectrum of frailty. These outcomes are consistent with quality palliative care intervention and likely useful in all but the final stages of frailty. Despite a general consensus that exercise interventions are beneficial, specific guidelines for exercise programs for frail, older adults have not been developed. The appropriate or targeted level or type of activity remains to be determined.[54]

Nutritional interventions

Although frail, older adults frequently are undernourished or frankly malnourished, increased nutritional supplementation by itself has not been demonstrated to increase lean body mass or strength in cachectic patients.[55] In hospitalized older patients, Plank et al.[56] were unable to demonstrate any difference in the decline in lean body mass in acutely ill patients when intravenous nutritional supplementation was used. In a study of frail nursing home patients, nutritional supplementation by itself had no effect on strength, gait, stair-climbing power, or spontaneous physical activity. In fact, these patients decreased

their oral, spontaneous intake so that total intake remained stable. However, when added to resistance exercise, there was an increase in total caloric intake and a further increase in lean body mass and strength.[50] The inability of nutritional supplementation as a solo intervention to increase total caloric intake or to have any impact on strength or function or on the signs or symptoms of frailty is most likely secondary to the physiologic processes that underlie frailty. These processes, including low-grade inflammation and neuroendocrine dysregulation, likely profoundly influence appetite regulatory mechanisms and the utilization of protein substrate and render intensive nutritional supplementation on its own ineffective in frail, older adults.[55]

Pain interventions

Because pain is such a common problem in frail, older adults, especially in those with multiple chronic medical conditions, appropriate pain management is a critical component of any palliative intervention. This area of medicine has been traditionally understudied and undertreated in older adults.[57] In fact, a recent analysis named pain management as one of the highest priorities for quality care improvement in vulnerable older adults.[58] In addition, the American Geriatrics Society published a supplement on pain management specifically targeting frail, older adults over age 75.[7]

For all painful conditions where the etiology is not clear, a comprehensive evaluation of the type and severity of symptoms is necessary for appropriate care.[7,59] Because pain may present atypically or frail, older adults may have more difficulty in describing the pain, it is important to have the appropriate tools at hand and to enlist family and caregiver support when identifying and treating pain.[60] It is important to utilize tools that go beyond the usual intensity scales because of the differences in presentation and symptoms that frail, older adults may experience.[8] For example, a measurement tool, the Geriatric Pain Measure, has been developed, validated, and tested for reliability. It utilizes measures of functional decline related to pain rather than pure intensity of pain, to express the severity and impact of pain. This tool can also be utilized to monitor treatment effectiveness.[59] Because pain is most effectively treated when its pathologic basis is understood, the assessment process must focus on etiology as well as severity.

When developing a comprehensive pharmacologic pain management plan in older adults or in palliative care, a stepped-care approach may be useful. This approach is modeled after the World Health Organization's treatment of cancer pain, which progresses from nonopioid analgesics, such as acetaminophen, to nonsteroidal anti-inflammatory drugs to corticosteroids. Further steps in this treatment pathway include neuotransmitter-modulating drugs such as nortriptyline, membrane-stabilizing drugs such as gabapentin, and opioid narcotics.[57] Concurrent treatment of anxiety and depression may also alleviate or attenuate many painful conditions.[9] Exercise interventions may also play an important role in the management of pain and may help to prevent functional decline related to severe or chronic pain;[61] physical or occupational therapies may also offer nonpharmacologic interventions that decrease pain and improve function.[10]

As with any pharmacologic intervention in frail, older adults, extreme caution must be utilized because of the very high risk of adverse effects, especially delirium and falls.[62] However, judicious use of these medications, along with patient, family, and caregiver education, will help to ensure that pain is appropriately addressed and monitored without unnecessary adverse effects.

Hormonal interventions

Several investigators have suggested that age-related declines in circulating levels of GH, sex steroids, and the adrenal androgen dehydroepiandrosterone sulfate may play roles in muscle mass decline and, hence, in the development of frailty. However, to date, no hormonal intervention is recommended for frail, older adults unless a clear, clinical deficiency is noted. For example, while the replacement of testosterone in hypogonadal younger and older men has proven effective at increasing muscle mass and strength, no study has clearly demonstrated a benefit of testosterone for the treatment of frail, older men with normal, age-related but not pathologic declines in testosterone.[23] A number of GH interventions have also been evaluated in older men. Again, while there is a clear indication for GH replacement therapy in those with pituitary deficiency, no study has yet demonstrated the efficacy of GH or GH-releasing factor at improving quality of life or function.[63] Further intervention studies may be useful for determining which frail, older adults may benefit most from interventions targeting weakness and fatigue.

Anti-inflammatory interventions

Although there is considerable evidence of a relationship between chronically elevated IL-6 and outcomes related to frailty in older adults, including muscle mass decline, anemia, disability, and early mortality, no treatment targeting inflammation has been developed or tested to date in frail, older adults. However, tumor necrosis factor-α inhibitors are currently in use for the adjuvant treatment of inflammation triggered by rheumatoid arthritis and other connective tissue disorders.[64,65] These agents have effects on several of the systemic symptoms of rheumatoid arthritis, which are similar to those of frailty, such as weakness, fatigue, and anemia.[65,66] Given our increasing understanding of the role of inflammation in the development of frailty, use of a more specific anti-inflammatory agent could delay the onset or progression of frailty while improving symptoms and quality of life. These goals are consistent with palliative care treatment plans and worthy of further study.

Palliative Care for Hospitalized Frail, Older Adults

Frail, older adults are hospitalized at higher rates than nonfrail adults, and the overall number of hospital admissions related to frailty is rapidly increasing.[1,67] This increasing frequency of hospitalization comes despite the fact that frail, older adults may be placed at risk by the hospitalization itself, may have increased vulnerability to adverse outcomes of invasive medical procedures, and are the most likely to suffer iatrogenic complications.[68] These most vulnerable older adults are more likely to develop delirium, lose function, fall, develop hospital-acquired infections, and die while hospitalized.[69] Because of the high risk of poor outcomes in frailty, careful consideration must be given to the benefit and burdens of hospitalization; and once admitted, their risk of adverse effects must be continuously monitored and minimized. Application of palliative care models to this group of individuals should focus on meticulous identification and treatment of symptom distress, preventing loss of function, preventing delirium, rapid return to the home setting, and coordination of outpatient or home care that may help prevent recurrent admissions and improve overall quality of life.

Identification of frail, older adults in the hospital setting

As with ambulatory patients, the identification of frailty in hospitalized patients is a necessary first step toward appropriate palliative care. Functional status before, during, and after hospitalization has been demonstrated to have important predictive value for outcomes.[70] Carlson et al.[71] identified change in functional status from acute illness as an independent predictor of adverse outcomes.[71] In the same study, change in function during hospitalization was a better predictor of poor outcomes than level of function at discharge.[71] Premorbid functional dependence and functional decline on admission were also predictive of worse outcomes in frail, hospitalized patients.[69] In the same study, frail compared to non-frail, older adults were far more likely to present with delirium (61% vs. 32%) and to have an atypical disease presentation (59% vs. 29%).[69] In summary, the results of these studies suggest the use of functional decline (especially during the hospital stay), delirium, and atypical disease presentation as markers of frailty and of risk for poor outcomes for hospitalized adults. These characteristics can then be utilized to appropriately target palliative care interventions toward frail patients who would most benefit.

Hospital-based palliative interventions for frail, older adults

As with outpatient care for frail, older adults, a multidisciplinary team consultation and care led by geriatricians appear to be among the most beneficial interventions to prevent iatrogenic complications, to improve clinical outcomes, and to improve quality of life.[49,72] The model most frequently applied to frail, older adults uses acute care of the elderly (ACE) units. These specialized units have been designed to target the most vulnerable older adults. Interventions have typically included a specially designed, more home-based environment;[9] patient-centered care plan, with focus on the prevention of disability and iatrogenic illness; and more intensive and comprehensive discharge planning and management.[73,74] These interventions have been demonstrated, through a randomized controlled study of 1531 community-dwelling individuals aged 70 and older, to be effective at reducing poor activities of daily living outcomes and decreasing nursing home placement goals that are consistent with palliative care.[73] In addition, ACE interventions do not increase costs or length of stay compared to usual hospital care.[73,75]

Alternative models for residential or hospital care in frail, older adults

Given that frail, older adults do suffer more comorbidities and adverse effects of hospitalization, alternative programs designed to provide comfort care and modest medical interventions in the home or in the outpatient clinic setting have been developed. The most widely utilized model is the Program for All-Inclusive Care of the Elderly (PACE). In this program, community-based primary care is delivered by interdisciplinary teams to provide targeted, thoughtful care in the appropriate setting, be it hospital, home, or nursing home.[76] This program is delivered on a capitated basis to participants who are eligible for nursing home placement. The model enables the participant to stay in the community setting through the establishment of a multidisciplinary care plan by a team that usually includes trained geriatrics providers, nurses, physical and occupational therapists, and social workers. The team, patient, and family develop a variety of patient-centered palliative interventions that decrease symptoms, improve function, overcome environmental challenges, and prevent hospital admissions.

Early studies of targeted delivery of hospital care in the home have demonstrated the potential utility of this delivery system within the spectrum of care of frail, older adults. In this developing model, community-dwelling persons aged 65 and older were enrolled for diagnoses of community-acquired pneumonia, CHF, chronic obstructive airways disease, and cellulitis.[77] Data from the pilot study have demonstrated that home hospital care was safe, effective, and highly satisfactory to those who participated.[77] Further trials in larger, older populations are under way to determine the safety and efficacy of this model in larger cohorts with a broader array of medical diagnoses and prognoses. If deemed safe and effective for a more frail cohort, this intervention may prove useful in the palliative care of frailty.

Family involvement
As older adults transition into frailty and are less able to tend to their needs, the family is typically mobilized to provide a broad range of informal services. This transition toward increased dependence on family or other caregivers is another marker for the increased need for palliative interventions. Most of this informal and unreimbursed care is performed by a spouse or an adult daughter and can be increasingly taxing both physically and psychologically as mobility and function decrease across the spectrum of frailty.[78] Following the identification of responsible caregivers, a number of practical family interventions may be useful in furthering any palliative treatment goals. Providing accurate and comprehensive information to the patient and family member and assessing their understanding of that information are a crucial first steps. The development of any comprehensive palliative treatment plan must include family and other caregivers to be effective. Defining end points and guidelines for symptom control and mechanisms for effective communication with health-care providers is crucial. Attention to the potential for caregiver burnout and options for caregiver support will help to ensure effective palliative treatment interventions.[78]

SUMMARY AND CONCLUSIONS

Frailty is an increasingly recognized clinical state of vulnerability with inherent increased risks of poor outcomes in a subset of older adults. Because of this vulnerability and the low probability of curing advanced frailty, this group is an excellent target for a broad range of palliative interventions. The recent development of conceptual models of frailty as well as investigation of the clinical syndrome and consequences of frailty have highlighted the need for further etiologic and intervention studies. Progress in the study of physiologic and etiologic factors that may influence frailty, including inflammation, neuroendocrine changes, and several specific disease states, may herald the introduction of new palliative treatments targeted at the symptoms of frailty. This new epidemiologic and biologic information together with the demonstrated efficacy of patient-centered, multidisciplinary treatment approaches across the spectrum of frailty provides the health-care worker with a wide variety of palliative treatment options for this most vulnerable subset of older adults.

REFERENCES

1. Fried LP, Tangen C, Walston J, Newman A, Hirsch CH, Gottdiener JS, Seeman T,

Tracy R, Kop WJ, Burke G, McBurnie MA. Frailty in older adults: evidence for a phenotype. J Gerontol 56A:M1–M11, 2001.

2. Walston J, McBurnie MA, Newman A, Tracy R, Kop WJ, Hirsch CH, Gottdiener JS, Fried LP. Frailty is associated with activation of the inflammation and coagulation systems, and with glucose intolerance, independent of clinical comorbidities: results from the Cardiovascular Health Study. Arch Intern Med 162(20):2333–41, 2002.

3. Newman AB, Gottdiener JS, Mcburnie MA, Hirsch CH, Kop WJ, Tracy R, Walston JD, Fried LP. Associations of subclinical cardiovascular disease with frailty. J Gerontol A Biol Sci Med Sci 56:M158–M166, 2001.

4. Fried LP, Walston J. Frailty and failure to thrive. In: Hazzard W (Ed.). Principles of Geriatric Medicine and Gerontology, New York, McGraw Hill, 1998, pp. 1387–1402.

5. Chin A, Paw MJ, Dekker JM, Feskens EJ, Schouten EG, Kromhout D. How to select a frail elderly population? A comparison of three working definitions. J Clin Epidemiol 52:1015–1021, 1999.

6. Hamerman D. Toward an understanding of frailty. Ann Intern Med 130:945–950, 1999.

7. AGS panel on persistent pain in older persons. The management of persistent pain in older persons. J Am Geriatr Soc 50(Supp 6):5205–5224, 2002.

8. Gloth FM III. Concerns with chronic analgesic therapy in elderly patients. Am J Med 101:19S–24S, 1996.

9. Gloth FM III. Geriatric pain. Factors that limit pain relief and increase complications. Geriatrics 55:46–48, 2000.

10. Gloth FM III. Pain management in older adults: prevention and treatment. J Am Geriatr Soc 49:188–199, 2001.

11. Leng S, Chaves P, Koenig K, Walston J. Serum interleukin-6 and hemoglobin as physiologic correlates in the geriatric syndrome of frailty: a pilot study. J Am Geriatr Soc 50(7):1268–1271, 2002.

12. Roubenoff R. Sarcopenia: a major modifiable cause of frailty in the elderly. J Nutr Health Aging 4:140–142, 2000.

13. Evans WJ. What is sarcopenia? J Gerontol A Biol Sci Med Sci 50:5–8, 1995.

14. Metter EJ, Conwit R, Tobin J, Fozard JL. Age-associated loss of power and strength in the upper extremities in women and men. J Gerontol A Biol Sci Med Sci 52:B267–B276, 1997.

15. Bassey EJ, Fiatarone MA, O'Neill EF, Kelly M, Evans WJ, Lipsitz LA. Leg extensor power and functional performance in very old men and women. Clin Sci (Colch) 82:321–327, 1992.

16. Rice CL, Cunningham DA, Paterson DH, Lefcoe MS. Arm and leg composition determined by computed tomography in young and elderly men. Clin Physiol 9:207–220, 1989.

17. Larsson L, Ramamurthy B. Aging-related changes in skeletal muscle. Mech Intervent Drugs Aging 17:303–316, 2000.

18. Morley JE, Kaiser FE, Sih R, Hajjar R, Perry HM III. Testosterone and frailty. Clin Geriatr Med 13:685–695, 1997.

19. Nourhashemi F, Andrieu S, Gillette-Guyonnet S, Vellas B, Albarede JL, Grandjean H. Instrumental activities of daily living as a potential marker of frailty: a study of 7364 community-dwelling elderly women (the EPIDOS Study). J Gerontol A Biol Sci Med Sci 56:M448–M453, 2001.

20. Morley JE, Kaiser FE, Perry HM III, Patrick P, Morley PM, Stauber PM, Vellas B, Baumgartner RN, Garry PJ. Longitudinal changes in testosterone, luteinizing hormone, and follicle-stimulating hormone in healthy older men. Metabolism 46:410–413, 1997.

21. O'Connor KG, Tobin JD, Harman SM, Plato CC, Roy TA, Sherman SS, Blackman MR. Serum levels of insulin-like growth factor-I are related to age and not to body composition in healthy women and men. J Gerontol A Biol Sci Med Sci 53:M176–M182, 1998.

22. Cappola AR, Bandeen-Roche K, Wand GS, Volpato S, Fried LP. Association of IGF-1 levels with muscle strength and mobility in older women. J Clin Endocrinol Metab 86:4139–4146, 2001.

23. Lamberts SW, van den Beld AW, van der Lely AJ. The endocrinology of aging. Science 278:419–424, 1997.

24. Lowy MT, Wittenberg L, Yamamoto BK. Effect of acute stress on hippocampal glutamate levels and spectrin proteolysis in young and aged rats. J Neurochem 65:268–274, 1995.

25. Sapolsky RM, Krey LC, McEwen BS. The neuroendocrinology of stress and aging: the glucocorticoid cascade hypothesis. Endocr Rev 7:284–301, 1986.

26. Seeman TE, Robbins RJ. Aging and hypothalamic–pituitary–adrenal responseto challenge in humans. Endocr Rev 15:233–260, 1994.

27. Van Cauter E, Leproult R, Kupfer DJ. Effects of gender and age on the levels and circadian rhythmicity of plasma cortisol. J Clin Endocrinol Metab 81:2468–2473, 1996.

28. Aasebo U, Bremnes RM, de Jong FH, Aakvaag A, Slordal L. Pituitary–gonadal dysfunction in male patients with lung cancer. Association with serum inhibin levels. Acta Oncol 33:177–180, 1994.

29. Morley JE, Melmed S. Gonadal dysfunction

in systemic disorders. Metabolism 28: 1051–1073, 1979.

30. Spector TD, Perry LA, Tubb G, Silman AJ, Huskisson EC. Low free testosterone levels in rheumatoid arthritis. Ann Rheum Dis 47:65–68, 1988.

31. Ershler WB, Keller ET. Age-associated increased interleukin-6 gene expression, late-life diseases, and frailty. Annu Rev Med 51:245–270, 2000.

32. Cohen HJ, Pieper CF, Harris T, Rao KM, Currie MS. The association of plasma IL-6 levels with functional disability in community-dwelling elderly. J Gerontol A Biol Sci Med Sci 52:M201–M208, 1997.

33. Harris TB, Ferrucci L, Tracy RP, Corti MC, Wacholder S, Ettinger WH Jr, Heimovitz H, Cohen HJ, Wallace R. Associations of elevated interleukin-6 and C-reactive protein levels with mortality in the elderly. Am J Med 106:506–512, 1999.

34. Buchner DM, Wagner EH. Preventing frail health. Clin Geriatr Med 8:1–17, 1992.

35. Lipsitz LA, Goldberger AL. Loss of "complexity" and aging. Potential applications of fractals and chaos theory to senescence. JAMA 267:1806–1809, 1992.

36. Evans WJ, Roubenoff R, Shevitz A. Exercise and the treatment of wasting: aging and human immunodeficiency virus infection. Semin Oncol 25(2 Suppl 6):112–122, 1998.

37. Margolick JB, Chopra RK. Relationship between the immune system and frailty: pathogenesis of immune deficiency in HIV infection and aging. Aging (Milano) 4:255–257, 1992.

38. Jorgensen JO, Vahl N, Hansen TB, Skjaerbaek C, Fisker S, Orskov H, Hagen C, Christiansen JS. Determinants of serum insulin-like growth factor I in growth hormone deficient adults as compared to healthy subjects. Clin Endocrinol (Oxf) 48:479–486, 1998.

39. Kanda N, Tsuchida T, Tamaki K. Testosterone suppresses anti-DNA antibody production in peripheral blood mononuclear cells from patients wth systemic lupus erythematosus. Arthritis Rheum 40:1703–1711, 1997.

40. Verdery RB. Failure to thrive in older people. J Am Geriatr Soc 44:465–466, 1996.

41. Verdery RB. Failure to thrive in the elderly. Clin Geriatr Med 11:653–659, 1995.

42. Berkman B, Foster LW, Campion E. Failure to thrive: paradigm for the frail elder. Gerontologist 29:654–659, 1989.

43. Epstein AM, Hall JA, Fretwell M, Feldstein M, DeCiantis ML, Tognetti J, Cutler C, Constantine M, Besdine R, Rowe J. Consultative geriatric assessment for ambulatory patients. A randomized trial in a health maintenance organization. JAMA 263: 538–544, 1990.

44. Reuben DB, Frank JC, Hirsch SH, McGuigan KA, Maly RC. A randomized clinical trial of outpatient comprehensive geriatric assessment coupled with an intervention to increase adherence to recommendations. J Am Geriatr Soc 47:269–276, 1999.

45. Boult C, Boult LB, Morishita L, Dowd B, Kane RL, Urdangarin CF. A randomized clinical trial of outpatient geriatric evaluation and management. J Am Geriatr Soc 49:351–359, 2001.

46. Stuck AE, Aronow HU, Steiner A, Alessi CA, Bula CJ, Gold MN, Yuhas KE, Nisenbaum R, Rubenstein LZ, Beck JC. A trial of annual in-home comprehensive geriatric assessments for elderly people living in the community. N Engl J Med 333:1184–1189, 1995.

47. Leveille SG, Wagner EH, Davis C, Grothaus L, Wallace J, LoGerfo M, Kent D. Preventing disability and managing chronic illness in frail older adults: a randomized trial of a community-based partnership with primary care. J Am Geriatr Soc 46:1191–1198, 1998.

48. Tinetti ME, Baker DI, McAvay G, Claus EB, Garrett P, Gottschalk M, Koch ML, Trainor K, Horwitz RI. A multifactorial intervention to reduce the risk of falling among elderly people living in the community. N Engl J Med 331:821–827, 1994.

49. Rubenstein LZ, Josephson KR, Wieland GD, English PA, Sayre JA, Kane RL. Effectiveness of a geriatric evaluation unit. A randomized clinical trial. N Engl J Med 311:1664–1670, 1984.

50. Fiatarone MA, O'Neill EF, Ryan ND, Clements KM, Solares GR, Nelson ME, Roberts SB, Kehayias JJ, Lipsitz LA, Evans WJ. Exercise training and nutritional supplementation for physical frailty in very elderly people. N Engl J Med 330:1769–1775, 1994.

51. Yarasheski KE, Pak-Loduca J, Hasten DL, Obert KA, Brown MB, Sinacore DR. Resistance exercise training increases mixed muscle protein synthesis rate in frail women and men ≥ 76 years old. Am J Physiol 277:E118–E125, 1999.

52. Province MA, Hadley EC, Hornbrook MC, Lipsitz LA, Miller JP, Mulrow CD, Ory MG, Sattin RW, Tinetti ME, Wolf SL. The effects of exercise on falls in elderly patients. A preplanned meta-analysis of the FICSIT trials. Frailty and Injuries: Cooperative Studies of Intervention Techniques. JAMA 273:1341–1347, 1995.

53. Schechtman KB, Ory MG. The effects of exercise on the quality of life of frail older

adults: a preplanned meta-analysis of the FICSIT trials. Ann Behav Med 23:186–197, 2001.

54. Spirduso WW, Cronin DL. Exercise dose-response effects on quality of life and independent living in older adults. Med Sci Sports Exerc 33:S598–S608, 2001.

55. Kotler DP. Cachexia. Ann Intern Med 133:622–634, 2000.

56. Plank LD, Connolly AB, Hill GL. Sequential changes in the metabolic response in severely septic patients during the first 23 days after the onset of peritonitis. Ann Surg 228:146–158, 1998.

57. Weiner DK, Hanlon JT. Pain in nursing home residents: management strategies. Drugs Aging 18:13–29, 2001.

58. Sloss EM, Solomon DH, Shekelle PG, Young RT, Saliba D, MacLean CH, Rubenstein LZ, Schnelle JF, Kamberg CJ, Wenger NS. Selecting target conditions for quality of care improvement in vulnerable older adults. J Am Geriatr Soc 48:363–369, 2000.

59. Ferrell BA. Pain management. Clin Geriatr Med 16:853–874, 2000.

60. Juarez G, Ferrell BR. Family and caregiver involvement in pain management. Clin Geriatr Med 12:531–547, 1996.

61. Gloth MJ, Matesi AM. Physical therapy and exercise in pain management. Clin Geriatr Med 17:525–535, 2001.

62. Inouye SK, Bogardus ST Jr, Baker DI, Leo-Summers L, Cooney LM Jr. The Hospital Elder Life Program: a model of care to prevent cognitive and functional decline in older hospitalized patients. J Am Geriatr Soc 48:1697–1706, 2000.

63. Lamberts SW. The somatopause: to treat or not to treat? Horm Res 53(Suppl 3):42–43, 2000.

64. Criscione LG, St Clair EW. Tumor necrosis factor-alpha antagonists for the treatment of rheumatic diseases. Curr Opin Rheumatol 14:204–211, 2002.

65. Gorman JD, Sack KE, Davis JC Jr. Treatment of ankylosing spondylitis by inhibition of tumor necrosis factor alpha. N Engl J Med 346:1349–1356, 2002.

66. Kietz DA, Pepmueller PH, Moore TL. Clinical response to etanercept in polyarticular course juvenile rheumatoid arthritis. J Rheumatol 28:360–362, 2001.

67. Haan MN, Selby JV, Quesenberry CP Jr, Schmittdiel JA, Fireman BH, Rice DP. The impact of aging and chronic disease on use of hospital and outpatient services in a large HMO: 1971–1991. J Am Geriatr Soc 45:667–674, 1997.

68. Fried TR, Mor V. Frailty and hospitalization of long-term stay nursing home residents. J Am Geriatr Soc 45:265–269, 1997.

69. Jarrett PG, Rockwood K, Carver D, Stolee P, Cosway S. Illness presentation in elderly patients. Arch Intern Med 155:1060–1064, 1995.

70. Covinsky KE, Palmer RM, Counsell SR, Pine ZM, Walter LC, Chren MM. Functional status before hospitalization in acutely ill older adults: validity and clinical importance of retrospective reports. J Am Geriatr Soc 48:164–169, 2000.

71. Carlson JE, Zocchi KA, Bettencourt DM, Gambrel ML, Freeman JL, Zhang D, Goodwin JS. Measuring frailty in the hospitalized elderly: concept of functional homeostasis. Am J Phys Med Rehabil 77:252–257, 1998.

72. Landefeld CS, Palmer RM, Kresevic DM, Fortinsky RH, Kowal J. A randomized trial of care in a hospital medical unit especially designed to improve the functional outcomes of acutely ill older patients. N Engl J Med 332:1338–1344, 1995.

73. Counsell SR, Holder CM, Liebenauer LL, Palmer RM, Fortinsky RH, Kresevic DM, Quinn LM, Allen KR, Covinsky KE, Landefeld CS. Effects of a multicomponent intervention on functional outcomes and process of care in hospitalized older patients: a randomized controlled trial of acute care for elders (ACE) in a community hospital. J Am Geriatr Soc 48:1572–1581, 2000.

74. Walter LC, Brand RJ, Counsell SR, Palmer RM, Landefeld CS, Fortinsky RH, Covinsky KE. Development and validation of a prognostic index for 1-year mortality in older adults after hospitalization. JAMA 285:2987–2994, 2001.

75. Covinsky KE, King JT Jr, Quinn LM, Siddique R, Palmer R, Kresevic DM, Fortinsky RH, Kowal J, Landefeld CS. Do acute care for elders units increase hospital costs? A cost analysis using the hospital perspective. J Am Geriatr Soc 45:729–734, 1997.

76. Wieland D, Lamb VL, Sutton SR, Boland R, Clark M, Friedman S, Brummel-Smith K, Eleazer GP. Hospitalization in the Program of All-Inclusive Care for the Elderly (PACE): rates, concomitants, and predictors. J Am Geriatr Soc 48:1373–1380, 2000.

77. Leff B, Burton L, Guido S, Greenough WB, Steinwachs D, Burton JR. Home hospital program: a pilot study. J Am Geriatr Soc 47:697–702, 1999.

78. Rapp S, Reynolds D. Families, social support, and caregiving. In: Hazzard W, Blass J, Ettinger W, Halter J, Ouslander J (Eds.). Principles of Geriatric Medicine and Gerontology, 4th ed. New York, McGraw-Hill, pp. 333–343, 1999.

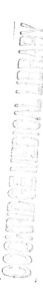

10

Heart Disease

JULIA M. ADDINGTON-HALL, ANGIE ROGERS,
ANNE McCOY, AND J. SIMON R. GIBBS

In this chapter, we focus on the application of palliative care to older people living with, and dying from, chronic heart failure (CHF). Older people with other heart conditions may also have needs within the remit of palliative care, particularly those with intractable angina. There is, however, some evidence, albeit limited, about the palliative care needs of people with CHF and the effectiveness of services at addressing these needs; but there is almost none outside of CHF. In addition, CHF is the only major cardiovascular disease with increasing incidence, and its incidence increases with age. By concentrating on CHF, we are making best use of the limited available evidence base, as well as addressing a condition that is particularly associated with aging.

CHRONIC HEART FAILURE

Chronic heart failure is a progressive disease that constitutes the final common pathway of many cardiovascular diseases. For clinical purposes, *heart failure* is defined by the European Society of Cardiology[1] as the symptoms of heart failure at rest or during exercise together with objective evidence of cardiac dysfunction, most commonly obtained by echocardiography. This evidence is important because heart failure is a clinical syndrome: the symptoms are nonspecific, and other conditions, such as circulatory, renal, or liver failure, may present with the same clinical picture as heart failure. A favorable response to heart failure treatment provides further evidence for the diagnosis. Identification of the etiology completes the diagnosis of heart failure, but it may not be possible or appropriate to pursue this, particularly in older, frail patients. The commonest cause of heart failure is coronary artery disease;[2] other causes include hypertension, valvular heart disease, arrhythmias, dilated cardiomyopathy, and alcohol.

Chronic heart failure is underdiagnosed in older people, particularly those aged 75 or older in whom nonspecific presentation is more common than in younger people.[3] Patients may present with confusion, depression, fatigue, weight loss, immobility, or a failure to cope at home. Up to half of patients in this age group who have activity-limiting CHF are undiagnosed and therefore untreated.[4] This may, at least in part, be due to older people themselves, their families, and on occasion their physicians attributing their symptoms to the normal effects of aging.[3]

Clinical Features

The clinical course of CHF is characterized by progressively worsening symptoms and frequent acute episodes of deterioration requiring hospitalization. Modern therapies slow but do not stop disease progression. The cardinal symptoms are breathlessness and fatigue. These are not a direct effect of poor cardiac function (the cause of heart failure), and the functional ability of CHF patients correlates poorly with left ventricular dysfunction.[5,6] Instead, the pathophysiological explanation for breathlessness and fatigue may involve deconditioning, wasting, and metabolic changes in skeletal muscle that activate ergo[7] and chemo[8] reflexes and influence sympathetic activation. Fluid retention is often evident at presentation or subsequently if deterioration occurs and is associated with breathlessness, cough, nocturia, swollen lower limbs/sacrum, anorexia, nausea, abdominal bloating, and liver capsular pain.

Drug Therapies

Advances in the pharmacological management of heart failure in the last 20 years may slow the progression of the disease and improve survival. Most research has, however, been conducted on the 17% of patients with CHF who are aged 65 or below, and the results have been extrapolated to older people.[3] It has been argued that, as a consequence, the benefits of β-blockers and spironolactone on those aged 75 and above are unknown.[3] Angiotensin-converting enzyme inhibitors (ACEIs) are, however, the cornerstone of therapy;[9] and there is evidence of their beneficial effects in older people, in whom they are probably underused.[3] The ACEIs produce consistent improve-

ments in symptoms and cardiac function and significantly reduce all-cause mortality by 20%–25% as well as recurrent hospital admissions for heart failure. They may, however, cause or contribute to renal failure, although the benefits of treatment may outweigh renal dysfunction, particularly in patients with severe heart failure. Their use in older patients needs to be carefully monitored, particularly during intercurrent disease. Randomized controlled trials of β-blockers (carvedilol, metoprolol, and bisoprolol) have shown that they reduce mortality and hospital admissions and improve functional class when added to ACEI therapy.[10] Spironolactone in low doses is indicated for severe CHF in addition to these therapies.[11] Digoxin, used in patients with sinus rhythm, may improve symptoms and reduce hospitalization but does not improve prognosis.[12] Diuretics are used to reduce fluid retention.

EPIDEMIOLOGY

Chronic heart failure is the only major cardiovascular disease with increasing incidence. It currently affects an estimated 3 million[13] to 4.7 million[14] people in the United States each year, and there are an estimated 400,000 new cases annually.[15] In the United Kingdom, the crude annual incidence rate is at least 1.3 cases per 1000 population for those aged 25 year or over[16] and the incidence is higher in men than in women (age-adjusted incidence ratio = 1.75).[17]

The incidence and prevalence of CHF increase with age. In the United Kingdom, the annual incidence rate in a community-based sample increased from 0.02 cases per 1000 population in those aged 25–34 years to 11.6 in those aged 85 years and over: the median age at presentation was 76 years.[16] In the United States, CHF is present in 2 in 100 people aged 40–59, more than 5 in 100 aged 60–69, and 10 in 100 aged 70 and older.[15] Only 17% of people with heart failure are aged 65 years or less.[3] With age-related mortality rates from cardiovascular disease declining and the size of the older population growing, the absolute number of people living with compromised cardiac function is expected to increase dramatically over the next few decades.[18] This has important consequences for health-care provision: hospital admissions and expenditure on heart failure have been increasing for over a decade,[15,19] CHF accounts for up to 2% of National Health Service costs in the United Kingdom, and care of CHF patients in the United States was estimated to cost $17.8 billion in 1993.[15]

Patients with CHF have high mortality rates. A population-based survey of newly diagnosed cases of heart failure in London found a mortality rate of 25% at 3 months and by 1 year 38% had died.[20] In hospital-based studies, CHF has a mortality rate of 31%–48% at 1 year and 76% at 3 years.[21–23] Age has an important effect on survival, with one-quarter (24%) of patients aged under 55 admitted with a principal diagnosis of heart failure dying within 1 year compared to 58% of those aged 85 or above.[24] It is estimated to account for at least 42,000 deaths each year in the United States, with another 219,000 related to the condition.[15]

Predicting Prognosis

Poor prognosis in CHF is predicted by poor left ventricular function, severe symptoms,[25] and metabolic markers.[26] While these factors may be useful in identifying groups of patients at increased risk of dying, they are less helpful in predicting individual prognoses. No prognostic models of CHF are as yet satisfactory, and a sizeable minority of patients die suddenly from a cardiac arrhythmia. There is no accepted marker to determine which patients are likely to do so.

The difficulties inherent in estimating prognosis in CHF are demonstrated powerfully by data from the Study to Understand Prognoses and Preferences for Outcomes and Risks of Treatments (SUPPORT), a prospective study undertaken in the United States in five academic medical centers. Multivariate computer models based on patient clinical and biochemical indices were developed to predict prognosis and found

to have a high degree of accuracy overall. Prognosis in CHF was much more difficult to predict than in cancer. On the day before death, lung cancer patients were estimated to have a <5% chance of surviving for 2 months while CHF patients had a >40% chance.[27]

Further analyses attempted to identify a population of patients with advanced lung, heart, or liver disease with a survival prognosis of 6 months or less using National Hospice Organisation guidelines.[28] These clinical prediction criteria were not effective at doing so, as the authors noted, "amongst patients meeting various combinations of criteria, 6-month survival ranged from 53% to 70%." One-quarter (655) of the 2607 patients who survived to hospital discharge died within 6 months. The criteria failed to correctly identify these patients; the most lenient criteria excluded 65% of them, while the most restrictive eliminated 99% of those who died within 6 months. The authors concluded that "the goal of determining in advance—with a high degree of accuracy—which individual patients with COPD, CHF or ESLD will die within six months is unrealistic." This has important implications for the development of appropriate services to address the palliative care needs of patients with CHF, and we will return to this later.

SYMPTOM CONTROL

Much of the evidence about the symptoms people with heart failure experience in the last months and weeks of life comes from two major contemporary studies of dying. The first is the Regional Study of Care for the Dying (RSCD), a population-based retrospective survey of a random sample of people who died in 20 English health districts in 1990. The study included 675 patients who died from heart disease of all causes.[29,30] Sudden deaths were excluded from the analysis of symptoms in the last year of life, so it is likely that many of these people died from heart failure. The second study is SUPPORT, which has already been mentioned. It included nine diagnostic groups of hospitalized patients with an aggregate mortality rate of 50% within 6 months. Out of the total of 9105 patients, 1404 had heart failure.[31]

In the RSCD, people who died from heart disease were reported by bereaved relatives and others who knew them to have experienced a wide range of symptoms in the last year of life. Many were reported to have found these symptoms distressing, and the symptoms often lasted more than 6 months. Pain was the most commonly reported symptom (78%) and was reported to have been very distressing for 50% of patients. This was surprising as pain has not been seen as a significant symptom in heart failure. We will return to pain in more detail below. Unsurprisingly, breathlessness was the second most commonly reported symptom (61%) and was reported to have been very distressing in 43% of patients. The survey did not ask about fatigue. More than half (59%) were reported to have had low mood and 45% anxiety. These symptoms were common in the last week of life as well as in the last year: 63% were reported to have had pain, 51% breathlessness, and 42% low mood. More than two-fifths (43%) of patients aged 85 and over were reported to have experienced confusion in the last year of life compared to 27% of those aged under 55 years. Quality of life was reported to have been poor in almost one-quarter of patients (24%), and a similar proportion (23%) was believed to have wanted to die earlier: this was associated with older age (75 or older), the number and severity of symptoms, and quality of life. Respondents reported low levels of symptom control: pain was reported to have been controlled partially or not at all in hospital by 34% of respondents, and 24% reported similar low levels of control in hospital of breathlessness. More than half (54%) of this sample died in hospital.

In SUPPORT, functional impairments, depression scores, and the percentage of patients reported by surrogates to have severe pain or breathlessness increased as death approached, with 41% of surrogates for patients who were conscious in the last 3 days reporting that the patient was in severe pain and 63% reporting that the patient experienced severe breathlessness during this period.[32]

Pain

Both the RSCD and SUPPORT identified pain as a significant problem for patients with heart disease/heart failure in the last days and months of life. As already indicated, this is surprising as pain is not normally regarded as an important symptom in heart failure. One explanation for this may be that both studies relied on retrospective proxy accounts of the patients' experiences. There is good evidence that proxy accounts of pain do not tally well with those of patients and may say more about the relatives' distress at watching their loved one in pain than about the patient's actual level of pain.[33] Proxies may be observing the patients' general distress and attributing it to pain. Prospective accounts of the pain experienced by patients living with severe CHF are therefore needed. Preliminary findings from a cohort study of 200 patients with CHF that we conducted suggest that pain is less prevalent than the retrospective studies suggest (27%) but that its prevalence increases with the severity of heart failure (J.M. Addington-Hall, et al., unpublished data). Pain may be caused by a variety of problems, including angina, liver capsular distension due to fluid retention, ankle swelling, and a comorbid disease such as arthritis. This is an important issue for older people with CHF, many of whom are likely to have musculoskeletal conditions. Nonsteroidal anti-inflammatories are contraindicated in CHF, and it was apparent in our prospective survey that a significant minority were taken off these drugs but not offered other analgesia. The principles of pain control developed within palliative care need to be applied to these patients, regardless of the cause of their pain.

DEPRESSION

Depression is a common problem among older people. Between 10% and 45% of hospitalized older people are clinically depressed.[34] It is commonly under-diagnosed, partly because depression is often accompanied by subjective memory loss and other signs of cognitive impairment, which may in older patients be wrongly attributed to dementia.[35,36] In addition, somatic symptoms are less helpful in diagnosing depression in older people, where disrupted sleep, fatigue, and constipation may be common in the non-depressed.[37] Early recognition and effective management of depression in older people are important if functional abilities are to be maintained and the heightened risk of mortality associated with depression avoided.[38]

Depression is also common in coronary heart disease (CHD): it has been identified in about 15% of patients following an acute myocardial infarction,[39-42] with comparable rates for CHD patients in outpatient clinics.[43,44,45] Again, depression is frequently underdiagnosed and undertreated. It has often been viewed as an inevitable consequence of coping with a cardiac event, and the somatic symptoms may be attributed to the impact of heart disease.[46] Detecting and treating depression is important in these patients because depressed post-myocardial infarction patients are at higher risk than those who are not depressed of reinfarction and hospitalization,[39,40] angina,[42] functional limitations,[47] reduced quality of life,[48] and death.[39,40]

As we have already seen, CHD accounts for more than half of all CHF cases,[49,50] and CHF is a disease of older age, with incidence rising with increasing age. Given the increased prevalence of depression in both older people and those with CHD, it is not surprising that depression is an important problem in CHF. A consecutive sample of medically ill patients aged over 60 years who were admitted to hospital were assessed for depression using the Diagnostic Interview Schedule.[51] Nearly two-fifths (36.5%) of those with a diagnosis of CHF had major depression, and one-fifth (21.5%) showed signs of minor depression. The rate of major depression was significantly higher than among comparable patients with other cardiac diseases. This was attributed to the greater severity of medical illness associated with CHF. Depressed CHF patients had a higher risk of death during follow-up. The relationship between depressive symptoms and poorer prognosis has been confirmed in subsequent studies of outpatient and hospitalized CHF patients.[52-54] The majority of depressed CHF patients did not receive treatment for their depression with either antidepressants or psychotherapy and did not see mental health specialists any more frequently than did the nondepressed.

In our recent cohort study of 200 CHF patients with a mean age of 74 years, 63% scored above the suggested cut-off on the 10-Item Geriatric Depression Scale.[55] When somatic symptoms that could be attributed to CHF rather than depression were removed, the proportion dropped to 29%, still indicative of a significant burden of depressive symptoms among these patients. High depression scores were associated with poor cognitive function, low social function, high levels of fatigue, and living in rented accommodation.

The management of depression in heart failure has not been investigated in clinical trials. Some major groups of drugs are contraindicated, and the safety of others is not well established. Tricyclic antidepressants mimic quinidine and affect cardiac conduction, cause orthostatic hypotension, may interact with concomitant drug therapy, and cause lethal cardiotoxicity in overdose. Sertraline has no clinically relevant effects on cardiac conduction, is unlikely to cause orthostatic hypotension, has a wide margin of safety in overdose, and has been used safely after myocardial infarction in a small number of patients.[56] The risks of not treating depression must, however, be weighed against the risk of cardiotoxic side effects. Successful management of heart failure depends in no small part on patients complying with complex drug regimes, abiding by dietary restrictions, and monitoring themselves for important changes, such as increased swelling and worsening breathlessness. Clinically significant levels of depression reduce motivation, cause memory deficits, and increase a sense of hopelessness. It is not surprising, therefore, that depression is associated with reduced survival in CHF patients.

Drug therapy is, of course, not the only treatment option in depression. Psychological therapies, such as cognitive-behavioral therapy and counseling, are effective in patients attending their family doctor because of depression.[57] Although there is currently no evidence of their benefits in CHF, there is some reason to believe they may be helpful. For example, patients with CHF who participated in a qualitative study on the impact of the disease in their lives highlighted the number of losses they had encountered because of the breathlessness and fatigue associated with their disease and because of the side effects of treatment, especially diuretics: loss of ability to work, to carry out household duties, to go on holiday, to walk to shops, to leave the house, to talk to family, and to do anything much beyond concentrating on breathing.[55] Loss is an important cause of depression, and these patients articulated that their feelings of depression were associated with these losses. Psychological therapies may well help patients come to terms with these losses and to find new sources of enjoyment. Research is urgently needed to investigate their impact on depression in CHF patients.

INFORMATION AND COMMUNICATION

Information about Treatment Regimes

We have already mentioned the importance of CHF patients complying with advice about lifestyle and with complex drug regimes if their symptoms are to be optimally controlled. Effective communication about treatment regimes is therefore essential. Non-compliance with treatment regimes is thought to account for between 20% and 58% of hospital admissions for heart failure.[58,59] Noncompliance is common among older CHF patients and has been associated with a lack of adequate knowledge about

their medication despite this information having been given to them.[60] In addition, older patients may be particularly likely not to appreciate the significance of their symptoms and to delay getting medical assistance, possibly because they attribute these symptoms to the normal effects of aging.[61] Other studies have also found that patients and their caregivers find it hard to retain information given to them about the disease and its treatment.[62,63] We found in a qualitative study that effective communication with patients was hampered by a number of disease-specific barriers, including short-term memory loss, confusion, and fatigue.[64] Patients in the study lacked a basic understanding of the purpose of their medications and found it hard to differentiate between symptoms and side effects of drugs. Interventions that have sought to improve patient knowledge with the expectation that this would improve compliance have found only short-term improvements despite the use of multidisciplinary approaches and enhanced contact between patients and health professionals.[65] All health professionals working with CHF patients need to be aware that these patients may find it especially difficult to take in the information they need to be active partners in their own care. This is likely to be a particular challenge for older patients, especially those who are depressed. Again, this highlights the importance of detecting and treating depression in these patients.

Information about Prognosis

Bereaved respondents in the RSCD reported that at least half of the patients who died from heart disease were thought to have known or probably known that they were likely to die.[29] Of these, 82% had worked this out for themselves rather than being told by a health professional. This suggests that although their prognosis may be no better than that of many cancer patients, they are unlikely to have discussed this openly with their physicians: the "open-awareness" context seen as desirable in cancer for the past three decades is not the norm in heart failure. Further evidence for this comes from a U.S. study that found that physicians were less likely to discuss resuscitation with CHF patients than with acquired immunodeficiency syndrome or non-small cell lung cancer patients.[66] This was despite the physicians having realistic ideas of the disease prognosis and patients experiencing similar levels of symptom burden.

Physicians in the United States hold powerful myths about the dangers of making prognostic judgments,[67,68] and it is likely that their colleagues in the United Kingdom and elsewhere hold similar views. This together with the undoubted difficulty of judging the likely survival of individuals with CHF (as opposed to the average survival of a group of patients) may account for the lack of open communication. Most older people with severe CHF, however, will have had a number of frightening severe exacerbations leading to emergency hospital admissions, will become progressively weaker, and will experience increased restrictions in their daily lives. These experiences are likely to lead many to wonder what the outcome will be and some at least to realize that their condition is terminal. We do not know what older people with CHF would like to know about their illness, but we suspect that the high levels of anxiety some experience are associated with the lack of open communication with their health-care providers. This is borne out by the findings of our recent qualitative study of CHF patients: some patients believed they were likely to die because of their heart problems and indicated that they would have valued the opportunity to discuss their prognosis with those caring for them. These patients expressed a desire to know more about their prognosis, to enable them to make provision for their relatives after their death. They seemed to be depressed because of the losses they had encountered but anxious about the future.

We hypothesize that patients may be seeking answers to a different question about prognosis from the question physicians think they want answered. Physicians think patients want to know when they will die and, because they cannot answer this question with any certainty in heart failure, avoid the issue or provide no information at all. Patients may, however, be able to accept that doctors cannot predict the timing of death precisely but still want to know as much about the likely outcome as possible, even if this is hedged in uncertainty; they may want to know that three-fifths of patients with similar problems will survive for 2 months, even if the physician cannot be more precise about their individual odds of doing so. This information would enable them to plan for their relatives after their death and to make plans about where and how they want to die. It would also enable them to share their fears and anxieties about the future. Further research is needed to find out which patients with CHF would like information about their prognosis and what information they would like. In the meantime, it is of concern that at least some, and probably many, patients with CHF are unable to access the open communication with health professionals which is now accepted as the norm in cancer and which is essential if patients are to make informed choices about their future.

ROLE OF PALLIATIVE CARE IN THE CARE OF OLDER PEOPLE WITH HEART DISEASE

Palliative and hospice care is associated with expertise in the control of distressing physical and psychological symptoms, with open communication between patients, families, and health-care providers, enhancing life in the face of death. We have established in this chapter that older people with CHF have a poor prognosis, have distressing symptoms, do not experience open communication about their prognosis, and experience diminishing quality of life. There is, therefore, prima facie a good case for palliative care involvement in the care of these patients. What might this involve in practice?

The difficulty in accurately judging the life expectancy of individuals with severe

CHF is a major barrier to them accessing care from hospice and palliative care services. In the United States, the Medicare Hospice Benefit is restricted to patients with a prognosis of 6 months or less, and programs can be penalized if patients survive for longer than this. There is no equivalent in the United Kingdom, but hospice and palliative care services are still reluctant to take patients with an uncertain prognosis because they fear their services being swamped by "long-stayers." Prognostic uncertainty is a major obstacle to hospice and palliative care services in the United Kingdom moving away from their focus on cancer: more than 95% of patients who receive care in the United Kingdom from inpatient hospices, community and hospital palliative care teams, and day hospices have cancer.[69]

One solution that has been proposed is for these services to offer three levels of care to patients: a consultancy service, short-term interventions, and full-scale palliative care.[70,71] It is argued that many noncancer patients would benefit from a one-off consultation between their health professionals and the specialist palliative care team to, for example, discuss a symptom control problem, provide encouragement and support when using opioids, or debate a difficult ethical dilemma. Other patients with "more complex needs" would have to be taken on by the hospice or palliative care team but for a time-limited period to sort out a particular problem, with re-referral if needed. Finally, a small number may have such complex needs that they require an open-ended commitment from the hospice or palliative care team. The effectiveness and acceptability of this model have yet to be tested, but the model offers U.K. hospice and palliative care services a way forward that reduces the risk involved in caring for patients with an uncertain prognosis while at the same time enabling these patients to access palliative care at whatever point in the disease trajectory they need it.

We think this model has particular benefits in older people with CHF. Many doctors and nurses working in hospice and pal-

liative care services in the United Kingdom and the United States have little experience outside of terminal cancer care. They need to work closely with health professionals who specialize in the care of CHF, especially as the use of diuretics, ACEI, digoxin, and other cardiac drugs is likely to be necessary to achieve optimal symptom control. Traditionally, hospice and palliative care has provided care for cancer patients who have moved beyond active treatment: this transition is enshrined in the Medicare legislation, which requires patients electing this benefit to forego active medical care. Such a transition is increasingly contested in cancer care but has even less relevance in the care of CHF patients. Partnership is therefore required between existing care providers and palliative care services.

This is particularly true in the United Kingdom when caring for older people with CHF. There is evidence that older people are less likely to access hospice and palliative care than younger patients with similar problems.[72,73] The reasons for this are not clear. It may be because they do not want to, but it may also reflect the focus of these services on terminal cancer: many older people with cancer also have other comorbidities, such as CHF, chronic obstructive pulmonary disease, arthritis, and dementia, and may be seen as unsuitable for palliative care unless cancer is their "main" problem, which can be difficult to establish in the face of complex disease interactions. Hospice and palliative care services in the United Kingdom therefore lack expertise not only in the care of CHF but also in the care of older people with multiple pathologies. This may be less of a problem in the United States, where there appears to be a greater involvement of geriatricians in hospice and palliative care. It does again, however, highlight the importance of developing models of care in which hospice and palliative care specialists work in partnership with the patient's existing care providers, rather than necessarily taking over care.

Educating all health professionals in the principles and practice of hospice and palliative care is central to meeting the palliative care needs of older people with CHF. The Department of Health in England and Wales has distinguished the "palliative care approach" from specialist hospice and palliative care.[74] It is argued that this should be part of all clinical practice whatever the illness or stage, informed by a knowledge of and practice of palliative care principles, and supported by specialist palliative care. The key principles are a focus on quality of life, including good symptom control; a whole-person approach, taking into account the person's past life experience and current situation; care that encompasses both the person with life-threatening disease and those who matter to that person; respect for patient autonomy and choice; and emphasis on open and sensitive communication. Progress is being made in both the United States and the United Kingdom in ensuring that all health professionals receive training in these principles in both undergraduate and postgraduate education, but there is still a long way to go before all health professionals caring for older people with CHF understand the basics of assessing and treating distressing symptoms, are alert to clinical depression and know how to treat it, and are comfortable talking about the uncertainty inherent in this condition and the likely prognosis.

Heart failure nurses have been effective at reducing hospital admissions in patients with severe CHF.[75–77] Their focus has been on improving patients' understanding of their condition and increasing compliance to dietary restrictions and medication regimes. A key way to address the palliative needs of older patients with CHF may be to equip these nurses to widen their gaze to include symptom control issues, depression and anxiety, and patient anxiety about prognosis. This will require training in the palliative care approach as well as support and encouragement from palliative care specialists as nurses put these principles into practice in their daily work.

The terms *hospice* and *palliative care* may, however, be barriers to heart failure

nurses and others seeing these principles as relevant to their work, especially given the well-rehearsed difficulty in identifying CHF patients with a limited prognosis. The term *supportive care* has begun to be used in the United Kingdom to describe interventions that address the psychological, social, information, and symptom-control needs of cancer patients throughout their disease journey, that is, any care not focused specifically on tumor control. While the relationship between supportive and palliative care is currently contested, we believe that use of the term *supportive care* may have particular benefits when applied to CHF. It does not require any consideration of prognosis but instead focuses attention on the support that patients need as they live (and die) with CHF. This is important because without some mechanism for enabling patients to access the care they need without first being categorized as having a limited prognosis, the vast majority of people with severe CHF will continue to receive care focused entirely, or almost entirely, on alleviating their cardiac symptoms. This problem has been addressed by Lynn,[78] who developed the concept of "Medicaring," which, they argue, is a way of funding and providing appropriate supportive care for patients living with chronic conditions who are not imminently dying.

Both the idea of supportive care in the United Kingdom and that of Medicaring in the United States are attempts to address the same fundamental issue: how, when the prognosis is unclear, to provide appropriate care for sick patients with CHF that is based on the principles of hospice and aimed at enhancing life. Further research is needed to develop and evaluate these models of care and to expand the limited evidence base on how to address the symptom-control, psychological, and informational needs of patients with severe CHF. We believe it is, however, clear that the answer to addressing the palliative care needs of older people with CHF lies in close partnerships between hospice and palliative care services and those currently caring for these patients, rather than in seeing these needs as lying solely within the domain of hospice and palliative care.

CONCLUSION

In this chapter, we have demonstrated that CHF is primarily a disease of older people and that its incidence and prevalence are increasing. It is a progressive, symptomatic disease; and the growing number of effective modern therapies slow, but do not stop, disease progression. Although it is difficult to judge prognosis in individuals, largely because of sudden deaths from cardiac arrythmias, the overall prognosis is poor. Breathlessness and fatigue are common, as is depression. There is growing evidence that older patients with CHF often experience inadequate symptom control, little psychological support, and limited open communication with health-care professionals. Those currently caring for these patients need to work closely with specialists in hospice and palliative care to develop and provide appropriate, acceptable, and effective services that improve the quality of life, and the quality of dying, of these patients and their families.

REFERENCES

1. Task Force for the Diagnosis and Treatment of Chronic Heart Failure, European Society of Cardiology. Guidelines for the diagnosis of chronic heart failure. Eur Heart J 16:741–751, 1995.
2. He J, Ogden LG, Bazzano LA, et al. Risk factors for congestive heart failure in US men and women: NHANES I epidemiologic follow-up study. Arch Intern Med 161:996–1002, 2001.
3. Lye M, Donnellan C. Heart disease in the elderly. Heart 84:560–566, 2000.
4. Luchi RJ, Taffet GE, Teasdale TA. Congestive heart failure in the elderly. J Am Geriatr Soc 39:810–825, 1991.
5. Franciosa JA, Dunkman WB, Wilen M, et al. Survival in men with severe chronic left ventricular failure due to either coronary artery disease or idiopathic dilated cardiomyopathy. Am J Cardiol 51:831–836, 1983.
6. Gorkin L, Norvell NK, Rosen RC, et al. Assessment of quality of life as observed from the baseline data of the Studies of Left Ventricular Dysfunction (SOLVD) trial quality of life substudy. Am J Cardiol 71:1069–1073, 1993.
7. Clark AL, Poole-Wilson P, Coats AJS. Exercise limitation in chronic heart failure: central role of the periphery. J Am Coll Cardiol 28:1092–1102, 1996.
8. Chua TP, Clark AL, Amadi AA, et al. Relationship between chemosensitivity and the ventilatory response to chronic heart failure. J Am Coll Cardiol 27:650–657, 1996.
9. Flather MD, Yusuf S, Kober L, et al. Long-term ACE-inhibitor therapy in patients with heart failure or left-ventricular dysfunction: a systematic overview of data from individual patients. ACE-Inhibitor Myocardial Infarction Collaborative Group. Lancet 355:1575–1581, 2000.
10. Shibata MC, Flather MD, Wang D. Systematic review of the impact of beta blockers on mortality and hospital admissions in heart failure. Eur J Heart Fail 3:351–357, 2001.
11. Pitt B, Zannad F, Remme WJ, et al. The effect of spironolactone on morbidity and mortality in patients with severe heart failure. Randomized Aldactone Evaluation Study investigators. N Engl J Med 341:709–717, 1999.
12. Digitalis Investigation Group. The effect of digoxin on mortality and morbidity in patients with heart failure. N Engl J Med 336:525–533, 1997.
13. Garg R, Packer M, Pitt B, et al. Heart failure in the 1990s: evolution of a major public health epidemic in cardiovascular medicine. Am J Coll Cardiol 22(Suppl A):3A–5A, 1993.
14. American College of Cardiology/American Heart Association Task Force on Practice Guidelines. Guidelines for the evaluation and management of heart failure. Circulation 92:2764–2784, 1995.
15. National Heart, Lung and Blood Institute, National Institutes of Health. Data Fact Sheet. Congestive Heart Failure in the United States: A New Epidemic. Bethesda, MD, National Heart, Lung and Blood Institute, National Institutes of Health, 1996.
16. Cowie MR, Wood DA, Coats AJ, et al. Incidence and aetiology of heart failure; a population-based study. Eur Heart J 20:421–428, 1999.
17. Department of Health. National Service Framework for Coronary Heart Disease—Modern Standards and Service Models. London, Department of Health, 2001.
18. Madsen BK, Hansen JF, Stokholm KH, et al. Chronic congestive heart failure: de-

scription and survival of 190 consecutive patients with a diagnosis of chronic congestive heart failure based on clinical signs and symptoms. Eur Heart J 15:303–310, 1994.

19. Haldeman G, Croft JB, Giles WH, et al. Hospitalisation of patients with heart failure: National Hospital Discharge Survey, 1985 to 1995. Am Heart J 137:352–360, 1999.

20. Cowie MR, Wood DA, Coats AJ, et al. Survival of patients with a new diagnosis of heart failure: a population based study. Heart 83:505–510, 2000.

21. Brophy JM, Deslauriers G, Rouleau JL. Long-term prognosis of patients presenting to the emergency room with decompensated congestive heart failure. Can J Cardiol 10: 543–547, 1994.

22. Bonneux L, Barendregt JJ, Meeter K, et al. Estimating clinical morbidity due to ischemic heart disease and congestive heart failure: the future rise of heart failure. Am J Public Health 84:20–28, 1994.

23. Franciosa JA, Dunkmen WB, Wilen M, et al. Survival in men with severe chronic left ventricular failure due to either coronary artery disease or idiopathic dilated cardiomyopathy. Am J Cardiol 51:831–836, 1983.

24. MacIntyre K, Capewell S, Stewart S, et al. Evidence of improved prognosis in heart failure: trends in case fatality in 66547 patients hospitalised between 1986 and 1995. Circulation 103:1126–1131, 2000.

25. Konstam MA, Rousseau MF, Kronenberg MW, et al. Effects of the angiotensin converting enzyme inhibitor enalapril on the long-term progression of left ventricular dysfunction in patients with heart failure. SOLVD investigators. Circulation 86:431–438, 1992.

26. Swedberg K, Eneroth P, Kjekshus J, et al. Hormones regulating cardiovascular function in patients with severe congestive heart failure and their relation to mortality. CONSENSUS Trial study group. Circulation 82:1730–1736, 1990.

27. Lynn J, Harrell F Jr, Cohn F, et al. Prognoses of seriously ill hospitalised patients on the days before death: implications for patient care and public policy. New Horiz 5:56–61, 1997.

28. Fox E, Landrum-McNift K, Zhong Z, et al. Evaluation of prognostic criteria for determining hospice eligibility in patients with advanced lung, heart or liver disease. JAMA 282:1638–1645, 1999.

29. McCarthy M, Addington-Hall JM, Ley M. Communication and choice in dying from heart disease. J R Soc Med 90:128–131, 1997.

30. McCarthy M, Lay M, Addington-Hall JM. Dying from heart disease. J R Coll Physicians Lond 30:325–328, 1996.

31. SUPPORT Principal Investigators. A controlled trial to improve care for seriously ill hospitalized patients. The Study to Understand Prognoses and Preferences for Outcomes and Risks of Treatments (SUPPORT). JAMA 274:1591–1598, 1995.

32. Lynn J, Teno JM, Phillips RS, et al. Perceptions by family members of the dying experience of older and seriously ill patients. SUPPORT investigators. Ann Intern Med 126:97–106, 1997.

33. Addington-Hall JM, McPherson C. Afterdeath interviews with surrogates/bereaved family members: some issues of validity. J Pain Symptom Manage 22:794–790, 2001.

34. Koenig HG, Meador KG, Cohen HJ, et al. Depression in elderly hospitalised patients with medical illness. Arch Intern Med 148:1929–936, 1988.

35. Kahn RL, Zaru SH, Hilbert NM, et al. Memory complaint and impairment in the aged: the effect of depression and altered brain function. Arch Gen Psychiatry 32: 1569–1573, 1975.

36. Small GW. Recognition and treatment of depression in the elderly. J Clin Psychiatry 52:11–22, 1991.

37. Coleman RM, Miles LE, Guilleminault CC, et al. Sleep–wake disorders in the elderly: a polysomnographic analysis. J Am Geriatr Soc 29:289–296, 1981.

38. Kivela S-L, Pahkala K. Depressive disorder as a predictor of physical disability in old age. J Am Geriatr Soc 49:290–296, 2001.

39. Frasure-Smith N, Lesperance F, Talajic M. Depression following myocardial infarction. Impact on 6 month survival. JAMA 270:1819–1829, 1993.

40. Frasure-Smith N, Lesperance F, Talajic M. Depression and 18-month prognosis after myocardial infarction. Circulation 91:999–1005, 1995.

41. Ladwig KH, Kieser M, Konig J, et al. Affective disorders and survival after acute myocardial infarction: results from the post-infarction late potential study. Eur Heart J 12:959–964, 1991.

42. Ladwig KH, Roll G, Breithwardt G, et al. Post-infarction depression and incomplete recovery 6 months after acute myocardial infarction. Lancet 43:20–23, 1994.

43. Lesperance F, Frasure-Smith N, Talajic M. Major depression before and after myocardial infarction: its nature and consequences. Psychosom Med 58:99–110, 1996.

44. Carney RM, Rich MW, Tevelde A, et al. Major depressive disorder in coronary artery disease. Am J Cardiol 60:1273–1275, 1987.

45. Schleifer SJ, Macari-Hinsom MM, Coyle DA, et al. The nature and cause of depression following myocardial infarction. Arch Intern Med 149:1785–1789, 1989.

45. Freedland K, Lustman PJ, Carney M, et al. Underdiagnosis of depression in patients with coronary artery disease: the role of nonspecific symptoms. Int J Psychiatry Med 22:221–229, 1992.

47. Ickovics JR, Viscoli CM, Horwitz RI. Functional recovery after myocardial infarction in men: the independent effects of social class. Ann Intern Med 127:18–25, 1997.

48. Lane D, Carroll D, Ring C, et al. Effects of depression and anxiety on mortality and quality of life 4 months after myocardial infarction. J Psychosom Res 49:229–238, 2000.

49. Cowie MR, Mosterd A, Wood DA, et al. The epidemiology of heart failure. Eur Heart J 18:208–225, 1997.

50. Kannel WB, Ho K, Thom T. Changing epidemiological features of cardiac failure. Br Heart J 72(Suppl):S3–S9, 1994.

51. Koenig HG. Depression in hospitalized older patients with congestive heart failure. Gen Hosp Psychiatry 20:29–43, 1998.

52. Murberg TA, Bru E, Suebak S, et al. Depressed mood and subjective health symptoms as predictors of mortality in patients with congestive heart failure: a two-year follow-up study. Int J Psychiatry Med 29:311–326, 1999.

53. Vaccarino V, Kasl SV, Abramson JKHM. Depressive symptoms and risk of functional decline and death in patients with heart failure. J Am Coll Cardiol 38:199–205, 2001.

54. Jiang W, Alexander J, Christopher E, et al. Relationship of depression to increased risk of mortality and rehospitalisation in patients with congestive heart failure. Arch Intern Med 161:1849–1856, 2001.

55. McCoy ASM, Addington-Hall JM, Rogers AE, Coats AJS, Gibbs JSR. Prevalence of depression in chronic heart failure. Palliat Med 15:524, 2001.

56. Shapiro PA, Lesperance F, Frasure-Smith N, et al. An open-label preliminary trial of sertraline for treatment of major depression after acute myocardial infarction (the SADHAT trial). Sertraline Anti-Depressant Heart Attack Trial. Am Heart J 137:1100–1106, 1999.

57. Ward E, King M, Lloyd M, et al. Randomised controlled trial of non-directive counselling, cognitive-behaviour therapy, and usual general practitioner care for patients with depression. I: Clinical effectiveness. BMJ 321:1383–1388, 2000.

58. Michalesen A, Koenig G, Thimme W. Preventable causative factors leading to hospital admission with decompensated heart failure. Heart 80:437–411, 1998.

59. Vinson JM, Rich MW, Sperry JC, et al. Early readmission of elderly patients with congestive heart failure. J Am Geriatr Soc 38:1290–1295, 1990.

60. Cline CM, Bjorck-Linne AK, Israelsson BY, et al. Non-compliance and knowledge of prescribed medication in elderly patients with heart failure. Eur J Heart Fail 1:145–149, 1999.

61. Friedman MM. Older adults' symptoms and their duration before hospitalisation for heart failure. Heart Lung 26:169–175, 1997.

62. Stull DE, Starling R, Haas G, et al. Becoming a patient with heart failure. Heart Lung 28:284–292, 1999.

63. Wehby D, Bremner PS. Perceived learning needs of patients with heart failure. Heart Lung 28:31–40, 1999.

64. Rogers AE, Addington-Hall JM, Abery AJ, et al. Knowledge and communication difficulties for patients with chronic heart failure: qualitative study. BMJ 321:605–607, 2000.

65. Rich MW, Gray DB, Beckham V, et al. Effect of a multidisciplinary intervention on medication compliance in elderly patients with congestive heart failure. Am J Med 101:270–276, 1996.

66. Wachter RM, Luce JM, Hearst N, et al. Decisions about resuscitation: inequalities among patients with different diseases but similar prognosis. Ann Intern Med 111:525–532, 1989.

67. Lamont EB, Christakis NA. Prognostic disclosure to patients with cancer near the end of life. Ann Intern Med 134:1096–1105, 2001.

68. Christakis NA, Lamont EB. Extent and determinants of error in doctors' prognoses in terminally ill patients: prospective cohort study BMJ 320:469–472, 2000.

69. Eve A, Higginson IJ. Minimum dataset activity for hospice and hospital palliative care services in the UK 1997/98. Palliat Med 14:395–404, 2000.

70. George R, Sykes J. Beyond cancer? In: Clark D, Hockley J, Ahmedzai S (Eds.). New Themes in Palliative Care. Buckingham, Open University Press, 1997.

71. Addington-Hall JM, Higginson IJ. Palliative Care for Non-cancer Patients. Oxford, Oxford University Press, 2001.

72. Addington-Hall JM, Altmann D, McCarthy M. Who gets hospice in-patient care? Soc Sci Med 46:1011–1016, 1998.

73. Addington-Hall JM, Altmann D. Which terminally ill cancer patients receive care from community specialist palliative care nurses? J Advanc Nurs 32:799–806, 2000.

74. National Health Service. A Policy Framework for Commissioning Cancer Services: Palliative Care Services. NHS Executive EL(96)85. London, NHS, 1996.

75. Blue L, Lang E, McMurray JJ, et al. Randomised controlled trial of specialist nurse intervention in heart failure. BMJ 323: 715–718, 2001.

76. Grady KL, Dracup K, Kennedy G, et al. Team management of patients with heart failure: a statement for healthcare professionals from the Cardiovascular Nursing Council of the American Heart Association. Circulation 102:2443–2456, 2000.

77. Rich MW, Beckham V, Wittenberg C, et al. A multidisciplinary intervention to prevent the readmission of elderly patients with congestive heart failure. N Engl J Med 333: 1190–1195, 1995.

78. Lynn J. Serving patients who may die soon and their families: the role of hospice and other services. JAMA 285:925–932, 2001.

11

Cancer

NATALIE R. SACKS AND JANET L. ABRAHM

The majority of cancer cases and cancer deaths occur in people over age 65, but both the cancers and the symptoms they cause are generally undertreated in the elderly. There is now an increased interest in understanding cancer in the elderly and an effort to correct biases that may adversely affect the care of older patients. Awareness of the heterogeneous physical, emotional, and social facets of this population will yield more appropriate treatment plans. Decisions about therapy will need to address the impact both of the disease and of the possible treatment-related side effects on these patients' autonomy, the possibility of increasing disability, and the pre-existing comorbid disease burden.[1] As this patient population grows, there will be an increased demand for oncologists and palliative care specialists who are informed and committed to weighing the risks, burdens, and benefits of various treatment modalities in the elderly.

This chapter provides a brief epidemiologic survey of cancer in the elderly, primarily to underscore the magnitude of disease that oncologists and palliative care specialists will be facing. We describe new approaches to the comprehensive assessment of the geriatric cancer patient. We review the medical oncologist's approach to several common tumors with emphasis on what, if any, data exist on the tolerability and efficacy of available cancer treatments for older patients. We also address the therapeutic modalities of surgery and radiation therapy, both of which play a central role in the palliation of cancer for elderly patients.

SCOPE OF THE PROBLEM

After heart disease, cancer is the second leading cause of death for both men and women.[2] It is a disease of the elderly, with 60% of all cancers and 69% of all cancer deaths occurring in people over 65 years old.[3] Current estimates indicate that by 2030 one in five people will be older than 65.[4] Since our population is both expanding and aging, oncologists and palliative care specialists will be facing an increasing number of patients with complex needs.

Figure 11–1 illustrates the incidence of common cancers in elderly women and men. For older women, the most common cancers are breast, colon, and lung.[5] Although lung cancer is the leading cause of cancer death in women of all ages, breast cancer is the leading cause in women older than 65.[2] For men, the most common cancers are prostate, colon, and lung, with the latter being responsible for the most deaths.

Incidence studies suggest that cancer is a less important cause of morbidity in the oldest old. An autopsy study of 350 people older than 94 years (of whom 99 were older than 100) revealed occult cancer in only 13%.[6] The greatest risk factor for cancer is aging. Figure 11–2 shows the proportion of persons with selected tumors who are at least 65 years old.[7] Older patients account for approximately three-quarters of all cases of colon cancer, and older men account for 80% of all prostate cancers. Unfortunately, most research in oncology has focused on younger people, who constitute the minority of cases. For instance, almost 30% of male leukemia cases occur in men older than 75 years, but this same cohort represents only 2% of the subjects enrolled in studies of this disease.

A recent study summarized the state of research in this area.[8] This retrospective analysis linked two large data sets: the Surveillance, Epidemiology, and End Results program of the National Cancer Institute, which collects and publishes cancer incidence and survival data, and the South-

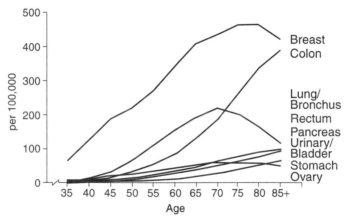

Cancer incidence rates in women.

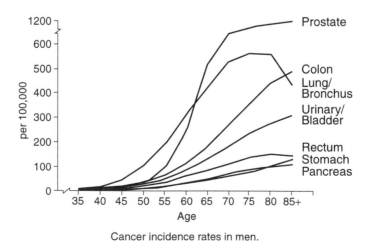

Cancer incidence rates in men.

Figure 11–1. Incidence rates of common cancers in elderly women *(A)* and men *(B)*.

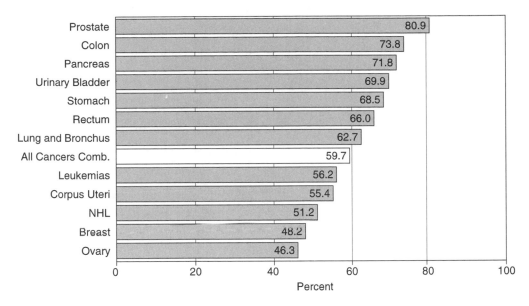

Figure 11–2. Proportion of individuals with selected tumor types who are at least 65 years old.

western Oncology Group data set, which contains information on all persons enrolled in treatment trials from 1993 through 1996 in that cooperative group. The authors compared rates of cancer in the general population with rates of enrollment in clinical trials and found significant discrepancies between cases and enrollment for all types of cancer except lymphoma. Specifically, patients who were over 65 years old accounted for 63% of patients in the national population with cancer but only 25% of patients in trials. Patients who were over 70 years old accounted for 47% of patients with cancer but only 13% of patients in trials. The reasons for this disparity are complex and include narrow study inclusion criteria, physician bias, and patient bias.

The lack of cancer research in persons over age 65 is a source of frustration for clinicians eager to provide optimal care for their older patients. Improvement in all aspects of care, ranging from appropriate use of proven chemotherapy regimens to more successful care of symptoms, both cancer- and treatment-related, will require broader inclusion of older patients. Fortunately, there has been a recent surge in research focusing on the barriers to research participation.[8] This work in combination with in-

creasing research into end-of-life care should improve our capacity to care for older adults with cancer.

Does cancer behave differently in older people? The data suggest a mixed picture. Older women with breast cancer are more likely to present with metastatic disease but also more likely to have tumors that are estrogen-receptor positive, which generally confers a better prognosis.[9] Thyroid cancer appears to be more aggressive in older patients, but the histologic subtype is more likely to be anaplastic.[10] Older persons with lung cancer present with less advanced disease than their younger counterparts.[11] These data may reflect timing of detection patterns more than absolute biology. In summary, clinicians cannot assume that tumors in older people are either more indolent or more aggressive. The data do not justify age-related conclusions about tumor behavior. In studies that control for tumor stage, age alone rarely affects outcome.[12]

COMPREHENSIVE GERIATRIC ASSESSMENT FROM AN ONCOLOGIST'S PERSPECTIVE

Traditionally, oncologists use the Eastern Cooperative Oncology Group Performance

Status score or the Karnovsky score to assess the overall health status of cancer patients.[13,14] Many oncology studies have validated both of these scores as predictors of survival and treatment tolerance. Unfortunately these scores are not as helpful in the evaluation of older patients because they under-represent impairments.

A profile of 200 older oncology patients presenting at one center revealed important discrepancies in the various assessment scores: only 17% of patients had a Performance Status score of 2 or more (2 = ambulatory and capable of self-care but cannot work; 3 = capable of limited self-care, confined to bed or chair at least 50% of waking hours; 4 = completely disabled, 100% confined to bed or chair), but 43% of these same patients had severe comorbidities (Cumulative Illness Rating Scale–Geriatric grade 3–4), 21% were dependent in the basic activities of daily living, and 56% were dependent in the instrumental activities of daily living.[15]

Why does this matter? Many studies of older patients have established correlations between baseline characteristics, such as comorbidity or functional status, and cancer outcomes. For breast cancer patients, risk of mortality has been correlated with the number of comorbid conditions.[16] Monfardini et al.[17] demonstrated that dependence in the instrumental activities of daily living increased the risk of complications from chemotherapy. Hence, the traditional performance scores may not capture the information that is critical to making appropriate therapeutic decisions for older cancer patients.

One of the most important developments in the field of geriatric oncology is the application of the Comprehensive Geriatric Assessment (CGA) to elderly patients with cancer. The CGA is comprised of validated health measures that are predictors of morbidity and mortality in the geriatric population.[18] The results of the CGA aid the clinician in identifying patients at risk for the classic geriatric syndromes: dementia, depression, delirium, falls, and failure to thrive. Although the screening tools vary across institutions, the basic package includes measures of functional status, cognitive function, affect, comorbid burden, nutrition, and socioeconomic status.

An example of a CGA is the National Comprehensive Cancer Network (NCCN) guidelines for assessment of an older cancer patient (Table 11–1).[19] Prospective clinical trials are ongoing to refine the tools for use in the oncology setting and to assess the role of the CGA as a predictor of treatment-related toxicity and survival.[20]

If proven to be predictive, the CGA would permit construction of the following management algorithm, which divides older cancer patients into three groups, as suggested by Balducci and Extermann:[21]

1. *Independent:* No functional impairments, no significant comorbidities. These patients could be candidates for standard chemotherapy with intent to cure.
2. *Partially Dependent:* Some functional impairment and fewer than three comorbid conditions. Treatment decisions should be made in the context of competing mortality risks.
3. *Frail:* Functionally dependent, multiple comorbidities, or at least one of the geriatric syndromes. These patients would not usually be considered candidates for life-prolonging treatment.

These components of the CGA provide objective measures that are independent of age and may help clinicians assess the therapeutic risk and benefit of pursuing chemotherapy. They would also guide detection of symptoms and problems that require attention and palliation.

The CGA also serves as a springboard to discussion about the patient's quality of life, health beliefs, and values about end-of-life care. This is an approach that recognizes and respects that "the elderly" represent a cohort of heterogeneous individuals who require multidimensional assessment to optimize their care, a principle that is highly consistent with the standard of practice of geriatricians and palliative care specialists.

Table 11–1. National Comprehensive Cancer Network Guidelines for Suggested Assessment of Older Cancer Patients

Realm	Screening	Confirmatory test
Mental status	Serial 3: Tell patient "I am going to name three objects (pencil, truck, book), and I am going to ask you to repeat them now and a few minutes from now."	Folstein Mini-Mental Status; if score <24, institute work-up for dementia
Emotional status/ depression	Do you often feel depressed or sad?	Geriatric Depression Scale; if positive (score >10), work-up for depression
Activities of daily living	Can you dress yourself? Do you need help going to the bathroom? Do you wet yourself? Can you eat without help? Can you move from one place to another without help? Do you need help taking a bath or a shower?	Formal Katz activities of daily living
IADL	Do you drive? Are you able to use public transportation? Do you prepare your own meals? Do you go shopping? Do you do your own checking? Can you call somebody with the telephone? Do you remember to take your medications?	Formal IADL scale
Home environment	Do you have trouble with stairs inside and outside the house? Do you trip often on rugs?	—
Social support	Who would be able to help you in case of emergency?	If no caregiver, try to arrange for one; if caregiver is a spouse, sibling, or friend of the same age as the patient, assess independence of caregiver
Comorbidity	Evaluate the presence of the following conditions from ROS: congestive heart failure, coronary artery disease, valvular heart disease, chronic lung disease (obstructive or restrictive), cerebrovascular disease, peripheral neuropathy, chronic renal insufficiency, hypertension, diabetes, coexisting malignancies, collagen vascular disease, incapacitating arthritis	Confirm the presence of the condition and grade the seriousness
Nutrition	Weigh patient, measure height, inquire about weight loss	Mini-Nutritional Assessment
Polypharmacy	Review number and type of medications	If more than three medications, look for duplications, interactions, and compliance

IADL, instrumental activities of daily living; ROS, review of systems.

USE OF CHEMOTHERAPY

Oncologists function in a framework that focuses on the goal of treatment: curative versus palliative. This dichotomy influences both the willingness of the physician to tolerate treatment side effects and the substance of advance care planning discussions. However, curative intent should not preclude attention to symptoms, due to either the cancer or the treatment. Whether curative or palliative, two questions arise about the use of chemotherapy in older individuals: Is it beneficial? Is it tolerable?

Fortunately, there is some evidence that chemotherapy is effective in older patients and can be well tolerated; specific examples will be illustrated below. These data should allow physicians caring for older patients with cancer to appreciate that chemotherapy has a role to play in a wide spectrum of patients. Both oral agents and less toxic novel molecular compounds that slow the progression of disease will have an increasing role in the late stages of disease, especially since they may palliate symptoms and improve quality of life. Chemotherapy may decrease symptoms of pain and improve quality of life despite a lack of a clinically objective tumor response. In a study of palliative chemotherapy for malignant mesothelioma, 62% of patients reported an overall improvement in symptoms, and this improvement rate was similar for patients who did and did not show a radiologic response.[22] In a trial of paclitaxel for metastatic breast cancer, 40% of patients reported improvement in symptoms but only 19% had an objective response to treatment.[23] Men with hormone-refractory prostate cancer treated with gemcitabine reported significant improvement in quality of life, especially in control of pain, despite no meaningful reduction in their level of prostate-specific antigen.[24] One possible explanation for this phenomenon is that chemotherapy inhibits the production of cytokines, which may be responsible for the pain and other symptom distress caused by the cancer.[25]

When reviewing the data on the use of chemotherapy in geriatric cancer patients, several other themes emerge: (1) age alone is not an independent predictor of outcome but, rather, tumor and patient characteristics determine the response to treatment; (2) although more study is required, preliminary results indicate that older people can both tolerate and benefit from chemotherapy; and (3) the strategy of dose reduction to avoid toxicity is ineffective. The following discussion of two prevalent tumor types in the elderly that are treated with chemotherapy will illustrate these points.

Colon Cancer

The incidence of colon cancer rises steadily with age for both men and women: 25% of patients are at least 80 years old.[26] Prognosis depends on stage, and stage depends on the extent of invasion by the tumor through the bowel wall and whether there is evidence of metastatic disease in lymph nodes or elsewhere in the body.[27] Tumors are treated by en-bloc surgical resection of the tumor and the draining lymph nodes, which is essentially curative for early-stage disease.

When all detectable tumor has been excised, adjuvant chemotherapy is offered for intermediate stages of colon cancer, to reduce the risk of recurrence. A recent meta-analysis of data from seven randomized clinical trials explored the effect of adjuvant chemotherapy in older cancer patients.[28] This analysis of 3351 patients included 1269 patients aged 61–70 years and 506 patients older than 70. The chance of being disease-free at 5 years was 69% for patients who received a 5-fluorouracil-containing regimen as adjuvant therapy compared to 58% for patients who had no additional treatment following surgery. The important finding from this study is that this therapeutic benefit was similar in all age groups.

In addition, the potential side effects of treatment (nausea, vomiting, stomatitis, and diarrhea) were not increased in patients over age 70 compared to younger patients. If the adjuvant therapy regimen included levamisole as opposed to leucovorin, older patients did have a higher rate of leukopenia, although this did not contribute to mortality. This type of analysis is critical for dispelling perceptions about the tolerability and efficacy of chemotherapy in older patients. Elderly people may choose not to pursue chemotherapy for a variety of reasons, but physicians should not discourage treatment based solely on concerns about increased toxicity or lack of efficacy.

In contrast to early-stage disease, the 5-year survival for stage IV metastatic colon cancer is only 5%, with 60% of deaths occurring in the first 12 months.[29] Chemotherapy can slow the progression of metastatic colon cancer and possibly add months to life.[30] Subset analyses from trials studying the combination of traditional 5-fluorouracil chemotherapy with a newer agent, irinotecan (CPT-11), showed that older patients had a similar beneficial effect of treatment without significant additional toxicity.[31] Trials are also ongoing to evaluate an oral 5-fluorouracil agent which may offer some palliative benefit and is easily administered.

Breast Cancer

Breast cancer is the leading cause of cancer-related death in woman over 65 years.[2] The incidence rises with age, peaks at about age 75, and then declines slightly. Early breast cancer is treated by modified radical mastectomy with axillary dissection or lumpectomy with axillary dissection plus radiation. Older women tolerate surgery well, and survival following surgery is similar in older and younger patients.[32] For women over age 70 with early-stage disease, the 5-year overall survival rate is 54%. The most commonly used adjuvant chemotherapy regimen for these older women is a combination of cytoxan, methotrexate, and 5-fluorouracil (CMF). This regimen carries a 0.1% risk of treatment-related mortality.[33] Studies of CMF have illustrated the futility of offering low-dose treatment to avoid toxicity. Bonadonna et al.[34] reported 20-year follow-up on 386 women treated with surgery who either did or did not receive adjuvant treatment. Survival was lengthened for the women who received the chemotherapy, except for the older women, who had received lower doses in the hope of diminishing toxicity.

For truly frail older women who cannot tolerate surgery, there is a proven benefit to treatment with tamoxifen and weekly radiation.[35] Tamoxifen is also the treatment of choice for women with metastatic disease who have hormone-responsive tumors.[36] This agent can produce a response rate of 30%–40%, with average response duration of 12 months. If hormonal agents stop working, cytotoxic chemotherapy can be used. Cytotoxic treatment can effectively palliate the symptoms of visceral metastatic disease, which can cause pain, nausea, vomiting, and other symptoms of biliary obstruction.

Use of Other Therapeutic Modalities: Radiation and Surgery

Radiation therapy is a critical component of the treatment of cancer and its symptoms. For situations that require urgent attention, radiation is more appropriate than chemotherapy because it provides a more rapid effect. Radiation is the primary modality for relief of pain from bony metastases, which are seen in prostate, breast, and other cancers. Meaningful pain relief can be achieved in 70% of patients with low-dose radiation treatments administered daily for 10 days.[37] Radiation in combination with steroids is the treatment of choice for spinal cord compression; this diagnosis should be considered in any older cancer patient who has back pain or any symptoms of lower extremity numbness or weakness.[38] The treatment consists of 10 daily treatments, totaling 30 Gy, and can be tolerated by older patients. Radiation can also be employed to treat liver metastases, which can cause symptoms of pain (especially when stretching Glisson's capsule), as well as nausea, anorexia, and jaundice. Symptoms of advanced lung tumors, including nerve, rib, and chest wall pain, and those due to obstructing mass effect, such as hemoptysis, dyspnea, and repeated pneumonias, are amenable to radiation.

In addition to these palliative benefits, radiation is part of the definitive treatment of some tumors. Unfortunately, in comparison with younger patients, elderly patients are less likely to undergo radiation therapy.[39] The reason for this discrepancy is unclear but may be bias regarding increased toxicity and decreased compliance. These perceptions may be unfair: some data suggest that the elderly are more compliant with radiation treatment.[40] Toxicity depends on the site of treatment; acute reactions include skin desquamation, mucositis, and diarrhea. Radiation reactions that appear months to years later include tissue fibrosis and necrosis as well as fistulae.

Elderly cancer patients are not necessarily at increased risk for toxicity. Larson et al.[41] studied 26 lung cancer patients whose average age was 70 years; all tolerated and completed radiotherapy and demonstrated improved functional status at 3 months compared to pretreatment status. In several large breast cancer series, containing hundreds of older breast cancer patients undergoing radiation treatment, older patients did not have more skin or hematologic toxicity than younger patients.[42,43] There are conflicting data on whether older patients experience a higher incidence of arm edema.[44] Newer technology yielding better definition of radiation fields will reduce toxicity for all patients. At present, age should not be considered an obstacle to radiation treatment, and cancer symptoms that can be devastating to the quality of life of older cancer patients can be ameliorated with radiation.

Surgery is the most important modality of treatment for many of the common tumors in the elderly. For instance, surgical resection is required for cure of early-stage colon cancer but is also frequently pursued for patients with metastatic disease, to prevent the likely complications of obstruction and bleeding. Studies in the surgical oncology literature demonstrate that advanced age does not preclude surgery; however, patients in these studies are usually selected carefully.[45] Mortality from elective surgery increases only minimally, if at all, with advancing age.[45]

However, if an older person requires emergency surgery, the operative risk can be at least twice as high.[46] Mortality rates for elective colon cancer resection range from 4% to 21% but rise to over 50% if the procedure is for an emergency. This illustrates the geriatric principle of *diminished functional reserve*, in which aging is associated with a diminution of the functional capacity of multiple organ systems

and the impact of a profound stress to the system is magnified compared to a younger person.

Nonetheless, surgery should be considered an important part of palliative treatment, even for older patients with poor prognosis. For example, patients with pancreatic cancer, of whom two-thirds are older than 65, have a 5-year survival of about 5%.[47] Approximately 50% of these patients will require surgery for biliary or gastric obstruction, which are the common complications of this disease.[48]

Performance status falls immediately after surgery for all patients, young and old. This status improves for younger patients, but older patients may not return to their functional baseline. Hence, surgical reports that describe short-term postoperative morbidity and mortality rates may be missing the outcomes that are most important for geriatric cancer patients: increasing dependence in activities of daily living, which leads to loss of autonomy. Some centers are exploring newer techniques, such as the role of laparoscopic surgery for colon resection in the elderly.[49] This may lead to less postoperative pain, diminution of postoperative ileus, and a shorter hospital stay.

CAREGIVERS

A cancer diagnosis affects the entire family and social system of the patient; this effect can be magnified for older patients, who may already be physically and economically dependent on others. For instance, one-third of people older than 65 are dependent for transportation, and that proportion rises to two-thirds of those older than 85.[50] Access to transportation influences care options, especially for travel-intensive treatments such as daily radiation. It is estimated that 26% of older cancer patients live alone and that one-third either do not have children or do not have children in the vicinity.[50]

When family members are involved, they must deal with the possibility of the patient's increasing dependence and impending death and must be included in the assessment and care plan. Anxiety and depression are more severe among family members of cancer patients than among patients themselves.[51]

Family members also bear the hidden costs of treatment. In a recent survey of more than 7400 people over age 70, those patients with cancer who underwent treatment received an average of 10 hours of informal caregiving each week, significantly greater than that received by cancer patients who did not receive treatment in the last year and those without cancer (6.9 and 6.8 hours, respectively).[52] The authors estimate that this incremental increase in hours translates to an average additional yearly cost for the cancer patients of $1200, which is over $1 billion nationwide.

The caregiver's role is particularly critical for patients with cognitive impairment who undergo treatment for cancer. These patients will need assistance to recognize and respond to adverse effects of treatment, such as mucositis, which can lead to dehydration and diarrhea, or fever, which can be life-threatening if a patient is myelosuppressed.

CONCLUSIONS

Large increases in the number of older patients with cancer demand a new paradigm for care. As with all illnesses in the older patient, the availability of caregiver support and attention to caregiver health are important elements of care. Further, the complexity of these patients requires formal and repeated multidimensional assessment, especially since chronologic age does not predict clinical response. Geriatric patients should not be denied potentially curative, life-prolonging, or palliative chemotherapeutic, radiation, or surgical treatments simply because of their chronologic age. Answers will come only if more focused research is conducted on the risks, burdens, and benefits of all modalities of cancer treatment in geriatric patients.

REFERENCES

1. Balducci L. Geriatric oncology: challenges for the new century. Eur J Cancer 36: 1741–1754, 2000.
2. American Cancer Society. Cancer Facts and Figures. Atlanta, American Cancer Society, 2000.
3. Ries LAG, Eisner MP, Kosary CL, Hankey BF, Miller BA, Clegg LX, Edwards BK (Eds.). SEER Cancer Statistics Review, 1973–1998. Bethesda, MD, National Cancer Institute, National Institutes of Health Publication 00-2789.
4. Yancik R, Ries LAG. Aging and cancer in America: demographic and epidemiologic perspectives. Hematol Oncol Clin North Am 14:17–23, 2000.
5. Yancik R, Ries LAG. Cancer in older persons. Magnitude of the problem: how do we apply what we know? Cancer 74:1995–2003, 1994.
6. Stanta G, Campagner L, Cavallieri F, et al. Cancer of the oldest old: what we have learned from autopsy studies. Clin Geriatr Med 13:55–69, 1997.
7. Yancik R. Cancer burden in the aged: an epidemiologic and demographic overview. Cancer 80:1273–1283, 1997.
8. Hutchins LF, Unger JM, Crowley JJ, Coltman CA, Albain KS. Underrepresentation of patients 65 years of age or older in cancer-treatment trials. N Engl J Med 341: 2061–2067, 1999.
9. Bernoux A, de Cremoux P, Laine-Bidron C, et al. Estrogen receptor negative and progesterone receptor positive primary breast cancer: pathologic characteristics and clinical outcome. Breast Cancer Res Treat 49: 219–225, 1998.
10. Schelfout LJ, Creutzberg CL, Hamming JF, et al: Multivariate analysis of survival in differentiated thyroid cancer: the prognostic significance of the age factor. Eur J Cancer 24:331, 1988.
11. O'Rourke MA, Feussner JR, Feigl P, Laszlo J. Age trends of lung cancer stage at diagnosis. Implications for lung cancer screening in the elderly. JAMA 258:921–926, 1987.
12. Balducci L. The geriatric cancer patient: equal benefit from equal treatment. Cancer Control 8(Suppl):1–25, 2001.
13. Zubrod CG, Schneiderman M, Frei E III, et al. Appraisal of methods for the study of chemotherapy in man: comparative therapeutic trial of nitrogen mustard and triethylene thiophosphoramide. J Chronic Dis 11:7–33, 1960.

14. Karnovsky DA, Abelman WH, Craver LF, Burchenal JH. The use of nitrogen mustards in the palliative treatment of carcinoma. Cancer 1:634–656, 1948.

15. Extermann M, Overcash J, Lyman GH, Parr J, Balducci L. Comorbidity and functional status are independent in older cancer patients. J Clin Oncol 16:1582–1587, 1998.

16. Satariano WA, Ragland DR. The effect of comorbidity on 3-year survival of women with primary breast cancer. Ann Intern Med 120:104–110, 1994.

17. Monfardini S, Ferruci L, Fratino L, Del Lungo I, Serraino D, Zagonel V. Validation of a multidimensional evaluation scale for use in elderly cancer patients. Cancer 77: 395–401, 1996.

18. Stuck AE, Siu AL, Wieland D, Adams J, Rubenstein LZ. Comprehensive geriatric assessment: a meta-analysis of controlled trials. Lancet 342:1032–1036, 1993.

19. Balducci L, Yates J. General guidelines for the management of older patients with cancer. NCCN Proceedings. Oncology 14:221–227, 2000.

20. Repetto L, Fratino L, Audisio RA, Venturino A, Gianni W, Vercelli M, et al. Comprehensive geriatric assessment adds information to Eastern Cooperative Oncology Group performance status in elderly cancer patients: an Italian Group for Geriatric Oncology study. J Clin Oncol 20:494–502, 2002.

21. Balducci L, Extermann M. Management of cancer in the older person: a practical approach. Oncologist 5:224–237, 2000.

22. Middleton GW, Smith JE, O'Brien ME, Norton A, Hickish T, et al. Good symptom relief with palliative MVP (mitomycin-C, vinblastine and cisplatin) chemotherapy in malignant mesothelioma. Ann Oncol 9: 269–273, 1998.

23. Geyer CE Jr, Green SJ, Moinpour CM, O'Sullivan J, Goodwin DK, Canfield VA, et al. Expanded phase II trial of paclitaxel in metastatic breast cancer: a Southwest Oncology Group study. Breast Cancer Res Treat 51:169–181, 1998.

24. Morant R, Bernhard J, Maibach R, Borner M, Fey MF, Thurlimann B, Jacky E, et al. Response and palliation in a phase II trial of gemcitabine in hormone-refractory metastatic prostatic carcinoma: Swiss Group for Clinical Cancer Research (SAKK). Ann Oncol 11:183–188, 2000.

25. Ellison NM. An overview of palliative chemotherapy. In: Berger AM, Portenoy RK, Weissman DE (Eds.). Updates Principles and Practice of Supportive Oncology, vol 4. pp. 1–12, 2001.

26. Miller BA, Ries LAG, Hankey BF, et al. SEER Cancer Statistics Review: 1973–1990. Bethesda, MD, National Cancer Institute, National Institutes of Health, 1993.

27. Cohen AM, Minsky BD, Schilsky RL. Cancer of the colon. In: DeVita VT, Hellman S, Rosenberg SA (Eds.). Cancer: Principles and Practice of Oncology, 5th ed. Philadelphia, Lippincott-Raven, pp. 1144–1197. 1997.

28. Sargent DJ, Goldberg RM, Jacobson SD, et al. A pooled analysis of adjuvant chemotherapy for resected colon cancer in elderly patients. N Engl J Med 345:1091–1097, 2001.

29. Greenlee RT, Hill-Harmon MB, Murray T, et al. Cancer Statistics, 2001. CA Cancer J Clin 51:15–36, 2001.

30. Popescu RA, Norman A, Ross PJ, Parikh B, Cunningham D. Adjuvant or palliative chemotherapy for colorectal cancer in patients 70 years or older. J Clin Oncol 17: 2412–2418, 1999.

31. Saltz LB, Cox JV, Blank C, et al. Irinotecan plus fluorouracil and leucovorin for metastatic colorectal cancer. N Engl J Med 343:905–914, 2000.

32. Masetti R, Antinori A, Terribile D, Marra A, Granone P, et al. Breast cancer in women 70 years of age or older. J Clin Oncol 13: 2722–2730, 1996.

33. Colleoni M, Price KN, Castiglione-Gertsch M, Gelber RD, Coates AS, Goldhirsh A. Mortality during adjuvant treatment of early breast cancer with cyclophosphamide, methotrexate, and fluorouracil. Lancet 352: 930–942, 1998.

34. Bonadonna G, Valagussa P, Moliterni A, Zambetti M, Brambilla C. Adjuvant cyclophosphamide, methotrexate, and fluorouracil in node-positive breast cancer: the results of 20 years of follow-up. N Engl J Med 332:901–906, 1995.

35. Rostom AY, Pradhan DG, White WF. Once weekly irradiation in breast cancer. Int J Radiat Oncol Biol Phys 13:551–555, 1987.

36. Kimmick G, Muss HB. Current status of endocrine therapy for metastatic breast cancer. Oncology 9:877–886, 1995.

37. Price P, Hoskin PJ, Easton D. Low dose single fraction radiotherapy in the treatment of metastatic bone pain: a pilot study. Radiother Oncol 12:297–301, 1988.

38. Janjan NA. Radiotherapeutic management of spinal metastases. J Pain Symptom Manage 11:47–56, 1996.

39. McKenna RJ. Clinical aspects of cancer in the elderly: treatment decisions, treatment choices and follow-up. Cancer 74:2107–2117, 1994.

40. Holland JC, Massie MJ. Pscyhosocial as-

pects of cancer in the elderly. Clin Geriat Med 3:2766–2770, 1987.

41. Larson PJ, Lindsey AM, Dodd MJ, Brecht ML, Packer A. Influence of age on problems experienced by patients with lung cancer undergoing radiation therapy. Oncol Nurs Forum 20:473–480, 1993.

42. Turesson I, Nyman J, Holmberg E, Oden A. Prognostic factors for acute and late skin reactions in radiotherapy patients. Int J Radiat Oncol Biol Phys 36:1065–1075, 1996.

43. Wyckoff J, Greenberg H, Sanderson R, Wallach P, Balducci L. Breast irradiation in the older woman: a toxicity study. J Am Geriatr Soc 42:150–152, 1994.

44. Mundt AJ. Radiation therapy and the elderly. In: Hunter CP, Johnson KA, Muss HB (Eds.). Cancer in the Elderly. New York, Marcel Dekker, pp. 187–216, 2000.

45. Busch-Deveaux E, Kemeny MM. Surgery in the elderly oncology patient. In: Hunter CP, Johnson KA, Muss HB (Eds.). Cancer in the Elderly. New York, Marcel Dekker, pp. 153–186, 2000.

46. Arnaud JP, Schoegel M, Ollier JC, Adloff M. Colorectal cancer in patients over 80 years of age. Dis Colon Rectum 34:896–898, 1991.

47. Niederhuber JE, Brennan MF, Menck HR. The National Cancer Data Base report on pancreatic cancer. Cancer 76:1671–1677, 1995.

48. Watanapa P, Williamson RCN. Surgical palliation for pancreatic cancer: developments during the past two decades. Br J Surg 79:8–20, 1992.

49. Peters WR, Fleshman JW. Minimally invasive colectomy in elderly patients. Surg Laparosc Endosc 5:477–479, 1995.

50. Goodwin JS, Hunt WC, Samet JM. Determinants of cancer therapy in elderly patients. Cancer 72:594–601, 1993.

51. Kozachik SL, Gicen CW, Given BA, et al. Improving depressive symptoms among caregivers of patients with cancer: results of a randomized clinical trial. Oncol Nurs Forum 28:1149–1157, 2001.

52. Hayman JA, Langa KM, Kabeto MU, et al. Estimating the cost of informal caregiving for elderly patients with cancer. J Clin Oncol 19:3219–3225, 2001.

12

Stroke: Prognosis, Treatment, and Rehabilitation

STEVEN R. FLANAGAN AND STANLEY TUHRIM

Stroke is a major public health problem, af-flicting primarily older adults. It is the third leading cause of death in the United States and is surpassed only by heart disease worldwide.[1,2] In the United States, over 700,000 new strokes occur annually.[3] Stroke is also the leading cause of disability in the United States, with an estimated 4 million stroke survivors living with stroke-related deficits.[1] Over 70% of stroke survivors remain vocationally impaired, over 30% require help with activities of daily living (ADL), and 20% walk only with assistance.[4] Approximately half of stroke survivors return to some form of employment, but this figure declines with age.[5] Although the potential impact of a stroke can be devastating, much can be done to mitigate its effects.

Stroke is actually a heterogeneous group of three distinct diseases: subarachnoid hemorrhage, intracerebral hemorrhage, and cerebral infarction. Although the epidemiology, clinical presentation, and initial treatment of these conditions may vary, the issues surrounding the palliation and reha-bilitation of patients suffering these types of stroke are more similar than different, de-pending more on the deficits incurred than the original pathophysiology of the ictus. The sections that follow provide a brief de-scription of each of these forms of stroke, followed by a detailed account of the reha-bilitation process common to all.

SUBARACHNOID HEMORRHAGE

Subarachnoid hemorrhage (SAH) is extra-vasation of blood at the brain surface into the cerebrospinal fluid, usually due to rup-ture of an aneurysm in an artery at the base of the brain. The majority of patients with SAH harbor saccular aneurysms as the cause of bleeding. Saccular aneurysms form at the bifurcation of large arteries and are probably caused by a combination of con-genital and degenerative changes in arter-ies. Less often, bleeding may be due to trauma to a surface vessel. Arteriovenous malformations can also cause SAH but rarely do so in the elderly.

Subarachnoid hemorrhage accounts for 5%–10% of all strokes. The incidence varies from 6 to 16 per 100,000 and increases with advancing age, with women affected more often than men by a ratio of 3:2.[6,7] Patients with SAH in the Framingham Study averaged 63 years of age.[8] Tobacco use and heavy alcohol consumption have been identified as risk factors for SAH.[9,10] Hypertension does not play as important a role in SAH risk as in other forms of stroke. The cause of SAH is more often undetermined in the elderly than in younger patients. Amyloid angiopathy, a degenerative condition of the arterial wall that markedly increases vessel fragility (see below), and/or unrecognized head trauma are often thought to be responsible.

Morbidity and mortality rates are high in SAH. About 12% of SAH patients die before receiving medical attention.[11,12] The 90-day mortality rate among those who do receive medical attention is about 25%, and 40% of survivors suffer residual cognitive, motor, and sensory deficits.[12] Early mortality results from the direct effects of the initial or recurrent bleeding, while delayed cerebral ischemia, secondary to vasospasm induced by subarachnoid blood, and medical complications that arise in the neurologically impaired patient are responsible for most deaths beyond the first week. Preventive treatment for delayed ischemia with nimodipine is begun as soon as aneurysmal SAH is recognized and continued for 21–28 days. Obliteration of the aneurysm is the key treatment for aneurysmal SAH. In the acute phase, this allows treatment of vasospasm (if ischemic symptoms develop) with hypervolemic, hypertensive therapy and in all patients removes the possibility of recurrent bleeding. Craniotomy and surgical clipping of the aneurysm are generally employed, but endovascular techniques currently being refined may provide a less invasive alternative, particularly in the elderly, where prolonged durability may be of secondary importance compared with the risk of acute morbidity.

INTRACEREBRAL HEMORRHAGE

Intracerebral hemorrhage (ICH) is localized bleeding into the brain parenchyma. It accounts for 10%–15% of all strokes and is associated with the highest mortality.[13] It can be classified into primary or secondary, on the basis of the underlying etiology of bleeding. Primary ICH accounts for about 80% of all cases[14] and is caused by spontaneous rupture of small vessels deep within the brain parenchyma that have been pathologically affected by chronic hypertension. Secondary ICH occurs in a minority of patients in association with structural vascular abnormalities, tumors, or impaired coagulation. Amyloid angiopathy occurs exclusively in older adults (age >60 years), affecting the cerebral vasculature selectively and favoring the lobar regions, while sparing deeper structures typically affected in hypertensive ICH. Incidence rises dramatically with age; in an autopsy series, it was present in 5% of those 60–69 years of age but rose to 50% in those over age 80.[15] Amyloid angiopathy also occurs with increased frequency in Alzheimer's disease patients, and at least 40% of patients with amyloid-related ICH have histological changes consistent with Alzheimer's disease at autopsy.[16]

The annual incidence of ICH is approximately 15 per 100,000 persons overall but increases with age to approximately 100 per 100,000 persons over age 75.[17–19] In younger groups, ICH is equally common in men and women; but it is more frequent in men after the age of 55.[19,20] It occurs more frequently in African Americans[17] and the Japanese.[21] For example, the incidence of ICH in the African-American cohort was 50 per 100,000, twice that of whites, in the National Health and Nutrition Examination Survey Epidemiologic Follow-up Study.[22] There are approximately 50,000 new cases of ICH in the United States every year, with a twofold increase expected in coming years due to increasing age and changes in the racial composition of the population.[23,24]

Hypertension is the most important risk factor for spontaneous ICH,[25,26], particularly in persons who are not compliant with antihypertensive medication,[27,28] while improved control of hypertension reduces the incidence of ICH.[18]

Mortality following spontaneous ICH ranges from 23% to 58%. Clinical severity, as measured by the initial Glasgow Coma Scale (GCS) score; hematoma volume; and presence of ventricular blood on initial computed tomographic scan have been consistently identified as predictive of high mortality.[29,30] Approximately 25% of patients who are alert when they reach the hospital deteriorate within the first 24 hours after onset. The presence of large hematomas and ventricular blood increases the risk for subsequent deterioration. Hematoma expansion is the most common cause underlying neurological deterioration within the first 3 hours. Worsening cerebral edema is also an important contributor in patients who deteriorate 24–48 hours after onset.[31,32] Knowledge of these accurately predictive variables and use of predictive instruments that can quantify the likelihood of mortality or long-term disability can guide the physician and family members or proxies in making decisions regarding life-prolonging therapies.

The long-term functional outcome in ICH survivors is similar to that observed with cerebral infarction. Approximately 40% of patients are functionally independent after 1 year.[33] Age, initial GCS, presence of ventricular blood, hematoma volume, and initial disability predict long-term outcome.[33,34] The likelihood of incurring a second ICH is about 2% annually, although the risk for recurrent ICH is much higher among lobar hemorrhages since these are more frequently the result of an underlying vascular anomaly (amyloid angiopathy in the elderly). The likelihood of recurrence is also much greater in those with persistently uncontrolled hypertension.[35] There is at least a 3% annual risk for ischemic stroke among survivors of primary ICH.[36]

ISCHEMIC STROKE

Infarction accounts for about 80% of strokes. There are three main subcategories of infarction: (1) cardioembolic, (2) large vessel atherothrombotic, and (3) small vessel or lacunar stroke.

Emboli from thrombi that form in the heart or that occur in large veins and pass through the heart via a right-to-left shunt account for approximately 30% of ischemic strokes. A variety of cardiac sources of embolism have been identified, but atrial fibrillation is the most frequent cardiac abnormality associated with ischemic stroke. It is a condition of the elderly, occurring in only 0.1% of those 50–59 years of age but increasing to 4% in those over age 80. The proportion of patients whose strokes are attributed to atrial fibrillation (AF) also increases with age, from 7% of those aged 50–60 to 36% for those over age 80.[37]

Lacunae are small, deep infarcts caused by degenerative changes within small penetrating arteries that arise from the large, circumferential arteries on the surface of the brain. Lacunar infarcts are the most common vascular lesions found within the brain at necropsy and account for at least 25% of ischemic strokes. The diagnosis of lacunar infarction is based on the presence of risk factors, the nature of the clinical signs and symptoms, and the results of neuroimaging tests. Most often, patients with lacunar infarction have a history of hypertension or diabetes.

Large vessel atherothrombotic stroke occurs when the large vessels that bring blood into the brain suffer atherosclerotic narrowing, most commonly at sites of origin or bifurcation. This is especially common at the bifurcation of the common carotid artery into the internal and external carotid arteries in the neck. Atherosclerotic stenosis leads to infarction by reducing blood flow distal to the point of stenosis and by acting as a nidus for the adhesion and aggregation of platelets, producing either thrombosis at that location or embolization to and occlusion of more distal arteries. Neurological symptoms and signs will depend on the affected artery. In general terms, symptoms of cerebral ischemia can be divided into those that arise from the anterior circulation, supplying the anterior three-fourths of each hemisphere, and the posterior circulation, supplying the occipital lobes, posterior thalamus, cerebellum, and brainstem. This distinction is important in determining recurrent stroke-prevention strategies because significant (>50%) narrowing of the cervical portion of the internal carotid artery should be treated surgically in most instances (see below).

ACUTE THERAPY

In June 1996, the U.S. Food and Drug Administration approved the use of tissue plasminogen activator in acute ischemic stroke if given within 3 hours of symptom onset. This remains the only treatment proven safe and effective for acute ischemic stroke. Although most patients who arrive in hospital within 3 hours of symptom onset will be candidates for intravenous thrombolysis, most (>90%) still arrive outside this time window. Improved educational efforts aimed at the population at risk are needed to improve recognition of the symptoms of stroke and the need for prompt treatment (Table 12–1). Intra-arterial thrombolysis, which may have a longer effective time window, requires that a microcatheter be advanced to, and sometimes through, the obstructing clot. A thrombolytic agent is then injected. This form of therapy is available only at selected centers but is gaining increased acceptance.[38]

Over the past 30 years, anticoagulation with unfractionated heparin has probably been the most widely used acute stroke treatment, yet no clinical trial has demonstrated its efficacy. In the International Stroke Trial,[39] there was an increased risk of hemorrhage in the high-dose heparin group that offset any decrease in the recurrent stroke rate, even in patients with AF. Outcome measures were similarly unaffected by anticoagulation. Low-molecular-weight heparins have been studied in several randomized trials, which have also been unable to demonstrate a benefit in acute stroke.[40,41] Early treatment with aspirin is common for patients not treated with thrombolysis or anticoagulation. This practice arose because aspirin was of proven benefit in secondary stroke prevention and in the acute management of myocardial ischemia, but recently two trials evaluated its benefit in over 40,000 patients treated within 48 hours of stroke onset. In the International Stroke Trial, although there was no difference in the primary outcome measures among treatment groups, secondary analyses demonstrated a small (2.8% vs. 3.9%) decrease in the rate of recurrent ischemic stroke in patients treated with aspirin. The Chinese Acute Stroke Trial randomized 21,106 patients to aspirin 160 mg or placebo for 4 weeks and demonstrated a slightly lower mortality rate (3.3% vs. 3.9%) and recurrent stroke rate (1.6% vs. 2.1%) in the aspirin group.[42]

The most widely applicable, effective acute stroke intervention is the use of dedicated acute stroke units. In randomized trials, this approach reduces death or dependency from stroke by as much as thrombolysis, but is applicable to all stroke patients.[43] Dedicated acute stroke units take various forms. Some focus on the initial 48 hours of care, while others include rehabilitation programs (discussed below); but numerous studies have demonstrated their effectiveness relative to general med-

Table 12–1. Effectiveness of Different Acute Stroke Interventions

Intervention	Stroke population treatable (%)	Absolute risk reduction (%)	Number needed to treat
Stroke unit	80	6.6	15
Aspirin	80	1.2	83
Thrombolysis	5	6.5	15

Source: Hankey.[43]

ical or neurological services. While the characteristics of these units may vary, they share an integrated approach to patient care in which an interdisciplinary team, including physicians, nurses, and therapists, works together to provide close monitoring and rapid assessment and treatment of the patient. As a result, short-term and long-term mortality rates are lower, hospitalizations are shorter, and patients are more likely to be discharged to home. The overall cost of the illness is also reduced.[44]

STROKE PREVENTION

Although effective treatment of acute stroke exists, it is far preferable to prevent its occurrence or recurrence. Effective prevention addresses general stroke risk factors and specific etiologies identified in a given individual.

Hypertension is the most important modifiable stroke risk factor. This was first demonstrated by investigators in the Framingham Heart Study, who found that stroke risk increased proportionally to both systolic and diastolic blood pressure throughout the measured range.[45] This effect has been found to be consistent across many populations.[46] Subsequent studies have demonstrated that reduction of blood pressure lowers initial stroke risk.[47] Treatment of isolated systolic hypertension is also clearly beneficial, especially in the elderly.[48] The Perindopril pROtection aGainst REcurrent Stroke Study (PROGRESS) trial demonstrated the benefit of blood pressure reduction with angiotensin-converting enzyme (ACE) inhibitor–based therapy in the secondary prevention of ischemic and hemorrhagic stroke among over 6100 subjects in 35 countries worldwide.[49] The choice of specific antihypertensive agent is probably less important than obtaining satisfactory blood pressure control and should be determined by individual patient characteristics, although a recent study suggested that an ACE inhibitor may provide stroke protection beyond its antihypertensive effect.[50] Since ACE inhibitors are generally well tolerated in the elderly, they should be con-

sidered as initial antihypertensive treatment in a stroke-prone individual. National guidelines suggest blood pressure of less than 140/85 (135/80 in diabetics) as the appropriate treatment goal.[51]

Elevated serum cholesterol is an important risk factor for coronary artery disease, but the evidence regarding its significance as a stroke risk factor is ambiguous. The Multiple Risk Factor Intervention Trial screened 351,000 men and demonstrated a curvilinear relationship, in which serum cholesterol more than approximately 240 mg/dl was associated with an increased risk of ischemic stroke mortality, while a level less than 140 mg/dl was associated with an increased risk of ICH.[52] However, the Prospective Studies Collaboration, a meta-analysis of 45 observational studies, failed to find a relationship between total cholesterol and stroke among 450,000 individuals.[53] Similarly, neither the Framingham Study[54] nor the Cardiovascular Health Study[55] demonstrated a relationship between cholesterol and stroke. Consistent with these primarily negative findings, early studies of cholesterol reduction failed to find a beneficial effect on stroke risk. However, more recent trials in patients with coronary artery disease and normal or elevated serum cholesterol levels using hydroxymethylglutaryl coenzyme A reductase inhibitors have consistently demonstrated a relative risk reduction of 20%–30% for stroke, similar to the risk reduction demonstrated for the various cardiovascular events studied.[56,57] This seemingly paradoxical finding may be explained by the putative effects of these "statins" on the stability of atherosclerotic plaques, smooth muscle cells, endothelial cell function, platelet adhesion, and inflammation, in addition to lowering low-density lipoprotein (LDL) cholesterol.[58] The effect of triglycerides on stroke risk is also unclear, but a recent study of gemfibrozil demonstrated a similar degree of stroke risk reduction with minimal effect on high-density or low-density lipoproteins but significant lowering of triglycerides, suggesting that triglycerides may also play a more significant role in stroke than previously recognized.[59] Current guidelines suggest treating individuals with coronary artery disease whose LDL cholesterol is >130 mg/dl with a target of <100 mg/dl. In view of the results of recent trials, extending this recommendation to patients with cerebrovascular disease seems prudent.

The Framingham Study was also among the first prospective cohort studies to demonstrate an increased stroke risk for cigarette smokers. Smokers had twice the risk of stroke as nonsmokers, but that risk was eliminated within about 2 years of cessation.[60] Most studies have shown an increased risk of stroke with heavy alcohol consumption, but moderate consumption (fewer than 2 drinks/day) has been shown to be protective against stroke.[61] While urging heavy drinkers to decrease or eliminate their alcohol consumption is advisable for many reasons, the idea of encouraging nondrinkers to begin is controversial. Among stroke survivors, results of attempts to encourage smoking cessation and decrease alcohol consumption among heavy drinkers have been mixed. Similarly, control of hypertension and hyperlipidemia has not been achieved consistently.[62]

Elevated levels of homocysteine in the blood, termed *hyperhomocysteinemia*, have been associated with increased risk of stroke and myocardial infarction.[63] Individuals with levels above 15 μmol/l appear to have five times the risk of stroke of those with levels below 10 μmol/l. The efficacy of reducing stroke risk by lowering blood homocysteine levels with a combination of vitamin B_6, vitamin B_{12}, and folic acid is currently being assessed, but recommending the use of a multivitamin containing these elements, especially in the elderly, appears prudent. Lower salt intake (accompanied by increased dietary potassium and calcium),[64] a diet high in folic acid and low in saturated fats, and no more than moderate alcohol consumption would likewise be advisable for elderly patients with cerebrovascular disease.

As mentioned above, AF is a particularly important risk factor in the elderly. Chronic AF in association with valvular heart disease increases stroke risk 17-fold, while in the absence of valvular disease stroke risk is still increased fivefold.[37] Recent studies have identified factors that increase stroke risk in nonvalvular AF, including old age, hypertension, recent onset of congestive heart failure, diabetes mellitus, a history of systemic embolism, or cerebral ischemia. Poor left ventricular function and increased left atrial size on echocardiogram also increase risk.[65]

Chronic anticoagulation with warfarin is very effective at reducing stroke risk in AF patients with or without a history of stroke. Anticoagulation should be prescribed for all patients who have had cerebral ischemic symptoms in the setting of AF, unless there is a specific contraindication.[66] In patients with noncardioembolic stroke, anticoagulation with an average international normalized ratio of 2.1 is equivalent (but not superior) in safety and efficacy of recurrent stroke prevention to antiplatelet therapy with aspirin 325 mg daily.[67]

Antiplatelet therapy is the most commonly prescribed stroke prevention remedy and is usually appropriate for any symptomatic individual who does not require anticoagulation. No consensus exists regarding the optimal dose, with recent recommendations suggesting a range of 50–325 mg,[68] although other authorities suggest that higher doses are more effective, if tolerated.[69] Analysis of stroke prevention among patients with cardiovascular disease indicated the superiority of aspirin 160 mg daily to the combination of aspirin 81 mg and warfarin 1 mg.[70] Newer medications, such as Aggrenox (a combination of 25 mg aspirin and 200 mg dipyridamole in a sustained-release formulation), ticlopidine, and clopidogrel, appear to have somewhat greater efficacy than aspirin alone in randomized trials;[68] but maintenance on these medications currently costs in excess of $1000/year in the United States for an individual purchasing the drug at a retail pharmacy. Elderly patients with vascular disease without prescription drug coverage have disproportionately large drug expenditures and are less likely to use preventive medications such as statins than those who have prescription coverage,[71] implying that cost is a significant contributor to lack of compliance. Since the differences among various antiplatelet agents are small compared with the effect of taking no anti-platelet agent and compliance is a major problem, attention should be directed to ensuring that patients are compliant with whatever regimen is prescribed.

Endarterectomy is the most widely used specific treatment for carotid stenosis. In both the European Carotid Stenosis Trial (ECST)[72] and the North American Symptomatic Carotid Endarterectomy Trial (NASCET),[73] individuals with symptoms referable to a highly stenotic (70%–90%) carotid artery randomized to the nonsurgical arms had an estimated 28% 2-year stroke rate. The ipsilateral stroke rate was 22% in ECST and 26% in NASCET. Individuals with moderate symptomatic stenosis had stroke rates approximately one-half those of the highly stenotic groups. The benefit of surgery at reducing subsequent stroke risk in the symptomatic highly stenotic groups was clear. This benefit disappeared once the degree of stenosis was <50% by NASCET criteria (comparable to approximately 75% by ECST criteria).

The benefit of surgery must be balanced against the risk for each individual. Life expectancy also plays a role in the decision-making process since there is early morbidity including stroke and death associated with the procedure. This should be <3% in experienced hands. When contemplating endarterectomy, the vascular territory at risk must also be considered. The benefit of endarterectomy is primarily in preventing strokes in the territory of the stenotic carotid artery. If that territory has already suffered a major infarction and recovery of functions it controls is deemed unlikely, there would be little potential benefit to surgery.

Opinions vary with regard to how long to wait after a stroke has occurred before performing an endarterectomy. Several case series suggest that in mild to moderate stroke immediate endarterectomy is safe,[74] while many experts recommend waiting 4–6 weeks to allow sufficient healing at the infarct site and return of cerebral autoregulation. In stable patients with fixed deficits and infarcts evident on imaging studies, waiting 4 weeks would seem prudent; but in unstable patients with fluctuating deficits and hemodynamically significant ipsilateral carotid stenoses, consideration should be given to immediate surgery.

A key element in post-stroke patient care is the prevention of recurrence. Recurrent strokes are more likely to be disabling than initial ones. Secondary prevention measures are effective and more likely to be utilized and tolerated if patients understand their importance. Physicians must recognize the importance and effectiveness of these measures and educate their patients in this regard. Given these caveats, endarterectomy can be performed safely even in the very elderly and should be recommended for appropriate individuals of any age whose life expectancy is great enough to anticipate benefit despite the risk of early perioperative morbidity (Table 12–2).

Table 12–2. Effectiveness of Different Secondary Stroke Prevention Strategies

Intervention	Transient ischemic attack/ischemic stroke eligible (%)	Absolute risk reduction	Relative risk reduction	Number needed to treat
Hypertension control	50	2.2	28	45
Cholesterol-lowering	40	1.7	24	60
Anticoagulation	20	8.0	67	12
Antiplatelet therapy*	75	1.2	23	83
Carotid endarterectomy	8	3.8	44	26

*Aspirin, clopidogrel, or aspirin + dipyridamole.
Source: Hankey.[43]

STROKE REHABILITATION

Medical advances have significantly improved survival after stroke, although afflicted individuals are often left with multiple disabling conditions in the realms of motor skills, mobility, self-care skills, communication, nutrition, and cognition. Physical and cognitive outcomes vary after stroke, with most individuals typically requiring some rehabilitation intervention, which is best initiated shortly after the onset of stroke to ensure a timely restoration of optimal functioning. The multitude of potential stroke-related impairments dictate that an interdisciplinary rehabilitation approach be initiated, optimally directed by a physiatrist. A *physiatrist* is a physician specifically trained in physical medicine and rehabilitation who works closely with other medical consultants and leads the rehabilitation team. Other members of the rehabilitation team vary depending on the specific needs of the patient (Table 12–3).

The physiatrist directs the rehabilitation team by prescribing specific treatments, monitoring the patient's progress over time, and anticipating and preventing secondary complications such as pressure sores, contractures, thrombophlebitis, and infection. Ideally, physiatrists are involved in patient care within the first few days following the stroke and follow the patient through acute neurological care and, as needed, through acute and subacute rehabilitation, outpatient rehabilitation, and lifelong management of disability-related conditions. Physiatrists also set specific goals for patients with stroke, which in general include maximizing mobility and self-care skills. Often, the use of various

adaptive aids, such as braces, canes, walkers, and long-handled reaches, are needed to achieve desired functional goals. Other goals include maximizing communication skills, ensuring safe and adequate nutrition, enhancing mood, and maximizing cognitive skills. Although many factors influence stroke recovery, including age, severity of impairments, and mood, the impact of specific impairments can be lessened by rehabilitation interventions, which are provided with the goal of enhancing independent living skills.

THE REHABILITATION PROCESS

Rehabilitation intervention should be initiated very shortly after a stroke, to begin the process of recovery and prevent secondary complications. A physiatry consultation should be sought within the first 2 days following a stroke to begin the process of rehabilitation. Other rehabilitation professionals are then involved under the direction of the physiatrist, as indicated by the patient's medical stability and neurological condition. Early physical therapy interventions are geared toward prevention of the deleterious effects of immobility, including joint contractures, thrombophlebitis, atelectasis, and pressure sores. Joints are ranged either passively by the therapist or by the patient using the nonparalyzed limbs. Regular mobilization of all joints through their full range of motion (ROM) is critically important as paralysis, spasticity, and general immobilization lead to joint contracture in a relatively short period of time, adversely impacting on mobility, self-care skills, skin health, and proper positioning. Maintenance of joint ROM will considerably ease the rehabilitation process during later stages of recovery, when therapists and patients can devote more time to re-attainment of functional skills rather than concentrating on limitations of joint ROM. The physical therapist should instruct the patient and family members in proper ROM exercises to enhance the beneficial effects of joint flexibility.

Table 12–3. Rehabilitation Team Members

Physiatrist	Vocational counselor
Medical consultants	Social worker
Physical therapist	Orthotist
Occupational therapist	Nutritionist
Neuropsychologist	Driving evaluator
Speech–language pathologist	Equipment coordinator
Recreational therapist	Rehabilitation engineer
	Patient and family

The early goals of occupational therapy are similar to those of physical therapy, particularly regarding upper limb flexibility and strengthening. Therapists will frequently utilize upper limb orthotics, such as resting hand or wrist splints, to prevent joint contractures. Speech–language pathologists often perform bedside swallowing evaluations during the first few days following a stroke to determine a patient's ability to swallow safely and maintain adequate nutrition and hydration. Additionally, simple communication devices can be provided to patients with impairments in either speech production or language.

Inpatient rehabilitation is required for individuals who have physical and/or cognitive impairments that persist beyond the acute stage. In general, patients are considered for acute inpatient rehabilitation following stroke if they can actively participate in at least 3 hours of daily rehabilitation 5 days per week, which is based on Medicare criteria. Individuals in acute inpatient rehabilitation should also have the potential to improve their functional skills in a reasonable amount of time. However, prediction of who will ultimately benefit from an intense rehabilitation program is difficult as generally accepted prognostic signs for poor recovery at the time of stroke are unreliable when applied to individual cases.[75] This suggests that most patients, regardless of age, level of disability, and sphincter control, should be given a trial of either acute or subacute rehabilitation. Therefore, if an individual does not meet the criteria for acute inpatient rehabilitation, subacute rehabilitation, which provides similar services but at a lower intensity level and over a longer period of time, should be considered. Conversely, if an individual has only mild impairments requiring less than 3 hours of daily therapy, either outpatient or home-based rehabilitation can be provided.

Once a patient is admitted to either an acute or a subacute rehabilitation setting, the physiatrist immediately performs a comprehensive evaluation. Documentation includes a detailed medical history, listing of premorbid functional skills, living arrangements, vocational and avocational endeavors, and a thorough neurological, musculoskeletal, and functional examination. The physiatrist then uses this information to predict functional outcomes and length of hospitalization, prescribe a detailed rehabilitation plan addressing the identified impairments and disabilities, and order appropriate diagnostic tests.

The rehabilitation prescription includes the patient's age, the location and type of stroke, related impairments and disabilities, all other medical conditions, as well as a listing of potential problems that may be encountered during the course of treatment, such as orthostasis, seizures, and hypoglycemia. The prescription identifies the rehabilitation services required by the patient and guides treatment, which ranges from general guidelines to specific interventions. All specified therapists are instructed to evaluate the patient and develop their own specific goals for the patient within their areas of expertise.

Bedside rounds are made daily for all inpatients on the rehabilitation medicine service and are ideally attended by physicians, rehabilitation nurses, and at least one representative from the therapy services. Within several days of admission, an initial conference is held to discuss the findings of all members of the interdisciplinary team, the patient's initial response to treatment, and the prognosis and timetable for inpatient rehabilitation. Rehabilitation goals are refined and options for posthospital care discussed. If a discharge to home is planned, arrangements are made for home care services, including attendant services and continued therapy, necessary equipment to ensure both safety and continued independence, and if needed, architectural modifications to make the home accessible. Additional team meetings are held weekly to discuss the patient's response to treatment, modify the program as needed, and update the discharge plan. If the patient's progress or other situations dictate that a safe discharge to the community is not feasible, alternative plans for longer-term care

are made, which may include transferring the patient to a subacute rehabilitation facility. The physiatrist meets with the patient and family after each team conference to discuss the patient's progress and address concerns.

THE REHABILITATION TEAM

Successful medical care results from a coordinated effort of multiple professionals, paraprofessionals, patients, and their loved ones, which is no more evident than in rehabilitation medicine. Effective rehabilitation is primarily dependent on the motivation of the patient to participate in therapy and the support received from loved ones. An integrated interdisciplinary team approach to rehabilitation is a prerequisite for a successful outcome (Table 12–3). The team is led by a physiatrist and typically includes a physical therapist, occupational therapist, rehabilitation psychologist, and social worker, with additional members included as deemed necessary by the patient's physical, cognitive, and emotional needs.

Physiatrist

A physiatrist provides medical care to individuals with physical and cognitive impairments. As the leader of the team, the physiatrist is responsible for overseeing all aspects of the rehabilitation process, including identifying which team members are needed, prescribing all treatments, and leading patient evaluation conferences. The physiatrist typically prescribes all medical care for patients on the inpatient rehabilitation medicine service, which requires a solid medical knowledge base. Good interpersonal skills are needed to lead the team effectively, including listening, motivating, negotiating, and mentoring. Physiatrists who provide care to individuals with stroke must be familiar with identifying and treating all stroke-related medical conditions and ensure that appropriate measures are taken to prevent stroke propagation, stroke re-occurrence, and all other stroke-related complications.

Physical Therapist

The goals of physical therapy are to maximize joint ROM, muscle strength, flexibility, coordination, balance, and mobility skills. This is achieved through therapeutic exercises as well as functional training in ambulation, curb and stair negotiation, transferring from various surfaces, and wheelchair propulsion. Frequently, adaptive devices are used to improve joint ROM or to ensure safety, including braces, walkers, and canes. Various physical modalities are available to the therapist to alleviate pain, including ultrasound, transcutaneous electrical nerve stimulation, electrical muscle stimulation, and deep or superficial heat and cold. As needed, a physical therapist will make a visit to a patient's home, often with an occupational therapist, to make recommendations to improve accessibility.

Occupational Therapist

The occupational therapist strives to improve a patient's skill in the performance of ADL (Table 12–4). This is achieved through strengthening and coordinating exercises for the upper limbs and functional activities, such as practicing transferring from various surfaces (e.g., tubs and commodes), dressing, and grooming. Instrumental ADLs, including housekeeping chores, shopping, and bill paying, are also addressed as needed. The occupational therapist assesses a patient's visual, perceptual, and cognitive abilities, particularly regarding their impact on the safe performance of ADLs, and provides treatment to lessen their impact. Adaptive devices are frequently used to promote upper limb flexibility and joint ROM as well as to aid in the safe and effective completion of ADLs. Adaptive aids frequently used following stroke include elevated toilet seats, tub

Table 12–4. Activities of Daily Living

Grooming	Home management
Hygiene	Transfers
Bathing	Toileting
Dressing	Feeding

transfer benches, grab bars, long-handled reachers, and eating utensils with large handles for easy gripping.

Rehabilitation Nurse

The rehabilitation nurse is an integral member of the team and is responsible not only for routine nursing care but also for additional care required by patients who often show severe physical and cognitive impairments. Rehabilitation nurses evaluate the specific needs of patients with stroke, develop an appropriate plan of care, and regularly assess the patient for developing complications, alerting other members of the rehabilitation team. Nurses are the only team members who regularly provide direct care around the clock. Therefore, they are often the first to notice complications and to initiate treatment. They are instrumental in insuring that skills learned during therapy sessions are carried through to the nursing unit. They provide valuable education to patients regarding medication, further stroke prevention, sexual dysfunction, mobility, positioning, and bowel and bladder management. Education is also provided to other nurses unfamiliar with specific stroke-related nursing issues. Emotional and behavioral issues are routinely assessed and information passed on to the team to ensure rapid and effective interventions. As patients prepare for discharge to their community, nurses ensure that all necessary nursing equipment is ordered and that patients and family members have been thoroughly trained on their proper use. Nursing care typically continues at home with regular assessments of the patient's condition and ability to function at home. The close working relationship that nurses require with their patients in order to ensure good care makes them invaluable members of the team as they often serve as the liaison for the patient to communicate with other team members.

Speech–Language Pathologist

Strokes often result in altered communication skills, in the form either of speech production or of producing or understanding language. Therapists provide treatment geared toward effective communication, either through vocal production or in some cases through augmentative communication techniques, such as communication boards or electronic devices. Swallowing disorders often result from stroke, which may place afflicted individuals at serious risk for aspiration. Speech–language pathologists evaluate patients' risks for aspiration at the bedside. If indicated, a videofluoroscopy of swallowing is evaluated by a speech–language pathologist, who then recommends both dietary modifications and specific techniques that minimize the risk of aspiration.

Rehabilitation Psychologist

The rehabilitation psychologist assesses the psychological condition of patients and assists them and their families to adapt to the new disability. Psychologists provide emotional support to both patients and their families and inform team members of pertinent psychological issues. The patient's cognitive abilities are assessed, and when needed, the psychologist provides remediation techniques to lessen the impact on ADL skills. When maladaptive behaviors arise as a result of stroke or trauma, psychologists assist with the development of a behavioral management plan to help promote adaptive behaviors.

Therapeutic Recreational Therapist

Recreational therapists are instrumental in assisting patients to return to their previous avocational pursuits. They are keenly aware of the provisions in the Americans with Disabilities Act, which they pass on to patients to help ensure that they are not limited by unnecessary barriers to community living. Therapists work closely with other rehabilitation team members to enhance the beneficial effects of skills learned in other areas. For instance, wheelchair mobility skills learned by a patient in physical or occupational therapy will be utilized by a recreational therapist to promote community excursions using public transportation. Innovative recreational therapy programs utilize a variety of modalities to promote socialization skills, ranging from computer training to pet-assisted therapy.

Vocational Counselor

The vocational counselor assists individuals with physical and/or cognitive impairments to return to either employment or school. This is achieved through assessment, counseling, skill training, supportive employment, and job placement. Often, modifications in the work place are recommended, which requires that the vocational counselor work closely with the patient, the rehabilitation team, and the employer.

Social Worker

The rehabilitation social worker helps patients and family members cope with the financial and emotional stress associated with stroke. Early involvement typically includes determining the extent of available financial support for rehabilitation services as well as providing emotional support for patients and family members. Assistance is provided by thoroughly assessing an individual's unique psychosocial needs, which helps the social worker predict the emotional, financial, and social needs of the patient throughout the course of rehabilitation. They are integrally involved with ensuring a smooth transition from acute inpatient rehabilitation to other settings, in either the community, a subacute rehabilitation facility, or a long-term-care facility.

Orthotist

An orthotist fabricates custom-molded splints and braces, also known as orthotic devices. Orthotics are generally indicated for weakened or paralyzed limbs and are designed to enhance strength, increase ROM, and improve function. Orthotic design is guided by the patient's physical condition and the ultimate goal of rehabilitation. For instance, an ankle–foot orthosis often helps a person with a paretic leg walk safely after a stroke by maintaining a paralyzed ankle in an appropriate position throughout the gait cycle. The components and design of the brace are discussed among the physiatrist, orthotist, and either the physical or occupational therapist but ultimately prescribed by the physiatrist.

REHABILITATION OF SPECIFIC IMPAIRMENTS

Paralysis and Immobility

Paralysis following stroke is typically manifested as hemiplegia, which in certain cases may be bilateral, as in locked-in syndrome. Motor impairments may improve over the first few weeks following a stroke, with a better prognosis for neurological recovery predicted the earlier that recovery begins. Many studies have suggested that most recovery of motor function occurs over the first few months after stroke, with motor skills stabilizing after 6–12 months, implying that further recover is unlikely. However, recent studies have challenged this premise, particularly as new treatments to improve function emerge and gain more widespread use. Currently, unpublished data strongly suggest that significant functional improvements can be realized with continued intensive rehabilitation well over 1 year after initial injury.

Traditional rehabilitation efforts should begin immediately after the onset of hemiplegia and ideally include participation by therapists, nurses, patients, and family members. Passive ROM is provided to prevent joint contractures in paralyzed limbs, which is typically accompanied by neurodevelopmental techniques provided by physical and occupational therapists to promote optimal motor recovery. Once medical stability is achieved, wheelchair and ambulation training may proceed. Orthostasis, a common problem resulting from prolonged bed rest, is generally easily managed with the use of lower-limb elastic stockings and abdominal binders. If needed, a tilt table may be used, which allows a therapist to slowly bring a patient from a supine to a fully upright position. Once the standing position has been achieved, balance and ambulation training commences, which may begin on the parallel bars and progress to a walker or cane. Orthotic devices are frequently used on weakened limbs to maintain ROM and improve function. An ankle–foot orthotic is among the most frequently prescribed orthotic device as it prevents foot drop in a paralyzed leg, enabling many patients with stroke to ambulate safely and efficiently.

Other than utilizing neurodevelopmental techniques, traditional rehabilitation efforts have been largely devoted to teaching stroke patients compensatory strategies to improve function. For instance, patients with a plegic upper limb are typically taught to perform ADL using one-handed techniques if there is insufficient motor recovery to use the involved arm functionally. However, therapy concentrating on compensatory strategies, rather than restorative techniques, may result in learned nonuse of the paralyzed limb and subsequently less motor recovery.[76–78] This theory of learned nonuse is the basis for a form of therapy known as constraint-induced movement therapy (CIMT).

In CIMT, the uninvolved upper limb is constrained for 14 hours daily, which is accompanied by an intensive 12-day therapy program consisting of specific activities to increase the use of the weakened arm and hand. Numerous studies have documented significant improvement in the function and strength of the plegic upper limb, even many years after stroke.[79,80] Such therapy may also result in some degree of neural reorganization, supporting the theory of cerebral plasticity.[81–82] Although CIMT appears promising and has received considerable attention in the media, it has been applied to only a select population of patients with stroke. Most studies to date have used CIMT on patients who had already achieved a considerable amount of motor recovery, limiting the generalization of results. Also, it requires highly motivated participants as it severely limits use of the uninvolved upper limb, making completion of ADL temporarily much more challenging.

Electrical stimulation of paralyzed muscles has also been used to enhance motor recovery after stroke, to some degree, for several decades.[83–85] Today, devices are commercially available that detect innate electrical activity in paretic muscles, which is then externally enhanced by a stimulator, resulting in improved motor function. Several studies have demonstrated that this system improves motor skills more than standard rehabilitation strategies alone.[86–89]

Spasticity

Spasticity, defined as a velocity-dependent increase in muscle tone, is a frequent impairment following stroke. It manifests as involuntary resistance to passive ROM accompanied by exaggerated deep tendon reflexes and, when present, typically impairs joint movement, mobility, and ADL. Its adverse impact on function is evident in that it often consumes a tremendous amount of treatment time during the rehabilitation process and can magnify the burden placed on care providers. When it develops, it needs to be addressed immediately to prevent joint contractures, which can seriously limit functional recovery. Traditional treatment has consisted largely of aggressive ROM exercises performed by health-care workers, family members, and when feasible the patients themselves. This is often accompanied by various modalities, such as the application of heat or cold to decrease muscle tone, or orthotic devices to either maintain or increase joint ROM. Plaster casts are often applied to spastic limbs across a contracted joint to maintain muscle stretch for prolonged periods of time, resulting in more effective and efficient improvement in ROM. More invasive methods are utilized as needed and may include pharmacological agents such as baclofen, benzodiazepines, muscle relaxers, and α_2 antagonists. However, most oral agents have other undesirable effects, such as lethargy, confusion, muscle weakness, and inhibition of functional recovery, which limit their usefulness in cerebrally mediated spasticity. Selective nerve blocks with either phenol or purified botulinum toxins are effective at reducing abnormal tone in individual muscles, but retreatment is often needed every few months. Also, antibodies to botulinum toxin may develop, limiting its effectiveness. Despite these drawbacks, considerable improvement in joint ROM and function can be achieved with motor point blocks.

Technological advances in the delivery of pharmacological agents have resulted in a relatively new method to treat spasticity with greater efficacy and fewer side effects. Baclofen is theorized to inhibit spasticity by agonism of γ-aminobutyric acid receptors in the spinal cord. However, large oral doses are typically needed to achieve therapeutic concentrations in the central nervous system, which are often accompanied by unacceptable side effects, including lethargy and confusion. Baclofen can now be provided via an intrathecal delivery system, which concentrates the drug at its site of action (i.e., in the spinal cord), greatly diminishing both the required therapeutic dose and the incidence of undesirable side effects while enhancing the beneficial effect of decreasing spasticity.[90,91] Another considerable advantage of this system is the ability to titrate the dose, enhancing the physician's ability to control the degree of spasticity reduction. This is an important consideration as some degree of spasticity may be used advantageously by patients to transfer, stand, or even ambulate.[92]

Prolonged spasticity typically results in joint contractures, seriously limiting functional skills. Surgical interventions, including tendon lengthening or tenotomy, are indicated in either longstanding untreated or refractory spasticity. Although neither surgery nor any of the other treatment options discussed cures spasticity, appropriate application of these modalities can result in significantly improved function following stroke or brain injury, even when used long after the initial event.

Post-Stroke Depression

Depression is a common comorbidity following stroke; however, its true incidence is not clearly delineated, with reported frequencies ranging from 25% to 79%.[93–104] Numerous methodological factors account for the extent of this range, including subject selection and the lack of reliable biochemical markers for post-stroke depression (PSD). Furthermore, accurately diagnosing PSD is complicated by the limitations of currently utilized instruments, which rely on physical and behavioral observations that may be attributable to stroke-related impairments rather than to depression.[105] For example, hypoarousal, aprosodic speech, and impaired concentration are symptoms of depression but are also directly attributable to stroke and, therefore, not necessarily a manifestation of affect.[105] Furthermore, external expression of affect is not necessarily an accurate representation of internal mood, as with emotional incontinence. Emotional incontinence is a perplexing condition following stroke and brain injury, which is manifested by uncontrolled outbursts of crying or laughing out of proportion to internal feelings of dysphoria or happiness. Lastly, diagnosis of PSD is complicated in patients with aphasia as they cannot verbally report their mood. Therefore, when making a diagnosis of PSD, behavioral observations must be made from multiple sources,[105,106] including the patient, family members, and all rehabilitation team members.

Despite these challenges, accurate and timely diagnosis of PSD is critically important as it has been repeatedly correlated with poorer functional outcomes compared to nondepressed stroke patients.[107–110] Furthermore, it continues to adversely impact on functional skills and the fulfillment of expected societal roles once an individual is discharged to the community and is associated with increased mortality. Therefore, symptoms of depression need to be recognized and treated, regardless of the time elapsed since the onset of stroke.[111–114] Early treatment with antidepressant medications appears to at least partially counter the adverse impact on recovery as several studies have shown that functional and cognitive skills improve with remission of PSD.[115–118] Pharmacological treatment is based largely on modifying central serotonergic systems, which may be injured following a stroke and thereby potentially play a significant role in the genesis of PSD.[119,120]

Subsequently, several studies have examined the effectiveness of various antidepressant medications on amelioration of PSD. Lipsey[121] found that nortriptyline significantly reduced depression scores compared to placebo in a group of stroke patients. However, tricyclic antidepressants are associated with numerous unacceptable side effects and contraindicated in several cardiac conditions that are frequent comorbidities of stroke. Trazodone is also an effective treatment for PSD,[115] although sedation may limit its use. Other studies examining the effectiveness of selective serotonin reuptake inhibitors (SSRIs) on PSD have demonstrated an overall favorable response.[116,122] Not surprisingly, SSRIs have become the preferred pharmacological treatment as they are effective and lack the cardiotoxic and anticholinergic effects of the tricyclic antidepressants.[123]

The use of psychostimulants, either alone or in combination with SSRIs, is becoming more prevalent and accepted as a means to treat PSD. Results of several studies support the use of either methylphenidate or dextroamphetamine to treat PSD.[124–127] Psychostimulants offer the advantage of speed over more traditional antidepressant medications. In a study comparing methylphenidate to nortriptyline, both agents were equally efficacious at remitting depression symptoms, but the response time was 2.4 days for methylphenidate compared to 27 days for nortriptyline.[128] The rapid treatment response of psychostimulants makes their use very advantageous, particularly as the length of inpatient rehabilitation hospitalization is likely to be dramatically reduced due to insurance pressures. Therefore, to enhance the likelihood of good rehabilitation outcomes, it is imperative that the symptoms of PSD be ameliorated as quickly as possible.

As the foregoing discussion demonstrates, the adverse impact of PSD on recovery dictates that it be diagnosed and treated rapidly after stroke. The difficulty in making an accurate diagnosis requires that physicians rely on many observations of patient behavior as depression may not always be obvious on a bedside evaluation. Depression may be manifested only as poor motivation for therapy, displays of dysphoria with family members, or other behaviors noted by other members of the rehabilitation team. Reliance solely on strict diagnostic criteria and available instruments is inadequate and may lead to nondiagnosis, ineffective treatment, and poor recovery. Early use of SSRIs and psychostimulants may ameliorate both the short- and long-term adverse impacts on recovery and subsequently improve quality of life.

PHARMACOLOGICAL INTERVENTIONS TO IMPROVE RECOVERY

The goals of stroke rehabilitation are to maximize mobility and ADL skills, enhance effective communication and cognition, and foster adaptive behaviors. This is typically a very time-consuming process, which combines an individual's natural ability to recover with the application of treatments that assist with the recovery of neurological function and the development of compensatory skills. Recent health-care trends demand that rising costs be curtailed, which for individuals with stroke typically means less time in formal rehabilitation. To achieve the desired rehabilitation goals, health-care providers can no longer rely solely on traditional methods of restoring function. Adjuvant treatments in stroke rehabilitation, either in the form of technological advances, novel pharmacological interventions, or new therapeutic exercise techniques, have been developed and are being used with greater frequency. These approaches are based on anatomical and physiological principles and are designed to not only increase the speed of recovery but to improve an individual's functional and cognitive abilities beyond that possible with traditional methods alone. As described in previous sections, CIMT, electrical stimulation, and intrathecal baclofen therapy are relatively new treatment modalities that have been utilized to enhance recovery after stroke. The following discussion will review data on the pharmacological enhancement of stroke recovery.

Over the past several decades, the role of pharmacological modification of recovery following brain injury has been widely studied. In one of the earliest studies, Feeney et al.[129] demonstrated that rats given a single dose of amphetamine following an experimentally induced cortical lesion recovered motor abilities more quickly than those given placebo, while animals given haloperidol experienced the poorest recovery. Since then, the beneficial role of adrenergic agonism and the adverse impact of both adrenergic and dopaminergic antagonism on recovery have been confirmed.[130–134] Today, pharmacological agents are used with increasing frequency to both enhance overall functional abilities and speed the process of recovery. Neurotransmitter systems that play a role in recovery after brain injury include, but are not limited to, the noradrenergic and dopaminergic systems. Although the cell bodies of these systems are fairly well localized to specific cerebral regions, they have widespread projections throughout the brain, which play an important role in their impact on recovery. Today, clinicians treating individuals with stroke or brain injury need to be familiar with agents that promote recovery and, equally important, with those commonly used agents that may have a detrimental impact on ultimate function.[135–136]

Human studies have essentially mirrored the results obtained on animals. Earlier human studies examining pharmacological intervention following traumatic brain injury (TBI) demonstrated a beneficial effect of amphetamines on recovery of motor skills, ADL, function, and cognition. For example, dextroamphetamine and methylphenidate diminished confusion and paranoia and improved short-term memory in young adults with TBI,[137,138] while methylphenidate enhanced attention compared to natural recovery following TBI and was

well tolerated.[139] Subacute administration of methylphenidate after moderately severe TBI significantly improved the rate, although not the overall level of recovery, in a small group of patients in a randomized, double-blind, placebo-controlled study.[140] While most studies examining the role of amphetamines on recovery have focused on TBI, several have studied their impact following stroke. Dextroamphetamine given to 10 hemiplegic patients at a prescribed time prior to physical therapy resulted in an increased rate and extent of motor recovery, which persisted up to 12 months despite discontinuation of the drug.[141] In a similar study, stroke patients receiving methylphenidate achieved greater motor recovery and were less depressed than subjects receiving placebo.[142] As stated previously, adrenergic antagonists have a detrimental impact on recovery after brain injury. To investigate this in humans, Goldstein[135] restrospectively examined the effects of various drugs on recovery following ischemic stroke. Motor and functional skills were significantly worse in subjects who received at least one of several drugs, including benzodiazepines, dopamine receptor antagonists (e.g., anti-emetics), α_2 agonists, α_1 antagonists, phenytoin, and phenobarbital. Despite their potentially detrimental impact on recovery, these drugs are frequently prescribed following stroke and brain injury.[136,143]

It is reasonable to expect that avoidance of these drugs may improve stroke outcomes, particularly since alternative rehabilitation strategies and numerous pharmacological agents can address the specific behaviors or medical conditions.

Several theories may account for amphetamine's beneficial impact after brain injury. The theory of *diaschisis* holds that an intact neural system that has lost afferent input from a distant and injured neural structure will not function properly. Therefore, administration of amphetamines may diminish a neurological impairment if the noradrenergic system was injured.[144] Amphetamines also increase metabolic activity in regions adjacent to injured cortex, which may result in enhanced functional activity.[145,146] Amphetamines potentially enhance long-term potentiation (LTP), which is a mechanism that may account for the neuronal basis of learning and memory. Norepinephrine enhances LTP, while neuroleptics inhibit it.[147] Lastly, amphetamine's beneficial effect on post-stroke depression likely plays a role in its positive impact on recovery.

Modulation of the dopaminergic system also impacts recovery after brain injury. Dopamine is involved in a wide array of neurological functions, including motor control, cognition, and arousal. Dopamine's role in recovery after brain injury was first inferred from animal studies, which demonstrated that dopaminergic antagonism resulted in poorer outcomes.[148–151] Most evidence supporting dopamine's role in brain injury recovery in humans comes from the TBI literature. Dopaminergic agonism improves the level of consciousness in patients in either a vegetative or a minimally conscious state,[152,153] as well as outcomes in patients with moderate to severe TBI.[154] Enhancement of the dopaminergic system also improves a wide spectrum of cognitive processes following brain injury, including attention, concentration, motor speed, visual/spatial skills, and executive function.[155–158]

Dopamine also plays a potential role in several stroke-related impairments, including hemispatial neglect, functional motor deficits, and aphasia. Hemispatial neglect is a common consequence of nondominant hemisphere strokes, described as an inability to attend to stimuli from the contralateral hemispace. Significant functional impairments typically result from hemispatial neglect, which complicates recovery. Although rehabilitation strategies to increase attention to the neglected hemispace have been shown to improve function,[159] they are frequently insufficient to counter the deleterious effects on mobility and ADL skills.

Injury to the dopaminergic system has been implicated in the genesis of hemispatial neglect,[160,161] although its exact role has not been fully delineated. Despite this, several trials have examined the role of dopaminergic agonism on neglect with mixed results. Treatment with various dopaminergic agonists has improved attention to the neglected hemispace, which in some cases persisted after discontinuation of the drug.[162,163] However, two other studies revealed that bromocriptine worsened the manifestation of neglect by increasing attention to the ipsilateral, rather than the contralateral, hemispace, possibly as a result of activating the noninvolved cerebral hemisphere.[164,165] Although results are mixed, clinicians may consider judicious use of dopaminergic agents given the detrimental effects of hemispatial neglect on both functional skills and ability to care for oneself independently.

Dopaminergic agonism enhances the level of functional motor recovery after stroke. A single daily dose of levodopa given at least 30 minutes prior to physical therapy in a group of stroke patients resulted in significantly improved functional motor abilities compared to patients receiving placebo, which persisted after discontinuation of the drug.[166] The treatment was well tolerated with very infrequent and minor side effects.

Dopaminergic agonism has also been explored as a means to improve communication skills in patients with aphasia. Bromocriptine has improved language function in subjects with nonfluent aphasia,[167–169] although the results of these studies were not confirmed in other trials.[170,171] The generalizability of these results is limited given a number of significant design flaws and the small number of subjects studied.[172] Dopamine also appears to play a role in motivation. Successful rehabilitation is dependent on the motivation of a stroke patient to participate in therapy. Lack of motivation, either due to depression or as a neurological consequence of stroke, severely inhibits rehabilitation. Several small studies and case reports support the theory that dopaminergic agonism improves motivation and initiation in various neurological conditions, including cerebral neoplasm, TBI, encephalitis, and stroke.[173–176] Given the need for active patient participation in rehabilitation to enhance successful outcomes, apathy and poor motivation must be addressed, which may necessitate the use of dopaminergic agonists. The majority of dopaminergic agonists are well tolerated, particularly when given in moderate doses. However, care should be taken in cases of psychosis, given their potential affinity for the mesolimbic and mesocortical systems. A general rule is to titrate the dose until maximum benefit is achieved without undesirable side effects. All drugs used to enhance stroke recovery should be withdrawn at various intervals to determine whether they continue to manifest their desired effect.

OUTCOMES

Financial resources for medical rehabilitation are limited, and efforts are under way to curtail rehabilitation costs further, both of which require that funds be allocated wisely. Predicting who will benefit from stroke rehabilitation is a seemingly integral component in determining how best to utilize these limited resources, which may determine where a patient will be treated (i.e., acute inpatient, subacute inpatient, home care, or outpatient settings). Over the past several decades, a multitude of studies have examined the impact of numerous variables on stroke recovery and effectiveness of rehabilitation, including age, stroke severity and location, initial functional impairment, and sphincter control. Outcomes are typically determined by standardized measures that quantify neurological and/or functional improvements as well as examining the disposition of patients after completion of inpatient rehabilitation. There is general agreement that various factors, such as age at onset and initial stroke severity, influence outcomes. However, the results of many studies examining recovery patterns cannot predict long-term outcomes as rehabilitation interventions continue over a longer period of time than formally studied. Therefore, it is reasonable to expect that determining the actual long-term outcomes of stroke survivors may be more difficult than the studies suggest. Furthermore, results of these studies cannot definitively predict an outcome for a single individual as they have been unable to account for all of the variance, even when considering multiple factors.

Despite this, efforts continue to classify stroke patients to determine the amount of resources dedicated to individuals receiving acute inpatient rehabilitation. Measures of functional ability have been developed for individuals receiving acute rehabilitation. The most widely used tool today is the Functional Independence Measure (FIM). The FIM is a minimum data set that describes the functional abilities of patients receiving inpatient rehabilitation. It consists of 18 items of motor, ADL, and cognitive abilities, each assessed on a seven-point scale, with higher scores indicating greater levels of independence. By 1995, it was used in more than 720 rehabilitation settings and accumulated outcome data on more than 800,000 discharges.[177] A modification of the FIM is currently used by the Commission of Medicare and Medicaid Services, formerly known as the Health Care Financing Administration, to prospectively determine payment to acute inpatient rehabilitation facilities, rather than the per diem basis used prior to January 1, 2002.

Of all the variables examined to date, age is among the most widely recognized factor that impacts on functional recovery.[178–183] Older age at onset is almost always associated with poorer outcome, although the relationship is complex. In one study examining several factors, age and admission FIM score retrospectively predicted discharge disposition and functional improvement. In this study, all subjects younger than 55 years were discharged home, as were most of those admitted with a modest functional disability regardless of age. For the remaining patients, age and level of initial disability interacted to determine discharge disposition.[183] However, in many studies examining age as a predictor, functional outcome and disposition assessments were made either at the time of hospital discharge[183] or several months later[178,182,184] and therefore could not account for additional recovery achieved with either outpatient, subacute, or home-based treatment. Furthermore, discharge disposition depends not only on functional skills and age but also on available community support systems, which vary greatly among stroke survivors. Initial level of stroke severity has also been correlated with outcomes, with more severe impairments associated with poorer outcomes.[183,185–187] However, as with age, the majority of these studies examined outcomes either at the time of discharge or several months later[183,185–187] and therefore could not assess improved functional skills achieved at a later time. Also, despite significant correlations between admission FIM score and rehabilitation discharge abilities and dispositions, FIM either alone or in combination with other factors has not accounted for all of the variance in outcomes.

Although multiple attempts to predict outcome have been made, studies to date have lacked sufficient accuracy to reliably predict stroke outcomes for individual patients. Mathematical formulae developed to predict stroke outcome based on retrospective review of various stroke factors[178,179,184] achieved greatly diminished accuracy when applied prospectively.[75] In another study using multiple regression analysis of 12 factors previously found to predict stroke, age, cognitive, and sphincter subitems on the admission FIM, neglect and ideomotor apraxia were significantly associated with outcomes but accounted for only 72% of the variance.[75] In this same study, 8.2% of patients with an admission FIM of <40, indicating a very severe disability, obtained good outcomes, in contrast to the results of other studies.[183,187] Furthermore, functional improvements continue after acute rehabilitation discharge, either with home-based, outpatient, or subacute rehabilitation. In one study examining functional skills 1 year after hospital discharge, patients receiving continued rehabilitation interventions after hospital discharge had improved mobility compared to their discharge status.[188]

Three large community-based studies, the Framingham Study, the Oxfordshire Community Stroke Project, and the Copenhagen Stroke Project, were reviewed by Gresham[189] to assess outcomes of a large number of individuals with stroke. These studies were selected for review based on the large number of subjects, methodological rigor, and inclusion of functional outcome data. While the analysis of these studies did not include prediction of outcome, survivors of stroke continued to regain functional abilities as time passed from stroke onset. For instance, in the Framingham Study, 52% of stroke survivors had no residual hemiparesis, while only 22% were dependent in mobility and 32% were dependent in ADL.[4,190] Furthermore, a 20-year follow-up study of 148 subjects and controls in the Framingham Study revealed that long-term stroke survivors maintained excellent levels of function.[191] Gresham[189] inferred that, in spite of significant mortality, stroke survivors as a group reach good levels of function. For example, four of five can ambulate and two of three regain independence in ADL.

As the previous discussion indicates, accurate prediction of outcome after stroke is difficult for any individual. Therefore, it is inappropriate to deny rehabilitation interventions to stroke survivors with persistent physical or cognitive impairments regardless of age and initial level of disability as function may improve, resulting in an improved quality of life and potentially decreased health-care costs. It is important, however, to select an appropriate setting for rehabilitation, either in an acute or a subacute facility or at home, or as an outpatient based on an individual's level of disability or ability to participate in 3 hours of intensive therapy per day and the amount of time needed to achieve rehabilitation goals.

ACKNOWLEDGMENTS

This work was supported by grant 2 RO1 29762 from the National Institutes of Health (National Institute of Neurological Disorders and Stroke).

REFERENCES

1. American Heart Association. 1999 Heart and Stroke Statistical Update. Dallas, American Heart Association, 1998.
2. Murray CJ, Lopez AD. Mortality by cause for eight regions of the world: Global Burden of Disease Study. Lancet 349:1269–1276, 1997.
3. Broderick J. The Greater Cincinnati/Northern Kentucky Stroke Study: preliminary first-ever and total incidence rates of stroke among blacks. Stroke 29:415–421, 1998.
4. Gresham GE. Residual disability in survivors of stroke—the Framingham Study. N Engl J Med 293:954–956, 1975.
5. Black-Schaffer RM, Osberg JS. Return to work after stroke: development of a predictive model. Arch Phys Med Rehabil 71:285–290, 1990.
6. Ingall TJ. Has there been a decline in subarachnoid hemorrhage mortality? Stroke 20:718–724, 1989.
7. Phillips LH. The unchanging pattern of subarachnoid hemorrhage in a community. Neurology 30:1034–1040, 1980.
8. Sacco RL. Subarachnoid and intracerebral hemorrhage: natural history, prognosis, and precursive factors in the Framingham Study. Neurology 34:847–854, 1984.
9. Longstreth WT Jr. Clinical course of spontaneous subarachnoid hemorrhage: a population-based study in King County, Washington. Neurology 43:712–718, 1993.
10. Juvela S. Cigarette smoking and alcohol consumption as risk factors for aneurysmal subarachnoid hemorrhage. Stroke 24:639–646, 1993.
11. Ingall T, Wiebers DO. National history of subarachnoid hemorrhage. In: Whismant JP (Ed.). Stroke: Populations, Cohorts and Clinical Trials. Oxford, Butterworth-Heinemann, pp. 174–186, 1993.
12. Kassell NF. The International Cooperative Study on the Timing of Aneurysm Surgery. Part 1: Overall management results. J Neurosurg 3:18–36, 1990.
13. Bamford J. A prospective study of acute cerebrovascular disease in the community: the Oxfordshire Community Stroke Project—1981–86. 2. Incidence, case fatality rates and overall outcome at one year of cerebral infarction, primary intracerebral and subarachnoid haemorrhage. J Neurol Neurosurg Psychiatry 3:16–22, 1990.
14. Foulkes MA. The Stroke Data Bank: design, methods, and baseline characteristics. Stroke 19:547–554, 1988.
15. Gilbert JJ, Vinters HV. Cerebral amyloid angiopathy: incidence and complications in the aging brain. I. Cerebral hemorrhage. Stroke 14:915–923, 1983.
16. Vinters HV. Cerebral amyloid angiopathy. A critical review. Stroke 18:311–324, 1987.
17. Broderick JP. The risk of subarachnoid and intracerebral hemorrhages in blacks as compared with whites. N Engl J Med 326:733–736, 1992.
18. Furlan AJ, Whisnant JP, Elveback LR. The decreasing incidence of primary intracerebral hemorrhage: a population study. Ann Neurol 25:367–373, 1979.
19. Giroud M. Cerebral haemorrhage in a French prospective population study. J Neurol Neurosurg Psychiatry 54:595–598, 1991.
20. Sacco R, Mayer S. Epidemiology of intracerebral hemorrhage. In: Feldmann E (Ed.). Intracerebral Hemorrhage. New York, Futura, pp. 3–23, 1994.
21. Suzuki K. Clinico-epidemiologic study of stroke in Akita, Japan. Stroke 18:402–406, 1987.
22. Qureshi AI, Giles WH, Croft JB. Racial differences in the incidence of intracerebral hemorrhage: effects of blood pressure and education. Neurology 52:1617–1621, 1999.
23. Taylor T, Davis P, Torner J. Projected number of strokes by subtypes in the year 2050 in the United States. [abstract] Stroke 29:322, 1998.
24. Broderick JP. Guidelines for the management of spontaneous intracerebral hemorrhage: a statement for healthcare professionals from a special writing group of the Stroke Council, American Heart Association. Stroke 30:905–915, 1999.
25. Brott T, Thalinger K, Hertzberg V. Hypertension as a risk factor for spontaneous intracerebral hemorrhage. Stroke 17:1078–1083, 1986.
26. Omae T, Ueda K. Risk factors for cerebral stroke in Japan: prospective epidemiologic study in Hisayama community. In: Katsuki S, Tsubaki T, Toyokura Y (Eds.). Proceedings of the 12th World Congress of Neurology. Amsterdam, Excerpta Medica, p. 119, 1982.
27. Thrift AG. Three important subgroups of hypertensive persons at greater risk of intracerebral hemorrhage. Melbourne Risk Factor Study Group. Hypertension 31:1223–1229, 1998.
28. Qureshi AI. Intracerebral hemorrhage in blacks. Risk factors, subtypes, and outcome. Stroke 28:961–964, 1997.
29. Broderick JP. Volume of intracerebral hemorrhage. A powerful and easy-to-use predictor of 30-day mortality. Stroke 24:987–993, 1993.
30. Tuhrim S. Validation and comparison of models predicting survival following intracerebral hemorrhage. Crit Care Med 23:950–954, 1995.

31. Qureshi AI. Predictors of early deterioration and mortality in black Americans with spontaneous intracerebral hemorrhage. Stroke 26:1764–1767, 1995.
32. Mayer SA. Neurologic deterioration in noncomatose patients with supratentorial intracerebral hemorrhage. Neurology 44:1379–1384, 1994.
33. Juvela S. Risk factors for impaired outcome after spontaneous intracerebral hemorrhage. Arch Neurol 52:1193–1200, 1995.
34. Tuhrim S. Intracerebral hemorrhage: external validation and extension of a model for prediction of 30-day survival. Ann Neurol 29:658–663, 1991.
35. Arakawa S. Blood pressure control and recurrence of hypertensive brain hemorrhage. Stroke 29:1806–1809, 1998.
36. Hill MD. Rate of stroke recurrence in patients with primary intracerebral hemorrhage. Stroke 31:123–127, 2000.
37. Wolf PA, Abbott RD, Kannel WB. Atrial fibrillation as an independent risk factor for stroke: the Framingham Study. Stroke 22:983–988, 1991.
38. Furlan A. Intra-arterial prourokinase for acute ischemic stroke. The PROACT II study: a randomized controlled trial. Prolyse in Acute Cerebral Thromboembolism. JAMA 282:2003–2011, 1999.
39. International Stroke Trial Collaborative Group. The International Stroke Trial (IST). a randomised trial of aspirin, subcutaneous heparin, both, or neither among 19435 patients with acute ischaemic stroke. Lancet 349:1569–1581, 1997.
40. Publications Committee for the Trial of ORG 10172 in Acute Stroke Treatment (TOAST) Investigators. Low molecular weight heparinoid, ORG 10172 (danaparoid), and outcome after acute ischemic stroke: a randomized controlled trial. JAMA 279:1265–1272, 1998.
41. Berge E. Low molecular-weight heparin versus aspirin in patients with acute ischaemic stroke and atrial fibrillation: a double-blind randomised study. HAEST Study Group. Heparin in Acute Embolic Stroke Trial. Lancet 355:1205–1210, 2000.
42. CAST (Chinese Acute Stroke Trial) Collaborative Group. CAST: randomised placebo-controlled trial of early aspirin use in 20,000 patients with acute ischaemic stroke. Lancet 349:1641–1649, 1997.
43. Hankey GJ. Stroke: how large a public health problem, and how can the neurologist help? Arch Neurol 56:748–754, 1999.
44. Stroke Unit Trialists Collaboration. How do stroke units improve patient outcomes? A collaborative systematic review of the randomized trials. Stroke 28:2139–2144, 1997.
45. Kannel WB. Epidemiologic assessment of the role of blood pressure in stroke. The Framingham Study. JAMA 214:301–310, 1970.
46. Collins R, MacMahon S. Blood pressure, antihypertensive drug treatment and the risks of stroke and of coronary heart disease. Br Med Bull 50:272–298, 1994.
47. Hypertension Detection and Follow-up Program Cooperative Group. Five-year findings of the Hypertension Detection and Follow-up Program. III. Reduction in stroke incidence among persons with high blood pressure. JAMA 247:633–638, 1982.
48. Staessen JA, Fagard R, Thijs L, et al. Randomised double-blind comparison of placebo and active treatment for older patients with isolated systolic hypertension. The Systolic Hypertension in Europe (Syst-Eur) Trial Investigators. Lancet 350:757–764, 1997.
49. Progress Collaborative Group. Randomised trial of a perindopril-based blood-pressure-lowering regimen among 6, 105 individuals with previous stroke or transient ischaemic attack. Lancet 358:1033–1041, 2001.
50. Yusuf S. Effects of an angiotensin-converting-enzyme inhibitor, ramipril, on cardiovascular events in high-risk patients. The Heart Outcomes Prevention Evaluation Study Investigators. N Engl J Med 342:145–153, 2000.
51. Joint National Committee on Prevention, Detection, Evaluation, and Treatment of High Blood Pressure. The sixth report of the Joint National Committee on Prevention, Detection, Evaluation, and Treatment of High Blood Pressure. Arch Intern Med 157:2413–2446, 1997.
52. Iso H, Jacobs D, Wentworth D. Serum cholesterol levels and six year mortality from stroke in 350,977 men screened for the MRFIT. N Engl J Med 320:9804–9810, 1989.
53. Prospective Studies Collaboration. Cholesterol, diastolic blood pressure, and stroke: 13,000 strokes in 450,000 people in 45 prospective cohorts. Prospective studies collaboration. Lancet 346:1647–1653, 1995.
54. Wolf PA. Secular trends in stroke incidence and mortality. The Framingham Study. Stroke 23:1551–1555, 1992.
55. Fried LP. The Cardiovascular Health Study: design and rationale. Ann Epidemiol 1:263–276, 1991.

56. Hebert PR. Cholesterol lowering with statin drugs, risk of stroke, and total mortality. An overview of randomized trials. JAMA 278:313–321, 1997.

57. The Long-Term Intervention with Pravastatin in Ischemic Disease (LIPID) Study Group. Prevention of cardiovascular events and death with pravastatin in patients with coronary heart disease and a broad range of initial cholesterol levels. N Engl J Med 339:349–357, 1998.

58. Furberg CD. Natural statins and stroke risk. Circulation 99:185–188, 1999.

59. Rubins HB. Gemfibrozil for the secondary prevention of coronary heart disease in men with low levels of high-density lipoprotein cholesterol. Veterans Affairs High-Density Lipoprotein Cholesterol Intervention Trial Study Group. N Engl J Med 341:410–418, 1999.

60. Wolf PA. Cigarette smoking as a risk factor for stroke. The Framingham Study. JAMA 259:1025–1029, 1988.

61. Sacco RL. The protective effect of moderate alcohol consumption on ischemic stroke. JAMA 281:53–60, 1999.

62. Joseph LN. Risk factor modification in stroke prevention: the experience of a stroke clinic. Stroke 30:16–20, 1999.

63. Giles WH. Total homocyst(e)ine concentration and the likelihood of nonfatal stroke: results from the Third National Health and Nutrition Examination Survey, 1988–1994. Stroke 29:2473–2477, 1998.

64. Sacks FM. Effects on blood pressure of reduced dietary sodium and the Dietary Approaches to Stop Hypertension (DASH) diet. DASH–Sodium Collaborative Research Group. N Engl J Med 344:3–10, 2001.

65. Atrial Fibrillation Investigators. Risk factors for stroke and efficacy of antithrombotic therapy in atrial fibrillation. Analysis of pooled data from five randomized controlled trials. Arch Intern Med 154:1449–1457, 1994.

66. Ezekowitz MD, Levine JA. Preventing stroke in patients with atrial fibrillation. JAMA 281:1830–1835, 1999.

67. Mohr JP. A comparison of warfarin and aspirin for the prevention of recurrent ischemic stroke. N Engl J Med 345:1444–1451, 2001.

68. Albers GW. Antithrombotic and thrombolytic therapy for ischemic stroke. Chest 114(Suppl 5):683S–698S, 1998.

69. Dyken ML. Low-dose aspirin and stroke. "It ain't necessarily so." Stroke 23:1395–1399, 1992.

70. O'Connor CM. Comparison of two aspirin doses on ischemic stroke in postmyocardial infarction patients in the warfarin (Coumadin) Aspirin Reinfarction Study (CARS). Am J Cardiol 88:541–546, 2001.

71. Federman AD. Supplemental insurance and use of effective cardiovascular drugs among elderly medicare beneficiaries with coronary heart disease. JAMA 286:1732–1739, 2001.

72. European Carotid Surgery Trialists' Collaborative Group. MRC European Carotid Surgery Trial: interim results for symptomatic patients with severe (70–99%) or with mild (0–29%) carotid stenosis. Lancet 337:1235–1243, 1991.

73. North American Symptomatic Carotid Endarterectomy Trial Collaborators. Beneficial effect of carotid endarterectomy in symptomatic patients with high-grade carotid stenosis. N Engl J Med 325:445–453, 1991.

74. Ricco JB. Early carotid endarterectomy after a nondisabling stroke: a prospective study. Ann Vasc Surg 14:89–94, 2000.

75. Giaquinto S. On the prognosis of outcome after stroke. Acta Neurol Scand 100:202–208., 1999.

76. Taub E, Crago JE, Burgio LD, Groomes TE, Look ED 3rd, DeLuca SC, Miller NE. An operant approach to rehabilitation medicine: overcoming learned nonuse by shaping. J Exp Anal Behav 61:281–293, 1994.

77. Wolf SLS, Lecraw DE, Burton LA, Jann BB. Forced use of hemiplegic upper extremities to reverse the effect of learned nonuse among chronic stroke and head-injured patients. Exp Neurol 104:125–132, 1989.

78. Taub E. Movement in non human primates deprived of somatosensory feedback. Exerc Sport Sci Rev 4:335–374, 1997.

79. Kunkel A, Kopp B, Miller G, Villringer K, Villringer A, Taub E, Flor H. Constraint-induced movement therapy for motor recovery in chronic stroke patients. Arch Phys Med Rehabil 80:624–628, 1999.

80. Miltner WH, Bauder H, Sommer M, Dettmers C, Taub E. Effects of constraint-induced movement therapy on patients with chronic motor deficits after stroke: a replication. Stroke 30:586–592, 1999.

81. Liepert J. Treatment-induced cortical reorganization after stroke in humans. Stroke 31:1210–1216, 2000.

82. Levy CEW, Nichols DS, Schmalbrock PM, Keller P, Chakeres DW. Functional MRI evidence of cortical reorganization in upper limbs stroke hemiplegia treated with

constraint-induced movement therapy. Am J Phys Med Rehabil 80:4–12, 2001.

83. Libeson WT. Functional electrotherapy: stimulation of peroneal nerve synchronized with swing phase of gait of hemiplegia patients. Arch Phys Med Rehabil 42:101–105, 1961.

84. Cozean CD, Pease WS, Hubbell SL. Biofeedback and functional electrical stimulation in stroke rehabilitation. Arch Phys Med Rehabil 69:401–405, 1988.

85. van Overeem HG. EMG-controlled functional electrical stimulation of the paretic hand. Scand J Rehabil Med 11:189–193, 1979.

86. Kraft GH, Fitts SS, Hammond MC. Techniques to improve function of the arm and hand in chronic hemiplegia. Arch Phys Med Rehabil 73:220–227, 1992.

87. Fields RW. Electromyographically triggered electrical muscle stimulation for chronic hemiplegia. Arch Phys Med Rehabil 68:407–414, 1987.

88. Francisco G, Chae J, Chawla H, Kirschblum S, Zorowitz R, Lewis G, Pang S. Electromyogram-triggered neuromuscular stimulation for improving the arm function of acute stroke survivors: a randomized pilot study. Arch Phys Med Rehabil 79:570–575, 1998.

89. Cauraugh J, Light K, Kim S, Thigpen M, Behrman A. Chronic motor dysfunction after stroke: recovering wrist and finger extension by electromyography-triggered neuromuscular stimulation. Stroke 31:1360–1364, 2000.

90. Rawicki B. Treatment of cerebral origin spasticity with continuous intrathecal baclofen delivered via an implantable pump: long-term follow-up review of 18 patients. J Neurosurg 91:733–736, 1999.

91. Meythaler JM, Guin-Renfroe S, Brunner RC, Hadley MN. Intrathecal baclofen for spastic hypertonia from stroke. Stroke 32:2099–2109, 2001.

92. Gerszten PC, Albright AL, Barry MJ. Effect on ambulation of continuous intrathecal baclofen infusion. Pediatr Neurosurg 27:40–44, 1997.

93. Gasparrini WG, Satz P, Heilman K, Coolidge FL. Hemispheric asymmetries of affective processing as determined by the Minnesota Multiphasic Personality Inventory. J Neurol Neurosurg Psychiatry 41:470–473, 1978.

94. Robinson RG, Price TR. Post-stroke depressive disorders: a follow-up study of 103 patients. Stroke 13:635–641, 1982.

95. Finklestein S, Benowitz LI, Baldessarini RJ, Arana GW, Levine D, Woo E, Bear D, Moya K, Stoll AL. Mood, vegetative disturbance, and dexamethasone suppression test after stroke. Ann Neurol 12:463–468, 1982.

96. Robinson RG. Mood changes in stroke patients: relationship to lesion location. Compr Psychiatry 24:555–566, 1983.

97. Finset A. Depressed mood and intra-hemispheric location of lesion in right hemisphere stroke patients. Scand J Rehabil Med 21:1–6, 1989.

98. Egelko S. First year after stroke: tracking cognitive and affective deficits. Arch Phys Med Rehabil 70:297–302, 1989.

99. Gordon WA, Hibbard MR. Poststroke depression: an examination of the literature. Arch Phys Med Rehabil 6:658–663, 1997.

100. Andersen G. Incidence of post-stroke depression during the first year in a large unselected stroke population determined using a valid standardized rating scale. Acta Psychiatr Scand 90:190–195, 1994.

101. Shima S. Poststroke depression. Gen Hosp Psychiatry 16:286–289, 1994.

102. Burvill PW. Prevalence of depression after stroke: the Perth Community Stroke Study. Br J Psychiatry 166:320–327, 1995.

103. Morris PL, Robinson RG, Raphael B. Prevalence and course of depressive disorders in hospitalized stroke patients. Int J Psychiatry Med 20:349–364, 1990.

104. Eastwood MR. Mood disorder following cerebrovascular accident. Br J Psychiatry 154:195–200, 1989.

105. Gordon WA, Hibbard MR. Poststroke depression: an examination of the literature. Arch Phys Med Rehabil 78:658–663, 1997.

106. Ross ED, Rush AJ. Diagnosis and neuroanatomical correlates of depression in brain-damaged patients. Implications for a neurology of depression. Arch Gen Psychiatry 38:1344–1354, 1981.

107. Robinson RG. The Clinical Neuropsychiatry of Stroke: Cognitive, Behavioral, and Emotional Disorders Following Vascular Brain Injury. Cambridge, Cambridge University Press, 1998.

108. Morris PL, Raphael B, Robinson RG. Clinical depression is associated with impaired recovery from stroke. Med J Aust 157:239–242, 1992.

109. Koivisto K, Viinamaki H, Riekkinen P. Post-stroke depression and rehabilitation outcome. Nord J Psychiatry 47:245–249, 1993.

110. Sharpe M. Depressive disorders in long-term survivors of stroke. Associations with demographic and social factors, functional status, and brain lesion volume. Br J Psychiatry 164:380–386, 1994.

111. Herrmann N. The Sunnybrook Stroke

Study: a prospective study of depressive symptoms and functional outcome. Stroke 29:618–624, 1998.

112. Parikh RM. The impact of poststroke depression on recovery in activities of daily living over a 2-year follow-up. Arch Neurol 47:785–789, 1990.

113. Morris PL. Association of depression with 10-year poststroke mortality. Am J Psychiatry 150:124–129, 1993.

114. Everson SA. Depressive symptoms and increased risk of stroke mortality over a 29-year period. Arch Intern Med 158:1133–1138, 1998.

115. Reding MJ. Antidepressant therapy after stroke. A double-blind trial. Arch Neurol 43:763–765, 1986.

116. Gonzalez-Torrecillas JL, Mendlewicz J, Lobo A. Effects of early treatment of poststroke depression on neuropsychological rehabilitation. Int Psychogeriatr 7:547–560, 1995.

117. Dam M. Effects of fluoxetine and maprotiline on functional recovery in poststroke hemiplegic patients undergoing rehabilitation therapy. Stroke 27:1211–1214, 1996.

118. Chemerinski E, Robinson RE, Arndt S, et al. The effect of remission of poststroke depression on activities of daily living in a double-blind randomized treatment study. J Nerv Ment Dis 189:421–425, 2001.

119. Mayberg HS. PET imaging of cortical S2 serotonin receptors after stroke: lateralized changes and relationship to depression. Am J Psychiatry 145:937–943, 1988.

120. Bryer JB. Reduction of CSF monoamine metabolites in poststroke depression: a preliminary report. J Neuropsychiatry Clin Neurosci 4:440–442, 1992.

121. Lipsey JR. Nortriptyline treatment of poststroke depression: a double-blind study. Lancet 1:297–300, 1984.

122. Andersen G, Vestergaard K, Riis JO. Citalopram for post-stroke pathological crying. Lancet 342:837–839, 1993.

123. Side-effects of nortriptyline treatment for post-stroke depression. Lancet 1:519–520, 1984.

124. Lingam VR. Methylphenidate in treating poststroke depression. J Clin Psychiatry 49:151–153, 1988.

125. Lazarus LW. Efficacy and side effects of methylphenidate for poststroke depression. J Clin Psychiatry 53:447–449, 1992.

126. Johnson ML. Methylphenidate in stroke patients with depression. Am J Phys Med Rehabil 71:239–241, 1992.

127. Masand P, Murray G, Pickett P. Psychostimulants in post-stroke depression. J Neuropsychiatry Clin Neurosci 3:23–27, 1991.

128. Lazarus LW. Methylphenidate and nortriptyline in the treatment of poststroke depression: a retrospective comparison. Arch Phys Med Rehabil 75:403–406, 1994.

129. Feeney DM, Gonzalez A, Law WA. Amphetamine, haloperidol, and experience interact to affect rate of recovery after motor cortex injury. Science 217:855–857, 1982.

130. Hovda DA, Fenney DM. Amphetamine with experience promotes recovery of locomotor function after unilateral frontal cortex injury in the cat. Brain Res 298:358–361, 1984.

131. Kline AE. Methylphenidate treatment following ablation-induced hemiplegia in rat: experience during drug action alters effects on recovery of function. Pharmacol Biochem Behav 48:773–779, 1994.

132. Goldstein LB, Davis JN. Clonidine impairs recovery of beam-walking after a sensorimotor cortex lesion in the rat. Brain Res 508:305–309, 1990.

133. Feeney DM, Westerberg VS. Norepinephrine and brain damage: alpha-noradrenergic pharmacology alters functional recovery after cortical trauma. Can J Psychol 44:233–252, 1990.

134. Stephens J, Gordberg G, Demopoulas JT. Clonidine reinstates deficits following recovery from sensorimotor cortex lesions in rats. Arch Phys Med Rehabil 67:666–667, 1986.

135. Goldstein LB. Common drugs may influence motor recovery after stroke. The Sygen in Acute Stroke Study Investigators. Neurology 45:865–871, 1995.

136. Goldstein LB, Davis JN. Physician prescribing patterns following hospital admission for ischemic cerebrovascular disease. Neurology 38:1806–1809, 1988.

137. Lipper S, Tuchman MM. Treatment of chronic post-traumatic organic brain syndrome with dextroamphetamine: first reported case. J Nerv Ment Dis 162:366–371, 1976.

138. Evans RW, Gualtieri CT, Patterson D. Treatment of chronic closed head injury with psychostimulant drugs: a controlled case study and an appropriate evaluation procedure. J Nerv Ment Dis 175:106–110, 1987.

139. Kaelin DL, Cifu DX, Matthies B. Methylphenidate effect on attention deficit in the acutely brain injured adult. Arch Phys Med Rehabil 1996:6–9, 1996.

140. Plenger PM. Subacute methylphenidate treatment for moderate to moderately severe traumatic brain injury: a preliminary double-blind placebo-controlled study. Arch Phys Med Rehabil 77:536–540, 1996.

141. Walker-Batson D. Amphetamine paired with physical therapy accelerates motor recovery after stroke. Further evidence. Stroke 26:2254–2259, 1995.
142. Grade C. Methylphenidate in early post-stroke recovery: a double-blind, placebo-controlled study. Arch Phys Med Rehabil 79:1047–1050, 1998.
143. Goldstein LB. Prescribing of potentially harmful drugs to patients admitted to hospital after head injury. J Neurol Neurosurg Psychiatry 58:753–755, 1995.
144. Feeney DM. Pharmacological modulation of recovery after brain injury: a recommendation of diaschisis. J Neurol Rehabil 5:113–128, 1991.
145. Dietrich WD. Influence of amphetamine treatment on somatosensory function of the normal and infarcted rat brain. Stroke 21(Suppl):47–50, 1990.
146. Goldstein LB. Pharmacology of recovery after stroke. Stroke 21(Suppl):139–142, 1990.
147. Dunwiddie TV, Roberson NL, Worth T. Modulation of long-term potentiation: effects of adrenergic and neuroleptic drugs. Pharmacol Biochem Behav 17:1257–1264, 1982.
148. Hovda DA, Sutton RL, Feeney DM. Amphetamine-induced recovery of visual cliff performance after bilateral visual cortex ablation in cats: measurements of depth perception thresholds. Behav Neurosci 103:574–584, 1989.
149. Hovda DA, Sutton RL, Feeney DM. Recovery of tactile placing after visual cortex ablation in cat: a behavioral and metabolic study of diaschisis. Exp Neurol 97:391–402, 1987.
151. Hovda DA, Feeney DM. Haloperidol blocks amphetamine induced recovery of binocular depth perception after bilateral visual cortex ablation in cat. Proc West Pharmacol Soc 28:209–211, 1985.
152. Haig AJ, Ruess JM. Recovery from vegetative state of six months' duration associated with Sinemet (levodopa/carbidopa). Arch Phys Med Rehabil 71:1081–1083, 1990.
153. Zafonte RD, Watanabe T, Mann NR. Amantadine: a potential treatment for the minimally conscious state. Brain Inj 12:617–621, 1998.
154. Lal S, Merbtiz CP, Grip JC. Modification of function in head-injured patients with Sinemet. Brain Inj 2:225–233, 1988.
155. Nickels JL. Clinical use of amantadine in brain injury rehabilitation. Brain Inj 8:709–718, 1994.
156. Edby K. Amantadine treatment of a patient with anoxic brain injury. Childs Nerv Syst 11:607–609, 1995.
157. Kraus MF, Maki PM. Effect of amantadine hydrochloride on symptoms of frontal lobe dysfunction in brain injury: case studies and review. J Neuropsychiatry Clin Neurosci 9:222–230, 1997.
158. McDowell S, Whyte J, D'Esposito M. Differential effect of a dopaminergic agonist on prefrontal function in traumatic brain injury patients. Brain 121:1155–1164, 1998.
159. Kalra L. The influence of visual neglect on stroke rehabilitation. Stroke 28:1386–1391, 1997.
160. Iversen SD. Behavioural effects of manipulation of basal ganglia neurotransmitters. Ciba Found Symp 107:183–200, 1984.
161. Vargo JM. D1-class dopamine receptor involvement in the behavioral recovery from prefrontal cortical injury. Behav Brain Res 72:39–48, 1995.
162. Fleet WS. Dopamine agonist therapy for neglect in humans. Neurology 37:1765–1770, 1987.
163. Geminiani G, Bottini G, Sterzi R. Dopaminergic stimulation in unilateral neglect. J Neurol Neurosurg Psychiatry 65:344–347, 1998.
164. Grujic Z. Dopamine agonists reorient visual exploration away from the neglected hemispace. Neurology 51:1395–1388, 1998.
165. Barrett AM. Adverse effect of dopamine agonist therapy in a patient with motor-intentional neglect. Arch Phys Med Rehabil 80:600–603, 1999.
166. Scheidtmann K. Effect of levodopa in combination with physiotherapy on functional motor recovery after stroke: a prospective, randomised, double-blind study. Lancet 358:787–790, 2001.
167. Albert ML. Pharmacotherapy for aphasia. Neurology 38:877–879, 1988.
168. Gupta SR, Mlcoch AG. Bromocriptine treatment of nonfluent aphasia. Arch Phys Med Rehabil 73:373–376, 1992.
169. Sabe L, Leiguarda R, Starkstein SE. An open-label trial of bromocriptine in nonfluent aphasia. Neurology 42:1637–1638, 1992.
170. Mackennan DL. The effects of bromocriptine on speech and language function in a man with transcortical aphasia. Clin Aphasiol 21:145–155, 1991.
171. Ozeren A. Bromocriptine is ineffective in the treatment of chronic nonfluent aphasia. Acta Neurol Belg 95:235–238, 1995.
172. Powell JH. Motivational deficits after brain injury: effects of bromocriptine in 11 patients. J Neurol Neurosurg Psychiatry 60:416–421, 1996.
173. Small SL. Pharmacotherapy of aphasia. A critical review. Stroke 25:1282–1289, 1994.
174. Ross ED, Stewart RM. Akinetic mutism from hypothalamic damage: successful

treatment with dopamine agonists. Neurology 31:1435–1439, 1981.

175. Van Reekum R. N of 1 study: amantadine for the amotivational syndrome in a patient with traumatic brain injury. Brain Inj 9:49–53, 1995.

176. Barrett K. Treating organic abulia with bromocriptine and lisuride: four case studies. J Neurol Neurosurg Psychiatry 54: 718–721, 1991.

177. Uniform Data System for Medical Rehabilitation. Getting Started with the Uniform Data Systems for Medical Rehabilitation. Buffalo, Center for Functional Assessment Research, State University of New York at Buffalo, 1995.

178. Wade DT, Wood VA, Hewer RL. Recovery after stroke—the first 3 months. J Neurol Neurosurg Psychiatry 48:7–13, 1985.

179. Lincoln NB. An investigation of factors affecting progress of patients on a stroke unit. J Neurol Neurosurg Psychiatry 52: 493–496, 1989.

180. Kalra L. Does age affect benefits of stroke unit rehabilitation? Stroke 25:346–351, 1994.

181. Nakayama H. The influence of age on stroke outcome. The Copenhagen Stroke Study. Stroke 25:808–813, 1994.

182. Lin JH, Hsiao SF, Chang CM, et al. Factors influencing functional independence outcome in stroke patients after rehabilitation. Kao Hsiung I Hsueh Ko Hsueh Tsa Chih 16:351–359, 2000.

183. Alexander MP. Stroke rehabilitation outcome. A potential use of predictive variables to establish levels of care. Stroke 25:128–134, 1994.

184. Wade DT, Hewer RL. Functional abilities after stroke: measurement, natural history and prognosis. J Neurol Neurosurg Psychiatry 50:177–182, 1987.

185. Inouye M. Influence of admission functional status on functional change after stroke rehabilitation. Am J Phys Med Rehabil 80:121–126, 2001.

186. Yavuzer G. Rehabilitation of stroke patients: clinical profile and functional outcome. Am J Phys Med Rehabil 80:250–255, 2001.

187. Ween JE. Factors predictive of stroke outcome in a rehabilitation setting. Neurology 47:388–392, 1996.

188. Paolucci S. Mobility status after inpatient stroke rehabilitation: 1-year follow-up and prognostic factors. Arch Phys Med Rehabil 82:2–8, 2001.

189. Gresham GE. Status of functional outcomes for stroke survivors. Phys Med Rehabil Clin N Am 10:957–966, 1999.

190. Gresham GE. Epidemiologic profile of long-term stroke disability: the Framingham Study. Arch Phys Med Rehabil 60: 487–791, 1979.

191. Gresham GE. Survival and functional status 20 or more years after first stroke: the Framingham Study. Stroke 29:793–797, 1998.

13

Dementia and Neurodegenerative Diseases

ELLEN OLSON

Chronic illness now accounts for approximately 70% of all deaths in the United States annually. Heart disease, cancer, emphysema, stroke, and dementia are the leading causes of death.[1] Between 1990 and 2040, annual neurodegenerative disease mortality is projected to increase between 119% and 231%. The major part of this increase is from deaths attributed to dementia.[2] When the same data are used to project neurodegenerative disease mortality specifically for minority populations, the numbers rise to 281% to 524%.[3] Despite the increasing prevalence of neurodegenerative disease, there is very little guidance in the leading neurology texts on how to deal with the palliative and end-of-life issues that these diseases present.[4]

Dementia is defined as a syndrome of acquired and persistent impairment in cognition and intellectual functioning. It must be differentiated from *delirium*, defined as a disturbance in consciousness and cognition that develops over a short period of time.[5] It is also differentiated from developmental disorders because it is preceded by a long period of normal cognitive functioning.[6]

The most common cause of dementia in the United States is Alzheimer's disease, accounting for approximately 50% of all cases.[7] This is true for most countries in the world, except Japan, China, and Russia, where the most common cause is felt to be vascular dementia.[8] It is estimated that the number of persons in the United States with Alzheimer's disease will rise from the current 4 million to 14 million in 2050, if the incidence remains unchanged and effective preventions or treatments remain elusive.[9] Multi-infarct dementia or vascular dementia is the next most common form. Together, Alzheimer's disease and vascular dementia account for 70%–90% of cases of dementia in the United States.[7,10,11] The remaining cases of dementia result from a number of diseases, including dementia with Lewy bodies, Parkinson's disease, and the frontotemporal degenerations, which include Pick's disease, supranuclear palsy, and Huntington's disease.

Dementia with Lewy bodies (DLB), another progressive dementing disorder, is either the second or third most common dementing disorder after AD.[12,13] First recognized as a pathological entity only 40 years ago, it is characterized by abundant Lewy bodies throughout the cerebral cortex and is often seen in combination with Alzheimer's disease. Parkinson's disease occurs when Lewy bodies are found only in the brain stem. Many patients with Parkinson's disease develop dementia, and most of these have either DLB or DLB and AD.[14] The incidence of Pick's disease is between 1% and 5%.[15] As many as 25% of dementias have multiple causes.[14]

Dementia can be classified into four stages, mild, moderate, severe, and terminal, each marked by progressive loss of independence. In early dementia, there are mild memory deficits and personality changes but the person can usually still function independently. The second, or moderate, stage is associated with the need for assistance in activities of daily living, such as bathing and dressing. Persons at this stage may also have significant cognitive impairment and judgment deficits that preclude them from living independently. In the severe stage of dementia, people can no longer eat or ambulate without assistance. In the terminal state, the individual can no longer ambulate, swallow safely, or communicate verbally.[9]

In the early stages, there may be certain characteristics and symptoms that are specific to the underlying etiology of the dementia. Behavioral problems may manifest before memory loss in the frontotemporal dementias, and hallucinations and extrapyramidal symptoms may present earlier in DLB. When dementia reaches the severe or terminal stage, there is not much difference in the clinical presentation between Alzheimer's disease and the other dementias.[9]

This chapter covers the symptoms common to end-stage dementia from all causes and the appropriate care for patients whether or not they have chosen in advance or through surrogates to limit life-prolonging therapies as their disease progresses. It is assumed that patients have sought out and been provided with the most recent and effective treatments for the specific diagnosis or diagnoses that underlie their dementia, to the extent that it was consistent with

their wishes. Wherever appropriate, symptoms specific to the disease processes responsible for the dementia will be discussed if they influence the comfort care needs of patients.

Dementia, along with Parkinson's disease, multiple sclerosis, and amyotrophic lateral sclerosis, is a progressive neurologic condition that will eventually contribute to or cause death.[16] Deaths associated with dementia come from impairments related to the dementia and not necessarily from the neurodegenerative diseases themselves. These impairments include immobility, eating difficulties, and associated infections.[9,16] Comorbid conditions, such as diabetes and heart disease, also contribute to progressive physical decline and death.[6] Demented individuals who are unable to ambulate are 3.4 times more likely to develop urinary tract infections and 6.8 times more likely to develop pneumonia than ambulators.[17] Immobility is associated with the development of pressure ulcers, another significant source of infection in dementia patients.[6,9] Pharmacological therapy can ameliorate many of the symptoms of the neurodegenerative diseases but cannot halt their progression.[18] Trigger events for discussions of the goals of care in persons with dementia include the time of diagnosis, progressive functional loss, difficulty swallowing, and pneumonia.[16]

Volicer and associates[19,20] pioneered the concept and practice of hospice care for dementia patients, based on the premise that if no treatment exists to reverse or arrest the progression of Alzheimer's disease, then treatment efforts should focus on providing maximal comfort. Much of their work will be reviewed in this chapter.

PROGNOSIS

The difficulty of prognostication in dementing illnesses remains a barrier to recognition by family and caregivers of the terminal nature of these diseases. It also acts as a barrier to the utilization of existing hospice and palliative care services and benefits that could be of assistance to patients and caregivers alike.[21] For example, Alzheimer's patients can live from 2 to 20 years after symptoms are first recognized and for as long as 3 years following admission to a nursing home.[22] Patients need to be given a prognosis of 6 months or less to qualify for the Medicare Hospice Benefit in the United States.

Several authors have addressed the issue of prognosis in end-stage dementia. Volicer and colleagues[23] noted in their early work that, based on a variety of behavioral and functional indicators, Alzheimer's patients who developed fevers had more advanced disease. With the need in mind to assign a 6-month or less survival time to advanced dementia patients so that they could receive the Medicare Hospice Benefit, they sought to determine what characteristics might be associated with Alzheimer's patients who developed fever and went on to live 6 months or less. Applying a logistic regression model, they showed that older age at the time of fever, severity of dementia, a

management strategy involving no antibiotics, and nursing home admission within 6 months were associated with a 6-month mortality.[23]

Following this work, Morrison and Siu[24] studied the survival of both cognitively intact and cognitively impaired individuals aged 70 or older who were hospitalized for either repair of a hip fracture or treatment of pneumonia. They found that patients with end-stage dementia who received routine care in a hospital setting for either pneumonia or a hip fracture had a four-fold increase in 6-month mortality compared to their cognitively intact counterparts.

Several groups have created guidelines to estimate the 6-month prognosis needed to qualify for the Medicare Hospice Benefit. The National Hospice and Palliative Care Organization has created guidelines that rely on the Functional Assessment Rating Scale, known as the FAST (Table 13–1).[25] The FAST consists of seven levels of functional decline that rate the progression of

Table 13–1. Functional Assessment Staging (FAST): Check Highest Consecutive Level of Disability

1. No difficulty either subjectively or objectively
2. Complaints that locations of objects have been forgotten, subjective work difficulties
3. Decreased job functioning evident to coworkers, difficulty in traveling to new locations, decreased organizational capacity*
4. Decreased ability to perform complex tasks (e.g., planning dinner for guests, handling personal finances such as forgetting to pay bills, difficulty marketing etc)
5. Required assistance in choosing proper clothing to wear for the day, season, or occasion (e.g., patients may wear the same clothing repeatedly unless supervised)*
6. A) Improperly putting on clothes without assistance or cuing (e.g., may put street clothes on over night clothes, put shoes on wrong feet, or have difficulty buttoning clothing) occasionally or more frequently over the past weeks*
   B) Unable to bathe properly (e.g., difficulty adjusting bath-water temperature) occasionally or more frequently over the past weeks*
   C) Inability to handle mechanics of toileting (e.g., forgets to flush toilet, does not wipe properly or properly dispose of toilet tissue) occasionally or more frequently over the past few weeks*
   D) Urinary incontinence (occasionally or more frequently over the past weeks)*
   E) Fecal incontinence (occasionally or more frequently over the past weeks)*
7. A) Ability to speak limited to approximately a half-dozen different intelligible words or fewer in the course of an average day or in the course of an intensive interview
   B) Speech ability limited to the use of a single intelligible word in an average day or in the course of an intensive interview (e.g., the person may repeat the word over and over)
   C) Loss of ambulatory ability (e.g., the individual cannot walk without personal assistance)
   D) Inability to sit up without assistance (e.g., the individual will fall over if there are not lateral rests [arms] on the chair)
   E) Loss of ability to smile
   F) Loss of ability to hold up head independently

*Scored primarily on the basis of information obtained from a knowledgeable informant and/or category.
Source: Reisberg.[25]

dementia. Stage 1 indicates that the patient is functioning without any subjective or objective difficulty. In stages 2–6, the patient progressively loses memory and organizational capacity, as well as the ability to dress, bathe, and toilet properly. Stage 7 is broken down further to six levels, A–F. At stage 7A, the patient's speech is limited to approximately a half-dozen different words or fewer in the course of an average day or intensive interview. By stage 7F, the person is nonambulatory, speech is limited to one intelligible word in a single day, and the person cannot hold up his or her head. Stage 7A is currently recommended by the National Hospice and Palliative Care Organization as an appropriate enrollment cut-off point for hospice care, in addition to the presence of medical complications related to the dementia and nonambulatory status (Table 13–2).[26]

Prior to the current recommendation regarding FAST criteria, the National Hospice and Palliative Care Organization suggested that stage 7C be the appropriate cut-off for hospice enrollment.[27] Luchins et al.[28] and Hanrahan et al.[29] studied these criteria in hospice patients in both the home and institutional settings. They determined that while the stage 7C FAST cut-off is an accurate predictor of 6-month survival for those dementia patients who follow the ordinal progression of functional loss as outlined by the FAST, a significant number of patients do not decline in such a stepwise manner and, therefore, cannot be assigned to a FAST category. In their two studies, 41% and 44% of patients, respectively, could not be characterized utilizing the FAST model. When they could be characterized, however, patients who had reached

Table 13–2. National Hospice and Palliative Care Organization Medical Guidelines for Determining Prognosis in Dementia

I. Functional Assessment Staging (FAST)
   A. May have a prognosis of up to 2 years. Survival time depends on variables such as the incidence of comorbidities and the comprehensiveness of care.
   B. Is at or beyond stage 7 of the FAST scale.
   C. Displays *all* of the following characteristics:
      1. Unable to ambulate without assistance
      2. Unable to dress without assistance
      3. Unable to bathe properly
      4. Urinary and fecal incontinence
         a. Occasionally or more frequently, over the past weeks
         b. Reported by knowledgeable informant or caregiver
      5. Unable to speak or communicate meaningfully
         a. Ability to speak is limited to approximately a half dozen or fewer intelligible and different words, in the course of an average day or in the course of an intensive interview

II. Presence of medical complications
   A. Has displayed comorbid conditions of sufficient severity to warrant medical treatment, documented within the past year.
   B. Comorbid conditions associated with dementia:
      1. Aspiration pneumonia
      2. Pyelonephritis or other upper urinary tract infection
      3. Septicemia
      4. Decubitus ulcers, multiple, stage 3–4
      5. Fever recurrent after antibiotics
   C. Difficulty swallowing food or refusal to eat, sufficiently severe that patient cannot maintain sufficient fluid and calorie intake to sustain life, with patient or surrogate refusing tube feeding or parenteral nutrition.
      1. Patients who are receiving tube feedings must have documented impaired nutritional status as indicated by:
         a. Unintentional, progressive weight loss of greater than 10% over the prior six months.
         b. Serum albumin less than 2.5 gm/dl may be a helpful prognostic indicator, but should not be used by itself.

Source: National Hospice & Palliative Care Organization.[26]

stage 7C had a mean survival of 4.1 months and 3.2 months in the two studies, respectively. As in the work of Volicer and colleagues cited above,[23] the level of medical care (tube feeding and antibiotics) also had some bearing on prognosis, depending on the degree of dementia. The results regarding antibiotics in the Hanrahan et al.[28] and Luchins et al.[29] studies have not been consistent, however, and research is required before they can be incorporated into specific guidelines. Other factors having a negative influence on survival in their two studies included mobility impairments, poor appetite, and functional impairment (poor activities of daily living scores), number of medical complications, and use of indwelling urethral catheters.

Regardless of attempts to create guidelines and facilitate the movement of appropriate patients into hospice, only about 15% of all terminal patients in the United States receive hospice services each year.[30] Only 1% of patients in hospice care have a diagnosis of dementia.[21] A more liberal benefit,[31] as well as more accurate guidelines, needs to be developed before hospice services become readily available to patients with advanced dementia.

SYMPTOM MANAGEMENT

Symptoms most commonly reported in the last year for dementia patients include mental confusion, urinary incontinence, pain, depression, constipation, and loss of appetite.[32] In Volicer's work,[9] managing behavioral symptoms, eating difficulties, and infection were the most problematic issues. These will be addressed in the following section.

Pain

Treatment of pain follows the same guidelines and is fraught with the same difficulties as treatment of pain in the elderly in general. Pain is under-reported and under-treated in the elderly. Older patients have many comorbid conditions associated with pain, such as osteoarthritis, which can be expected to cause discomfort even as demen-

tia progresses.[33] There is evidence that the presence of dementia results in undertreatment of pain.[34] Demented patients with frontal lobe involvement have reduced capacity to report pain because of reduced verbal abilities, motivation, and complex thinking. Pain in advanced dementia may present as agitation, social withdrawal, or other changes in behavior. Tachypnea, vocalizations, facial grimacing, agitation, posturing, or splinting may represent pain and not simply agitated delirium in severely demented patients. Pain perception may be intact but not pain behaviors. Memory deficits can block the memory of pain but not the actual experience of it. Some dementing diseases, such as multi-infarct dementia or Parkinson's disease, are associated with their own pain syndromes, including musculoskeletal pain, neuritic or radicular pain, pain associated with dystonia, central pain, and akathitic discomfort.[6,35]

The Discomfort Scale for Dementia of the Alzheimer's Type (DS-DAT) was developed by Hurley et al.[36] to assess pain and discomfort in advanced Alzheimer's disease patients who have lost the ability to communicate. It is a reliable and validated instrument which assesses nine categories of behavior that have been observed in advanced dementia patients and are felt to be associated with the patient's physical and emotional state. These include noisy breathing, negative vocalization, content facial expression, sad facial expression, frightened facial expression, frown, relaxed body language, tense body language, and fidgeting. Each item is scored on a four-point Likert scale, based on a 5-minute observation period, with lower scores being associated with greater comfort levels. It has proven to be a useful instrument in monitoring the comfort level of end-stage dementia patients who can no longer communicate their discomfort.[36,37]

When pain is identified in end-stage dementia patients, treatment should follow the stepwise recommendations put forth by the World Health Organization, starting with acetaminophen and nonsteroidal anti-inflammatory drugs for mild pain and progressing to opioids for more severe pain.[38] As swallowing difficulties ensue with advancing dementia, the oral route of treatment can be problematic. In cases where there is significant chronic pain, morphine is available in a concentrated liquid form (20 mg/ml) that allows the administration of significant oral or sublingual doses. Morphine serves the additional role of ameliorating the discomfort of dyspnea. In treating symptoms of end-stage dementia, as well as symptoms of other terminal illness, medications should be chosen that address multiple symptoms, if possible. It is very easy to create a situation of polypharmacy in palliative care, especially if patients have comorbidities for which ongoing treatment is a part of the plan. This is particularly common in patients with congestive heart failure or Parkinson's disease, when multiple medications may still be indicated in the patient who is not yet at the end stage and maintaining maximal functional status is important.

In treating pain in elderly demented patients, it must be remembered that constipation is already an issue. If opioid medication is added, meticulous preventive attention must be paid to bowel hygiene. Fecal impaction is extremely common, painful, and a frequent source of agitated behavior in elderly patients. It is also associated with fever, urinary tract infection, bowel obstruction, and colonic perforation. Difficulty swallowing often complicates the treatment of constipation in demented patients. Oral laxatives and adequate fluids and fiber by mouth become impractical. In these cases, the regular use of rectal suppositories and enemas is indicated. Dulcolax suppositories (1–2 10 mg) followed in approximately 30 minutes with a sodium biphosphate (Fleet®) or oil retention enema several times a week can be a safe and effective regimen for patients who cannot predictably take oral preparations or dietary supplements.

As will be further discussed in the next section, agitated behaviors are often the first sign of pain in an advanced dementia patient. Dementia patients have comorbidities associated with pain, as discussed above; and dementia itself is associated with painful conditions, such as pressure ulcers and immobility. When a dementia patient becomes agitated or has a change in baseline agitation, a thorough investigation for any potentially painful conditions must be undertaken before a presumptive diagnosis of delirium is made. Low-dose opioids should be considered when the source of the patient's agitated behavior could be pain or when the patient exhibits any of the negative signs or symptoms described above in the DS-DAT.

Dementia patients also respond to nonpharmacological pain treatment modalities. Soothing and supportive communication, music therapy, sensory stimulation, "busy hand" activities, soothing and supportive touch, therapeutic message, physical exercise and movement, and cold and heat therapy have been described as helpful in treating pain and discomfort in patients with late-stage dementia.[39] As with pain management in general, an interdisciplinary approach can best serve the needs of a patient with advanced dementia.

The evaluation and treatment of pain is discussed in more detail in Chapter 16.

Agitation and Delirium

As stated above, discomfort can manifest as agitation and delirium in patients with dementia. Although dementia renders older patients more susceptible to delirium from infection, electrolyte abnormalities and medication side effects, pain and discomfort must be ruled out when evaluating agitation in a patient with dementia. Untreated pain and discomfort may be the most important cause of agitated behavior in patients with advanced dementia.[9]

Delirium is very common at the end of life, occurring in as high as 85% of cases in the days before death.[6] Dementia makes patients more susceptible to delirium of any cause, as well as to side effects from anticholinergic and opioid medications. Opiates are more likely to be the source of delirium in the setting of renal insufficiency. When opioid medications are felt to be the cause of an acute delirium, opioid rotation, addition of a neuroleptic, or reduced opiate dose plus adjuvant analgesics may be helpful.[40,41] The rule is to try to minimize or change to other categories of drugs when delirium is felt to be drug-induced. In dementia, as with other conditions in the elderly, this is often impractical. When medications are felt to be necessary for comfort, such as scopolamine for increased secretions, but could also contribute to agitated behavior, a risk–benefit assessment must be made. An antipsychotic drug such as haloperidol can be added to treat the symptoms of delirium if the benefit gained from the potentially offending agent is felt to be worthwhile. Haloperidol is the first-line agent for delirium because of its low cost and ease of administration. However, it may not be the best medication when dementia is accompanied by parkinsonian symptoms. Risperidone and olanzapine appear to be equally effective, although there are fewer options for their route of administration. Suggested doses are risperidone 0.5–1.0 mg po bid/tid and olanzapine 2.5–5.0 mg po qd.[6] Chlorpromazine can also be used for agitated delirium as it is more sedating than haloperidol. Both chlorpromazine and haloperidol have the advantage of coming in concentrated oral solutions that can be administered by mouth or sublingually to patients with impaired swallowing. If doses in the range of 2 mg of haloperidol tid or risperidone 1 mg qid are inadequate, a benzodiazepine may be added, keeping in mind the possibility of paradoxical agitation with this class of medication in the elderly. However, lorazepam is a short-acting and well-tolerated drug in the elderly and comes in a concentrated solution for oral or sublingual administration. Doses of up to 1–2 mg q 6 hours in addition to haloperidol or risperidone usually result in quieting even the most agitated patient.

Whenever possible, delirium should be anticipated and diagnosed as early as possible. It is much easier to treat delirium in its earlier stages than to wait until patients need significant sedation to control symptoms.

A supportive environment is also important in the control of problem behaviors in dementia. Both overstimulation and isolation are detrimental to the delirious demented patient. If the patient cannot be at home, the environment should be filled with as many familiar items as possible. Room temperature should be neither too hot nor too cold, and excessive noise should be avoided. Staff should provide gentle redirection and orientation. Having family members or other persons around with whom the patient is familiar can be helpful.[6] Providing the opportunity for meaningful activities can lessen agitation and repetitive vocalizations.[14] Physical restraints should be avoided if at all possible. Restraints have been associated with increased agitation, discomfort,[14,42] increased falls,[43] and death.[44]

Delusions and Hallucinations

Delusions and hallucinations are closely linked to the agitated behaviors that make the care of end-stage dementia so challenging. Hallucinations are shared by many diagnoses, including Alzheimer's disease and Parkinson's disease. In one study, half of all patients with clinically diagnosed Alzheimer's disease manifested hallucinations or delusions within 4 years of diagnosis.[45] Hallucinations occur in 20% of Parkinson's patients, the incidence increasing with age and severity of cognitive impairment. Parkinsonian medications, anxiolytics, sedatives, antidepressants, and other neuropsychiatric drugs are associated with hallucinations in Parkinson's patients.[46] Hallucinations can be made worse by opioids; however, the association in one study of hospice patients was not strong.[47] In a study by Manfredi et al.[48] on the use of naloxone in this setting, opiates were not the cause of cognitive impairment in the majority of cases. Other causes include sepsis, subarachnoid hemorrhage, and meningitis.[49] When patients with advanced disease need significant doses of opioids for comfort but are experiencing untoward psychiatric side effects, a neuroleptic may need to be added to minimize the cognitive impairment.[49]

Delusional thinking can make dementia patients resistant to care. Caregivers need to be educated on techniques for handling patients who exhibit resistive behaviors.[14] A supportive environment and antipsychotic medications are the mainstay of therapy for these symptoms. As extrapyramidal symptoms often accompany psychotic symptoms, the newer antipsychotic medications already mentioned should be used to minimize extrapyramidal side effects.

Depression

Depression is the most common mood disorder in demented individuals. Depression is reported to be present in 15%–57% of patients with Alzheimer's disease and does not change with disease progression.[9] The wide variation in frequency is related to the difficulty in diagnosing this disease in patients with impaired language and communication skills. Untreated depression may lead to other symptoms of dementia, including the inability to engage in meaningful activities, increased dependence on others for activities of daily living, agitation, repetitive vocalization, apathy, insomnia, food refusal, and resistance to care. Often, these symptoms manifest late in the course of the disease, making it unlikely that treatment will make a significant impact in the patient's quality of life. Given the burden of depressive illness, a trial of a standard antidepressant is indicated. Antidepressants improve the mood of even patients with advanced dementia and increase intake in people who previously refused food.[50] If time is of the essence or apathy is the predominant symptom, a psychostimulant such as methylphenidate (Ritalin) is indicated.[6] The selective serotonin reuptake inhibitors are the drugs of choice, given their decreased anticholinergic and cardiovascular side effects. There is still a role, however, for the more sedating antidepressants such as trazodone, especially in the treatment of insomnia or where mild sedation is desirable.[51]

Insomnia

Insomnia and disrupted sleep accompany the aging process for many people, and dementia compounds this problem. Sleep disturbances are even more common in Parkinson's disease, where more than 75% of patients have some form of sleep disorder. Pain, dyspnea, and nausea, as well as medications, can disrupt sleep. Other factors known to affect sleep are depression, restless leg syndrome, periodic limb movements of sleep, rapid eye movement behavior disorder, and sleep apnea. A detailed review of sleep disorders in the elderly is beyond the scope of this chapter. However, fragmented sleep and the reversal of the sleep–wake cycle that is seen in dementia can be a source of significant discomfort for patient and caregiver alike. Addressing sleep hygiene issues can be very helpful in caring for the elderly patient with dementia. A regular bedtime should be established, to set and maintain the circadian clock. Alcohol, caffeine, and tobacco should be avoided at the end of the day, as well as large quantities of liquids. A nighttime condom catheter could prove useful if nighttime awakenings are related to need to void. Patients should be kept busy during the day, with daytime napping kept to a minimum. If the sleep disorder cannot be reversed with nonpharmacotherapeutic options and other treatable sleep disorders, such as restless leg syndrome, are not felt to be the cause, then sedating medications may be necessary. Benzodiazepines to aid sleep should be avoided as they may produce a paradoxical agitation instead. Low-dose trazodone (25–100 mg qhs) or small doses of an antipsychotic medication are considered better alternatives for demented patients.[6,46,52]

Fever and Infection

Infection is an inevitable consequence of severe and terminal dementia. Predisposing factors are impaired immune function, incontinence, immobility, pressure sores, and aspiration.[53] Pneumonia is the most common cause of death in demented individuals, almost regardless of the cause of the dementia, and reflects the limited usefulness of antibiotics in a population where normal host defense mechanisms are impaired.[9] One of the most difficult decisions faced by clinicians and families is how long to provide antibiotic treatments for recurrent infections in demented individuals, by what route, and in what setting. Hospitalization for nursing home patients with pneumonia has not been shown to improve outcomes and often results in more functional deterioration.[54] Treatment with intravenous antibiotics also places additional burdens on demented patients, who often need to be restrained so as not to interfere with treatments. One study suggested that antibiotic treatment of fevers accelerated the progression of Alzheimer's disease.[55] Several studies have shown that antibiotic therapy does not prolong survival in advanced dementia.[28,56] Patient comfort with and without antibiotics has also been studied; and analgesics, antipyretics, and oxygen result in the same or a better level of comfort compared to antibiotics in advanced dementia.[37] Forgoing antibiotic treatment of infections, especially pneumonia, in advanced dementia, where the causes of infection are irreversible and the patient's ability to understand the nature of his or her illness and the tests and treatments it involves is limited, seems most prudent, given the evidence to date. The challenge remains when to make the determination that the burdens of treatment outweigh the benefits.

Skin Care

Pressure ulcers can be a significant source of morbidity for patients with advanced disease of any kind. Hanson et al.[57] reported a 13% incidence of pressure sores among hospice patients, with more than half occurring within 2 weeks of death.[56] Pressure sores can be the source of local and systemic infection, as well as pain. Recognizing the risk factors for the development of pressure sores and addressing them prior to their development are key to the successful management of this difficult problem. Pressure relief is the most important preventive modality, and this is best achieved with frequent turning and positioning and the use of air mattresses or air-fluidized beds at the first signs of any skin breakdown (stage II or greater), if at all possible. Painful dressing changes require pretreatment with analgesics.

Incontinence

Urinary incontinence is an inevitable problem with progressive dementia. Its treatment often involves anticholinergic medications, which can exacerbate other symptoms in patients with dementia, such as agitation and delirium. Incontinence predisposes to skin breakdown and urinary tract infection. Reversal of incontinence is often impossible, and successful management requires protective garments that involve meticulous skin care to avoid breakdown or indwelling internal or external catheters, which are associated with increased risk of serious infection. When urinary retention is the cause of incontinence, another choice is intermittent catheterization. This approach may be problematic for the patient with advanced dementia, who has little understanding of the reasons for such a frequent, uncomfortable, and invasive procedure.

Other Symptoms

Other symptoms that may present in the very end stages of dementia include dry mouth, from mouth breathing or poor oral intake, and dyspnea, which may accompany the dying process. Treatment of these symptoms is the same as for any other terminal illness. Dry mouth responds to frequent oral hygiene with artificial saliva or mouthwash sponges, as well as sips of water or ice chips as tolerated. Some patients who can still report symptoms find the lemon-glycerin sponges too drying. They can be rinsed in cold water to lessen this response. Artificial saliva can also be used in conjunction with the sponges. Oral care is something family caregivers can be taught and allows them to feel as though they are doing something for the patient, especially in situations where the plan of care does not involve oral or tube feeding. Dyspnea can occur in the setting of infection or as a part of the dying process in end-stage dementia and responds to supplemental oxygen, low doses of morphine, and room fans. When morphine seems ineffective, low doses of benzodiazepines, such as lorazepam, can be useful. Morphine in the form of liquid concentrate (20 mg/ml) can be given at a starting dose of 5–10 mg orally or sublingually every 3–4 hours, titrated as indicated. Lorazepam can be given, also in concentrated liquid form, 0.5–2 mg every 6 hours. Lorazepam tablets have also been used sublingually but dissolve less well in patients who are dehydrated. Where intravenous access is in place, these drugs may also be given by this route. Doses of lorazepam remain the same. Intravenous doses of morphine should begin at 2 mg q 4 hours in opioid-naive patients and be titrated upward, depending on patient response. Higher doses of morphine can result in involuntary motor activity, at which point the opiate should be rotated or the dose lowered and a benzodiazepine added.[49]

End-stage dementia patients may also manifest noisy breathing, also known as the "death rattle," in the terminal stage of their disease. This is presumed to be secondary to pooled respiratory secretions that the patient can no longer clear. It is best managed by atropine or scopolamine patches. Death rattle is not felt to cause significant discomfort to the patient but can be a significant source of distress to family and caregivers.[49]

NUTRITIONAL ISSUES

Eating difficulties develop in all individuals as dementia progresses, regardless of the original etiology of the dementia. Whether to provide artificial nutrition and hydration to dementia patients who can no longer be adequately nourished by mouth continues to be a difficult decision for families and health-care providers alike. Two excellent review articles summarized the evidence of the risks and benefits of tube feeding in advanced dementia and found no evidence of benefit in terms of survival or comfort to individuals with advanced dementia.[58,59] The emotional context of forgoing nutrition remains, however.

Good palliative care of all terminal patients, especially those with dementia, dictates that all reversible causes of poor oral intake be adequately addressed before a decision is made to use or to forgo artificial nutrition and hydration. Decreased appetite can be a side effect of constipation, fecal impaction, urinary retention, untreated pain, infection, medications, depression, changing food preferences, problems with consistency in patients who have developed dysphagia, or poor oral hygiene or dentition. Poor appetite is a symptom of advanced dementia itself and may respond transiently to appetite stimulants such as megestrol and dronabinol. Tube feedings should never be instituted as a substitute for oral feeding, even when this becomes a very time-consuming process. If all reversible causes of inadequate nutritional intake have been addressed and the demented patient still refuses to eat, caregivers and family members alike need to be reassured that refusal of food and fluids is part of the natural dying process and not associated with the symptoms of hunger and thirst experienced by healthy individuals. A study of dying cancer patients showed that the only discomfort experienced by individuals who were not eating or drinking was dry mouth, which can successfully be treated with ice chips, sips of water, and artificial saliva, as previously described.[60] For a more comprehensive discussion of artificial nutrition and hydration at the end of life, please see Chapter 5.

FAMILY ISSUES

As previously mentioned, prognostic uncertainty in dementing illness contributes to caregiver distress. Knowing when treatment of intercurrent illnesses will return the patient to an acceptable level of functioning or when it will only prolong a painful dying process remains a challenge. Failure to acknowledge that a particular patient has entered the terminal phase of his or her disease prevents the patient and family alike from receiving the supportive services that could be provided by hospice agencies. Families are often asked to make decisions for patients who have not previously expressed treatment preferences. Out of guilt or uncertainty, families may make decisions to provide life-prolonging medical treatments even when the likelihood of any benefit to the patient is minimal.

As early as possible, families of dementia patients should be informed of the typical but uncertain course of dementia and the treatment decisions they will face as the disease progresses. They should also be educated as to some of the difficult symptoms they may encounter, such as agitation or combativeness, and how to deal with them. They should be ensured a close and continuing relationship with professional caregivers who can guide them throughout the entire course of their loved one's illness and address any symptoms of discomfort that should arise. It is estimated that caregivers of dementia patients spend between 60 and 100 hours each week in caregiving responsibilities. This can lead to physical, mental, and emotional exhaustion[61] and puts caregivers at risk for clinical depression and impaired health. Information regarding local services and support groups for patients with dementia and their families should be made available.[6,14]

ADVANCE CARE PLANNING

Advance care planning is covered in detail in Chapter 21. However, the importance of advance care planning for patients who will experience progressive cognitive decline cannot be overstated. The family and caregivers of patients with advanced dementia will face with certainty decisions regarding nursing home placement, transfer to an acute-care setting for ongoing care, resuscitation, antibiotic treatment, and tube feeding. To the extent possible, these decisions should be driven by the treatment preferences of the patient. This cannot be done in patients with dementia unless these discussions are held early enough in the disease process that decision-making capacity is preserved. As soon as a diagnosis of dementia, regardless of the cause, is certain, discussions should begin with the patient and family about the expected course of the disease and the treatment options they will face as the dementia progresses.

SUMMARY

The provision of palliative care for end-stage dementia presents unique challenges for all involved. The uncertain course of the disease, as well as the inability to communicate with the patient in the terminal and most symptomatic stages, when communication would be most helpful, are two significant factors with which families and caregivers deal. Given the increasing numbers of patients who will suffer from progressive dementia unless new treatments are found, we need to continue to work on better systems of hospice care for patients with dementia as well as tools to assess the symptoms associated with end-stage dementia and the response to treatments.

REFERENCES

1. Foley KM, Carver AC. Palliative care in neurology: an overview. Neurol Clin 19: 789–799, 2001.
2. Lilienfeld DE, Perl DP. Projected neurodegenerative disease mortality in the United States, 1990–2040. Neuroepidemiology 12: 219–228, 1993.
3. Lilienfeld DE. Projected neurodegenerative disease mortality among minorities, 1990–2040. Neuroepidemiology 13:179–186, 1994.
4. Rabow MW, Fair JM, Hardie GE, McPhee SJ. An evaluation of the end-of-life content in leading neurology textbooks. Neurology 55:893–894, 2000.
5. American Psychiatric Association. Diagnostic and Statistical Manual of Mental Disorders, 4th ed. Washington DC, American Psychiatric Press, 1994.
6. Shuster JL. Palliative care for advanced dementia. Clin Geriatr Med 16:373–386, 2000.

7. Gray KF, Cummings JL. Dementia. In: The American Psychiatric Press Textbook of Consultation-Liaison Psychiatry. Washington DC, American Psychiatric Press, pp. 277–309, 1996.

8. Markesbery WR (ed). Neuropathology of Dementing Disorders. New York: Oxford University Press, 1998.

9. Volicer L. Management of severe Alzheimer's disease and end-of-life issues. Clin Geriatr Med 17:377–391, 2001.

10. Evans DA, Funkenstein HH, Albert MS, et al. Prevalence of Alzheimer's disease in a community population of older persons: higher than previously reported. JAMA 262:2551–2556, 1989.

11. Tomlinson BE, Blessed G, Roth M. Observations on the brains of demented old people. J Neurol Sci 11:205–242, 1970.

12. Byrne EJ, Lennox G, Lowe J, Godwin-Austen RB. Diffuse Lewy body disease: clinical features in 15 cases. J Neurol Neurosurg Psychiatry 52:709–717, 1989.

13. McKeith IG, Galasko D, Kosaka K, et al. Consensus guidelines for the clinical and pathological diagnosis of dementia with Lewy bodies (DLB): report of the consortium on DLB international workshop. Neurology 47:1113–1124, 1996.

14. Volicer L, McKee A, Hewitt S. Dementia. Neurol Clin 19:867–885, 2001.

15. Heston LL, White JA, Mastri AH. Pick's disease: clinical genetics and natural history. Arch Gen Psychiatry 44:409–411, 1987.

16. McGrew DM. Chronic illnesses and the end of life. Prim Care 28:339–347, 2001.

17. Magaziner J, Tenney JH, DeForge B, et al. Prevalence and characteristics of nursing home-acquired infections in the aged. J Am Geriatr Soc 39:1071–1078, 1991.

18. Doody RS, Stevens JC, Beck C, et al. Practice parameter: management of dementia (an evidence-based review). Report of the Quality Standards Subcommittee of the American Academy of Neurology. Neurology 56:1154–1166, 2001.

19. Volicer L, Rheaume Y, Brown J, Fabiszewsky K, Brady R. Hospice approach to the treatment of patients with advanced dementia of the Alzheimer type. JAMA 256:2210–2213, 1986.

20. Volicer L. Need for hospice approach to treatment of patients with advanced progressive dementia. J Am Geriatr Soc 34:655–658, 1986.

21. Hanrahan P, Luchins DJ. Access to hospice programs in end-stage dementia: a national survey of hospice programs. J Am Geriatr Soc 43:56–59, 1995.

22. Volicer L, Seltzer B, Rheaume Y, et al. Progression of Alzheimer-type dementia in institutionalized patients: a cross-sectional study. J Appl Gerontol 6:83–94, 1987.

23. Volicer BJ, Hurley A, Fabiszewski KJ, Montgomery P, Volicer L. Predicting short-term survival for patients with advanced Alzheimer's disease. J Am Geriatr Soc 41:535–540, 1993.

24. Morrison RS, Siu AL. Survival in end-stage dementia following acute illness. JAMA 284:47–52, 2000.

25. Reisberg B. Functional Assessment Staging (FAST). Psychopharm Bull 24:653–659, 1988.

26. National Hospice Organization, Stuart B, Herbst L, Kinzbrunner B, et al. Hospice Care: A Physician's Guide. Published by National Hospice and Palliative Care Organization, Arlington, VA, 1998.

27. National Hospice Organization, Stuart B, Herbst L, Kinzbrunner B, et al. Medical guidelines for determining prognosis in selected non-cancer diseases. Hospice J 11: 47–63, 1996.

28. Luchins DJ, Hanrahan P, Murphy K. Criteria for enrolling dementia patients in hospice. J Am Geriatr Soc 45:1054–1059, 1997.

29. Hanrahan P, Raymond M, McGowan E, Luchins DJ. Criteria for enrolling dementia patients in hospice: a replication. Am J Hospice Palliat Care 16:395–400, 1999.

30. Mahoney JJ, Miller G. What Does Hospice Offer Alzheimer's Patients and Families? Hastings Center Conference on Dying with Dementia. Briarcliff Manor, NY, Hastings Center, 1996.

31. Lynn J. Caring at the end of our lives. N Engl J Med 335:201–202, 1996.

32. McCarthy M, Addington-Hall J, Altmann D. The experience of dying with dementia: a retrospective study. Int J Geriatr Psychiatry 12:404–409, 1997.

33. Ferrell BA, Stein WM. Pain. In: Yoshikawa TT, Cobbs EL, Brummel-Smith K (Eds.). Practical Ambulatory Geriatrics, 2nd ed. St. Louis, Mosby Year Book, pp. 331–341, 1998.

34. Farrell MJ, Katz B, Helme RD. The impact of dementia on the pain experience. Pain 67:7–15, 1996.

35. Ford B. Pain in Parkinson's disease. Clin Neurosci 5:63–72, 1998.

36. Hurley AC, Volicer BJ, Hanrahan P, et al. Assessment of discomfort in advanced Alzheimer's patients. Res Nurs Health 15: 369–377, 1992.

37. Hurley AC, Volicer B, Mahoney MA, et al. Palliative fever management in Alzheimer patients: Quality plus fiscal responsibility. Adv Nurs Sci 16:211–232, 1993.

38. World Health Organization. Cancer Pain Relief and Palliative Care. Technical Report Series 804. Geneva, World Health Organization, 1990.

39. Kovach CR, Weissman DE, Griffie J, Matson S, Muchka S. Assessment and treatment of discomfort for people with late-stage dementia. J Pain Symptom Manage 18:412–419, 1999.

40. Bruera E, Schoeller T, Montejo G. Organic hallucinosis in patients receiving high doses of opiates for cancer pain. Pain 48:397–399, 1992.

41. Maddocks I, Somogyi A, Abbott F, et al. Attenuation of morphine-induced delirium by substitution with infusion of oxycodone. J Pain Symptom Manage 12:182–189, 1996.

42. Morrison RS. Pain and discomfort associated with common hospital procedures and experiences. J Pain Symptom Manage 15:91–101, 1998.

43. Tinetti ME, Liu WL, Ginter SF. Mechanical restraints use and fall-related injuries among residents of skilled nursing facilities. Ann Intern Med 116:369–374, 1992.

44. Miles SH, Irvine P: Deaths caused by physical restraints. Gerontologist 32:762–766, 2001.

45. Paulsen JS, Salmon DP, Thal LJ, et al. Incidence of and risk factors for hallucinations and delusions in patients with probable AD. Neurology 54:1965–1971, 2000.

46. Olanow CW, Watts RL, Koller WC. An algorithm (decision tree) for the management of Parkinson's disease (2001): treatment guidelines. Neurology 56(Suppl 5):S1–S88, 2001.

47. Fountain A. Visual hallucinations: a prevalence study among hospice inpatients. Palliat Med 15:19–25, 2001.

48. Manfredi PL, Ribeiro S, Chandler SW, et al. Inappropriate use of naloxone in cancer patients with pain. J Pain Symptom Manage 11:131–134, 1996.

49. Carver AC, Foley KM. Symptom assessment and management. Neurol Clin 19:921–947, 2001

50. Volicer L, Rheaume Y, Cyr D. Treatment of depression in advanced Alzheimer's disease using sertraline. J Geriatr Psychiatry Neurol 7:227–229, 1994.

51. Volicer L, Hurley AC, Mahoney E. Behavioral symptoms of dementia. In: Volicer L, Hurley A (Eds.). Hospice Care for Patients with Advanced Progressive Dementia. New York, Springer, p. 68–87, 1988.

52. Singer C. Sleep disorders. In: Yoshikawa TT, Cobbs EL, Brummel-Smith K (Eds.). Practical Ambulatory Geriatrics, 2nd ed. St. Louis, Mosby Year Book, pp. 496–505, 1998.

53. Volicer L, Brandeis GH, Hurley AC. Infections in advanced dementia. In: Volicer L, Hurley A (Eds.). Hospice Care for Patients with Advanced Progressive Dementia. New York, Springer, p. 30, 1998.

54. Fried TR, Gillick MR, Lipsitz LA. Short-term functional outcomes of long-term care residents with pneumonia treated with and without hospital transfer. J Am Geriatr Soc 45:302–306, 1997.

55. Hurley AC, Volicer BJ, Volicer L. Effect of fever-management strategy on the progression of dementia of the Alzheimer type. Alzheimer Dis Assoc Disord 10:5–10, 1996.

56. Fabiszewski KJ, Volicer B, Volicer L. Effect of antibiotic treatment on outcome of fevers in institutionalized Alzheimer patients. JAMA 263:3168–3172, 1990.

57. Hanson D, Langemo DK, Olson B, et al. The prevalence and incidence of pressure ulcers in the hospice setting: analysis of two methodologies. Am J Hosp Palliat Care 8:18–22, 1991.

58. Finucane TE, Christmas C, Travis K. Tube feeding in patients with advanced dementia: a review of the evidence. JAMA 282:1365–1370, 1999.

59. Gillick MR. Rethinking the role of tube feeding in patients with advanced dementia. N Engl J Med 342:206–210, 2000.

60. McCann RM, Hall WJ, Groth-Juncker A. Comfort care for terminally ill patients: the appropriate use of nutrition and hydration. JAMA 272:1263–1266, 1994.

61. Dunkin JJ, Anderson-Hanley C. Dementia caregiver burden: a review of the literature and guidelines for assessment and intervention. Neurology 51(Suppl 1):S53–S60, 1998.

14

Chronic Lung Disease and Lung Cancer

JOHN P. KRCMARIK, THOMAS J. PRENDERGAST,
E. WESLEY ELY, AND JAMES R. RUNO

Chronic lung disease presents a twofold challenge. First, it is a common problem. Lung cancer is the leading cause of cancer death in both men and women in the United States. There were 169,400 new diagnoses and 154,900 deaths from lung cancer in the United States in 2002, accounting for 12.8% of new cancer diagnoses and 28% of all cancer deaths. More Americans now die of lung cancer than of colon, breast, and prostate cancers combined. The National Heart, Lung, and Blood Institute estimates that over 16 million Americans have been diagnosed with chronic obstructive pulmonary disease (COPD). A greater number is thought to be afflicted but undiagnosed. The American Lung Association reports 119,524 deaths from COPD in 1999, making this the fourth leading cause of death in the United States. Both lung cancer and COPD are more prevalent among older patients.

The second challenge is that both malignant and nonmalignant advanced lung disease (ALD) convey a heavy burden of symptoms. In particular, the latter kills very

slowly. Long before patients with COPD or pulmonary fibrosis succumb to respiratory failure, their activities are progressively circumscribed by breathlessness or dyspnea. During this period of progressive, disabling symptoms, exacerbations are common and frequently result in hospitalization, intubation, and mechanical ventilation. This predictable pattern should afford health-care providers multiple opportunities to intervene, both to treat symptoms and to address goals of care with this group of slowly dying patients. Interestingly, in both malignant[1] and nonmalignant ALD,[2] neither of these opportunities seems to be seized consistently. The reasons are complex, but several issues stand out. Symptom control is poor because dyspnea is subjective and frustratingly difficult to treat.[3] Goals of care are not addressed because death, unlike dying, is unpredictable, especially in nonmalignant ALD.[4]

As will become obvious in the literature review that follows, much of the research into chronic lung disease measures objective outcomes, e.g., the forced expiratory volume in 1 second (FEV_1) in COPD and survival in lung cancer, despite clear evidence that dyspnea is a much better indicator of health-related quality of life than pulmonary function tests[5] and that lung cancer patients value quality at least as much as quantity of life.[6] One obvious key to appropriate palliative care in elderly patients with chronic lung disease is to inquire about and address patients' genuine concerns. A second, subtler key is to understand how prognosis affects decision making. Medicine has a very clear understanding of disease progression in groups of patients over the long term, but short-term prognostication in individual patients is extremely difficult (Table 14–1).

These two facts place providers in the awkward position of having to advise patients of what to expect from their chronic lung disease without knowing when to expect it. Toward the end of life, most patients develop serious progressive illnesses that interfere with their daily functioning and worsen until the point of death. The trajectory from chronic illness to death is different in different diseases, but the common pattern is that people do not simply die but, rather, die of acute illnesses or acute complications of chronic illnesses after a considered, deliberate decision to stop, to limit, or not to pursue some form of medical therapy. Treatment options that help control the tremendous symptom burden in end-stage lung disease tend to become less and less efficacious as the illness progresses. This effectively means that at some point in the course of illness, most patients or their surrogates have to accept or to make an affirmative judgment that "today is the day" when they will acknowledge not the

theoretical possibility of dying but their own imminent death. Success at facilitating such decisions demands insight into patients' genuine needs, empathy for their suffering, the trust that comes from aggressive management of physical symptoms, and appropriate end-of-life planning to improve the quality of the dying process.

BURDEN OF DYSPNEA IN ADVANCED LUNG DISEASE

Dyspnea is one of the most common symptoms experienced by patients with all types of ALD, including lung cancer, interstitial lung disease, and particularly COPD.[7,8] In the Study to Understand Prognoses and Preferences for Outcomes and Risks of Treatments (SUPPORT),[9] severe dyspnea occurred in 56% and 32% of patients with severe COPD or stage III/IV non-small cell lung cancer, respectively, while severe pain was experienced in 21% and 28%, respectively.[6] Dyspnea is common among patients with lung cancer and increases with the approach of death.[10,11] Uncontrolled dyspnea can be extremely distressing for patients and their caretakers.

Dyspnea is analogous to pain in that sensory input from multiple sites is integrated in the cerebral cortex to produce a subjective sensation that is not closely tied to easily measured objective correlates. Neither spirometric abnormalities nor disturbances in arterial blood gases predict the severity of dyspnea.[12] The American Thoracic Society (ATS) defines *dyspnea* as "a subjective experience of breathing discomfort that derives from interactions among multiple physiological, psychological, social, and en-

Table 14–1. Median Predicted 2-Month Mortality in the Study to Understand Prognoses and Preferences for Outcomes and Risks of Treatments

Patient population	1 week prior to death	1 day prior to death
All deaths	51%	17%
Coma	27%	5%
Congestive heart failure	62%	42%
Chronic obstructive pulmonary disease	41%	21%

Source: Lynn et al.[4]

vironmental factors."[13–16] This elaborate definition reflects the complex mechanisms that underlie dyspnea.

The most important contributor to dyspnea in patients with ALD is the increased respiratory effort that accompanies the underlying disease: airflow obstruction in COPD, impaired pulmonary compliance in interstitial disease or chest wall compliance in pleural disease, intrinsic respiratory muscle weakness from cancer-related inanition, respiratory muscle dysfunction from the mechanical disadvantage of hyperinflation in COPD. This sensation of increased effort is magnified by the increased respiratory drive that is ubiquitous in ALD and modulated by various psychological and environmental stimuli. Thus, it is not surprising that the perception of dyspnea varies greatly among ALD patients.

For therapeutic purposes, it is most helpful to think of dyspnea as a mechanical mismatch between afferent information from receptors in respiratory muscles, airways, and the thoracic cage and their corresponding motor activity. If an individual does not have the ventilatory capacity to meet demand, dyspnea results. To decrease dyspnea, one may aim to increase ventilatory capacity, decrease ventilatory demand, or alter the central perception of dyspnea.

PHARMACOLOGICAL APPROACHES TO DYSPNEA IN ADVANCED LUNG DISEASE

Increase Ventilatory Capacity

Bronchodilator therapy

Inhaled β_2-agonists (e.g., albuterol, metaproterenol) and the anticholinergic ipratropium bromide (Atrovent®) are the most important agents in the pharmacological management of dyspnea in patients with COPD. They reduce the work of breathing by reducing airway resistance and the associated hyperinflation that compromises diaphragmatic function.[17] Bronchodilators offer improvement in dyspnea, exercise tolerance, and overall health status but do not alter the inexorable decline in lung function

that is the hallmark of COPD.[18] Their efficacy in patients with interstitial lung disease or respiratory compromise from lung cancer is anecdotal at best.

Ipratropium bromide is generally preferred to the short-acting β_2 agonists as a first-line agent due to its longer duration of action and absence of sympathomimetic side effects.[19] Some studies have suggested that ipratropium achieves superior bronchodilation in COPD patients.[20] Short-acting β_2 agonists are less expensive than ipratropium and have a more rapid onset of action, commonly leading to greater patient satisfaction. Use of both short-acting β_2 agonists and ipratropium at submaximal doses leads to improved bronchodilation compared to use of either agent alone, but the combination does not further reduce dyspnea.[21–23] Long-acting β_2 agonists (e.g., formoterol, salmeterol) and anticholinergics (tiotropium) appear to achieve equivalent or superior bronchodilation to ipratropium in addition to similar improvements in dyspnea and overall health status.[24–26] Both short- and long-acting bronchodilators have been reported to reduce dyspnea in ALD independent of their effects on FEV_1.[12,27]

Patients with dyspnea and COPD should receive a clinical trial of bronchodilator medications, even in the absence of documented reversal of airflow obstruction. Patients with interstitial lung disease or lung cancer in the absence of COPD do not generally benefit from bronchodilators, but a clinical trial may be appropriate. Bronchodilators should be discontinued in patients who do not experience a clear symptomatic benefit. Long-acting bronchodilators simplify dosing, improve compliance, and may offer improved symptom control. Medications can be delivered through metered-dose inhalers, dry powder inhalers, and updraft nebulizers. There are no data to support greater efficacy of nebulized medications over metered-dose inhaler delivery, although nebulizers may be more convenient and effective in patients who are immobile and/or have difficulty mastering inhaler technique.[28]

Theophylline

Theophylline has fallen out of favor because of its narrow toxic–therapeutic window, significant drug interactions, and the availability of more potent and better-tolerated bronchodilators. Nonetheless, theophylline has been shown to improve respiratory muscle function,[29,30] increase minute ventilation,[31] reduce pulmonary vascular resistance, improve cardiac output and myocardial perfusion,[32] improve mucociliary clearance,[33,34] and reduce airway inflammation[35,36] in addition to its beneficial effects on bronchomotor tone.[37] There is also a well-recognized propensity for stable COPD patients maintained on theophylline to decompensate when theophylline is withdrawn.[38]

Several studies have documented improvement in dyspnea and morning symptoms in association with theophylline.[39,40] Recent data from a randomized controlled trial of 943 patients with COPD showed significantly greater improvement in dyspnea, pulmonary function, and exacerbation frequency in patients receiving both inhaled salmeterol and theophylline (200 mg/day) than either agent alone.[41] Similar reductions in dyspnea with the combination of theophylline and short-acting β_2 agonists have been documented.[42] Overall, it appears that some patients with COPD may receive additional dyspnea relief and improved exercise tolerance from the addition of theophylline to their bronchodilator regimen. In appropriate patients, a short-term (2–4 weeks) trial of long-acting theophylline preparations in doses that achieve a serum drug level of 10–12 mcg/ml is recommended. As always with symptomatic therapy, the drug should be discontinued in nonresponders.

Corticosteroids

The use of oral steroids in exacerbations of COPD is well supported[43] despite various doses and durations of treatment studied and the increased rates of steroid-related side effects reported, particularly hyperglycemia.[44] The role of oral steroids in stable COPD is less clear. Only 10% of sta-ble outpatients with COPD given oral corticosteroids have a $\geq20\%$ increase in FEV_1 compared to patients receiving placebo.[45] Recent studies challenge even these limited data.[46,47] Side effects of systemic corticosteroid therapy are significant; therefore, any spirometric gain must be weighed against steroid-related complications such as diabetes, cataracts, osteoporosis, and others.[48] Observational data suggest an association between corticosteroid use and increased mortality.[48] Finally, the effect of oral steroids on dyspnea and functional status has not been well characterized.

An evidence-based approach to corticosteroid therapy in stable outpatients is very limited. Empirical trials of oral corticosteroids should be guided by the following principles. The baseline FEV_1 should be stable, i.e., not measured during an exacerbation; and taken on maximal bronchodilator therapy; the postbronchodilator value is considered the appropriate baseline. Corticosteroid therapy equivalent to 0.5 mg/kg daily of prednisone is given for 14–21 days. The drug should be discontinued unless there is a $\geq20\%$ increase in FEV_1. Patients with subjective benefit without spirometric improvement or a clear change in functional status are nonresponders. They should be continued on treatment only if symptomatic benefit is clear and life expectancy is short. In patients who require maintenance therapy, the lowest dose and/or alternate-day dosing should be used in conjunction with measures to reduce the risk of osteoporosis.[49] Responders are often switched to inhaled corticosteroids, but there are few data to guide this practice (see below). Patients with COPD should not be treated with inhaled corticosteroids simply because these agents lack the full toxicity of oral preparations.

Inhaled corticosteroids have beneficial effects on the health status and exacerbation rate in some stable COPD patients, although they do not affect the decline of lung function over time. Recent data from a multicenter, randomized, placebo-controlled trial of over 1100 patients with

COPD found no effect of chronic inhaled triamcinolone (600 mcg bid) on the rate of FEV_1 decline over a mean 40-month period.[50] However, there were significant reductions in dyspnea, other respiratory symptoms, and hospitalizations. These gains were accompanied by a significant loss of bone density in the treatment group. In another study, more severe, non-asthmatic COPD patients randomized to inhaled fluticasone (500 mcg bid) showed no significant improvement in FEV_1 over 36 months compared to placebo. However, fluticasone was associated with a significant reduction in COPD exacerbations and an improved standardized measurement of health status found to correlate with dyspnea intensity.[51]

Given the heterogeneity of patients studied, there is no way to predict which COPD patients will respond to inhaled corticosteroids. Therefore, short-term trials are appropriate in patients who are dyspneic despite optimal bronchodilation. The inhaled route may be preferable to systemic use because of a lower incidence of side effects. However, inhaled corticosteroids, especially newer, high-potency agents, are systemically absorbed and do have the potential for significant adverse effects.[52–54]

Oral steroids have been used to treat many types of interstitial lung disease (ILD, also termed *diffuse parenchymal lung disease*). No randomized trial has demonstrated that any proposed therapy improves survival or quality of life compared with no treatment. Some forms of ILD appear to be prednisone-responsive, e.g., acute sarcoidosis, bronchiolitis obliterans organizing pneumonia, and some forms of ILD with histological patterns of nonspecific interstitial pneumonitis or desquamative interstitial pneumonitis.[55–61] Treatment of such patients is appropriate if not based on good outcome data. However, the most common clinical presentation of ILD in geriatric patients is idiopathic pulmonary fibrosis (IPF) with the histological subtype of usual interstitial pneumonitis (UIP), which typically presents in patients in their sixth or seventh decade. UIP is marked by progressive fi-

brosis of the basal and peripheral lung parenchyma. The associated scarring reduces pulmonary compliance, leading to pulmonary restriction and increased work of breathing manifesting as progressive dyspnea. Median survival of IPF/UIP is less than 3 years from diagnosis.

Decrease Ventilatory Demand

Oxygen therapy

Supplemental oxygen is one of the few clearly life-prolonging therapies available for ALD patients, specifically for those with advanced COPD complicated by resting hypoxemia. In the Nocturnal Oxygen Therapy Trial (NOTT), 203 patients with severe COPD and hypoxemia at rest were randomized to 12 or 24 hours of oxygen therapy.[62,63] These studies did not assess the effect of supplemental oxygen on dyspnea.

Supplemental oxygen therapy has multiple physiological effects. It variably depresses carotid body output and respiratory drive, improves respiratory muscle function, decreases respiratory system impedance, decreases pulmonary artery pressures, and improves oxygen delivery and cardiac function. Supplemental oxygen usually causes an increase in arterial partial pressure of CO_2 (PCO_2) by reducing the ventilatory response to CO_2.[28] Rarely, it may cause a significant increase in PCO_2 by altering ventilation–perfusion relationships or reducing respiratory drive.[64] This effect is almost exclusively seen in patients with resting hypercapnia. The effects of supplemental oxygen on arterial PCO_2 levels should be monitored on initiation of therapy in patients with ALD, particularly in those with significant hypercapnia.

The physiological effects of supplemental oxygen predictably improve exercise capacity in patients with ALD, but this change is generally modest.[65–67] The effect of supplemental oxygen on dyspnea is less consistent. In a randomized, double-blind, crossover trial of severely disabled hypoxemic patients with COPD and ILD, Swinburn and colleagues[68] reported significant reductions in rest dyspnea using 28% oxygen versus compressed air. This was not corroborated in a single-blind trial of eight patients with moderate to severe COPD and rest dyspnea.[69] Similarly, in patients with terminal cancer and rest dyspnea, some investigators have found that supplemental oxygen reduces rest dyspnea,[70] while others have found no difference between oxygen and compressed air delivered by nasal cannula.[71] This latter finding may reflect the presence of extrathoracic receptors on the face and in the nasal passages that mitigate the sensation of breathlessness.[72] Open windows and a fan to circulate air across the face frequently improve breathlessness. Oxygen may also act synergistically with opioids to relieve exertional dyspnea, as demonstrated by a reduced dyspnea score among 12 moderate to severe COPD patients during exercise, compared to opioid therapy alone.[73]

Medicare reimbursement for home oxygen therapy is based on the enrollment criteria of the NOTT and not on symptomatic dyspnea (Table 14–2). However, the Medicare Hospice Benefit will pay for home oxygen therapy for dyspnea.

Independent of the important issue of reimbursement, patients who do not meet Medicare criteria for home oxygen but who suffer from dyspnea refractory to standard therapy should be offered a trial of supplemental oxygen therapy. A letter to insurance companies documenting improved symptoms (some authors recommend a blinded trial of oxygen as evidence) and failure of other therapies to control dyspnea may result in reimbursement of long-term oxygen therapy for this purpose. Although no optimal flow rate of oxygen has been defined, it seems reasonable to titrate the flow rate to achieve effective palliation of dyspnea and/or improved exercise capacity while avoiding symptomatic hypercapnia.

Most patients receive supplemental oxygen through a nasal cannula. Face masks can be used but tend to interfere with speaking and eating and may contribute to a sense of suffocation. Transtracheal delivery through a percutaneous catheter may improve comfort, reduce nasal mucosal desiccation, and produce superior oxygen saturation at lower flow rates than nasal delivery. Direct flow into the trachea may also reduce inspired minute ventilation[74] and in one small study improved morale, depression, and exercise capacity compared to nasal administration.[75] Conflicting data, along with the increased maintenance requirement and risk of infection or dis-

Table 14–2. Criteria for Medicare Reimbursement of Home Oxygen Therapy

I. Continuous therapy, either of the following:
    A. $PaO_2 \leq 55$ mm Hg or $SpO_2 \leq 88\%$ taken at rest or while awake and breathing room air
    B. $PaO_2 \leq 59$ mm Hg or $SpO_2 \leq 89\%$ taken at rest or while awake and breathing room air if there is evidence of any one or more of the following:
        1. Dependent edema suggesting congestive heart failure
        2. p pulmonale on electrocardiogram (P wave > 3 mm in standard leads II, III, or aVF).
        3. Hematocrit $> 56\%$
II. Prescription for nocturnal oxygen use only, either of the following
    A. $PaO_2 \leq 55$ mm Hg or $SpO_2 \leq 88\%$ while asleep and breathing room air, resting $PaO_2 \geq 59$ mm Hg or $SpO_2 \geq 89\%$ in a patient who is awake
    B. A decrease while asleep in $PaO_2 > 10$ mm Hg or in $SpO_2 > 5\%$ associated with symptoms or signs reasonably attributed to nocturnal hypoxemia (e.g., impaired cognitive functioning, nocturnal restlessness, insomnia)
III. Prescription for use only during exercise, both of the following:
    A. $PaO_2 \leq 55$ mm Hg or $SpO_2 \leq 88\%$ during exercise for a patient who is awake, resting $PaO_2 \geq 59$ mm Hg or $SpO_2 \geq 89\%$
    B. Evidence that use of supplemental oxygen during exercise improves the hypoxemia that was demonstrated during exercise while breathing room air

PaO_2, partial pressure of arterial O_2; SpO_2, pulse oximeter oxygen saturation; aVF, augmented voltage unipolar left foot lead.

lodgement with a transtracheal catheter, probably account for its lack of widespread use despite the potential advantages.

Alter Central Perception

When measures to improve ventilatory capacity or to reduce ventilatory drive cannot be achieved in the setting of ALD, interfering with neural pathways that give rise to the sensation of breathlessness may be an alternate way to palliate dyspnea. Several classes of drugs have been used for this purpose, including opioids, benzodiazepines, and neuroleptics.

Opioid therapy

Opioids are potent analgesics and mild sedatives and have powerful effects on respiration to decrease ventilatory drive while facilitating higher tolerance to resultant hypoxemia and hypercapnia.[76] This combination of physiological effects in a familiar class of medications makes opioids attractive therapeutic agents for dyspnea. Clinical trials have yielded inconsistent results, however. In patients with severe COPD, multiple trials suggest improvement in refractory dyspnea in patients given dihydrocodeine (15–60 mg tid),[73,77,78] morphine sulfate (0.8 mg/kg/qd)[79] and hydromorphone (3 mg qid rectally).[80] In general, opioid use was associated with decreased minute ventilation but hypercapnia and hypoxemia were well-tolerated. Two of these trials reported significant incidence of opioid-related side effects, such as nausea, constipation, and drowsiness, which resulted in a 30% discontinuation rate in one study.[73]

Multiple studies have come to the opposite conclusion. One randomized, placebo-controlled trial of codeine (30 mg qid) failed to demonstrate improved dyspnea or exercise tolerance among 11 patients with severe COPD while reporting significant drowsiness.[81] A randomized, double-blind, placebo-controlled study using diamorphine at two doses (2.5 and 5 mg q 6 hours for 2 weeks) in the setting of severe emphysema, failed to show significant dyspnea reduction or improvement in exercise tolerance.[82] In a more recent randomized, double-blind, placebo-controlled crossover study of sustained-release morphine in severe COPD patients, a mean dose of 25 mg daily over 6 weeks did not improve quality of life, exercise tolerance, dyspnea, or oxygen saturation, with a trend toward increased opioid-related side effects.[83]

In addition to subcutaneous, oral, and rectal administration of opioids to dyspneic COPD patients, nebulized delivery has been studied. In a double-blind, placebo-controlled trial, Young and colleagues[84] reported that nebulized morphine (mean nebulized dose 1.7 mg) significantly improved dyspnea-limited exercise times without untoward side effects in nine patients with severe COPD. In contrast, four subsequent trials of similar design in patients with multiple forms of ALD failed to demonstrate significant improvement in rest or exertional dyspnea despite nebulized doses ranging from low (1–2 mg) to high (10–25 mg).[85–88]

The literature shows more consistent improvements in dyspnea in terminally ill cancer patients. Bruera and colleagues[89] reported favorable effects of subcutaneous morphine in 19 of 20 terminally ill cancer patients without significant respiratory or hemodynamic changes. This finding was reproduced in a placebo-controlled trial by the same author of 10 terminally ill patients with dyspnea already receiving daily morphine with reported "good" control of pain. Patients receiving a 50% increase in their morphine dose reported an average 50% reduction in their dyspnea without significant effects on respiration or hemodynamics.[90] Cohen and colleagues studied terminal lung cancer patients who lacked adequate pain control despite oxygen and intermittent dosing of opioids.[91] Employing continuous intravenous morphine after 5- to 10-minute bolusing to achieve complete pain relief, six of eight patients reported complete relief of dyspnea within 16–87 hours. Sedation was a significant side effect but was tempered by reducing the hourly amount without loss of effective analgesia.

In summary, opioids are effective agents to treat dyspnea but have a high incidence of side effects, particularly dysphoria and sedation. Tolerance of these side effects tends to be poor among ambulatory outpatients. For patients who have pain in addition to dyspnea and those with refractory dyspnea in the setting of terminal cancer, a trial of opioids is clearly indicated. A careful reading of the literature does not support the routine use of oral opioid therapy in ambulatory outpatients with nonmalignant ALD and dyspnea, and there is no good evidence to support that inhaled opioids alleviate dyspnea in patients with nonmalignant ALD. Nonetheless, therapeutic options are very limited, and clinical experience suggests that there are some patients who may benefit from opioid therapy. Therefore, a trial of opioids may be worthwhile, to reduce ventilatory drive when supplemental oxygen and pharmacological therapies fail to palliate dyspnea. The lowest dose should be employed to minimize side effects when opioids provide effective dyspnea relief.

Anxiolytics, neuroleptics, and antidepressants

Benzodiazepines are generally ineffective at relieving dyspnea in ALD and have also been shown to reduce exercise tolerance,[92] worsen oxygenation,[93] and increase sedation.[94] Buspirone is an anxiolytic structurally and pharmacologically distinct from the benzodiazepines. In one study,[95] but not another,[96] buspirone (20 mg qd) significantly reduced dyspnea and anxiety and improved exercise tolerance without changes in blood gases.

There is conflicting evidence for the use of neuroleptic medications to relieve dyspnea in ALD. Woodcock and colleagues[92] reported promethazine, a phenothiazine derivative with potent H_1 blocking and sedative properties, at a total dose of 125 mg/day, had a modest effect on dyspnea while producing less sedation than valium. Rice and colleagues[81] failed to confirm a benefit of promethazine at a dose of 25 mg qid. One uncontrolled study of 20 terminally ill cancer patients reported that chlorpromazine, given intravenously or rectally at a dose of 12.5–25 mg every 4–12 hours, reduced restlessness and dyspnea in 18 of 20 patients.[97] Trials in ALD patients who are not actively dying are needed to corroborate this finding. There may be a synergistic role of neuroleptics when used with opioids. Light and colleagues[98] reported improved dyspnea and exercise tolerance in seven stable patients with COPD taking 30 mg morphine combined with either promethazine or prochlorperazine but not with morphine alone.

Overall, there are scant and conflicting data among a relatively small number of patients to suggest that monotherapy with benzodiazepines or neuroleptics provides predictable relief of dyspnea or improved functional capacity in the setting of ALD. These agents are not recommended for relief of dyspnea in patients with ALD, although specific symptoms such as restlessness, anxiety, and insomnia may merit a clinical trial in individual patients. We suggest a trial of buspirone in preference to benzodiazepines. When used in conjunction with opioids, promethazine or prochlorperazine may act synergistically to palliate refractory dyspnea in ALD.

NONPHARMACOLOGICAL APPROACHES TO DYSPNEA IN ADVANCED LUNG DISEASE

Pulmonary Rehabilitation

Integrated programs for patients with ALD include exercise training, breathing strategies, disease-specific education, and psychosocial support. In stable ALD patients with compensated comorbidities, such programs have been shown to improve dyspnea, exercise tolerance, and quality of life, independent of effects on pulmonary function.[99–101] As little as 3 hours a week for 6 weeks was found to increase quality of life on standardized measurement in 65 COPD patients for at least as long as the 6-month study period.[102] Pulmonary rehabilitation incorporating exercise and specific inspiratory muscle training may provide synergistic improvement in dyspnea and exercise capacity superior to long-acting bronchodilator therapy alone in the setting of moderate to severe COPD.[103] These programs are individualized to patient needs, environment, and level of function. Although most studies have been reported in COPD patients, the principles seem applicable to other groups of ambulatory ALD patients who might benefit. The goal of rehabilitation is to restore individuals with ALD to the highest level of independent function possible, but may it not be indicated for patients with decompensated lung disease or comorbidities that may cause an undue burden of symptoms without restoration of function. Nonetheless, most ambulatory ALD patients should be considered for pulmonary rehabilitation.

Noninvasive Positive Pressure Ventilation

Data from multiple prospective, randomized trials convincingly support the use of noninvasive positive pressure ventilation (NPPV) in patients with acute exacerbations of COPD. It has been shown to reduce intubation rates, length of intensive care unit and hospital stays, nosocomial infection rates, and in-hospital mortality rates.[104–107] The benefits of NPPV in patients with advanced, stable COPD are less clear. Randomized trials comparing oxygen plus NPPV to oxygen therapy alone in stable COPD patients have shown conflicting results,[108,109] with some[108] demonstrating significant improvements in sleep, daytime and nocturnal gas exchange, and quality-of-life scores and others failing[109] to confirm these benefits. Considering additional, unfavorable results of smaller, controlled trials of NPPV in stable COPD patients over shorter treatment periods, there are scant data to support its use in ALD outside of COPD with marked hypercapnia. Even in this subset of patients, no trial has convincingly demonstrated a survival advantage over long-term oxygen therapy. Practically, use of NPPV is tempered by the high financial cost and high noncompliance rate associated with the home setting.

Noninvasive positive pressure ventilation has become an accepted therapy for chronic respiratory failure secondary to neuromuscular disease, thoracic deformity, and idiopathic hypoventilation. Uncontrolled cohort studies have shown that NPPV improves gas exchange, nocturnal hypoventilation, and daytime symptoms (cognitive dysfunction, morning headache, daytime hypersomnolence, and sleep difficulties) and reduces the need for tracheotomy. Despite the lack of prospective controlled trials addressing the use of NPPV in other forms of ALD, consensus opinion favors initiating it in symptomatic patients, when $PaCO_2$ is >45 mm Hg, or when there is significant nocturnal desaturation.[110]

SURGICAL APPROACHES TO ADVANCED LUNG DISEASE

Bullectomy

Bullectomy, or the surgical removal of lung bulla(e), is distinct from lung volume reduction surgery (see below). A minority of COPD patients have relatively normal pulmonary parenchyma apart from their bullae, which cause airflow obstruction through compression of normal bronchi and the mechanical disadvantages of hyperinflation. In these patients, removal of bullae and re-expansion of normal lung may improve both pulmonary function and symptoms. There are no controlled trials, but multiple case series of COPD patients support subjective and objective improvements in lung function, with the magnitude of improvement (FEV_1 increases of 50%–200 %) greatest in those whose bullae occupy up to 50% of the hemithorax.[111] Results are less favorable in those whose bullae occupy <30% of the hemithorax and in those with diffuse emphysema. In one of the largest case series to date, operative mortality was 2.1% while improvement in pulmonary function persisted up to 20 years. Thus, bullectomy is an option for COPD patients with large bullae not associated with wide-spread emphysema, although these are by far the minority of COPD patients.[112]

Lung Volume Reduction Surgery

Lung volume reduction surgery (LVRS) is an option for patients dyspneic from advanced emphysema and hyperinflation. It involves removal of 20%–30% of apical emphysematous lung tissue to allow re-expansion of more normal lung, leading to improved expiratory airflow and respiratory mechanics.[113,114] Variable effects on lung function, exercise capacity, and quality of life have been reported, while surgical mortality has varied from 4% to 15%.[115] Based on conflicting clinical trial data, the National Heart, Lung, and Blood Institute and the Center for Medicare and Medicaid services recently sponsored the National Emphysema Treatment Trial,[116] a multicenter, randomized clinical trial in patients with advanced emphysema randomized to LVRS versus medical management. Patients must be nonsmoking for a minimum of 4 months and must complete 6–10 weeks of pulmonary rehabilitation, following which they must be able to walk more than 140 meters in 6 minutes. Additional entry criteria include clinical and radiographic evidence of bilateral emphysema, FEV_1 <45% predicted, PO_2 > 45 mm Hg, and PCO_2 < 60 mm Hg. The primary outcome measure is survival over a 2-year minimum follow-up. Secondary outcome measures include exercise capacity measured by distance walked in 6 minutes, pulmonary function, oxygen requirement, quality of life, respiratory symptoms, and health-care utilization and costs.

The trial is still enrolling patients. However, the safety monitoring board stopped enrollment in one group of patients with an unacceptably high mortality. In patients with FEV_1 < 20% predicted and either homogeneous distribution of emphysema or a single breath-diffusing capacity of <20% predicted, 30-day mortality was 16% versus 0% in the medically treated group, with an overall 3-year relative risk of death of 3.9 (confidence interval 1.9–9.0).[117] Despite relatively small, but significant gains in pulmonary function and exercise capacity in LVRS survivors, there were no dif-ferences in standardized measurements of health-related quality of life compared to medical patients. Until a particular subtype of COPD patient is identified for whom LVRS is predictably safe and effective at improving pulmonary function and symptoms, this operation cannot be recommended outside the ongoing research trial.

Lung Transplant

Lung transplant remains an option for patients with chronic ALD for whom medical and surgical therapies fail and who are expected to die soon enough that transplant offers a potential survival advantage. Survival following lung transplantation at 1, 3, and 5 years is 70%, 55%, and 42%, respectively, with median survival of approximately 3.8 years.[118] Transplants are typically limited to patients under age 65 (single lung) or age 60 (double lung). Therefore, they are not currently a realistic therapeutic option for the geriatric patient.

Other Surgical Options

Surgical procedures aimed at palliating refractory dyspnea include vagal nerve transection and carotid body resection, with the goal of decreasing ventilatory drive by reducing chemoreceptor stimulus in the setting of hypoxemia. Bradley et al.[119] described five COPD patients with intractable dyspnea undergoing unilateral right vagotomy under local anesthesia. Two patients markedly improved, while three patients died within a year of the operation, two of whom developed respiratory infections possibly related to depressed cough reflex dampened by the operation. In another uncontrolled case series, three COPD patients underwent bilateral carotid body resection resulting in long-lasting, subjective dyspnea relief associated with decreased minute ventilation, oxygen consumption, and CO_2 production.[120] However, all died within 2 years of the procedure, with two patients dying from severe respiratory insufficiency thought to be secondary to decreased hypoxemic ventilatory drive. The potential role of these therapies in palliative care has not been pursued in larger, controlled trials due to poor outcomes in small case series.

DYSPNEA IN LUNG CANCER PATIENTS

Some causes of dyspnea are either exclusively seen in cancer patients or more common in this population (Table 14–3). Approximately 40% of all pleural effusions result from cancer, and lung cancer accounts for almost one-third of all malignant pleural effusions.[121] Pleural disease represents a significant cause of dyspnea in patients with cancer. *Thoracentesis* is the percutaneous drainage of pleural fluid. This can be done safely at the bedside with local anesthesia only and is effective at relieving dyspnea in the short term. Recurrence of pleural fluid is common. *Pleurodesis* is a technique of draining an effusion, then instilling a sclerosing agent into the pleural space with the goal of adhering the parietal and visceral pleural surfaces, to prevent accumulation of fluid in the pleural space.[122,123] Fever and pain are the most common side effects of pleurodesis and can be tempered with antipyretics, analgesics, and the instillation of local anesthetic. Talc is superior to other sclerosing agents used in chemical pleurodesis of malignant pleural effusions, with a reported success rate (nonrecurrence after initial drainage) of 93% compared to 72%, 67%, and 54% with doxycycline, tetracycline, and bleo-

Table 14–3. Causes of Dyspnea in Patients with Lung Cancer

Pleural effusions
Endobronchial obstruction, causing atelectasis and affecting gas exchange or post-obstructive pneumonia
Superior vena cava syndrome
Phrenic nerve dysfunction
Pulmonary embolism, with thrombus or tumor
Lymphangitic spread of cancer with altered gas exchange and increased work of breathing
Radiation fibrosis
Anemia
Generalized weakness from inanition

mycin, respectively.[124] Sterile, asbestos-free talc may not be readily available, however.

Pleurodesis is not usually performed following thoracentesis because success depends on draining the pleural space completely. Pleurodesis usually involves a chest tube and a 3- to 7-day inpatient hospitalization. An alternative to pleurodesis is the outpatient placement of a small-bore, biocompatible pleural catheter, which may be left in place for months.[125] This approach avoids hospitalization, facilitates repeated drainage at home through a special collection bottle, has a low rate of complications, and is at least as effective at causing pleural sclerosis as standard pleurodesis.[126]

Medical thorocoscopy, which employs local or conscious sedation in the ambulatory setting, may be used to manage pleural effusions refractory to chest tube drainage and pleurodesis. Unlike standard thoracoscopy and open thorocotomy, medical thorocoscopy does not require general anesthesia and can be performed in the outpatient setting. As such, it may be particularly useful for palliation of symptomatic cancer patients who are poor operative candidates.[127]

Interventional pulmonology employs several effective bronchoscopic and pleuroscopic techniques as alternatives to surgery for the management of dyspnea, lung collapse, and/or pneumonia secondary to tumors causing endobronchial obstruction. Laser therapy, cryotherapy, electrocautery, brachytherapy, and photodynamic therapy are bronchoscopic treatments of airway lesions causing significant obstruction. Endobronchial stents yield effective, short-term palliation of symptomatic airway narrowing caused by extrinsic compression from tumors.[128] Referral to specialized centers is appropriate when these techniques promise effective palliation, even in advanced disease.

Both chemotherapy and radiation therapy are effective palliative therapies in patients with advanced lung cancer. An extensive literature exists on the role of chemotherapy in inoperable non-small cell lung cancer. A meta-analysis published in 1995 reported that, in patients with stage IIIB or IV disease and good performance status (World Health Organization performance status 0–1, <5% weight loss in the past 6 months), multidrug, platinum-based chemotherapy led to improved survival equivalent to a mean gain of 6 weeks at 1 year.[129] There was no survival benefit in patients with poor performance status. Older trials using alkylating agents (cyclophosphamide) were associated with decreased survival. More recent clinical trials have addressed the issue of quality of life as well as survival. Some show improved survival without any change in quality of life,[130–132] some show improved quality of life without any change in survival,[133] and others show variable effects on quality of life with improvement in some areas but impairment in others related to medication effects.[134] These outcomes are seen in all age groups.[135,136] It is difficult to make an unequivocal recommendation in a field under such intensive investigation. It seems safe to say that all patients, including the elderly, with inoperable non-small cell lung cancer and good performance status should be offered palliative chemotherapy. It remains to be seen which patients benefit most from what combination of agents. Patients with poor performance status should not routinely be given chemotherapy but may be appropriate candidates in individual circumstances. Accurate and complete information is essential to informed consent to proceed.[137]

Radiotherapy is an effective tool for palliation of symptoms, though it may be more effective for pain and hemoptysis than for dyspnea.[138] There is no strong evidence that any regimen gives greater palliation, although higher-dose regimens are associated with more acute toxicity. There is evidence for a small increase in survival (6% at 1 year and 3% at 2 years) in patients with better performance status given higher-dose radiation therapy.[139] A recent report used the technique of quality-adjusted life days to quantify the impact of targeted, high-dose radiotherapy for symptomatic non-small cell lung cancer.[140] The authors calculate that patients receiving palliative radiotherapy gained one-third of their quality-adjusted life days to radiotherapy. There is retrospective evidence to suggest that patients age 75 and older have responses similar to younger patients.[141]

PSYCHOLOGICAL BURDEN OF ADVANCED LUNG DISEASE

Depression and Anxiety

Psychiatric symptoms are common in patients with ALD. An estimated 45% of patients with moderate to severe COPD suffer from depression, a rate higher than that reported in other populations of chronically ill patients[142] or the estimated 10% among age-matched controls.[143] Anxiety has been reported in up to 34% of hospitalized COPD patients.[144] One-third of patients with inoperable lung cancer self-reported depression in a recent study. The most important risk factor was the patient's degree of functional impairment.[145] When associated with ALD, depression and anxiety may amplify somatic symptoms, threaten quality of life, and increase disability.[146] Improvements in depression and anxiety may improve function independent of spirometry.[147] Left untreated, psychological comorbidity may interfere with effective patient interaction with loved ones or threaten the integrity of established relationships. The urgency of treating depression and anxiety is proportional to the degree that it causes functional and emotional impairment. Emotional and physical withdrawal may lead to isolation, which may be complicated by substance abuse and suicide. Pharmacotherapy and supportive counseling, specifically cognitive behavioral therapy, are available treatments.

Pharmacological Approaches

Multiple classes of drugs are available to treat depression, panic, and anxiety. Among antidepressant drug classes, the selective serotonin reuptake inhibitors have the fewest side effects, despite drug interactions with tricyclic antidepressants and cardiac medications such β-blockers, calcium channel blockers, and antiarrythmics frequently taken by older ALD patients whose course is complicated by cardiac illness. Among the selective serotonin reuptake inhibitors, sertraline, paroxetine, and the phenylpiperazine nefazodone have fewer side effects and drug interactions and may be better tolerated in elderly populations. Nefazodone and trazodone, when administered at bedtime, may improve sleep in ALD patients who suffer concomitant insomnia. If these agents fail to improve symptoms after time-limited trials of 1–2 months, other drug classes may be of benefit as monotherapy or as adjunctive medication. Use of tricyclic antidepressants (amitriptyline) is complicated in the geriatric population by anticholinergic side effects, typically confusion, constipation, hypotension, or urinary retention, which may be slightly lessened with second-generation formulations such as nortriptyline. Benzodiazepines may prove useful for panic and anxiety, though they carry the risk of causing respiratory depression, dependence, and withdrawal. Nonetheless, moderate doses under appropriate monitoring can be effective in patients with anxiety complicating ALD.[148] Buspirone, a novel anxiolytic, may be of benefit in that, unlike benzodiazepines, it does not depress ventilation and may actually have a respiratory stimulant effect.

Cognitive Behavioral Therapy

In some patients with ALD, fearful thoughts such as suffocation related to disease-specific symptoms of dyspnea may lead to panic, which can cause increased autonomic arousal and variable amounts of hyperventilation. The result is dynamic hyperinflation and an increase in the work of breathing, creating a positive feedback cycle for the intensification of dyspnea.[148] Cognitive behavioral therapy, a time-limited form of psychotherapy including disease-specific education, thought restruc-

turing, relaxation techniques, and guided therapy, may reduce panic sensations as effectively as drug therapy in ALD patients.[149] With or without pharmacotherapy, it may help to reduce stimulus severity and provide enough mental desensitization to break a potentially deleterious cycle of fearful cognitions driving dyspnea intensification. Referral to a behavioral therapist is appropriate when a patient's cognition about the disease amplifies, leading to somatic symptoms and functional decline.

REFERENCES

1. Escalante CP, Martin CG, Elting LS, et al. Dyspnea in cancer patients. Etiology, resource utilization, and survival—implications in a managed care world. Cancer 78:1314–1319, 1996.
2. Lynn J, Ely EW, Zhong Z, et al. Living and dying with chronic obstructive pulmonary disease. J Am Geriatr Soc 48:S91–S100, 2000.
3. LeGrand SB, Walsh D. Palliative management of dyspnea in advanced cancer. Curr Opin Oncol 11:250–254, 1999.
4. Lynn J, Harrell F Jr, Cohn F, et al. Prognoses of seriously ill hospitalized patients on the days before death: implications for patient care and public policy. New Horiz 5:56–61, 1997.
5. Ferrer M, Alonso J, Morera J, et al. Chronic obstructive pulmonary disease stage and health-related quality of life. The Quality of Life of Chronic Obstructive Pulmonary Disease Study Group. Ann Intern Med 127:1072–1079, 1997.
6. Claessens MT, Lynn J, Zhong Z, et al. Dying with lung cancer or chronic obstructive pulmonary disease: insights from SUPPORT. Study to Understand Prognoses and Preferences for Outcomes and Risks of Treatments. J Am Geriatr Soc 48:S146–S153, 2000.
7. Rousseau P. Nonpain symptom management in terminal care. Clin Geriatr Med 12:313–327, 1996.
8. Hansen-Flaschen J. Advanced lung disease. Palliation and terminal care. Clin Chest Med 18:645–655, 1997.
9. SUPPORT Principal Investigators. A controlled trial to improve care for seriously ill hospitalized patients. The Study to Understand Prognoses and Preferences for Outcomes and Risks of Treatments (SUPPORT). JAMA 274:1591–1598, 1995.

10. Reuben DB, Mor V. Dyspnea in terminally ill cancer patients. Chest 89:234–236, 1986.

11. Vainio A, Auvinen A. Prevalence of symptoms among patients with advanced cancer: an international collaborative study. Symptom Prevalence Group. J Pain Symptom Manag 12:3–10, 1996.

12. Wolkove N, Dajczman E, Colacone A, Kreisman H. The relationship between pulmonary function and dyspnea in obstructive lung disease. Chest 96:1247–1251, 1989.

13. Manning HL, Schwartzstein RM. Pathophysiology of dyspnea. N Engl J Med 333:1547–1553, 1995.

14. O'Donnell DE, Bertley JC, Chau LK, Webb KA. Qualitative aspects of exertional breathlessness in chronic airflow limitation: pathophysiologic mechanisms. Am J Respir Crit Care Med 155:109–115, 1997.

15. O'Donnell DE, Chau LK, Webb KA. Qualitative aspects of exertional dyspnea in patients with interstitial lung disease. J Appl Physiol 84:2000–2009, 1998.

16. American Thoracic Society. Dyspnea. Mechanisms, assessment, and management: a consensus statement. Am J Respir Crit Care Med 159:321–340, 1999.

17. Belman MJ, Botnick WC, Shin JW. Inhaled bronchodilators reduce dynamic hyperinflation during exercise in patients with chronic obstructive pulmonary disease. Am J Respir Crit Care Med 153:967–975, 1996.

18. Anthonisen NR, Connett JE, Kiley JP, et al. Effects of smoking intervention and the use of an inhaled anticholinergic bronchodilator on the rate of decline of FEV_1. The Lung Health Study. JAMA 272:1497–1505, 1994.

19. Colice GL. Nebulized bronchodilators for outpatient management of stable chronic obstructive pulmonary disease. Am J Med 100:11S–18S, 1996.

20. Tashkin DP, Ashutosh K, Bleecker ER, et al. Comparison of the anticholinergic bronchodilator ipratropium bromide with metaproterenol in chronic obstructive pulmonary disease. A 90-day multi-center study. Am J Med 81:81–90, 1986.

21. Dorinsky PM, Reisner C, Ferguson GT, et al. The combination of ipratropium and albuterol optimizes pulmonary function reversibility testing in patients with COPD. Chest 115:966–971, 1999.

22. COMBIVENT Inhalation Aerosol Study Group. In chronic obstructive pulmonary disease, a combination of ipratropium and albuterol is more effective than either agent alone. An 85-day multicenter trial. Chest 105:1411–1419, 1994.

23. Campbell S. For COPD a combination of ipratropium bromide and albuterol sulfate is more effective than albuterol base. Arch Intern Med 159:156–160, 1999.

24. Rennard SI, Anderson W, ZuWallack R, et al. Use of a long-acting inhaled beta2-adrenergic agonist, salmeterol xinafoate, in patients with chronic obstructive pulmonary disease. Am J Respir Crit Care Med 163:1087–1092, 2001.

25. Cazzola M, Donner CF. Long-acting beta2 agonists in the management of stable chronic obstructive pulmonary disease. Drugs 60:307–320, 2000.

26. Vincken W, van Noord JA, et al. Improved health outcomes in patients with COPD during 1 yr's treatment with tiotropium. Dutch Belgian Tiotropium Study Group. Eur Respir J 19:209–216, 2002.

27. Hay JG, Stone P, Carter J, et al. Bronchodilator reversibility, exercise performance and breathlessness in stable chronic obstructive pulmonary disease. Eur Respir J 5:659–664, 1992.

28. Berry RB, Shinto RA, Wong FH, et al. Nebulizer vs spacer for bronchodilator delivery in patients hospitalized for acute exacerbations of COPD. Chest 96:1241–1246, 1989.

29. Murciano D, Auclair MH, Pariente R, Aubier M. A randomized, controlled trial of theophylline in patients with severe chronic obstructive pulmonary disease. N Engl J Med 320:1521–1525, 1989.

30. Grazzini M, Stendardi L, Rosi E, Scano G. Pharmacological treatment of exercise dyspnoea. Monaldi Arch Chest Dis 56:43–47, 2001.

31. Sherman MS, Lang DM, Matityahu A, Campbell D. Theophylline improves measurements of respiratory muscle efficiency. Chest 110:1437–1442, 1996.

32. Matthay RA. Favorable cardiovascular effects of theophylline in COPD. Chest 92:22S–26S, 1987.

33. Wanner A. Effects of methylxanthines on airway mucociliary function. Am J Med 79:16–21, 1985.

34. Ziment I. Theophylline and mucociliary clearance. Chest 92:38S-43S, 1987.

35. Minoguchi K, Kohno Y, Oda N, et al. Effect of theophylline withdrawal on airway inflammation in asthma. Clin Exp Allergy 28:57–63, 1998.

36. Rabe KF, Dent G. Theophylline and airway inflammation. Clin Exp Allergy 28:35–41, 1998.

37. Wolfe JD, Tashkin DP, Calvarese B, Simmons M. Bronchodilator effects of terbu-

taline and aminophylline alone and in combination in asthmatic patients. N Engl J Med 298:363–367, 1978.

38. Kirsten DK, Wegner RE, Jorres RA, Magnussen H. Effects of theophylline withdrawal in severe chronic obstructive pulmonary disease. Chest 104:1101–1107, 1993.

39. Mahler DA, Matthay RA, Snyder PE, et al. Sustained-release theophylline reduces dyspnea in nonreversible obstructive airway disease. Am Rev Respir Dis 131:22–25, 1985.

40. Martin RJ, Pak J. Overnight theophylline concentrations and effects on sleep and lung function in chronic obstructive pulmonary disease. Am Rev Respir Dis 145:540–544, 1992.

41. ZuWallack RL, Mahler DA, Reilly D, et al. Salmeterol plus theophylline combination therapy in the treatment of COPD. Chest 119:1661–1670, 2001.

42. Guyatt GH, Townsend M, Pugsley SO, et al. Bronchodilators in chronic air-flow limitation. Effects on airway function, exercise capacity, and quality of life. Am Rev Respir Dis 135:1069–1074, 1987.

43. Niewoehner DE, Erbland ML, Deupree RH, et al. Effect of systemic glucocorticoids on exacerbations of chronic obstructive pulmonary disease. Department of Veterans Affairs Cooperative Study Group. N Engl J Med 340:1941–1947, 1999.

44. Snow V, Lascher S, Mottur-Pilson C. Evidence base for management of acute exacerbations of chronic obstructive pulmonary disease. Joint Expert Panel on Chronic Obstructive Pulmonary Disease of the American College of Chest Physicians and the American College of Physicians–American Society of Internal Medicine. Ann Intern Med 134:595–599, 2001.

45. Callahan CM, Dittus RS, Katz BP. Oral corticosteroid therapy for patients with stable chronic obstructive pulmonary disease. A meta-analysis. Ann Intern Med 114:216–223, 1991.

46. Rice KL, Rubins JB, Lebahn F, et al. Withdrawal of chronic systemic corticosteroids in patients with COPD: a randomized trial. Am J Respir Crit Care Med 162:174–178, 2000.

47. Weiner P, Weiner M, Rabner M, et al. The response to inhaled and oral steroids in patients with stable chronic obstructive pulmonary disease. J Intern Med 245:83–89, 1999.

48. Schols A, Wesseling G, Kester A, et al. Dose dependent increased mortality risk in COPD patients treated with oral glucocorticoids. Eur Respir J 17:337–342, 2001.

49. Libanati CR, Baylink DJ. Prevention and treatment of glucocorticoid-induced osteoporosis. A pathogenetic perspective. Chest 102:1426–1435, 1992.

50. The Lung Health Study Research Group. Effect of inhaled triamcinolone on the decline in pulmonary function in chronic obstructive pulmonary disease. N Engl J Med 343:1902–1909, 2000.

51. Burge PS, Calverley PM, Jones PW, et al. Randomised, double blind, placebo controlled study of fluticasone propionate in patients with moderate to severe chronic obstructive pulmonary disease: the ISOLDE trial. BMJ 320:1297–1303, 2000.

52. Nielsen LP, Dahl R. Therapeutic ratio of inhaled corticosteroids in adult asthma. A dose-range comparison between fluticasone propionate and budesonide, measuring their effect on bronchial hyperresponsiveness and adrenal cortex function. Am J Respir Crit Care Med 162:2053–2057, 2000.

53. Meibohm B, Hochhaus G, Mollmann H, et al. A pharmacokinetic/pharmacodynamic approach to predict the cumulative cortisol suppression of inhaled corticosteroids. J Pharmacokinet Biopharm 27:127–147, 1999.

54. Toogood JH. Side effects of inhaled corticosteroids. J Allergy Clin Immunol 102:705–713, 1998.

55. Zisman DA, Lynch JP 3rd, Toews GB, et al. Cyclophosphamide in the treatment of idiopathic pulmonary fibrosis: a prospective study in patients who failed to respond to corticosteroids. Chest 117:1619–1626, 2000.

56. Kolb M, Kirschner J, Riedel W, et al. Cyclophosphamide pulse therapy in idiopathic pulmonary fibrosis. Eur Respir J 12:1409–1414, 1998.

57. Douglas WW, Ryu JH, Schroeder DR. Idiopathic pulmonary fibrosis: impact of oxygen and colchicine, prednisone, or no therapy on survival. Am J Respir Crit Care Med 161:1172–1178, 2000.

58. Lynch JP 3rd, White E, Flaherty K. Corticosteroids in idiopathic pulmonary fibrosis. Curr Opin Pulm Med 7:298–308, 2001.

59. Baughman RP, Alabi FO. Nonsteroidal therapy for idiopathic pulmonary fibrosis. Curr Opin Pulm Med 7:309–313, 2001.

60. Flaherty KR, Toews GB, Lynch JP 3rd, et al. Steroids in idiopathic pulmonary fibrosis: a prospective assessment of adverse reactions, response to therapy, and survival. Am J Med 110:278–282, 2001.

61. Ziesche R, Hofbauer E, Wittmann K, et al. A preliminary study of long-term treat-

ment with interferon gamma-1b and low-dose prednisolone in patients with idiopathic pulmonary fibrosis. N Engl J Med 341:1264–1269, 1999.

62. Nocturnal Oxygen Therapy Trial Group. Continuous or nocturnal oxygen therapy in hypoxemic chronic obstructive lung disease: a clinical trial. Ann Intern Med 93:391–398, 1980.

63. Report of the Medical Research Council Working Party. Long term domiciliary oxygen therapy in chronic hypoxic cor pulmonale complicating chronic bronchitis and emphysema. Lancet 1:681–686, 1981.

64. Robinson TD, Freiberg DB, Regnis JA, Young IH. The role of hypoventilation and ventilation-perfusion redistribution in oxygen-induced hypercapnia during acute exacerbations of chronic obstructive pulmonary disease. Am J Respir Crit Care Med 161:1524–1529, 2000.

65. Dewan NA, Bell CW. Effect of low flow and high flow oxygen delivery on exercise tolerance and sensation of dyspnea. A study comparing the transtracheal catheter and nasal prongs. Chest 105:1061–1065, 1994.

66. Garrod R, Paul EA, Wedzicha JA. Supplemental oxygen during pulmonary rehabilitation in patients with COPD with exercise hypoxaemia. Thorax 55:539–543, 2000.

67. McDonald CF, Blyth CM, Lazarus MD, et al. Exertional oxygen of limited benefit in patients with chronic obstructive pulmonary disease and mild hypoxemia. Am J Respir Crit Care Med 152:1616–1619, 1995.

68. Swinburn CR, Mould H, Stone TN, et al. Symptomatic benefit of supplemental oxygen in hypoxemic patients with chronic lung disease. Am Rev Respir Dis 143:913–915, 1991.

69. Liss HP, Grant BJ. The effect of nasal flow on breathlessness in patients with chronic obstructive pulmonary disease. Am Rev Respir Dis 137:1285–1288, 1988.

70. Bruera E, Schoeller T, MacEachern T. Symptomatic benefit of supplemental oxygen in hypoxemic patients with terminal cancer: the use of the N of 1 randomized controlled trial. J Pain Symptom Manage 7:365–368, 1992.

71. Booth S, Kelly MJ, Cox NP, et al. Does oxygen help dyspnea in patients with cancer? Am J Respir Crit Care Med 153:1515–1518, 1996.

72. Schwartzstein RM, Lahive K, Pope A, et al. Cold facial stimulation reduces breathlessness induced in normal subjects. Am Rev Respir Dis 136:58–61, 1987.

73. Woodcock AA, Gross ER, Gellert A, et al. Effects of dihydrocodeine, alcohol, and caffeine on breathlessness and exercise tolerance in patients with chronic obstructive lung disease and normal blood gases. N Engl J Med 305:1611–1616, 1981.

74. Couser JI Jr, Make BJ. Transtracheal oxygen decreases inspired minute ventilation. Am Rev Respir Dis 139:627–631, 1989.

75. Bloom BS, Daniel JM, Wiseman M, et al. Transtracheal oxygen delivery and patients with chronic obstructive pulmonary disease. Respir Med 83:281–288, 1989.

76. Weil JV, McCullough RE, Kline JS, Sodal IE. Diminished ventilatory response to hypoxia and hypercapnia after morphine in normal man. N Engl J Med 292:1103–1106, 1975.

77. Bar-Or D, Marx JA, Good J. Breathlessness, alcohol, and opiates. N Engl J Med 306:1363–1364, 1982.

78. Johnson MA, Woodcock AA, Geddes DM. Dihydrocodeine for breathlessness in "pink puffers." BMJ 286:675–677, 1983.

79. Light RW, Muro JR, Sato RI, et al. Effects of oral morphine on breathlessness and exercise tolerance in patients with chronic obstructive pulmonary disease. Am Rev Respir Dis 139:126–133, 1989.

80. Robin ED, Burke CM. Single-patient randomized clinical trial. Opiates for intractable dyspnea. Chest 90:888–892, 1986.

81. Rice KL, Kronenberg RS, Hedemark LL, Niewoehner DE. Effects of chronic administration of codeine and promethazine on breathlessness and exercise tolerance in patients with chronic airflow obstruction. Br J Dis Chest 81:287–292, 1987.

82. Eiser N, Denman WT, West C, Luce P. Oral diamorphine: lack of effect on dyspnoea and exercise tolerance in the "pink puffer" syndrome. Eur Respir J 4:926–931, 1991.

83. Poole PJ, Veale AG, Black PN. The effect of sustained-release morphine on breathlessness and quality of life in severe chronic obstructive pulmonary disease. Am J Respir Crit Care Med 157:1877–1880, 1998.

84. Young IH, Daviskas E, Keena VA. Effect of low dose nebulised morphine on exercise endurance in patients with chronic lung disease. Thorax 44:387–390, 1989.

85. Noseda A, Carpiaux JP, Markstein C, et al. Disabling dyspnoea in patients with advanced disease: lack of effect of nebulized morphine. Eur Respir J 10:1079–1083, 1997.

86. Leung R, Hill P, Burdon J. Effect of inhaled morphine on the development of

breathlessness during exercise in patients with chronic lung disease. Thorax 51: 596–600, 1996.

87. Masood AR, Reed JW, Thomas SH. Lack of effect of inhaled morphine on exercise-induced breathlessness in chronic obstructive pulmonary disease. Thorax 50:629–634, 1995.

88. Beauford W, Saylor TT, Stansbury DW, et al. Effects of nebulized morphine sulfate on the exercise tolerance of the ventilatory limited COPD patient. Chest 104:175–178, 1993.

89. Bruera E, Macmillan K, Pither J, MacDonald RN. Effects of morphine on the dyspnea of terminal cancer patients. J Pain Symptom Manage 5:341–344, 1990.

90. Bruera E, MacEachern T, Ripamonti C, Hanson J. Subcutaneous morphine for dyspnea in cancer patients. Ann Intern Med 119:906–907, 1993.

91. Cohen MH, Anderson AJ, Krasnow SH, et al. Continuous intravenous infusion of morphine for severe dyspnea. South Med J 84:229–234, 1991.

92. Woodcock AA, Gross ER, Geddes DM. Drug treatment of breathlessness: contrasting effects of diazepam and promethazine in pink puffers. BMJ 283:343–346, 1981.

93. Man GC, Hsu K, Sproule BJ. Effect of alprazolam on exercise and dyspnea in patients with chronic obstructive pulmonary disease. Chest 90:832–836, 1986.

94. Eimer M, Cable T, Gal P, et al. Effects of clorazepate on breathlessness and exercise tolerance in patients with chronic airflow obstruction. J Fam Pract 21:359–362, 1985.

95. Argyropoulou P, Patakas D, Koukou A, et al. Buspirone effect on breathlessness and exercise performance in patients with chronic obstructive pulmonary disease. Respiration 60:216–220, 1993.

96. Singh NP, Despars JA, Stansbury DW, et al. Effects of buspirone on anxiety levels and exercise tolerance in patients with chronic airflow obstruction and mild anxiety. Chest 103:800–804, 1993.

97. McIver B, Walsh D, Nelson K. The use of chlorpromazine for symptom control in dying cancer patients. J Pain Symptom Manage 9:341–345, 1994.

98. Light RW, Stansbury DW, Webster JS. Effect of 30 mg of morphine alone or with promethazine or prochlorperazine on the exercise capacity of patients with COPD. Chest 109:975–981, 1996.

99. Ries AL, Kaplan RM, Limberg TM, Prewitt LM. Effects of pulmonary rehabilitation on physiologic and psychosocial outcomes in patients with chronic obstructive pulmonary disease. Ann Intern Med 122: 823–832, 1995.

100. Lacasse Y, Wong E, Guyatt GH, et al. Meta-analysis of respiratory rehabilitation in chronic obstructive pulmonary disease. Lancet 348:1115–1119, 1996.

101. Griffiths TL, Burr ML, Campbell IA, et al. Results at 1 year of outpatient multidisciplinary pulmonary rehabilitation: a randomised controlled trial. Lancet 355: 362–368, 2000.

102. Finnerty JP, Keeping I, Bullough I, Jones J. The effectiveness of outpatient pulmonary rehabilitation in chronic lung disease: a randomized controlled trial. Chest 119:1705–1710, 2001.

103. Weiner P, Magadle R, Berar-Yanay N, et al. The cumulative effect of long-acting bronchodilators, exercise, and inspiratory muscle training on the perception of dyspnea in patients with advanced COPD. Chest 118:672–678, 2000.

104. Kramer N, Meyer TJ, Meharg J, et al. Randomized, prospective trial of noninvasive positive pressure ventilation in acute respiratory failure. Am J Respir Crit Care Med 151:1799–1806, 1995.

105. Brochard L, Mancebo J, Wysocki M, et al. Noninvasive ventilation for acute exacerbations of chronic obstructive pulmonary disease. N Engl J Med 333:817–822, 1995.

106. Antonelli M, Conti G, Rocco M, et al. A comparison of noninvasive positive-pressure ventilation and conventional mechanical ventilation in patients with acute respiratory failure. N Engl J Med 339: 429–435, 1998.

107. Celikel T, Sungur M, Ceyhan B, Karakurt S. Comparison of noninvasive positive pressure ventilation with standard medical therapy in hypercapnic acute respiratory failure. Chest 114:1636–1642, 1998.

108. Meecham Jones DJ, Paul EA, Jones PW, Wedzicha JA. Nasal pressure support ventilation plus oxygen compared with oxygen therapy alone in hypercapnic COPD. Am J Respir Crit Care Med 152:538–544, 1995.

109. Strumpf DA, Millman RP, Carlisle CC, et al. Nocturnal positive-pressure ventilation via nasal mask in patients with severe chronic obstructive pulmonary disease. Am Rev Respir Dis 144:1234–1239, 1991.

110. Robert D, Willig TN, Leger P. Long-term nasal ventilation in neuromuscular disorders: report of a consensus conference. Eur Respir J 6:599–606, 1993.

111. Sung DT, Payne WS, Black LF. Surgical management of giant bullae associated

with obstructive airway disease. Surg Clin North Am 53:913–920, 1973.

112. Benditt JO, Albert RK. Surgical options for patients with advanced emphysema. Clin Chest Med 18:577–593, 1997.

113. Flaherty KR, Martinez FJ. Lung volume reduction surgery for emphysema. Clin Chest Med 21:819–848, 2000.

114. Stirling GR, Babidge WJ, Peacock MJ, et al. Lung volume reduction surgery in emphysema: a systematic review. Ann Thorac Surg 72:641–648, 2001.

115. Flaherty KR, Kazerooni EA, Curtis JL, et al. Short-term and long-term outcomes after bilateral lung volume reduction surgery: prediction by quantitative CT. Chest 119:1337–1346, 2001.

116. National Emphysema Treatment Trial Research Group. Rationale and design of the National Emphysema Treatment Trial: a prospective randomized trial of lung volume reduction surgery. Chest 116:1750–1761, 1999.

117. National Emphysema Treatment Trial Research Group. Patients at high risk of death after lung-volume-reduction surgery. N Engl J Med 345:1075–1083, 2001.

118. Hosenpud JD, Bennett LE, Keck BM, et al. The Registry of the International Society for Heart and Lung Transplantation: eighteenth official report–2001. J Heart Lung Transplant 20:805–815, 2001.

119. Bradley GW, Hale T, Pimble J, et al. Effect of vagotomy on the breathing pattern and exercise ability in emphysematous patients. Clin Sci (Colch) 62:311–319, 1982.

120. Stulbarg MS, Winn WR, Kellett LE. Bilateral carotid body resection for the relief of dyspnea in severe chronic obstructive pulmonary disease. Physiologic and clinical observations in three patients. Chest 95:1123–1128, 1989.

121. American Thoracic Society. Management of malignant pleural effusions. Am J Respir Crit Care Med 162:1987–2001, 2000.

122. Rodriguez-Panadero F, Antony VB. Pleurodesis: state of the art. Eur Respir J 10:1648–1654, 1997.

123. Sahn SA. Malignancy metastatic to the pleura. Clin Chest Med 19:351–361, 1998.

124. Walker-Renard PB, Vaughan LM, Sahn SA. Chemical pleurodesis for malignant pleural effusions. Ann Intern Med 120:56–64, 1994.

125. Putnam JB Jr, Walsh GL, Swisher SG, et al.: Outpatient management of malignant pleural effusion by a chronic indwelling pleural catheter. Ann Thorac Surg 69:369–375, 2000.

126. Putnam JB Jr, Light RW, Rodriguez RM, et al. A randomized comparison of indwelling pleural catheter and doxycycline pleurodesis in the management of malignant pleural effusions. Cancer 86:1992–1999, 1999.

127. Seijo LM, Sterman DH. Interventional pulmonology. N Engl J Med 344:740–749, 2001.

128. Vonk-Noordegraaf A, Postmus PE, Sutedja TG. Tracheobronchial stenting in the terminal care of cancer patients with central airways obstruction. Chest 120:1811–1814, 2001.

129. Non-small Cell Lung Cancer Collaborative Group. Chemotherapy in non-small cell lung cancer: a meta-analysis using updated data on individual patients from 52 randomised clinical trials. BMJ 311:899–909, 1995.

130. Cullen MH, Billingham LJ, Woodroffe CM, et al. Mitomycin, ifosfamide, and cisplatin in unresectable non-small-cell lung cancer: effects on survival and quality of life. J Clin Oncol 17:3188–3194, 1999.

131. Ranson M, Davidson N, Nicolson M, et al. Randomized trial of paclitaxel plus supportive care versus supportive care for patients with advanced non-small-cell lung cancer. J Natl Cancer Inst 92:1074–1080, 2000.

132. Roszkowski K, Pluzanska A, Krzakowski M, et al. A multicenter, randomized, phase III study of docetaxel plus best supportive care versus best supportive care in chemotherapy-naive patients with metastatic or non-resectable localized non-small cell lung cancer (NSCLC). Lung Cancer 27:145–157, 2000.

133. Anderson H, Hopwood P, Stephens RJ, et al. Gemcitabine plus best supportive care (BSC) vs BSC in inoperable non-small cell lung cancer—a randomized trial with quality of life as the primary outcome. UK NSCLC Gemcitabine Group. Non-Small Cell Lung Cancer. Br J Cancer 83:447–453, 2000.

134. Gridelli C. The ELVIS trial: a phase III study of single-agent vinorelbine as first-line treatment in elderly patients with advanced non-small cell lung cancer. Elderly Lung Cancer Vinorelbine Italian Study. Oncologist 6:4–7, 2001.

135. Hickish TF, Smith IE, O'Brien ME, et al. Clinical benefit from palliative chemotherapy in non-small-cell lung cancer extends to the elderly and those with poor prognostic factors. Br J Cancer 78:28–33, 1998.

136. Earle CC, Tsai JS, Gelber RD, et al. Effectiveness of chemotherapy for advanced lung cancer in the elderly: instrumental

variable and propensity analysis. J Clin Oncol 19:1064–1070, 2001.

137. Silvestri G, Pritchard R, Welch HG. Preferences for chemotherapy in patients with advanced non-small cell lung cancer: descriptive study based on scripted interviews. BMJ 317:771–775, 1998.

138. Langendijk JA, ten Velde GP, Aaronson NK, et al. Quality of life after palliative radiotherapy in non-small cell lung cancer: a prospective study. Int J Radiat Oncol Biol Phys 47:149–155, 2000.

139. Macbeth F, Toy E, Coles B, et al. Palliative radiotherapy regimens for non-small cell lung cancer. Cochrane Database Syst Rev CD002143, 2001.

140. Schaafsma J, Coy P. Response of global quality of life to high-dose palliative radiotherapy for non-small-cell lung cancer. Int J Radiat Oncol Biol Phys 47:691–701, 2000.

141. Patterson CJ, Hocking M, Bond M, Teale C. Retrospective study of radiotherapy for lung cancer in patients aged 75 years and over. Age Ageing 27:515–518, 1998.

142. Katon W. The epidemiology of depression in medical care. Int J Psychiatry Med 17:93–112, 1987.

143. McSweeney AJ, Heaton RK, Grant I, et al. Chronic obstructive pulmonary disease; socioemotional adjustment and life quality. Chest 77:309–311, 1980.

144. Yellowlees PM, Alpers JH, Bowden JJ, et al. Psychiatric morbidity in patients with chronic airflow obstruction. Med J Aust 146:305–307, 1987.

145. Hopwood P, Stephens RJ. Depression in patients with lung cancer: prevalence and risk factors derived from quality-of-life data. J Clin Oncol 18:893–903, 2000.

146. Greenberg GD, Ryan JJ, Bourlier PF. Psychological and neuropsychological aspects of COPD. Psychosomatics 26:29–33, 1985.

147. Light RW, Merrill EJ, Despars J, et al. Doxepin treatment of depressed patients with chronic obstructive pulmonary disease. Arch Intern Med 146:1377–1380, 1986.

148. Smoller JW, Pollack MH, Otto MW, et al. Panic anxiety, dyspnea, and respiratory disease. Theoretical and clinical considerations. Am J Respir Crit Care Med 154:6–17, 1996.

149. Corner J, Plant H, A'Hern R, Bailey C. Non-pharmacological intervention for breathlessness in lung cancer. Palliat Med 10:299–305, 1996.

15

End-Stage Renal Disease and Discontinuation of Dialysis

LEWIS M. COHEN, MICHAEL J. GERMAIN,
AND MAURA J. BRENNAN

End-stage renal disease (ESRD) has become a geriatric disease, and the discipline of nephrology increasingly appreciates the need to institute palliative medicine innovations in the management of these patients. In the late 1960s and early 1970s, when dialysis was first being developed and the technology rationed, treatment was restricted to young, nondiabetic individuals who were predominantly Caucasian, male, and middle class, not unlike the physicians who were caring for them. However, the 1973 United States Medicare ESRD Program resulted in nearly universal access to dialysis treatment. Subsequently the patient population receiving dialysis support has steadily grown and aged. There are now approximately 300,000 individuals with ESRD, and 45% are over the age of 65.[1]

According to the *United States Renal Data System 2000 Annual Data Report*, the average age of the incident population has increased yearly; in 1986, the mean age was 56 years while this increased to 60 years by 1995.[2] The fastest growth has occurred among the oldest age groups: 46% of incident patients in 1996 were 65 years old or greater and 20% were over 75 years of age; in 1999, 58% of the newly diagnosed chronic ESRD patients in New England were 65 years or older and 17% 80 years or older.[3]

Patients are not only older but also sicker. Acceptance of people whose renal disease results from, or is associated with, more severe comorbid conditions has also increased. In particular, diabetes has become an accelerating cause of renal failure, and patients with diabetes now represent 39% of the ESRD population. In 1999,[2] other comorbid disorders of incident patients included congestive heart failure (34%), coronary artery disease (25%), peripheral vascular disease (15%), and cerebrovascular disease (10%). It is no exaggeration to claim that even young patients with ESRD have old bodies.

While dialysis sustains life by substituting for the kidneys, the underlying systemic diseases responsible for causing renal failure usually continue to progress. For example, a person with ESRD and diabetes may be sustained for years on dialysis, but also experience blindness, amputations, painful neuropathies, and other severe complications. Under such circumstances, dialysis supports life, but not necessarily what the individual considers quality of life (QOL). In some surveys, almost two-thirds of ESRD patients rate their QOL as being less than good.[4,5] In our own survey, which took place in 2002 at nine New England dialysis clinics and involved 619 patients, 57% of the sample reported that physical health problems during the past 4 weeks had forced them to cut down on the amount of time spent on work or other activities, 69% accomplished less than they would have preferred, and 71% were limited in the kind of work or activities that they could pursue. For some patients, treatment becomes a Sisyphean ordeal.

As the population has aged and grown sicker, it should come as no surprise that death is a regular specter at dialysis facilities. Despite technological advances, the annual mortality rate of patients maintained with dialysis in the United States is now approximately 23%. Cardiovascular complications account for at least half of the deaths. The expected lifetime of a dialysis patient is between 16% and 37% that of an age- and sex-matched general population. The risk of death for a 45-year-old patient is 20 times that of a person of the same age not receiving dialysis. Although the techniques of dialysis care have improved, the 5-year survival rate remains low.[2,3] Only 27.5% of the 1980 incident cohort survived 5 years, while 29.4% of the 1990 cohort remained alive after 1995. For patients between the ages of 65 and 74, the 5-year survival rate drops to 21%.

Elderly patients are more likely to start dialysis in a debilitated state compared to younger patients. This is partly related to decreased muscle mass, which gives them a lower serum creatinine at any given glomerular filtration rate (GFR) compared to a younger person. This can falsely reassure the medical team and delay recognition of the severity of renal failure. It is not unusual for a woman in her 70s to have a serum creatinine of 2.0 and a GFR <10 to require dialysis. When patients start dialysis at lower GFRs, they are more malnourished and debilitated. It is often impossible for elderly patients to regain their former strength and nutritional state. A late start to dialysis is associated with more hospitalizations, worse QOL scores, and higher morbidity and mortality.

Elderly dialysis patients face special challenges that impact on QOL. They have more dialysis-related symptoms, such as cramps, nausea and vomiting, hypotension, and postdialysis "washout." The latter consists of subjective feelings of weakness and can persist in an elderly patient until the next dialysis treatment. They also have more side effects from medications due to decreased hepatic metabolism and decreased renal clearance.

Because of its slow and continuous nature, peritoneal dialysis avoids the dialysis-related symptoms that can occur with hemodialysis and can be quite effective for the geriatric patient. However, the basic requirements of peritoneal dialysis can be overwhelming for a patient who is living at home alone or with an equally elderly, and often debilitated, spouse. Consequently, most geriatric patients with ESRD are forced to rely on hemodialysis.

Nursing home placement carries its own treatment considerations. Peritoneal dialysis is available at only a few nursing homes throughout the country. Patients residing in nursing homes generally are sustained with hemodialysis, and this requires attention to the logistics involved in transporting the patient to the dialysis unit three times per week. This can be physically taxing. Furthermore, many common medications used in the nursing home are problematic. Magnesium-containing laxatives and aluminum-containing antacids are two such examples. They are frequently written as "standing orders" in nursing homes, but can accumulate and cause serious complications.

WITHDRAWAL AND WITHHOLDING OF DIALYSIS

It is not unusual for nephrologists to offer geriatric patients with renal failure the "fourth option," i.e., to not start dialysis at all and to instead receive comfort/hospice care. Another approach is a limited trial of 3–6 months' dialysis to see if the QOL is acceptable to the patient. If the patient and family decide that the suffering outweighs the benefits of life prolongation, dialysis can be withdrawn.

Withdrawal of dialysis has been almost completely ignored as a geriatric issue, but the mean age of patients in our research sample was 70 years. Retrospective studies in the 1980s recognized that ethnicity (Caucasian), diagnosis (diabetes), and age all increased the likelihood that life-support treatment would be terminated.[6] This last factor has become increasingly important as the elderly constitute a larger proportion of the ESRD population. Also, while the possibility of transplantation is held out to the young, geriatric patients face the more limited options of continuing dialysis, termination, or death by other causes.

Between 1990 and 1995, there were over 20,000 deaths in the United States preceded by dialysis discontinuation;[7] and in 1997, the well-publicized demise of Pulitzer Prize–winning novelist James Michener gave a human face to this phenomenon.[8] During the 10 years that our group has been studying dialysis discontinuation, the rates have nearly tripled. When we started our research, between 8% and 10% of ESRD deaths were preceded by decisions to stop treatment. During the past year in New England, this rate has risen to 28%. Discontinuation rates vary widely between dialysis clinics; in our research, they ranged from 8% to 53%. The study site with the highest rate underwent subsequent scrutiny, but was found to have normal mortality rates and other indices of care. We suspect that the culture of the individual dialysis clinics as shaped by their nephrologists determines discontinuation. This is likely to change in the future as the National Kidney Foundation, Renal Physicians Association, and other groups within the ESRD community have issued guidelines concerning initiation and discontinuation of dialysis.[9]

Dialysis discontinuation is an example of cessation of life support. It is but one of numerous life-limiting options in the context of physical and terminal illness that are increasingly available to patients, including do-not-treat orders, withholding life-saving interventions, and withdrawal of fluid and nutrition.[10] Citing studies that found decisions hastening death in 90%–95% of intensive care unit patient samples, Emanuel concluded that "the good news is that the withdrawal or withholding of life-sustaining treatments is now standard practice."[11] The contemporary bioethical approval of these planned deaths is driven by a growing respect for patient autonomy and what Thomson et al. call "the sanctity of patient choice."[12]

Until 1995, the Health Care Financing Administration Death Certificate form, which is completed by ESRD providers, listed "withdrawal of dialysis" as a potential cause of death. After that year, it was removed from the list, but separate questions are asked as to whether renal replacement therapy was discontinued prior to death and the reason for withdrawal. The choices for the latter question include access failure, transplant failure, chronic failure to thrive, and acute medical complications. Most instances of dialysis discontinuation are prompted by the latter two situations.

Termination of dialysis can be seen as an appropriate decision for situations in which dialysis is prolonging suffering rather than prolonging life. Alternately, it can be viewed as a public health problem that contributes to the high mortality of ESRD. Although dialysis discontinuation represents an ideal opportunity to study cessation of life support, methodological obstacles abound and there have only been a few prospective investigations.[13,14] We conducted the first of these, exploring decision making and the ensuing quality of dying at a single dialysis clinic.[15] The study was followed by a more ambitious endeavor at eight dialysis clinics in the United States and Canada and involved 131 patients, 79 of whom were interviewed along with their families.[16,17]

PSYCHOSOCIAL CONSIDERATIONS AND COMMON SYMPTOMS

In the multicenter study, patients who withdrew from treatment were severely ill; three-quarters of the sample had between three and seven comorbid conditions.[16] Half of the subjects had inanition or failure-to-thrive syndromes, while other problems included neuropathies (34%), blindness (18%), gastroparesis (14%), and malignancies (12%). Forty-eight hours after withdrawal, mental status was alert (43%), somnolent (46%), or comatose (11%); only one-third of the subjects could meaningfully participate in an interview. Although we concluded that terminal treatment was generally satisfactory and most (85%) people had good or even very good deaths, pain and agitation were not uncommon during the last day of life. The symptoms present in the final 24 hours of life are summarized in Table 15–1.

THE FAMILIES

Families are intimately affected by dialysis discontinuation decisions.[18] In about half of the cases, they are the primary decision makers when patients lack the capacity to speak for themselves due to cognitive impairment.[6] Even if older patients are mentally competent, they often defer to younger relatives and staff to help make these difficult decisions. Advance care planning is especially important and needs to take into account religious beliefs and cultural factors within families. It is best to discuss these issues when patients are physically and mentally stable. Otherwise, families may feel the burden of such a decision is too great. The default decision is then to provide full technological treatment, and this is often futile, against patient values, and associated with needless suffering.

In cases in which the patient initiates the decision, families may be troubled at first by this wish to hasten death. Sometimes the adult child or relative who has been most emotionally and geographically distant from the patient, surfaces and proceeds to object to withdrawal of dialysis. In these instances, the family member may feel guilt over having neglected the patient and now want to "make it up" by insisting on every available treatment. In large families, it is not uncommon for there to be conflict. Gentle but firm diplomacy is necessary and helpful. It has been our experience that tincture of time and the opportunity to more fully see and acknowledge suffering will allow most families to achieve unanimity in their support of the patient and the decision. We agree with the description by Rosenfeld and associates[19] of collaborative surrogate decision making by families and physicians. This model has emerged from a qualitative study of elderly individuals and encourages physicians to assume responsibility for recommending the difficult treatment plans, such as discontinuation of dialysis, when such recommendations are consistent with patient and family goals for care.

PSYCHOSOCIAL ISSUES

We have written about the complex relationship between depression, competence, and withdrawal of life-saving medical treatments.[10,20] Depression can interfere with

Table 15–1. Symptoms during the Last 24 Hours ($n = 79$)

Symptom	Present	Severe
Pain	42%	5%
Agitation	30%	1%
Myoclonus or muscle twitching	28%	4%
Dyspnea or agonal breathing	25%	3%
Fever	20%	
Diarrhea	14%	1%
Dysphagia	14%	
Nausea	13%	1%

decision-making capacity and should be suspected in any patient who refuses medical treatment.[21-23] The effect of depression on the rate of dialysis withdrawal is unknown, but it presumably has a powerful influence.[24] Recently published guidelines on the initiation and discontinuation of treatment suggest use of depression screening tools (e.g., the Beck Depression Inventory) to rule out this possibility, but at the present time it is unlikely that these are being widely employed.[25]

On occasion, we have found patients who request discontinuation of dialysis to be in the midst of a major depression or bipolar affective disorder.[26] Consultation is helpful in these complex situations, and the nephrologists can refuse to discontinue dialysis while psychiatric treatment is provided. This may include commitment of delusional patients to a psychiatric facility. Several of our patients have had excellent responses to antidepressant and neuroleptic medications and have no longer expressed interest in terminating dialysis. Critical examination of the ESRD literature suggests that moderate depressive syndromes are likely in about 25% of patients and major depression in 5%–22% of patients.[27,28] In our multicenter study, we found approximately the same range of depression for the ESRD patient population who terminate dialysis as the overall ESRD population and, therefore, do not believe in most cases that depression is a primary factor. Interestingly, 9% of the patient sample (according to both their own and family reports) had made a suicide attempt in the past, and there was a family history of suicide attempts in 14% of the families. By comparison, National Institute of Mental Health Epidemiologic Catchment Area data suggest a lifetime prevalence of suicide attempts in the general population of about 3%.[29] Accordingly, we suspect that termination of dialysis may be considered a more likely option by individuals who have made a suicide attempt or have family members who have tried to end their lives.

Another psychosocial consideration that bears mention is the issue of deathbed vigils. Dialysis discontinuation offers families and loved ones an opportunity to communicate with the patient and achieve reconciliation and closure.[15] For some families, it may become a vigil, in which they set a goal of being present at the exact moment when the last breath is drawn. We have found it necessary to challenge the wisdom of making that goal the ultimate determinant of quality of dying. Some patients have died while relatives stepped out for a bite or a trip to the bathroom, and anticipation and discussion of this possibility with families is essential. However, we have also needed to discuss this matter with nursing staff, who on at least one occasion ushered the family out of the room (with them loudly protesting) so that the patient (who had soiled himself) could be cleaned up. Naturally, it was at that awkward moment that death arrived.

PAIN

Pain is the most common and distressing physical problem for dying older adults who discontinue dialysis.[17,18] Pain is not caused by the progression of uremia following cessation of dialysis but, rather, preexisting conditions, such as diabetic neuropathy. A little known but severe pain disorder associated with long-term dialysis is calciphylaxis. Calciphylaxis is a particularly troublesome complication that is being diagnosed in an increasing number of patients with ESRD.[30] The diagnosis is suspected when the patient has skin induration and severe pain, which usually appear on the inner thighs or abdominal wall. The skin transdermal oxygen content is almost always low. Skin necrosis is followed by a poorly healing eschar. Predisposing factors include obesity (abdominal wall pannus), extreme parathyroid hormone elevation, and calcium phosphate product >70. The possible etiological role of increased use of calcium as a phosphate binder and intravenous iron administration is being studied. Hyperbaric oxygen has been used with limited successes. Calciphylaxis pain is excruciating and difficult to manage; it has prompted several of our patients to discontinue dialysis to put an end to unremitting suffering.

General principles of pain management for the geriatric patient are discussed in Chapter 16. However, medical management is invariably complicated for this group by the concomitant renal failure. Over 90% of most opioids are excreted through the kidneys, and many have active metabolites that may accumulate and cause distressing symptoms. This difficult situation is worsened by a paucity of hard data on the use of analgesics in ESRD.[31]

Morphine is the mainstay of pain control for most palliative care programs, and we have generally achieved good pain control with intravenous pumps in our population. Theoretically, morphine can prove problematic. Its metabolite, morphine-6-glucuronide, is a more potent analgesic than morphine itself and equilibrates very slowly across the blood–brain barrier. The associated sedation may be beneficial if the patient is agitated or in intractable pain but could also deny a patient the level of alertness necessary to achieve spiritual and interpersonal goals.[32–34]

Several drugs are best avoided altogether. Meperidine use results in accumulation of normeperidine, which is only half as potent an analgesic as the parent compound but two to three times more likely to cause seizures.[35] This year, one of our patients received a prescription through the emergency room and was promptly admitted later that day with his first seizure episode. Toxicity can occur even in younger patients with normal renal function, but the elderly renal patient is especially likely to have central nervous system toxicity (agitation, myoclonus, and seizures).[36–39]

Propoxyphene is doubly undesirable. Levels of both the parent compound and the active metabolites rise in renal failure with an increased risk of cardiac and neurological sequelae. Even for older patients with normal renal function, the relatively low level of analgesia that is provided at a high cost of toxicity has led a panel of geriatric experts to conclude that it should not be used.[40,41] Essentially the same could

be said of pentazocine. Adverse reactions can be further reduced by avoiding the use of mixed agonist/antagonist agents with strong psychotomimetic propensities, such as nalbuphine and butorphanol.

Nonsteroidal anti-inflammatory drugs are also not without their own hazards. For the patient whose kidneys have already failed, the renal threat is inconsequential. However, patients with uremia are already plagued by gastrointestinal symptoms and are prone to bleeding from platelet dysfunction. One New Zealand study found dyspepsia, nausea, vomiting, and bleeding to be among the prime causes of a "bad" death identified by survivors/caregivers in end-of-life patients.[42]

So what is a sensible approach to pain control for this vulnerable group, and how can the adverse drug effects be minimized? It is distressing to note that families and caregivers of nearly half of the patients in our series felt that pain was present in the final hours. It is likely that psychic distress or agitated delirium was interpreted as pain by some observers; nonetheless, it is clear that we must do a better job at providing analgesia in the last hours of life. A fundamental principle of palliative care is that constant pain needs to be treated with a constant supply of drug. Aggressive titration to effect with needed dosing and a morphine pump will likely best preserve QOL in the last days. Rotating or substituting opioids is another intuitively attractive approach, which may limit the buildup of toxic metabolites. Unfortunately, data are limited and largely anecdotal for functionally anephric older adults.[43] The same considerations obviously apply if opiates are used for other indications, such as dyspnea. In the last analysis, constant vigilance to shifting pain control needs and early identification of side effects are required for palliative success.

GASTROINTESTINAL SYMPTOMS

Geriatric renal failure patients are particularly prone to constipation, dyspepsia, and nausea. Contributing factors include comorbidities such as diabetes, autonomic dysfunction, and congestive heart failure, which can delay gastric emptying. In addition, complex drug regimens often include cardiovascular drugs, analgesics, and psychoactive agents, which can affect the gastrointestinal tract. Finally, uremia causes nausea by both stimulating the chemoreceptor trigger zone and acting as a direct mucosal irritant. Symptom management is similar to that undertaken in older adults without renal failure.

Metoclopramide can be tried at low doses if gastric motility is felt to be a major factor. However, there are high rates of dystonia and movement disorders in both the renal and geriatric populations.[44,45] If possible, its use should be limited and patients closely monitored. Aluminum-, magnesium-, and phosphate-containing compounds present problems for patients wishing to prolong life; but they may be useful after dialysis discontinuation when goals have shifted. If the patient is agitated and delirious, haloperidol may simultaneously target both the nausea and the confusion of uremia. Alternatively, ondansetron may be the drug of choice for the patient with both pruritus and nausea.[46] Most geriatricians shun cimetidine because of its increased risk of delirium. Renal patients have an elevated incidence of confusion on the drug, and it should not be used in older adults with ESRD.[47]

THE SKIN AND MOUTH

Even healthy older adults may be troubled by a dry mouth. Renal patients are often on drugs such as anticholinergics, narcotics, and β-blockers, which may exacerbate the problem. Adjusting the drug regimen, providing assiduous mouth care, offering small amounts of fluid or ice chips, and humidifying the air may improve comfort and the ability to speak and swallow.

Skin care is of critical importance. Patients with ESRD frequently have a combination of peripheral vascular disease, dementia, visual impairment, pruritus, dia-

betes, decreased mobility, peripheral neuropathy and poor nutrition. Many have already had amputations, and a decision to discontinue dialysis often follows a recommendation for an additional amputation. This obviously places patients at high risk for skin breakdown and pressure ulcers. In addition to pain, there is an increased physical and emotional toll on patients, families, and caregivers. If a patient develops a foul-smelling sacral pressure ulcer, serious issues arise with regard to body image, modesty, and dignity. When a patient is likely to live more than a few days, careful attention to repositioning, use of pressure relief systems, lubricating the skin, controlling moisture, and educating caregivers in appropriate techniques to avoid shear forces and relieve pressure is beneficial. Many products exist for the topical treatment of existing ulcers. All patients should be premedicated for wound care. Comfort and dignity can be enhanced using products that do not require frequent dressing changes. It may also make sense to simplify or eliminate dressing changes in the last few days of life, if as death approaches the patient has disturbance pain.

PRURITUS

Itching, like xerostomia, is common even in healthy older adults. In uremic geriatric patients the problem is magnified. The pathophysiology is poorly understood, but renal itch is likely transmitted by a specific subset of polymodal C fibers. Endogenous opioids; dry skin; hyperparathyroidism; defective cutaneous innervation; abnormal fatty acid metabolism; altered serum levels of calcium, magnesium, phosphate, vitamin A, histamine, and/or serotonin; increased serum bile acids; and aluminum toxicity have been proposed as causative factors.[48–52]

Antihistamines have limited utility, and some (notably hydroxyzine and diphenhydramine) are profoundly anticholinergic with a high incidence of confusion, constipation, urinary retention, and dry mouth. More selective agents, such as fexofenadine, may help; but since peak plasma levels and half-life are prolonged in both geriatric and renal patients, once-daily dosing seems judicious. Supplementation with fish oil or primrose oil may yield some modest benefit, but these require 6–10 weeks of therapy.[53] In one small trial, erythropoietin treatment over several weeks lowered histamine levels and improved uremic itch.[54] There have also been reports of response to naltrexone, orally activated charcoal, ultraviolet B phototherapy, and other agents, although there are practical problems when using these modalities in patients in the last weeks of their lives.[48] A small study of chronic ambulatory peritoneal dialysis patients (including some octogenarians) showed prompt resolution of itch within 1–2 weeks when treated with twice-daily ondansetron.[46] If both topical treatment and a course of selective antihistamines fail, particularly if the patient also has nausea, ondansetron may be a good, although expensive, choice.

DELIRIUM, MYOCLONUS, AND AGITATION

There has been little research on the prevalence, causes, and treatment of agitated delirium in the ESRD patient. Delirium and dementia are common around the time of dialysis discontinuation; as illustrated in Table 15–1, agitation and myoclonus are frequent in the terminal stage. In fact, this is twice the frequency of myoclonus reported in the general palliative care population.[42] One can suspect that the percentage would be higher if restricted to the older adults in the cohort. Myoclonus is likely due to drug metabolites (primarily opioids) and the effects of uremic encephalopathy.[55] In the face of progressing uremia, dehydration, and other medical problems, it is virtually certain that all of these patients were delirious prior to death. The appropriate goal is to maintain alertness and the ability to interact while disturbing symptoms are controlled. The majority of patients in our series gradually

became less responsive and more peaceful as stupor deepened. However, the subset with agitated delirium was very distressing to families, and terminal sedation may be necessary.[56,57]

If the patient approaching death becomes agitated, it does the patient a disservice to launch an extensive work-up. Neither is it correct to reflexively push sedatives without considering possible precipitants.[58] Is the patient's catheter blocked? Is there a fecal impaction? Is pain poorly controlled? Alternatively, is the patient suffering a buildup of opiate metabolites or the effects of digoxin toxicity? The patient with pre-existing cognitive deficits and visual impairment is most likely to become agitated.[59] If the clinical situation and the drug regimen are continuously monitored, the patient's chances for the maximum amount of "good" time is optimized. If symptomatic drug therapy is needed for the agitation, antipsychotics may ease the delusions and disorganized thought. If the goal is control of agitated delirium, sedating antipsychotic agents, such as chlorpromazine and thioridazine, are effective. Haloperidol (though not sedating) is frequently used since it can be given intramuscularly, intravenously, as well as orally. If that fails or if anxiety, myoclonus, and seizures are prominent, benzodiazepines can be added.

AFTER THE DEATH: BEREAVEMENT

Dame Cicely Saunders, the founder of the hospice movement, has said "How people die remains in the memories of those who live on." We do not know the impact of dialysis discontinuation on the bereaved loved ones, and it remains for future research to explore the prevalence of traumatic grief and major depression in this population. In the meantime, we have begun to encourage dialysis facilities to screen families for bereavement problems, arrange for the necessary grief counseling referrals, and sponsor an annual service of remembrance.

Memorial services are commonplace at

hospice programs but virtually unknown at dialysis facilities. The services are a means to allow families, friends, and staff to say good-bye and to acknowledge the reality of loss.[60] They provide an opportunity to support bereaved relatives; permit communication with staff, who are often unaware of the circumstances of the deaths; allow different families to grieve together; and facilitate the achievement of much needed closure. They embody the need for both families and staff to heal after a death and to recognize the intimate relationship established between them. They also fulfill a basic tenet of palliative medicine in the extension of care to families and loved ones, both around the time of death and in the period afterward. Our annual dialysis memorial services have been extremely well attended and are of considerable solace to the families of elderly patients. We are convinced that there is a need for comprehensive bereavement programs to address these issues in ESRD and hope that this will become integral to the practice of nephrology.

SUMMARY AND CONCLUSION

Elderly patients with renal failure who are nearing death present many challenges to the care team, particularly regarding psychosocial issues and symptom management. While there is a growing awareness that patients benefit from palliative care throughout the spectrum of life-threatening illness, dialysis discontinuation is clearly one of those circumstances that call for a maximal palliative medicine approach.

The ESRD population is ideal for research into geriatric palliative care. Nephrology is a protocol-driven specialty that makes considerable use of benchmarks and quality-control tools.[1] Accordingly, it presents an opportunity for symptom management studies, such as the treatment of nausea or itching, which can be relevant to other geriatric patients. Dialysis discontinuation can also be a paradigm for research into the bioethical and physiological aspects of cessation of life support. Since patients live an average of 8 days following

the decision to stop dialysis, and during that time many are able to fully communicate (unlike patients on ventilators), they are in a unique position to teach us about these matters. Sir Thomas Browne has pointed out that "Many have studied to exasperate the ways of Death, but fewer hours have been spent to soften that necessity." Geriatric and palliative medicine are already aware of the truth of this statement, nephrology is coming to recognize its veracity, and all three specialties are likely to benefit from future collaborative clinical and research endeavors.

ACKNOWLEDGMENTS

Dr. Cohen was supported by the Greenwall Foundation and the Promoting Excellence in End-of-Life Care Program of the Robert Wood Johnson Foundation.

REFERENCES

1. Zabetakis PM, Sasak C, Callahan C, Gutzmer L, Tozzi MJ, Balter P, Michelis MF. Improving clinical outcomes through internal benchmarking and quality targets. Dialysis Transplant 29:130–135, 2000.
2. National Institutes of Health, NIDDK/DKUHD. Excerpts from the United States Renal Data System 2000 Annual Data Report. Am J Kidney Dis 36(Suppl 2):S1–S239, 2000.
3. Network of New England Inc. End Stage Renal Disease 1999 Annual Report. New Haven, Health Care Financing Administration. p. 84, 1999.
4. Roberts JC, Kjellstrand CM. Choosing death: withdrawal from chronic dialysis without medical reason. Acta Med Scand 223:181–186, 1988.
5. Levy WB, Wynbrandt GD. The quality of life on maintenance haemodialysis. Lancet 1:1328–1330, 1975.
6. Neu S, Kjellstrand CM. Stopping long-term dialysis: an empirical study of withdrawal of life-supporting treatment. N Engl J Med 314:14–20, 1986.
7. Leggat JE Jr, Bloembergen WE, Levine G, Humbert-Shearon TE, Port FK. An analysis of risk factors for withdrawal from dialysis before death. J Am Soc Nephrol 8:1755–1763, 1997.
8. Krebs A. James Michener, author of novels that sweep through the history of places, is dead. New York Times 17 October 1997, p. C31.

9. Moss AH, RPA and ASN Working Group. A new clinical practice guideline on initiation and withdrawal of dialysis that makes explicit the role of palliative medicine. J Palliat Med 3:253–260, 2000.

10. Cohen LM. Suicide, hastening death, and psychiatry. Arch Intern Med 158:1973–1976, 1998.

11. Emanuel JE. Care for dying patients. Lancet 349:1714, 1997.

12. Thomson GE, Hurzeler RJ, Fraunhar G, Howe K. Physician assisted living: the PAL partner initiative. Conn Med 61:775–778, 1997.

13. Bajwa K, Szabo E, Kjellstrand CM. A prospective study of risk factors and decision making in dialysis discontinuation. Arch Intern Med 156:2571–2577, 1996.

14. Sekkarie MA, Moss AH. Withholding and withdrawing dialysis: the role of physician specialty and education and patient functional status. Am J Kidney Dis 31:464–472, 1998.

15. Cohen LM, McCue JD, Germain M, Kjellstrand CM. Dialysis discontinuation: a good death? Arch Intern Med 155:42–47, 1995.

16. Cohen LM, Germain M, Poppel DM, Woods A, Pekow PS, Kjellstrand CM. Dying well after discontinuing the life-support treatment of dialysis. Arch Intern Med 160:2513–2518, 2000.

17. Cohen LM, Germain M, Poppel DM, Woods A, Kjellstrand CM. Dialysis discontinuation and palliative care. Am J Kidney Dis 36:140–144, 2000.

18. Woods A, Berzoff J, Cohen LM, Cait CA, Pekow P, Germain M, Poppel D. The family perspective of end-of-life care in endstage renal disease: the role of the social worker. J Nephrol Social Work 19:9–21, 1999.

19. Rosenfeld KE, Wenger NS, Kagawa-Singer M. End-of-life decision making: a qualitative study of elderly individuals. J Gen Intern Med 15:620–625, 2000.

20. Levy NB, Cohen LM. End-stage renal disease and its treatment: dialysis and transplantation. In: Stoudemire A, Fogel BS, Greenberg D (Eds.). Psychiatric Care of the Medical Patient, 2nd ed. London, Oxford University Press, pp. 791–800, 2000.

21. Sullivan MD, Youngner SJ. Depression, competence, and the right to refuse lifesaving medical treatment. Am J Psychiatry 151:971–978, 1994.

22. Leeman CP. Depression and the right to die. Gen Hosp Psychiatry 21:112–115, 1999.

23. Beck DA, Koenig HG, Beck JS. Depression. Clin Geriatr Med 14:765–786, 1998.

24. Kimmel PL, Weihs K, Peterson RA. Survival in hemodialysis patients: the role of depression. J Am Soc Nephrol 3:12–27, 1993.

25. Renal Physicians Association and American Society of Nephrology. Shared Decision-Making in the Appropriate Initiation of and Withdrawal from Dialysis: Clinical Practice Guideline: Washington DC, 2000.

26. Levy NB, Cohen LM. Central and peripheral nervous systems in uremia. In: Massry SG, Glassock R (Eds.). Textbook of Nephrology, 4th ed. Philadelphia, Williams and Wilkins, pp. 1279–1282, 2001.

27. Craven JL, Rodin GM, Johnson L, Kennedy SH. The diagnosis of major depression in renal dialysis patients. Psychosom Med 49:482–492, 1987.

28. Israel M. Depression in dialysis patients: a review of psychological factors 31:445–451, 1986.

29. Moscicki EK. Epidemiology surveys as tools for studying suicidal behavior: a review. Suicide Life Threat Behav 19:131–146, 1989.

30. Coates, T, Kirkland GS, Dymock RB, Murphy BF, Brealey JK, Mathew TH, Disney AP. Cutaneous necrosis from calcific uremic arteriolopathy. Am J Kidney Dis 32:384–391, 1998.

31. Davies G, Kingswood C, Street M. Pharmacokinetics of opioids in renal dysfunction. Clin Pharmacokinet 6:410–422, 1996.

32. Angst MS, Buhrer M, Lotsch J. Insidious intoxication after morphine treatment in renal failure: delayed onset of morphine-6-glucuronide action. Anesthesiology 92:1473–1476, 2000.

33. Dubs A, Wiedemeier P, Caduff B. Morphinintoxikation bei chronischer niereninsuffizienz. Morphin-6-glucuronid als pharmakologisch aktiver morphin-metabolit. Dtsch Med Wochenschr 124:896–898, 1999.

34. Chauvin M, Sandouk P, Schermann JM, et al. Morphine pharmacokinetics in renal failure. Anesthesiology 66:327–331, 1987.

35. Pellegrini JE, Paice J, Faut-Callahan M. Meperidine utilization and compliance with Agency for Health Care Policy and Research guidelines in a tertiary care hospital. The Clinical Forum for Nurse Anesthetists 10:174–180, 1999.

36. Szeto HH, Inturrisi CE, Houde R, et al. Accumulation of normeperidine, an active metabolite of meperidine, in patients with renal failure or cancer. Ann Intern Med 86:738–741, 1977.

37. Marinella MA. Meperidine-induced generalized seizures with normal renal function. South Med J 90:556–558, 1997.

38. Hagemeyer KO, Mauro LS, Mauro VF. Meperidine-related seizures associated with patient-controlled analgesia pumps. Ann Pharmacother 27:29–32, 1993.

39. Hassan H, Bastani B, Gellens M. Successful treatment of normeperidine neurotoxicity by hemodialysis. Am J Kidney Dis 35: 146–149, 2000.

40. Giacomini KM, Gibson TP, Levy G. Effect of hemodialysis on propoxyphene and norpropoxyphene concentrations in blood of anephric patients. Clin Pharmacol Ther 27:508–514, 1980.

41. Wilcox SM, Himmelstein DU, Woolhandler S. Inappropriate drug prescribing for the community-dwelling elderly. JAMA 272: 292–296, 1994.

42. Lichter L, Hunt E. The last forty-eight hours of life. J Palliat Care 6:7–15, 1990.

43. Ashby MA, Martin P, Jackson KA. Opioid substitution to reduce adverse effects in cancer pain management. Med J Aust 170:68–71, 1999.

44. Caralps A. Metoclopramide and renal failure. Lancet 1:554, 1979.

45. Miller LG, Jankovic J. Metoclopramide-induced movement disorders. Arch Intern Med 149:2486–2492, 1989.

46. Balaskas EV, Bamihas G, Karamouzis M, et al. Histamine and serotonin in uremic pruritus: effect of ondansetron in CAPD-pruritic patients. Nephron 78:395–402, 1998.

47. Schentag JJ, Calleri G, Rose JQ, et al. Pharmacokinetic and clinical studies in patients with cimetidine-associated mental confusion. Lancet 1:177–181, 1979.

48. Murphy M, Carmichael AJ. Renal itch. Clin Exp Dermatol 25:103–106, 2000.

49. Peck LW. Essential fatty acid deficiency in renal failure: can supplements really help? J Am Diet Assoc 10:S150–S153, 1997.

50. Mamianetti A, Tripodi V, Vescina C, et al. Serum bile acids and pruritus in hemodialysis patients. Clin Nephrol 53:194–198, 2000.

51. Friga V, Linos A, Linos D. Is aluminum toxicity responsible for uremic pruritus in chronic hemodialysis patients? Nephron 75:48–53, 1997.

52. Goicoechea M, de Sequera P, Ochando A, et al. Uremic pruritus: an unresolved problem in hemodialysis patients. Nephron 82: 73–74, 1999.

53. Yoshimoto-Furuie K, Yoshimoto K, Tanaka T, et al. Effects of oral supplementation with evening primrose oil for six weeks on plasma essential fatty acids and uremic skin symptoms in hemodialysis patients. Nephron 81:151–159, 1999.

54. De Marchi S, Cecchin E, Villalta D, et al. Relief of pruritus and decreases in plasma histamine concentrations during erythropoietin therapy in patients with uremia. N Engl J Med 326:969–974, 1992.

55. Burn DJ, Bates D. Neurology and the kidney. J Neurol Neurosurg Psychiatry 65: 810–821, 1998.

56. Fainsinger RL, DeMoissac D, Mancini I, et al. Sedation for delirium and other symptoms in terminally ill patients in Edmonton. J Palliat Care 16:5–10, 2000.

57. Fainsinger RL, Waller A, Bercovici M, et al. A multicentre international study of sedation for uncontrolled symptoms in terminally ill patients. Palliat Med 14:257–265, 2000.

58. Breitbart W, Strout D. Delirium in the terminally ill. Clin Geriatr Med 16:257–372, 2000.

59. Inouye SK, Charpentier PA. Precipitating factors for delirium in hospitalized elderly persons: predictive model and interrelationship with baseline vulnerability. JAMA 275:852–857, 1996.

60. Worden WJ. Grief Therapy, Grief Counselling. London, Tavistock, 1992.

III

SYMPTOM DISTRESS IN OLDER PATIENTS

16

Pain

BRUCE A. FERRELL AND J. ELIZABETH WHITEMAN

Pain is the most feared complication of disease and the most distressing symptom near the end of life. It is common in persons with chronic illness, and the prevalence increases in older populations. Severity of pain often correlates with advancing disease and always signals the need for attention and relief. Pain can be a diagnostic sign of critical importance, necessitating acute life-saving intervention. It may represent a cry for help by patients with more emotional than physical illness, or it may serve absolutely no good purpose for patients near the end of life. For the latter patients, unrelieved pain often results in rapid deterioration of functional status, poor quality of life, psychological distress, and unnecessary suffering. Unrelieved pain may hasten death through its effects on physiological and neuropsychological systems. With no objective biological markers for pain, inadequate training in most schools, and professional fear of liabilities associated with the use of potent analgesic drugs, assessment and management of pain often remain perplexing for clinicians.

Pain assessment and management have reached a high level of sophistication and are usually successful. The publication of clinical practice guidelines, the focus of quality review organizations, and moral outrage over unnecessary suffering have fueled rapid development of new strategies, products, and technologies. Descriptions of the pathophysiological mechanisms of pain have helped to effectively target existing pain management strategies, further enhanced by new drugs and interventions with lower side-effect profiles. However, substantial barriers to treatment of pain still exist. Zealous regulation of opioid drugs and prejudicial attitudes about the patients who need them, health systems that still emphasize cure over care, and financial incentives that favor high-tech pain management strategies over other conventional approaches remain all too common.

Pain management is different in older compared to younger persons.[1] Older persons may under-report pain for a variety of reasons, despite functional impairment, psychological distress, and needless suffering related to pain.[2] They often present with concurrent illnesses and multiple problems, making pain evaluation and treatment more difficult. Elderly persons have a higher incidence of side effects to medications and a greater potential for complications and adverse events related to many treatment procedures. Despite these challenges, pain can be effectively managed in most elderly patients. Moreover, clinicians have an ethical and moral obligation to prevent needless suffering and provide effective pain relief, especially for those nearing the end of life.[3]

EPIDEMIOLOGY OF PAIN IN OLDER PERSONS

The precise incidence and prevalence of pain in older populations is not known. Pain is a universal sensation. Every individual has an occasional experience of pain, such as a headache or muscle or joint pain from overexertion. Studies have suggested that the prevalence of significant pain in community-dwelling older persons may be as high as 25%–56%.[4] Prevalence rates have been reported for back pain of 21%–49.5%, for joint pain of 20.5%–71%, and for headache of 1.2%–50% in persons over the age of 65 years.[5] In 1997, a Harris telephone poll reported that 18% of elderly people take analgesic medications on a regular basis (several times a week or daily).[6] Of those who took analgesic drugs regularly, more than 70% reported taking over-the-counter analgesics and more than 70% took prescription analgesics, indicating that most patients took both sources of medication simultaneously. In general, the most common causes of pain in elderly persons are related to musculoskeletal disorders, such as back pain and arthritis. Neuralgia or neuropathic pain is also common, stemming from diseases such as diabetes, herpes zoster, trauma, amputation, and other nerve injuries. Nighttime leg pain (e.g., cramps, restless legs) is also common, as is claudication. Cancer is a cause of severe pain that is distressing to patients, families, and health-care professionals. The distress

of pain from any source has brought attention to the medical, ethical, and recently legal obligations of clinicians to provide effective pain and symptom management near the end of life, even if doing so may hasten death by a few hours or days.[3]

Pain is also common in nursing homes. It has been suggested that 45%–80% of nursing home residents may have substantial pain.[7] Many of these patients have multiple pain complaints and multiple potential sources of pain. Our studies have suggested that 70% of nursing home patients' pain results from arthritis and other musculoskeletal causes.[2,8]

A number of studies have suggested that pain is often under-recognized and undertreated. Those with cancer pain in nursing homes,[9] cognitive impairment,[10,11] postoperative pain,[10,11] or a history of substance abuse or major psychiatric disorders are particularly vulnerable. These groups represent particular difficulties in assessment and treatment that may require specialized expertise and unique strategies to improve pain mangement.

Unrelieved pain is associated with a number of negative outcomes in elderly people.[12] Depression, decreased socialization, sleep disturbance, impaired ambulation, and increased health-care utilization and costs have been associated with the presence of pain in older people. Other outcomes less thoroughly explored include gait disturbances, slowed rehabilitation, and adverse effects of analgesic medications.[13] Older patients rely heavily on family and other caregivers near the end of life. For these patients and their caregivers, pain can be especially distressing. Caregiver strain and caregiver attitudes can have substantial impact on pain.

PHYSIOLOGY OF PAIN

Pain is an unpleasant sensory and emotional experience.[14] It is derived from complex physiological processes that include elements of neural sensation and nerve transmission integrated with central nervous system processing of memory, expectations, and emotions. Pain may be initiated by cellular organs excited by tissue damage or by neuropathic mechanisms arising from peripheral nerves or the central nervous system itself. Unfortunately, there are no reliable biological markers of the pain experience. There are no measurements in blood, electroencephalographic, or other imaging devices that accurately reflect the intensity or character of pain. The most accurate and reliable evidence for the existence and intensity of pain is the patient's description.[15] Patient reports of pain are often quite variable in description, character, and intensity.

Clinicians may find it helpful to classify pain by its physiological mechanism.[16,17] Treatment targeted by specific physiological pain mechanisms may be more effective. Pain problems can be categorized into one of four basic physiological mechanisms. Pain that results largely from stimulation of pain receptors is called *nociceptive pain*.[18] Nociceptive pain may arise from tissue injury, inflammation, or mechanical deformity. Examples include trauma, burns, infection, arthritis, ischemia, and tissue distortion. Pain from nociception usually responds well to common analgesic medications or relief of the underlying cause. *Neuropathic pain* results from pathophysiological processes that arise in the peripheral or central nervous system.[19,20] Examples include diabetic neuralgia, postherpetic neuralgia, and post-traumatic neuralgia (postamputation or "phantom limb" pain). In contrast to nociceptive pain, neuropathic pain syndromes respond best to nonconventional analgesic medications, such as tricyclic antidepressants and anticonvulsant drugs. *Mixed pain syndromes* are often thought to have multiple or unknown pathophysiological mechanisms. Treatment is more problematic and often unpredictable. Examples include recurrent headaches and some vasculitic syndromes. Finally, there are some *psychological pain* disorders (e.g., conversion reactions) where psychological factors may be responsible for the pain experience. These patients may benefit from specific psychiatric interven-

tion, but traditional pain strategies are probably not indicated.

In clinical settings, most pain arises from multiple mechanisms. Cancer, for instance, may cause nociceptive pain from tumor distention and deformation of surrounding tissues. It may also come from neuropathic mechanisms caused by tumor invasion of peripheral nerves or the central nervous system. Arthritis may cause nociceptive pain from joint inflammation, joint distortion, strain on associated muscles and connective tissue, and microfracture from eroded cartilage or bone. Unfortunately for many diseases, the physiological basis of pain is only partially understood.

In this discussion, it is important to remember that there is a psychological and interpretive component to every pain experience. When psychological factors are thought to play a major role in perpetuating or masking complications associated with pain, a multidisciplinary and multimodal treatment strategy is often required.[21] Anxiety and depression are common problems associated with chronic pain, which often interfere with and complicate simple pain management strategies. When psychological problems resulting from pain syndromes coexist simultaneously with pain, psychological interventions alone are not likely to yield pain relief. Likewise, pain interventions alone are not likely to be successful in the absence of simultaneous psychological interventions.

AGE-RELATED CHANGES IN PAIN PERCEPTION

Elderly persons are known to have altered presentations of disease. Elderly persons may have apparently painless myocardial infarction and painless intra-abdominal catastrophies. The extent to which these observations are attributable to age-related changes in pain perception remains uncertain.[22,23] Studies of pain sensitivity across the life span have shown mixed results.[22] If more recent observations are correct, overall pain perception may not change much with aging.[23] Clearly, additional studies are needed to better define age-related changes specific to nervous system function and pain perception.

ASSESSMENT OF PAIN IN ELDERLY PEOPLE

Pain assessment is the most critical part of pain management. Accurate pain assessment is important to identify the underlying cause and to choose the most effective treatment. Pain management is most effective when the underlying cause has been identified and eliminated. Inherent in pain assessment is the need to evaluate acute pain for which the cause can be eliminated and distinguish this from exacerbations of chronic pain. Chronic pain for which the cause is not reversible or only partially treatable requires a palliative approach to symptom management. In this case, the goals of care include the prevention of or rehabilitation from complications such as functional decline, social isolation, depression, and resulting impairment in quality of life.

Compared to younger patients, older persons often present with unique challenges to pain assessment. Elders tend to under-report pain despite substantial functional impairment. Multiple concurrent medical problems and multiple sources of pain make assessment more difficult. Finally, cognitive impairment, impaired sensory function, and denial and avoidance behaviors may all contribute to under-reporting.[24]

Pain History and Physical Examination

Assessment of pain should begin with a thorough history and physical examination to help establish a diagnosis of underlying disease and form a baseline description of pain experiences. Many older persons do not use the word *pain* but may refer to their problems as "hurting" or "aching," or use other synonyms or descriptive words. It is important to probe for and identify pain in the patient's own words so that references for subsequent follow-up evaluations are clearly established.[25] The history should include questions to elicit details of the pain onset, location, and character. Aggravating and relieving influences and the outcomes of previous treatments should be recorded. Past medical and surgical history is important to define coexisting disease and previous experience with pain and analgesic use. The review of systems should include special focus on the musculoskeletal and nervous systems. Any history of trauma should be thoroughly investigated because falls, occult fractures, and other injuries are common in this age group. In this setting, care must be taken to avoid attributing acute pain to pre-existing conditions. Making this problem worse is the fact that chronic pain does fluctuate with time. Injuries from minor trauma and acute disease, such as gout or calcium pyrophosphate crystal arthropathy, can be easily overlooked.

A thorough physical examination should confirm any suspicions suggested by the history. Because of the frequency with which problems are often identified, the physical exam should focus on the musculoskeletal and nervous systems. Tender points of inflammation, muscle spasm, and trigger points should be palpated. Observation of abnormal posture, gait impairment, and limitations in range of motion may indicate a need for physical therapy and rehabilitation. Evidence of kyphosis, scoliosis, and abnormal joint alignments should be identified. A systematic neurological exam is also important, to identify potential sources of neuropathic pain. Focal muscle weakness, atrophy, abnormal reflexes, or sensory impairments may indicate peripheral or central nervous system injury. Mottled skin in a denervated extremity, presence of a Charcot joint, orthostatic hypotension, impaired gastric emptying, or incontinence may indicate autonomic nervous system dysfunction, which can imply sympathetically maintained pain or a complex regional pain syndrome.[24,25,26]

It is important to assess functional status to identify self-care deficits and formulate treatment plans that maximize independence and quality of life. Functional status can also represent an important outcome measure of overall pain management. Functional status can be evaluated from information taken from the history and physical examination as well as one or several formal functional status assessment scales validated in elderly people.[27,28]

A brief psychological and social evaluation is also important. Depression, anxiety, social isolation, and disengagement are all common in patients with chronic pain.[29] There is clearly a significant association between chronic pain and depression, even when controlling for overall health and functional status.[30] Therefore, assessment should always include a screen for depression. The simple question "Are you depressed?" has been shown to be a sensitive and specific screening tool for depression in medically ill patients.[31] Psychological evaluation should also include consideration of anxiety and coping skills. Anxiety is common among patients with acute and chronic pain and requires extra time and frequent reassurance from health-care providers. Pain management often requires effective coping skills for anxiety and other emotional feelings that can be learned.[32] For those with significant psychiatric symptoms, referral for formal psychiatric evaluation and management may be required. Specific counseling, supportive group therapy, biofeedback, or psychoactive medications may be necessary for developing and maintaining effective coping strategies as well as management of major psychiatric complications. Social networks should also be explored for availability and involvement of family and other caregivers. It has been shown that care settings, family, and informal caregivers can have a substantial impact on overall pain management.[7,33] Evaluation of caregivers is particularly necessary when complicated or high-tech pain management strategies are contemplated, such as continuous analgesic infusions. Some pain management strategies can place substantial demands on caregivers, resulting in additional caregiver stress. The need for frequent transportation, continuous reassessment of the need for administration of pain treatments, and technical training to identify and respond to treatment effects and side effects may result in substantial stress for nonprofessional caregivers, which can result in work absence, emotional and physical illness, and collapse of the home-care environment.

Pain Assessment Scales

A variety of pain scales are available to help categorize and quantify the magnitude of pain complaints in elderly persons. Results of these scales are helpful in the documentation and communication of pain experiences as well. It is helpful to evaluate pain using an appropriate pain scale initially and periodically to maximize treatment outcomes. Results can be recorded in a flow chart or graph, making it easy to identify stability or changes in pain over time.[16]

Pain scales can be grouped into multidimensional and unidimensional scales. In general, multidimensional scales with multiple items often provide more stable measurement and evaluation of pain in several domains.[34] For example, the McGill Pain Questionnaire captures pain in terms of intensity, affect, sensation, location, and several other domains, which are not possible to evaluate with a single question.[35–37] At the same time, multidimensional scales are often long and time-consuming and can be difficult to score at the bedside, making them difficult to use in a busy clinical setting. Unfortunately, few data are available on the use of many of these scales, specifically in elderly populations.

Unidimensional scales usually consist of a single item that relates to pain intensity. These scales are familiar to many people and easy to administer. They require little time or training to produce reasonably valid and reliable results. They have found widespread use in many clinical settings to monitor treatment effects and for quality-assurance indicators. Table 16–1 describes some unidimensional scales that are commonly used, but a large number of variants are available that have similar characteristics and produce similar results. It is important to remember that unidimensional pain scales often require framing the pain question appropriately for maximum relia-

Table 16–1. Comparison of Selected Pain Scales

Scale	Description	Advantages	Disadvantages	References
Visual analogue	100 mm line, vertical or horizontal	Continuous scale	Requires pencil and paper	Acute Pain Management Guideline Panel,[15] American Geriatric Society (AGS) Panel on Chronic Pain in Older Persons[16]
Present pain intensity	Six-point 0–5 scale with word descriptors (subscale of McGill Pain Questionnaire)	Easy to understand, word anchors decrease clustering toward middle of scale	Usually requires visual cue	Melzack[35]
Functional pain scale	Six-point word descriptor scale	Ease of administration	Equates pain with function	Gloth[27]
Graphic pictures	Happy faces, others	Amusing	Requires vision and attention	(AGS) Panel on Persistent Pain in Older Persons,[17] Herr et al.[38]
Sloan Kettering Pain Card	Seven words randomly distributed on a card	Ease of administration	Requires visual cue	Ferrell et al.,[8] Fishman et al.[39]
Verbal 0–10 scale	"On a scale of 0 to 10, if 0 means no pain and 10 means the worst pain you can imagine, how much is your pain now?"	Probably easiest to use	Requires hearing	Ferrell et al.[8]

Source: Ferrell.[24]

bility. Subjects should be asked about pain in the present tense (here and now). For example, the interviewer should frame the question "How much pain are you having right now?" Questions that require long-term memory or integration over time such as "How much pain have you had over the last week?" or "On average, how much pain have you had in the last month?" are more difficult for most patients. Recent studies in those with cognitive impairment have shown that pain reports requiring recall are influenced by pain at the moment.[40] Thus, it may be better to assess pain frequently, similar to the concept of monitoring vital signs, than to rely on patients' memory, especially among those with any degree of cognitive impairment.

Pain Assessment in Cognitively Impaired Patients

Pain assessment can be particularly challenging in patients with Alzheimer's disease, stroke, or other forms dementia and cognitive impairment. Fortunately, it has been shown that pain reports from those with mild to moderate cognitive impairment are no less valid than those from other patients with normal cognitive function.[41] Weiner and associates[40] have shown that these reports are usually stable over time as well. Our experience has shown that commonly available instruments, such as those in Table 16–1, are feasible for use in most patients.[8]

Patients with severe cognitive impairment coma may present pain assessment problems for which results often remain ambiguous. Although it has been assumed that those in deep coma do not experience pain, it is not clear that such brain damage necessarily results in complete anesthesia. Patients with locked-in syndrome (having intact perception and cognitive function but no purposeful motor function and no means of communication) may suffer severely. Unfortunately, no reliable methods exist to assess pain in these individuals. Health-care providers must be aware of these situations and provide analgesia empirically, especially during procedures or for conditions known to be uncomfortable or painful. More often, the majority with severe cognitive impairment can and do make their needs known in simple yes-or-no answers communicated in various ways. For example, those with profound aphasia can often provide accurate and reliable answers to yes-or-no questions when confronted by a sensitive and skilled interviewer. For these patients, it is important to be creative in establishing communication methods for the purpose of pain assessment.

Although pain is an individual experience, the use of family and caregivers in the assessment of pain can sometimes be helpful.[42] Among patients with cognitive impairment, the history is often obtainable only from family or close caregivers. Family and caregivers are an excellent source of qualitative information about general behavior, medication usage, actions that seem to reduce pain, and actions that seem to aggravate pain. It is important to remember, however, that family and caregivers are limited in their interpretation of events and behaviors. Indeed, evidence has suggested that when it comes to estimating pain intensity, proxies are not always very accurate or reliable. Studies of elderly cancer patients suggest that caregivers may overestimate pain intensity and distress.[33] Both physicians and nurses have been found to underestimate pain as well as provide inadequate pain medication.[43,44] In the final analysis, family and close caregivers can be valuable sources of qualitative information, but they probably should not be relied on entirely for quantitative assessment of pain intensity or distress, especially with patients who are able to communicate their own pain experiences.

Of particular interest in geriatric patients is the Hurley Discomfort Scale.[45] This instrument was developed for the assessment of discomfort in patients with severe dementia. The scale consists of items scored by a trained examiner after observation of a non-communicative patient. Behavioral observations such as breathing, vocalization, facial expression, body language, and restlessness are included. Testing of the scale has demonstrated reasonable reliability and stability over time.[45,46] Unfortunately, the scale requires some skill and experience to administer, which may be problematic for some clinical settings.

PAIN MANAGEMENT

Pain management, especially for those near the end of life, often requires a multimodal approach of drug and nondrug strategies. Although analgesic medications are the most common strategy employed, the concurrent use of cognitive-behavioral therapy and other nondrug strategies may be essential to reduce long-term reliance on medications alone, which may have substantial side effects. It is important to consider that pain management is often a labor-intensive effort. Not unlike the effort required to provide anticoagulation therapy, pain management requires frequent monitoring and dose adjustments. Indeed, elderly patients with pain benefit particularly from physicians, nurses, and restorative personnel who are able to employ an interdisciplinary approach to complex problems.

The most common approach to treating pain near the end of life relies on the World Health Organization (WHO) recommendations for choosing an initial treatment based on the intensity of pain.[47–49] Figure 16–1 provides an illustration of this approach. Pain of mild intensity usually responds to nonopioid drugs used alone or in combination with other physical and cognitive-behavioral interventions. Pain of moderate intensity often requires stronger efforts using weak opioids or low doses of stronger opioid drugs. Many of these drugs are compounded with acetaminophen or nonsteroidal anti-inflammatory drugs (NSAIDs) to achieve enhanced relief with only modest exposure to the risks and side effects. In the elderly, the hepatic, renal, gastrointestinal, and hemorrhagic toxicities of long-term acetaminophen or NSAIDs may pose more serious risks than the manageable side effects of opiate therapy. Severe pain usually requires strong opioid analgesic medications in higher doses given alone or in combination with other analgesic strategies. For some patients, continuous intravenous infusions, spinal anesthesia, nerve block, or neurosurgical approaches may be required. Although initially designed as a stepwise ap-

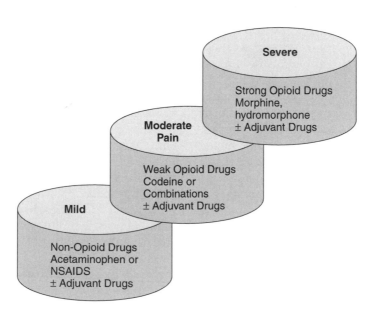

Figure 16–1. World Health Organization stepwise approach to cancer pain mangement. NSAID, non-steroidal anti-inflammatory drug.

proach to cancer pain managment, the WHO approach has become an acceptable one to other persistent pain problems as well, with only a few caveats.[17] First, it is important to remember that the model does not imply that severe pain should be shown to fail initial steps before escalation to higher steps. When patients present with severe pain, they should be initially treated with strong medications. Second, when pain rapidly escalates from mild to severe, analgesia should be rapidly escalated to stronger medications with or without other combined strategies (e.g., it may be appropriate to skip steps). Third, adjuvant drugs and combined treatments should be used early for mild to moderate pain, especially in pain of the neuropathic type. Finally, when patients present with acute pain, even though establishing a diagnosis is a priority, symptomatic management should be initiated while investigations proceed. It is rarely justified to defer analgesia until a definitive diagnosis is made. In fact, a comfortable patient is better able to cooperate with diagnostic procedures.

Although complete pain relief is often difficult to achieve, pain can always be reduced. The goals of medical care and the trade-offs of possible side effects need to be discussed openly. Patients should be given an expectation of pain control, but for some patients it is unrealistic to promise an expectation of complete relief. A period of trial and error should be anticipated when new medications are initiated and titration occurs. Review of medications, doses, use patterns, efficacy, and adverse effects should be a part of the routine process of care. Side effects must be meticulously managed, and ineffective drugs should be tapered and discontinued. [17]

Economic issues are also important in the management of pain. It is appropriate to consider economic issues and make balanced decisions while basic principles of assessment and treatment are followed. Health-care professionals should be aware of the costs and economic barriers that patients and families may encounter with the expensive strategies often prescribed. These issues include lack of Medicare reimbursement for prescription medications, limited formularies, delays in referrals in some managed-care environments, delays from mail-ordered pharmacies, and limited availability of strong opioid medications in some pharmacies. Long-acting oral and transdermal opiates, with the exception of methadone, are expensive. Short-acting generic morphine is the least expensive opiate analgesic.

ANALGESIC MEDICATIONS

Any patient who has pain that impairs functional status or quality of life is a candidate for analgesic drug therapy.[17] When properly prescribed and managed, analgesic medications are both safe and effective in elderly people. All analgesic interventions carry a balance of benefits and burdens. For some classes of pain-relieving medications (e.g., opioids), elderly patients have increased analgesic sensitivity and may require lower doses than younger patients.[48] However, elderly people are a heterogenous population; thus, optimum dosage and side effects are difficult to predict. Recommendations for age-adjusted dosing are not available for most analgesics. In reality, dosing for most patients requires beginning with low doses and careful upward titration based on clinical effectiveness.

The least invasive route of drug administration should be used.[17,47] Some drugs can be administered from a variety of routes, such as subcutaneous, intravenous, transcutaneous, sublingual, and rectal; but most are limited to only a few safe routes of administration. The oral route is preferable because of its convenience and production of relatively steady blood levels. Significant drug effects are often seen in 30 minutes to 2 hours for most analgesics given orally, which may be a drawback in acute, rapidly fluctuating pain. Intravenous bolus provides the most rapid onset and shortest duration of action, which often requires inpatient care, technical skill, and monitoring. Subcutaneous and intramuscular injection have the disadvantages of uncomfortable or painful administration, wider fluctuations in absorption, and rapid fall-off of action compared to the oral route. Transcutaneous, rectal, and sublingual routes are possible for some drugs, and they may be essential for those with difficulty swallowing.[47]

Timing of medications is also important. Fast-onset, short-acting analgesic drugs should be used for episodic or intermittent pain. For intermittent or episodic pain, medications can usually be prescribed as needed.[17] For continuous pain, medications should be provided around the clock.[47] In these situations, a steady-state analgesic blood level is more effective at maintaining comfort and results in a lower 24-hour dose requirement than sporadic administration of as-needed analgesia. Most patients with continuous pain also need fast-onset, short-acting rescue drugs for breakthrough pain. There are at least three types of breakthrough pain: (1) end-of-dose failure as a result of decreased blood levels of analgesic with a concomitant increase in pain prior to the next scheduled dose; (2) incident pain, usually caused by activity such as transfers or dressing changes that can be anticipated and pretreated; and (3) spontaneous pain, common with neuropathic pain, which is often fleeting and difficult to predict.[16,17]

The use of placebos is unethical in clinical practice, and there is no place for them in the management of acute or chronic pain. Placebos, in the form of inert oral medications, sham injections, or other fraudulent procedures, are justified only in certain research designs, where patients have given informed consent and understand that they may be receiving a placebo as a part of the research design.[50] In research, placebos help identify and measure random or uncontrollable events that may confound results.[51] In clinical settings, placebo effects are common, but they are neither diagnostic of pain nor indicative of a therapeutic response.[52] The effects of placebos are short-lived, and most patients eventually learn the truth, resulting in pro-

found loss of trust in the medical profession and more needless suffering.

Acetaminophen

Acetaminophen is the drug of choice for elderly persons with mild to moderate pain, especially that of osteoarthritis and other musculoskeletal problems.[17] As an analgesic and antipyretic, acetaminophen acts in the central nervous system to reduce pain perception. Despite the lack of anti-inflammatory activity, studies have shown that acetaminophen is as effective as most NSAIDs.[53] Given in a dose of 650–1000 mg qid it remains the safest analgesic medication compared to traditional NSAIDs and other analgesic drugs for most patients. Unfortunately, overdose or long-term use of high-dose acetaminophen can result in irreversible hepatic necrosis. Therefore, the maximum daily dose should never exceed 4000 mg, and those with hepatic dysfunction or alcoholism should have doses reduced by 50%–75% to avoid liver damage.[17] Patients on long-term, high-dose acetaminophen (4 g/day) should probably undergo periodic monitoring of liver function.

Non-Steroidal Anti-Inflammatory Drugs

The NSAIDs have analgesic activity both peripherally and centrally. They are potent inhibitors of prostaglandin synthesis, which have effects on inflammation, pain receptors, and nerve conduction and may have central effects as well.[54] For inflammatory arthritis or when maximum safe doses of acetaminophen do not adequately control pain, NSAID therapy may be beneficial.[17] However, the long-term use of traditional NSAIDs is associated with an unacceptable rate of life-threatening gastrointestinal bleeding.[55] Although the risk is reduced with the concomitant use of misoprostol or proton pump inhibitors, these additional agents also may not be well tolerated in elderly persons.[56–59] Therapy with NSAIDs is also associated with a propensity to cause renal impairment, particularly in patients with diabetes, gout, or diuresis. Many of these drugs also have substantial effects on platelet function, resulting in prolonged bleeding times.[60,61] Many NSAIDs have been noted to occasionally have drug–drug and drug–disease interactions, which may adversely affect the treatment of hypertension and other common chronic diseases.[62] It is important to note that all NSAIDS have a ceiling to their effects and limited potency for patients with moderate to severe pain problems. For some patients, chronic opioid therapy, low-dose or intermittent corticosteroid therapy, or other non-opioid analgesic drug strategies may have fewer life-threatening risks compared to long-term NSAID use.[7]

For patients with mild to moderate pain who require long-term NSAID therapy and have no specific contraindications, the current evidence, weighing efficacy versus adverse effects, supports the use of cyclo-oxygenase-2 (COX-2)–selective agents such as rofecoxib and celecoxib.[17,63–65] Unfortunately, the cost of these agents is prohibitive for many patients. The nonacetylated salicylates (e.g., choline magnesium trisalicylate, salsalate) may provide a relatively safe and less expensive alternative to the newer agents.[17] The COX-2-selective agents appear to have a dramatically lower incidence of gastrointestinal bleeding and perhaps less antiplatelet effect, but other properties appear to be similar to traditional nonselective NSAIDs. Of recent concern is a possible adverse effect of these agents on cardiovascular events in persons at risk for stroke or heart attack.[66] Studies suggest that patients at risk for stroke or heart attack should continue to take aspirin or other antiplatelet agents to reduce the risk of cardiovascular events.[17] It is important to understand that the nuances of NSAID therapy continue to be researched, and clinicians are advised to watch the current literature and other sources for the most current information on NSAID therapy. Table 16–2 lists the COX-2-selective agents and other examples of NSAIDs for pain.

Opioid Analgesic Medications

Opioid analgesic medications act by blocking receptors in the central nervous system (brain and spinal cord), resulting in decreased perception of pain. Many opioids also have a similar mode of action as local anesthetics and have recently found widespread use in epidural anesthesia. Selected opioid analgesic medications are listed in Table 16–3. Opioid drugs have no ceiling to their analgesic effects and have been shown to relive all types of pain. Short-term studies have suggested that elderly people, compared to younger people, may require lower doses of these drugs for pain relief.[67–70]

It is important for clinicians who prescribe opioid analgesics to understand issues of tolerance, dependence, and addiction. *Tolerance* is a pharmacological phenomenon that occurs with many drugs, defined by diminished effect of a drug associated with constant exposure to the drug over time.[71] Opiate drugs have a number of side effects, most of which resolve over hours to days as tolerance develops. Tolerance develops rapidly to the side effects of sedation, associated respiratory depression, and nausea. Informing patients and families in advance of the possibility of these effects, how to manage them effectively, and their short-term nature contributes to the adherence to and long-term success of analgesic therapy. Unfortunately, tolerance does not develop to constipation, and aggressive pre-emptive management of this uncomfortable and at times life-threatening side effect is a mandatory component of rational opiate analgesic therapy. Tolerance rarely develops to the analgesic effects of opiates; if pain escalates while opiates are used, it is most often due to progression of underlying disease.[72,73]

Opioid drugs have the potential to cause cognitive disturbances, respiratory depression, and constipation; and when used chronically, they can cause physical symptoms on abrupt cessation in older people. Drowsiness, performance-based measures of cognitive impairment, and respiratory depression associated with opioids should be anticipated when opioids are initiated and doses are escalated rapidly. Drowsiness, cognitive impairment, and respiratory depression occur in a dose-dependent fash-

Table 16–2. Acetaminophen and Selected Non-Steroidal Anti-Inflammatory Drugs (NSAIDs) for Pain*

Drug	Maximum dose	Description	Comments
Acetaminophen (Tylenol)	4000 mg/qd	Drug of choice for mild to moderate pain	Adjust dose by 50% in patients with impaired hepatic metabolism
Aspirin	4000 mg/qd (q4–6h dosing)	Prototype NSAID, non-selective COX enzyme inhibitor	Salicylate levels may be helpful in monitoring
Celecoxib (Celebrex)	200 mg bid	Selective COX-2 inhibition, pain and anti-inflammatory activity similar to other NSAIDs	Less gastric toxicity, less platelet inhibition
Refocoxib (Vioxx)	50 mg qd	Selective COX-2 inhibition. pain and anti-inflammatory activity similar to other NSAIDs	Less gastric toxicity, less platelet inhibition
Nabumetone (Relafen)	2000 mg qd	Partially COX-2-selective, gastric toxicity may be less, occasionally requires q12h dosing	Avoid maximum dose for prolonged periods
Salsalate (Disalcid)	3000 mg qd h (q6–8h dosing)	Hydrolyzed in small intestine to aspirin	Elderly may require dose adjustment downward to avoid salicylate toxicity, salicylate levels may be helpful in monitoring
Ibuprofen (Motrin by prescription; Advil, Nuprin, and others otc†)	2400 mg qd (q6–8h dosing)	Gastric, renal, and abnormal platelet function may be dose-dependent; constipation, confusion, and headaches may be more common in older persons	Avoid high doses for prolonged periods of time
Naproxen (Naprosyn by prescription, Aleve and others otc)	1000 mg qd (q8–12h dosing)	Same as ibuprofen, may require a loading dose	Same as ibuprofen
Diflunisal (Dolobid)	1000 mg qd maximum dose, loading = 1000 mg then 500 q12h or 750 mg then 250 mg q8h in small patients or frail elderly	Relatively good analgesic properties but requires loading dose	Dose may need downward adjustment for small patients or frail elderly
Ketorolac (Toradol)	Only NSAID approved for IM administration, –120 mg qd (30–60 mg loading dose, followed by half the loading dose, 15–30 mg q6h, limited to not more than 5 days) po 60 mg qd (q6h dosing limited to not more that 14 days)	Substantial gastrointestinal toxicity as well as renal and platelet dysfunction, relatively high postoperative complications documented	Duration of treatment limited because of high toxicity, reduce dose by half for those <50 kg or >65 years of age

*Limited number of examples provided. For comprehensive lists of other available NSAIDs and a host of brand names, clinicians should consult other sources. COX, cyclo-oxygenase. †otc, over-the-counter or available without prescription.

Table 16–3. Selected Opioid Analgesic Medications for Pain*

Drug	Starting dose (oral)	Description	Comments
Tramadol (Ultram)	25 mg (q4–6h dosing)	Weak opioid, mixed opioid and CNS neurotransmitter mechanisms, has ceiling limitations.	Monitor for opioid side effects, drowsiness, nausea, etc.
Codeine (plain codeine, Tylenol 3, other combinations with acetaminophen or NSAIDs)	30–60 mg (q4–6h dosing)	Acetaminophen or NSAIDs limit dose, nausea and constipation are major issues with acetaminophen or NSAIDs	Begin bowel program early, do not exceed maximum dose for
Hydrocodone (Norco, Vicodin, Vicoprofen, others)	5–10 mg (q3–4h dosing)	Toxicity similar to morphine, acetaminophen or NSAID combinations limit maximum dose	Same as above
Oxycodone (Roxicodone, OxyIR, or in combinations with acetaminophen or NSAIDs such as Percocet, Tylox, Percodan, others)	20–30 mg (q3–4h dosing)	Toxicity similar to morphine, acetaminophen or NSAID combinations limit maximum dose, available generically as a single agent	Same as above
Sustained-release oxycodone (Oxicontin)	15–30 mg (q12h dosing)	Similar to sustained-release morphine	Similar to sustained-release morphine
Morphine (Roxanol, morphine sulfate immediate-release)	30 mg (q4h dosing)	Short to intermediate half-life, older people more sensitive than younger people to side effects	Titrate to comfort, continuous use for continuous pain, intermittent use for episodic pain, anticipate and prevent side effects
Hydromorphone (Dilaudid)	4 mg (q3–4h dosing)	Half-life may be shorter than morphine, toxicity similar to morphine	Similar to morphine
Sustained-release morphine (MS Contin, Oramorph, Kadian)	MS Contin: 30–60 mg (q12h dosing) Oramorph: 30–60 mg (q12h dosing) Kadian: 30–60 mg (q24h dosing)	Morphine sulfate in a wax matrix tablet or sprinkles, MS Contin and Oramorph should not be broken or crushed, Kadian capsules can be opened and sprinkled on food but should not be crushed	Titrate dose slowly because of drug accumulation, immediate-release opioid analgesic always necessary for breakthrough pain
Transderm fentanyl (Duragesic)	25 μg patch (q72h dosing)	Reservoir for drug is in the skin, not in the patch; equivalent dose compared to other opioids is not very predictable (see package insert); effective activity may exceed 72 h in older patients	Titrate slowly using immediate-release analgesics for breakthrough pain, peak effect of first dose may take 18–24 h, not recommended for opioid-naive patients
Fentanyl lozenge on an applicator stick	Rub on bucal mucosa until analgesia occurs, then discard	Short half-life, useful for acute and breakthrough pain when oral route is not possible	Absorbed via bucal mucosa, not effective when swallowed

*Limited number of examples are provided. For comprehensive lists of other available opioids, clinicians should consult other sources. CNS, central nervous system; NSAID, nonsteroidal anti-inflammatory drug.

ion and can be used to judge dose escalations. If patients have unrelieved pain with little drowsiness or cognitive impairment, doses may be escalated without much fear of sudden respiratory depression. When drowsiness does occur, tolerance to these side effects usually develops in a few days, at which time patients usually return to an alert status and baseline cognitive function. Until this adjustment takes place, patients should be instructed not to drive and to take precautions against falls or other accidents. Once tolerance to these effects has developed, patients can return to normal activities, including driving and other demanding tasks despite the regular use of opioid drugs. In fact, cancer patients are often observed to have improved physical function, alertness, and mood once pain is adequately relieved on opioid analgesics.[47]

Constipation is a side effect of opioid drugs to which older patients do not develop tolerance. The management of constipation usually includes increasing fluid intake, maintaining mobility, and use of multiple cathartic medications. Some patients find relief with remedies like prune juice or other natural laxatives. Most patients require osmotic laxatives such as milk of magnesia, lactolose, or sorbitol and many also require simultaneous use of potent stimulant laxatives such as senna or biscodyl. Stimulants should not be used until distal fecal impactions have been removed through digital rectal exam or enemas and obstruction has been ruled out. Finally, some patients require regular enemas to ensure bowel evacuation during high-dose opioid administration for severe pain.[16,74]

Nausea also occasionally complicates opioid therapy. Nausea from opioid medications may result from several mechanisms (gastroparesis, constipation, and central nervous system) and usually wanes as tolerance develops. Rapid development of nausea postopiate administration is often associated with gastroparesis, and a prokinetic agent such as metoclopramide may be most effective. Centrally mediated opiate-induced nausea is best treated with antidopaminergic agents, such as prochlorper-

azine or haloperidol. Antihistamines such as diphenhydramine orally or intravenously may also be effective. Aggressive identification and treatment of constipation is a mainstay of therapy for opiate-associated nausea. It should be remembered that antinausea agents have high side-effect profiles in elderly patients, including movement disorders, delirium, and anticholinergic effects. Thus, clinicians should choose antiemetic medications with the lowest side effects and monitor patients frequently.[17]

Dependence is also a pharmacological phenomenon associated with many drugs, such as corticosteroids and β-blockers. Dependence is present when patients experience uncomfortable or dangerous side effects when the drug is withheld abruptly. For example, abrupt discontinuation of corticosteroids can lead to adrenal crisis, and steroids are carefully tapered to prevent this. Drug dependence from opiates or develops after constant exposure to the agent for days to weeks. Symptoms associated with overly rapid opioid taper may include anorexia, nausea, diaphoresis, tachycardia, hypertension, and fever. Worsening symptoms may including skin mottling, gooseflesh, and frank autonomic crisis.[71] Fortunately, these symptoms can be easily prevented by tapering opioids at a rate of 50% per day over a few days. Clonidine given short term in titrated doses will usually control serious autonomic or uncomfortable symptoms associated with abrupt discontinuation or overly rapid taper of opiates. The physiological effects of opioid withdrawal are usually not life-threatening compared to the serious abrupt withdrawal complications common with corticosteroids, β-blockers, alcohol, benzodiazepines, or barbiturates.[71]

Addiction is a psychiatric and behavioral problem. Addictive behavior is defined by compulsive drug seeking and use despite negative physical and social consequences and the craving for effects other than pain relief. Addicted patients often have erratic behavior that can be observed in a clinical setting in the form of selling, buying, and procuring drugs on the street and the use of medication by bizarre means, such as dis-

solving tablets for self-intravenous administration. It is now clear that prior exposure to opiates is not the major factor in
the development of addiction. Other psychiatric, medical, social, and economic factors play immense roles in addictive behavior.[75] It is also important to not
construe all drug-seeking behaviors as necessarily addictive behaviors. In undertreated medically ill patients with pain,
hoarding of medications, persistent or
worsening pain complaints, frequent office
visits, requests for dose escalations, and
other behaviors associated with unrelieved
pain point to the syndrome of iatrogenic
pseudoaddiction.[76] Laws, regulations, and
unintentionally inadequate or underpre-
scribing behavior by clinicians may require
patients to hoard medication and turn to
other physicians for additional help in
achieving appropriate pain relief. In fact,
true psychiatric addiction is rare among patients taking opioid analgesic medications
for medical reasons. This is not meant to
imply that opioid drugs can be used indis-
criminately, only that fear of opiate addiction and side effects does not justify failure
to effectively treat pain in elderly patients,
especially those near the end of life.

Fear of addiction has been identified as
a major barrier to pain management in elderly people.[77] Unfortunately, fears by clinicians and patients have been overinfluenced
by social pressures to reduce illegal drug
use among younger people and those that
take opiate drugs for psychiatric and emotional, rather than medical, reasons. Regulation of controlled substances by state and
federal authorities as well as scrutiny of
physician practices by state license boards
have intimidated clinicians, so many will
not prescribe potent analgesic medications
even for those with severe pain in the context of serious medical illness. Real and
imagined fear of undertreatment of pain
and other symptoms may actually contribute in cases where patients seek suicide
rather that endure inadequately managed
pain. Many organizations, such as the
American Medical Association, the American College of Physicians, and the American Geriatrics Society, have released posi-

tion statements supporting comfort and the
control of pain in patients with serious
medical illness and for those near the end
of life. As emphasized by these organizations, clinicians have an obligation to provide comfort, pain relief, and dignity for
patients even if such interventions may
shorten life by a few hours or days.[3,78,79]

It is beyond the scope of this chapter to
review individual analgesic drugs. However, a few drugs with special problems in
elderly persons should be discussed.
Meperidine (Demerol) should be avoided
because it has an active metabolite
(normeperidine) that accumulates in renal
impairment and can cause neuroexcitatory
toxicity and seizures.[80] Pentazocine (Tal-
win) has both agonist and antagonist opiate receptor activity and is associated with
a high incidence of delirium in elderly people.[81] Like pentazocine, butorphanol (Sta-
dol) has mixed opiate receptor activity and
can displace other opioid analgesic compounds from the receptor, resulting in immediate withdrawal symptoms, including
autonomic crisis.[82] Methadone is a potent
opiate receptor agonist whose use for pain
control has gone in and out of fashion over
the years. It has regained the interest of pain
management physicians recently because it
is inexpensive, long-acting, and thought to
be effective for both neuropathic and nociceptive pain. It may also slow the development of opioid tolerance through partial N-
methyl-D-aspartate receptor activity.[83]
However, methadone is difficult to titrate
because of its long and variable half-life.
This property is onerous in older persons
because the analgesic half-life may be substantially shorter than the serum half-life,
resulting in a propensity for both under-
dosing and overdosing, with the risk of
late development of sedation. Methadone
should be used very carefully in elderly persons by clinicians with substantial experience in closely monitored settings.

Other Nonopioid Medications for Pain

A variety of other medications not formally
classified as analgesics have been found to
be helpful in certain specific pain problems. The term *adjuvant analgesic drugs*, al-

though frequently used, is a misnomer in that some of these nonopioid drugs may be the primary pain-relieving pharmacological intervention in certain cases. Table 16–4 provides some examples of nonopioid drugs that may help certain kinds of pain. The largest body of evidence available relates to the use of these drugs for neuropathic pain, such as diabetic neuropathies, postherpetic neuralgia, and trigeminal neuralgia. These drugs have also had limited success in pain syndromes that are not associated with neuropathic mechanisms.[84,85] Fifty to seventy percent of patients have a measurable response but only partial pain relief.[84–86] One exception may be trigeminal neuralgia, where carbamazepine is probably the drug of choice.[16] Usually, these agents work best in combination with other traditional drug and non-drug strategies, to improve pain and keep drug doses and toxicities at a minimum. Failure of response to one particular class of drugs does not necessarily predict failure of another class of agents. In general, nonopioid medications for neuropathic pain should be chosen according to side-effect profile.[17] Treatment should start with lower doses than those recommended for younger patients, and doses should be escalated slowly based on the known pharmacokinetics of individual drugs, drug–drug interaction, renal and hepatic function, as well as appropriate knowledge of disease-specific treatment strategies. Unfortunately, most of the nonopioid medications for pain management have high side-effect profiles in elderly people and must be monitored carefully.

Tricyclic antidepressants have been the most widely studied class of nonopioid medications for pain. The mechanism of action for these drugs is not entirely known but probably has to do with interruption of norepinephrine- and serotonin-mediated mechanisms in the brain.[84] For neuropathic pain, the major effect of these drugs is not their mood-altering capacity, although this may also be helpful in those with concurrent depression. A randomized placebo-controlled trial of amitriptyline, desipramine, and fluoxetine indicated that desipramine may be as effective as amitriptyline but fluoxetine is no better than placebo for the treatment of diabetic neuropathy.[86] Thus, desipramine may be a better choice because it has fewer anticholinergic side effects than amitriptyline. Other studies of the selective serotonin reuptake inhibitors, which have lower side-effect profiles for elderly people, have had mixed reviews; and most have not been effective for pain management.[17]

It has been known for many years that antiepileptic medication may relieve the pain of trigeminal neuralgia (tic douloureux).[87] Compounds such as diphenylhydantoin, carbamazepine, and valproic acid may also help diabetic neuralgia and other neuropathic pain in some patients. The usefulness of these drugs has been limited by their high side-effect profiles in elderly people and the fact that most patients respond only partially, making the overall risk/benefit ratio rather large in this population. Indeed, these drugs are not simple analgesics and should not be used for the relief of trivial aches and pains.[16] Of recent interest has been the effectiveness of gabapentin for the treatment of diabetic neuralgia and postherpetic neuralgia.[88,89] Clinical observations suggest that this agent has a significant analgesic effect on neuropathic pain with a much lower side-effect profile compared to other antiepilepic drugs and most tricyclic antidepressants. The major side effect of gabapentin is sedation and dizziness.

Several local anesthetics have also been shown to relieve neuropathic pain when administrated systemically in addition to their known local anesthetic effects. Successful analgesia with intravenous lidocaine has been found to sometimes predict response to other anticonvulsant and systemically administered local anesthetics.[87] Mexiletine (Mexil), similar to lidocaine but active orally, has also shown some activity against neuropathic pain of diabetic neuralgia. Although this drug also has a high risk/benefit ratio, some studies have reported response rates at lower doses than are often recommended for cardiac arrhythmias.[90]

Finally, chronic pain associated with osteoporotic fractures may improve with cal-

Table 16–4. Selected Nonopioid Medications for Pain*

Drug	Description	Comments
Tricyclic antidepressants (amitriptyline, desipramine, nortriptyline, others)	Anticholinergic effects may outweigh benefits in many older patients; desipramine or nortriptyline is a better choice than amitriptyline	Complete relief unusual, used best as adjunct to other strategies, start low and increase slowly every 3–5 days, SSRI antidepressants may have no effect on pain but may be helpful in management of concurrent depression
Anticonvulsants gabapentin, carbamazepine	Gabapentin may have more favorable side-effect profile over other anticonvulsans and tricyclic antidepressants	Start low and increase slowly
Anti-arrhythmics (mexiletine [Mexitil])	Common side effects include tremor, dizziness, paresthesias; rarely may cause blood dyscrasias and hepatic damage	Avoid use in patients with pre-existing heart disease, start low and titrate slowly, monitor EKGs
Local anesthetics (lidocaine intravenous or transdermal patch [Lidoderm], capsaicin)	IV lidocaine associated with delirium, transdermal patch may have systemic absorption, Capsaicin depletes nerve endings of substance P	IV lidocaine may predict response to anticonvulsants and anti-arrhythmics; may apply up to three patches; alternating 12 h intervals may improve pain, reduce denervation hypersensitivity, and decrease systemic absorption; may take 2 weeks to peak effect
Muscle-relaxants (baclofen, chlorzoxazone [Paraflex], cyclobenzaprine [Flexaril])	Sedation, anticholinergic effects, abrupt withdrawal of baclofen may cause CNS irritability	Mechanism of action nct precisely known, monitor for sedation and anticholinergic effects, taper baclofen on discontinuation
Substance P inhibitors (capsaicin available otc, for topical use only)	Burning pain during depletion of substance P may be intolerable by as many as 30% of patients, may take 14 days for maximum response, avoid eye contamination	Start with small doses, can be partially removed with vegetable oil
NMDA inhibitors (ketamine dextromethorphan)	N-Methyl-D-aspartate antagonists, ketamine is a potent anesthetic, dextromethorphan is a common cough-suppressant	Ketamine only available IV, both may cause delirium
Drugs for osteoporosis (calcitonin, bisphosphonates)	Pain-relief mechanisms unknown	Not effective on pain other than osteoporosis
Corticosteroids (prednisone dexamethasone)	Decrease inflammation in many tissues	Classic corticosteroid side effects limit overall usefulness in chronic pain

*Limited number of examples provided. For comprehensive lists of other available medications for pain clinicians should consult other sources. CNS, central nervous system; otc, over the counter; SSRI, selective serotonin reuptake inhibitor; EKG, electrocardiogram.

citonin.[91] Most investigators of the effects of calcitonin on osteoporosis have anecdotally reported that pain improves significantly. These studies were not designed to assess pain, but results thus far are encouraging.

ANESTHETIC AND NEUROSURGICAL APPROACHES TO PAIN MANAGEMENT

A wide variety of anesthetic and neurosurgical approaches are available for recalcitrant pain, and some require highly specialized skills.[92] Table 16–5 lists some common anesthetic and neurosurgical interventions for severe pain. Although it is beyond the scope of this chapter to review the details of all of these techniques, a few deserve mention.

Trigger point injections have been used extensively for the treatment of myofascial pain syndromes. Myfascial pain with trigger points were first recognized more than 50 years ago.[93] In a relatively high percentage of cases, trigger points may initiate a reflex mechanism that produces referred pain, tenderness, and muscle spasm. With local injection of the trigger point followed by stretching and reconditioning of the muscles, the myofascial pain syndrome usually subsides. Similar results have been obtained using ice massage or vapocoolant spray applied topically, followed by specific muscle-stretching and physical therapy techniques.[94]

Continuous drug infusions are highly effective for providing steady-state analgesic drug levels. Continuous infusions can be maintained by implantable pumps or external devices to deliver intravenous, subcutaneous, intrathecal, or epidural medications. Continuous infusions of opioid drugs have found widespread use in severe chronic cancer pain, especially among those near the end of life. Other uses have included continuous infusion of muscle-relaxants for patients with severe muscle spasm from spinal injury, multiple sclerosis, or end-stage Parkinson's disease.

Whether these invasive hi-tech strategies are appropriate for patients with all kinds of chronic pain remains unclear. Use of these techniques is very expensive but often reimbursed by third-party payers, including Medicare. These issues have raised ethical questions about the application of high-tech strategies for patients who might be equally well managed using oral medications that are not reimbursable.[95,96] In general, these methods should be used only when oral medications become ineffective or the oral route of administration is no longer viable. More work needs to be done to justify these risky and expensive techniques that need to be carefully monitored in nursing homes, home care, and other low-tech, long-term care settings.

NONDRUG STRATEGIES FOR PAIN MANAGEMENT

Nondrug strategies, used alone or in combination with appropriate analgesic medications, should be an integral part of the care plan for most elderly patients with significant pain problems. Nondrug strategies for pain management encompass a broad range of treatments and physical modalities, most of which carry low risks for adverse effects (Table 16–6). Used in combination with appropriate drug regimens, these interventions often enhance therapeutic effects while allowing medication doses to be kept low to prevent side effects.[17]

Among the nondrug interventions, the importance of patient education cannot be overstated. Studies have shown that patient education programs alone significantly improve overall pain management, but they often work even better with accompanied by actual practice of self-management and coping strategies.[97,98] Such programs often include content about the nature of pain, how to use pain diaries and pain assessment instruments, how to use medications appropriately, and how to use self-help nondrug strategies. Whether conducted in groups or individually, education should be tailored for individual patient needs and

Table 16–5. Anesthetic or Neurosurgical Pain Management Techniques

Procedure	Possible indications	Comments
Continuous-infusion opioids (morphine, hydromorphone, fentanyl)	Perioperative pain; severe cancer pain when oral, transdermal, rectal routes have failed	Subcutaneous infusions usually well tolerated by patients in nursing homes or home care, IV infusions require more skilled monitoring
Implantable pumps or reservoirs (sufentanil, muscle-relaxants, others)	Severe recalcitrant pain, severe spastic paralysis, other rare conditions	Expensive; a variety of highly reliable and programmable pump is available for epidural, intrathecal, or intraventricular delivery
Epidural analgesia (intermittent local anesthetics or opioids or continuous opioids)	Perioperative pain, severe cancer pain when oral route has failed	Can be supplied by external or internally implanted pumps, does not avoid constipation and occasional delirium, serious complications are rare but can be devastating
Nerve blocks	Mononeuropathies, postherpetic neuralgia, intercostal nerve pain	Usually temporary relief limited to a few days or weeks
Intrathecal analgesia	Perioperative pain	Can cause respiratory depression
Stellate ganglia blockade	Sympathetically mediated pain of the upper extremity	Not to be confused with complex regional pain syndromes
Lumbar sympathetic blockade	Sympathetically mediated pain of the lower extremity, peripheral vascular disease	May cause orthostatic hypotension
Celiac plexus blockade	Severe pain from carcinoma of pancreas	Requires substantial skill
Neuroablation (permanent nerve destruction)	Severe recalcitrant mononeuropathic pain	May recur after several years
Cordotomy	Severe recalcitrant cancer pain	May not relieve all pain
Neurostimulation (dorsal column or thalamic)	Severe recalcitrant pain usually following thalamic stroke or spinal cord injury	Requires substantial skill

Source: Ferrell.[105]

Table 16–6. Selected Nondrug Strategies for Pain Management

Intervention	Comments	Limitations
Education	Content should include basic knowledge about pain (diagnosis, treatment, complications, and prognosis), other available treatment options, and information about over-the-counter medications and self-help strategies	May require substantial time, may be enhanced by association with actual practice of self-management and coping strategies
Exercise	Can be tailored for individual patient needs and lifestyle, moderate-intensity exercise should be maintained for 30 minutes or more 3–4 times a week and continued indefinitely	Maintenance is critical, but difficult to continue indefinitely
Cognitive-behavioral therapy	Should be conducted by a trained therapist	Requires substantial cognitive function
Physical modalities (heat, cold, and massage)	A variety of techniques are available for application	Heat and cold should be used with caution in those with cognitive impairment to avoid thermal injuries
Physical or occupational therapy	Should be conducted by a trained therapist; physical therapy for transfer, gait, and balance training; occupational therapy for activities of daily living	Can be expensive if not reimbursed, usually limited to periods of recovery and not maintenance therapy
Chiropractic	As effective as other treatments for acute back pain	Potential spinal cord or nerve root impingement should be ruled out prior to any spinal manipulation
Acupuncture	Should be provided only by a qualified acupuncturist	Effects may be short-lived and require repetitive treatments
Transcutaneous electrical nerve stimulation (TENS)	Should initially be applied and adjusted by an experienced professional	Effects are often short-lived, clear placebo effects have been observed
Relaxation and distraction techniques	Therapeutic modalities require individual buy-in and substantial training	Patients with cognitive impairment may not be good candidates

Source: Ferrell.[105]

level of understanding. Written materials and methods of reinforcement are important to the overall success of the program.

Physical exercise is important for most patients with pain. A program of exercise can be tailored to most patients' needs and is extremely important for rehabilitation and the maintenance of mobility, strength, and endurance. Clinical trials of older patients with chronic musculoskeletal pain have shown that moderate levels of exercise (aerobic and resistance training) on a regular basis are effective at improving pain and functional status.[99–101] Initial training for chronic pain patients usually requires 8–12 weeks with supervision by a professional who can focus on the needs of older people with musculoskeletal disorders. There is no evidence that one form of exercise is better than another, so programs can be tailored for the individual's needs, lifestyle, and preferences. The intensity of exercise along with frequency and duration must be adjusted to avoid exacerbation of the underlying condition while gradually increasing and later maintaining overall conditioning. It is important to remember that feeling better often gives rise to a false impression that the discipline of regular exercise is not necessary. Continued encouragement and reinforcement are often required. Unless complications arise, the program of exercise should be maintained indefinitely to prevent deconditioning and deterioration.

Psychological strategies are also helpful for some with significant pain. Cognitive therapies aim at altering belief systems and attitudes about pain and suffering and include various forms of improving coping skills, distraction, relaxation, biofeedback, and hypnosis. Behavioral therapies aim at enhancing healthy behaviors and discouraging behaviors that are unpredictable and self-defeating. Cognitive therapy can be combined with behavioral approaches, and together they are known as cognitive-behavioral therapy. Cognitive-behavioral therapy in its purest form includes a structured approach to teaching coping skills that might be used alone or in combination with analgesic medications and other non-drug strategies for pain control. Effective programs can be conducted by trained professionals with individual patients or in groups, and there is some evidence that the effect is enhanced with caregiver involvement.[102,103] Although it may not be appropriate for those with significant cognitive impairment, there is evidence from randomized trials to support the use of cognitive-behavioral therapy for many patients with chronic pain.

Finally, a variety of alternative therapies are also used by many patients. Many patients seek alternative medicine approaches with or without the knowledge or recommendation of their physician or other primary-care provider. Alternative medicine approaches to chronic pain may include homeopathy, spiritual healing, or the growing market of vitamin, herbal, and natural remedies. Although there is little scientific evidence to support these strategies for pain control, it is important that health-care providers not abandon patients or leave them with a sense of hopelessness[104] as a consequence of their use of complementary and alternative modalitites.

REFERENCES

1. Ferrell BA. Overview of aging and pain. In: Ferrell BR, Ferrell BA (Eds.). Pain in the Elderly. Seattle, IASP Press, pp. 1–10, 1996.
2. Ferrell BA, Ferrell BR, Osterweil D. Pain in the nursing home. J Am Geriatr Soc 38:409–414, 1990.
3. AGS Ethics Committee. The care of dying patients: a position statement. J Am Geriatr Soc 43:577–578, 1995.
4. Helm RD, Gibson SJ. Pain in older people. In: Cronbie IK, Croft R, Linton SJ, Leresche L, Von Dorff M (Eds.). Epidemiology of Pain. Seattle, IASP Press, Chapter 8, pp. 103–112, 2000.
5. Helm RD, Gibson SJ. Epidemiology of pain in elderly people. Clin Geriatr Med 17:417–431, 2001.
6. Cooner E, Amorosi S. The Study of Pain and Older Americans. New York, Louis Harris and Associates, 1997.
7. Ferrell BA. Pain evaluation and management in the nursing home. Ann Intern Med 123:681–687, 1995.

8. Ferrell BA, Ferrell BR, Rivera L. Pain in cognitively impaired nursing home patients. J Pain Symptom Manage 10: 591–598, 1995.

9. Bernabei R, Bambassi G, Lapane K, et al. Management of pain in elderly patients with cancer. JAMA 279:1877–1882, 1998.

10. Morrison RS, Sui AL. A comparison of pain and its treatment in advanced dementia and cognitively intact patients with hip fracture. J Pain Symptom Manage 19:240–248, 2000.

11. Feldt KS, Ryden MB, Miles S. Treatment of pain in cognitively impaired compared to cognitively intact older patients with hip fracture. J Am Geriatr Soc 46: 1079–1085, 1998.

12. Reyes-Gibby CC, Aday L, Cleeland C. Impact of pain on self-rated health in the community-dwelling older adults. Pain 95:75–82, 2002.

13. Ferrell BA. Pain management in elderly people. J Am Geriatr Soc 39:64–73, 1991.

14. Merskey H, Bogduk N (Eds.). Classification of Chronic Pain, 2nd ed. Seattle, IASP Press, 1994.

15. Acute Pain Management Guideline Panel. Acute Pain Management: Post-operative or Medical Procedures and Trauma. Clinical Practice Guideline. #1 AHCPR Publication 92-0032. Rockville, MD, Agency for Health Care Policy and Research, Public Health Service, US Department of Health and Human Services, 1993.

16. AGS Panel on Chronic Pain in Older Persons. The management of chronic pain in older persons. J Am Geriatr Soc 46:635–651, 1998.

17. AGS Panel on Persistent Pain in Older Persons. The management of persistent pain in older persons. J Am Geriatr Soc, in press.

18. Max MB, Payne R (Eds.). Principles of Analgesic use in Treatment of Acute Pain and Cancer Pain, 4th ed. Glenview, IL, American Pain Society, 1999.

19. Myer RA, Campbell JN, Raja SN. Peripheral and neural mechanisms of nociception. In: Wall PD, Melzack R (Eds.). Textbook of Pain, 3rd ed. New York, Churchill Livingstone, pp. 13–44, 1994.

20. Bennett GF. Neuropathic pain. In: Wall PD, Melzack R (Eds.). Textbook of Pain, 3rd ed. New York, Churchill Livingstone, pp. 201–224, 1994.

21. Craig KD. Emotional aspects of pain. In: Wall PD, Melzack R (Eds.). Textbook of Pain, 3rd ed. New York, Churchill Livingstone, pp. 261–274, 1994.

22. Gibson SJ, Helme RD. Age differences in pain perception and report: a review of

23. Gibson SJ, Helme RD. Age related differences in pain perception and report. Clin Geriatr Med 17:433–456, 2001.

24. Ferrell BA. Pain assessment. In: Osterweil D, Brummel Smith K, Beck JC (Eds.). Comprehensive Geriatric Assessment. New York, McGraw-Hill, pp. 381–397, 2000.

25. Herr KA, Garand L. Assessment and measurement of pain in older adults. Clin Geriatr Med 17:457–478, 2001.

26. Nishikawa ST, Ferrell BA. Pain assessment in the elderly. Clin Geriatr Issues Long Term Care 1:15–28, 1993.

27. Gloth FM III. Pain management in older adults: prevention and treatment. J Am Geriatr Soc 40:188–199, 2001.

28. Gloth FM III, Scheve AA, Stober CV, et al. The functional pain scale: reliability, validity and responsiveness in an elderly population. J Am Med Dir Assoc 2: 110–114, 2001.

29. Kerns RD, Jacob MC. Assessment of the psychosocial context of the experience of pain. In: Turk DC, Melzack R (Eds.). Handbook of Pain Assessment. New York, Guilford Press, pp. 235–253, 1992.

30. Parmalee PA, Katz IR, Lawton MP. The relation of pain to depression among institutionalized aged. J Gerontol 46:15–21, 1991.

31. Chochinov HM, Wilson KG, Enns M, Lander S. "Are you depressed?" Screening for depression in the terminally ill. Am J Psychiatry 154:674–676, 1997.

32. Keefe FJ, Beaupre PM, Weiner DK, Siegler IC. Pain in older adults: a cognitive behavioral perspective. In: Ferrell BR, Ferrell BA (Eds.). Pain in the Elderly. Seattle, IASP Press, pp. 11–19, 1996.

33. Ferrell BR, Ferrell BA, Rhiner M, et al. Family factors influencing cancer pain. Postgrad Med J 67(Suppl 2):654–669, 1991.

34. Ferrell BA, Stein WM, Beck JC. The Geriatric Pain Measure: validity, reliability and factor analysis. J Am Geriatr Soc 48: 1669–1673, 2000.

35. Melzack R. The McGill Pain Questionnaire: major properties and scoring methods. Pain 1:277–299, 1975.

36. Melzack R. The Short-Form McGill Pain Questionnaire. Pain 30:191–197, 1987.

37. Melzack R, Katz J. The McGill Pain Questionnaire: appraisal and current status. In: Turk D, Melzack R (Eds.). Handbook of Pain Assessment. New York, Guilford Press, pp. 152–168, 1992.

38. Herr KA, Mobily PR, Kohour FJ, et al.

Evaluation of the Faces Pain Scale for use with the elderly. Clin J Pain 14:1–10, 1998.

39. Fishman B, Pasternak S, Wallenstein SL, Houde RW, Holland JC, Foley KA. The Memorial Pain Assessment Card: a valid instrument for the evaluation of cancer pain. Cancer 60:1151–1158, 1987.

40. Weiner DK, Peterson BL, Logue P, et al. Predictors of self-report in nursing home residents. Aging Clin Exp Res 10:411–420, 1998.

41. Parmelee AP, Smith BD, Katz IR. Pain complaints and cognitive status among elderly institutional residents. J Am Geriatr Soc 41:517–522, 1993.

42. O'Brien J, Francis A. The use of next-of-kin to estimate pain in cancer patients. Pain 35:171–178, 1988.

43. Von Roenn JH, Cleeland CS, Gonin R, Hatfield AK, Pandya KJ. Physician attitudes and practice in cancer pain management. A survey from the Eastern Cooperative Oncology Group. Ann Intern Med 119:121–126, 1993.

44. Camp DL. A comparison of nurses' assessments of pain as described by cancer patients. Cancer Nurs 11:237–243, 1988.

45. Hurley AC, Volicer BJ, Hanrahan PA, Houde S, Volicer V. Assessment of discomfort in advanced Alzheimer patients. Res Nurs Health 15:369–377, 1992.

46. Fabinszewiski KL, Folicer B, Volicer L. Effect of antibiotic treatment on outcomes of fevers in the institutionalized Alzheimer patients. JAMA 263:3168–3172, 1990.

47. Jocox A, Car DB, Payne R, et al. Management of Cancer Pain. Clinical Practice Guideline 9. AHCPR Publication 94-0592. Rockville, MD, Agency for Health Care Policy and Research, US Department of Health and Human Services, Public Health Service, 1994.

48. Foreman WB. Opioid analgesic drugs in the elderly. Clin Geriatr Med 12:489–500, 1996.

49. World Health Organization. Cancer Pain Relief, 2nd Ed. WHO Technical Report Series 804. Geneva, WHO, 1996.

50. Temple R, Ellenberg SS. Placebo-controlled trials and active control trials in the evaluation of new treatments: Part 1. Ethical and scientific issues. Ann Intern Med 133:455–463, 2000.

51. Turner JA, Deyo RA, Losser JD, et al. The importance of placebo effects in pain treatment and research. JAMA 271:1609–1614, 1994.

52. Hrobjartsson A, Totzsche PC. Is the placebo powerless? An analysis of clinical trials comparing placebo with no treatment. N Engl J Med 344:1594–1602, 2001.

53. Bradley JD, Brandt KD, Katz BP, et al. Comparison of an anti-inflammatory dose of ibuprofen, an analgesic dose of ibuprofen and acetaminophen in treatment of patients with osteoarthritis of the knee. N Engl J Med 325:87–91, 1991.

54. Roth SH. Merits and liabilities of NSAID therapy. Rheumatol Dis Clin North Am 15:479–498, 1989.

55. Griffin MR, Piper JM, Daugherty JR, et al. Nonsteroidal anti-inflammatory drug use and increased risk for peptic ulcer disease in elderly persons. Ann Intern Med 114:257–263, 1991.

56. Graham DY, White RH, Foreland LW, et al. Duodenal and gastric ulcer prevention with misoprostol in arthritis patients taking NSAIDs: Misoprostol Study Group. Ann Intern Med 119:257–262, 1993.

57. Ehsanullah RS, Page MC, Tildesley G, Wood JR. Prevention of gastroduodenal damage induced by non-steroidal anti-inflammatory drugs: controlled trial of ranitidine. BMJ 297:1017–1021, 1988.

58. Taha AS, Hudson N, Hawkey CJ, et al. Famotidine for the prevention of gastric and duodenal ulcers caused by nonsteroidal anti-inflammatory drugs. N Engl J Med 334:1435–1449, 1996.

59. Stucki J, Hohannesson M, Liang MH. Use of misoprostol in the elderly: is the expense justified? Drugs Aging 8:84–88, 1996.

60. Perneger TV, Shelton PK, Klag MJ. Risk of kidney failure associated with use of acetaminophen, aspirin and nonsteroidal antiinflammatory durgs. N Engl J Med 331:1675–1679, 1994.

61. Gurwitz JH, Avorn J, Ross-Degnan D, Sipsitz LA. Nonsteroidal anti-inflammatory drug associated azotemia in the very old. JAMA 264:471–475, 1990.

62. Pope JE, Anderson JJ, Felson DT. A meta-analysis of the effects of nonsteroidal anti-inflammatory drugs on blood pressure. Arch Intern Med 153:477–484, 1993.

63. Geba GP, Weaver AL, Polis AB, et al. Efficacy of rofecoxib, celecoxib and acetaminophen in osteoarthritis of the knee: a randomized trial. JAMA 287:64–71, 2002.

64. Bombardier C, Laine L, Reicin A, et al. Comparison of upper gastrointestinal toxicity of rofecoxib and naproxen in patients with rheumatoid arthritis. VIGOR Study Group. N Engl J Med 343:1520–1528, 2000.

65. Silverstein FE, Faich G, Golstein JL, et al. Gastrointestinal toxicity with celecoxib vs. nonsteroidal anti-inflammatory drugs for

osteoarthritis and rheumatoid arthritis. The CLASS study: a randomized controlled trial. Celecoxib Long-term Arthritis Safety Study. JAMA 284:1247–1255, 2000.

66. Mukherjee D, Nissen SE, Topol EJ. Risk of cardiovascular events associated with selective COX-2 inhibitors. JAMA 286: 954–959, 2001.

67. Kaiko RF. Age and morphine analgesia in cancer patients with postoperative pain. Clin Pharmacol Ther 28:823–826, 1980.

68. Bellville WJ, Forrest WH Jr, Miller E, Brown BW Jr. Influence of age on pain relief from analgesics: a study of postoperative patients. JAMA 217:1835–1841, 1971.

69. Kaiko RF, Wallenstein SL, Rogers AG, et al. Narcotics in the elderly. Med Clin North Am 66:1079–1089, 1982.

70. Ready BL, Chadwick HS, Ross B. Age predicts effective epidural morphine dose after abdominal hysterectomy. Anesth Analg 66:1215–1218, 1987.

71. Jaffe JH. Drug addiction and drug abuse. In: Goodman SLA, Gilman AG, Rall TW, Murad F (Eds.). Goodman and Gilman's The Pharmacological Basis of Therapeutics, 7th ed. New York, MacMillian, pp. 532–581, 1985.

72. Melzack R. The tragedy of needless pain. Sci Am 262:27–33, 1990.

73. Portenoy RK. Opiate therapy for chronic noncancer pain: can we get past the bias? Am Pain Soc Bull 1:4–7, 1991.

74. Derby S, Portenoy RK. Assessment and management of opioid-induced constipation. In: Portenoy RK, Bruera E (Eds.). Topics in Palliative Care, vol 1. New York, Oxford University Press, pp. 95–112, 1997.

75. Obrien CP. Drug addiction and drug abuse. In: Hardman JG, Limbird LE, Molinoff PB, Ruddon RW, Gilman AG (Eds.). Goodman and Gilman's The Pharmacological Basis of Therapeutics, 9th ed. New York, McGraw-Hill, pp. 557–580, 1996.

76. Weisman DE, Haddox JD. Opioid pseudo-addiction—an iatrogenic syndrome. Pain 36:363–366, 1989.

77. Portenoy RK. Opioid therapy for chronic non-malignant pain: current status. In: Fields HL, Libeskind JC (Eds.). Pharmacological Approaches to the Treatment of Chronic Pain. New Concepts and Critical Issues: Progress in Pain Research and Management, vol 11. Seattle, IASP Press, pp. 247–288, 1994.

78. Council on Scientific Affairs, American Medical Association. Good care of the dying patient. JAMA 275:474–478, 1996.

79. American College of Physicians and the ACP Ethics and Human Rights Committee. Ethics Manual, 4th ed. Ann Intern Med 128:576–594, 1998.

80. Kaiko RF, Foley KM, Gabinski PY, et al. Central nervous system excitatory effects of mepridine in cancer patients. Ann Neurol 13:180–185, 1983.

81. Hanks GW. The clinical usefulness of agonist-antagonist opioid analgesics in chronic pain. Drug Alcohol Depend 20: 339–346, 1987.

82. Nagashima H, Karamanian A, Malovany R, et al. Respiratory and circulatory effect of intravenous butorphanol and morphine. Clin Pharmacol Ther 19:738–745, 1976.

83. Fainsinger R, Schoeller T, Bruera E. Methadone in the management of cancer pain: a review. Pain 52:137–147, 1993.

84. Max MB. Antidepressants and analgesics. In: Fields HL Leibeskind JC (Eds.). Progress in Pain Research and Management, vol I. Seattle, IASP Press, pp. 229–246, 1994.

85. Onghena P, Van Houdenhove B. Antidepressant-induced analgesia in chronic nonmalignant pain: a metanalysis of 39 placebo-controlled studies. Pain 49:205–219, 1992.

86. Max MB, Lynch SA, Muir J, et al. Effects of desipramine, amytriptyline, and fluoxetine on pain in diabetic neuropathy. N Engl J Med 326:1250–1256, 1992.

87. Swerdlow M. The use of local anesthetics for relief of chronic pain. Pain Clinic 2:3–6, 1988.

88. Backonja M, Beydoun A, Edwards KR, Schwartz SL, Fonseca V, Hes M, LaMoreaux L, Garofalo E. Gabapentin for the symptomatic treatment of painful neuropathy in patients with diabetes mellitus: a randomized controlled trial. JAMA 280:1831–1836, 1998.

89. Rowbotham M, Harden N, Stacey B, Bernstein P, Magnus-Miller L. Gabapentin for the treatment of postherpetic neuralgia: a randomized controlled trial. JAMA 280:1837–1842, 1998.

90. Stracke H, Myer UE, Schumacher HE, Federlin K. Mexiletine in the treatment of diabetic neruopathy. Diabetes Care 15: 1550–1555, 1992.

91. Gennari C, Agnusdei D, Camporeale A. Use of calcitonin in the treatment of bone pain associated with osteoporosis. Calcif Tissue Int 49(Suppl 2):s9–s13, 1991.

92. Prager JP. Invasive modalities for the diagnosis and treatment of pain in the elderly. Clin Geriatr Med 12:549–561, 1996.

93. Bonica JJ, Sola AE. Other painful disorders of the low back. In: Bonica JJ (Ed.). The Management of Pain. Philadelphia, Lea & Febiger, pp. 1484–1514, 1990.

94. McCain GA. Fibromyalgia and myofascial pain syndromes. In: Wall PD, Melzack R (Eds.). Textbook of Pain, 3rd ed. New York, Churchill Livingstone, pp. 475–493, 1994.

95. Ferrell BR, Griffith H. Cost issues related to pain management: report from the Cancer Pain Panel of the Agency for Health Care Policy and Research. J Pain Symptom Manage 9:221–234, 1994.

96. Wedon M, Ferrell BR. Professional and ethical considerations in the use of high-tech pain management. Oncol Nurs Forum 18:1135–1143, 1991.

97. Ferrell BR, Rhiner M, Ferrell BA. Development and implementation of a pain education program. Cancer 72(Suppl):3426–3432, 1993.

98. Rhiner M, Ferrell BR, Ferrell BA, Grant MM. A structured nondrug intervention program for cancer pain. Cancer Pract 1:137–143, 1993.

99. Ferrell BA, Josephson KR, Pollan AM, et al. A randomized trial of walking versus physical methods for chronic pain management. Aging (Milano) 9:99–105, 1997.

100. Ettinger WH Jr, Burns R, Messier SP, et al. A randomized trial comparing aerobic exercise and resistance exercise with a health education program in older adults with knee osteoarthritis: the Fitness Arthritis and Seniors Trial (FAST). JAMA 277:25–31, 1997.

101. Kovar PA, Allegrante JP, MacKenzie CR, et al. Supervised fitness walking in patients with osteoarthritis of the knee: a randomized trial. Ann Intern Med 116:529–534, 1992.

102. Keefe FJ, Caldwell DS, Williams DA, et al. Pain coping skills training in the management of osteoarthritic knee pain: a comparative study. Behav Ther 21:49–62, 1990.

103. Pruder RS. Age analysis of cognitive-behavioral group therapy for chronic pain outpatients. Psychol Aging 3:204–207, 1988.

104. Eisenberg, Kessler RC, Foster C, et al. Unconventional medicine in the United States: prevalence, costs and patterns of use. N Engl J Med 328:246–252, 1993.

105. Ferrell BA. Pain management. In: Hazzard WR, Blass JP, Ettinger WH Jr, et al. (Eds.). Principles of Geriatric Medicine and Gerontology. New York, McGraw-Hill, Chapter 30, pp. 413–433, 1999.

17

Dyspnea

CYNTHIA X. PAN

Dyspnea is one of the most common symptoms experienced by patients with cancer and other incurable, progressive illnesses. Dyspnea affects patients' sense of well-being, anxiety, relationships with others, self-perception, ability to function, and sense of hope, thereby compounding the suffering associated with life-threatening illness. Like pain, dyspnea is what the patient says it is since it is a subjective experience. In palliative care, it is of value to understand the experience of dyspnea within a range of patient populations, disease states, and stages of illness.

DEFINITION OF DYSPNEA

The term *dyspnea* is derived from the Greek *dys*, meaning "bad" or "difficult," and *pneo*, meaning "breathing." Dyspnea is a subjective experience of breathing discomfort, which consists of qualitatively distinct sensations that vary in intensity.[1] It is thought to occur when the brain detects a mismatch between the central respiratory motor output and the feedback from afferents in the lung and peripheral receptors.

Dyspnea may occur at rest or with exertion and usually compels the person to increase ventilation or reduce activity.

Patients with dyspnea may describe it in unique ways, such as shortness of breath, a smothering feeling, a tightness in the chest, a need to gasp or pant, inability to get enough air, or a feeling of suffocation or drowning.[2,3]

Dyspnea is sometimes mistakenly used to describe disturbed patterns of breathing, such as the following:

- *Tachypnea:* increased rate of breathing caused by elevated by metabolic rate, e.g., with fever
- *Hyperpnea:* increased ventilation through metabolic acidosis, e.g., with diabetic ketoacidosis
- *Hyperventilation:* psychologically induced increased respiration

MULTIDIMENSIONAL ASPECTS OF DYSPNEA

Dyspnea, like pain, is a multidimensional, subjective experience that can have multiple layers of meaning for the person. A complex phenomenon, dyspnea has physiological, emotional, cognitive, and behavioral dimensions.

Physiologically, dyspnea results when the demands on the lungs are out of proportion to their capacity to respond.[4] Thus, dyspnea should be viewed as a warning sign of disease, a call to investigate and treat underlying medical conditions. Such conditions or etiologies can be related to the underlying disease itself (primary or metastatic lung cancer, congestive heart failure, pleural effusions), a side effect of treatment of disease (chemotherapy, radiation, surgery, biological response modifiers), intercurrent systemic disorders (anemia, infection, pulmonary disorders, hepatic failure, heart failure, renal failure, neuromuscular disorders), thick secretions, sleep disorders, chronic pain, use of centrally acting drugs, as well as lack of mobility and lack of exercise.

Emotionally and psychologically, dyspnea can be associated with increased levels of anxiety and depression, which can be further exacerbated by functional losses. Dyspnea can bring up fears of what it might mean in terms of disease type, recurrence, and prognosis. Feeling short of breath can also bring up existential feelings such as "Why is this happening to me?" and "What have I done to deserve this?" Having difficulty breathing can certainly impair quality of life.[5] Other consequences of dyspnea may include decreased functional status and socialization. For all of these reasons, dyspnea should be assessed and treated aggressively, by both investigating the underlying etiologies and treating symptomatically.

PREVALENCE OF DYSPNEA

Dypsnea is a highly prevalent symptom in older adults, regardless of the type of illness or community in which they live.

The prevalence of dyspnea appears to increase with age. In the Personnes âgées QUID (PAQUID) cohort of 3777 persons >65 years of age and living at home in the southwest of France, the prevalence of dys-

pnea was 25% and increased progressively with age.[6] In a cross-sectional study done on a representative systematic sample ($n = 1148$, 521 males, 627 females) of 70-year-old Swedes between 1971 and 1977, the prevalence among males was 30.5% and that among females, 36.1%; 44% of those with dyspnea had no evidence of cardiac failure or pulmonary disease.[7]

Dyspnea is one of the most common symptoms experienced by patients with all types of advanced lung disease, including lung cancer, interstitial lung disease, and particularly chronic obstructive pulmonary disease (COPD).[8,9] In the Study to Understand Prognoses and Preferences for Outcomes and Risks of Treatments (SUPPORT)[10] severe dyspnea occurred in 56% and 32% of patients with severe COPD or stage III/IV non-small cell lung cancer, respectively, while severe pain was experienced in 21% and 28%, respectively.[11] Dyspnea is common among patients with lung cancer and increases with the approach of death.[12,13] Uncontrolled dyspnea is extremely distressing for patients and their caretakers.

As a symptom in patients with advanced malignancy, dyspnea is very common. According to the National Hospice Study, dyspnea occurred in 70% of terminal cancer patients. Dyspnea was rated as at least "moderate" in severity by more than 28% of patients who were able to describe it. Prevalence rates were also noted to increase toward death.[12] In a study examining symptoms at the end of life of persons dying of cancer versus nonmalignant causes, "trouble breathing" was reported in 47% of persons dying with cancer and in 49% of those dying with other illnesses.[14]

In a study of patients with congestive heart failure (CHF) during their last 6 months of life, 63% of patient surrogates reported that the patient was severely short of breath during the 3 days before death.[15]

DYSPNEA IN THE OLDER ADULT

When treating the older adult in palliative care, the potential for confounding pathology secondary to the patient's age cannot be ignored. It can be difficult to discern if the dyspnea is secondary to deconditioning, CHF, anemia, hypothyroidism, various treatment modalities, or chronic pulmonary disease, to name but a few conditions in the differential. Many older adults erroneously consider dyspnea to be inevitable and, therefore, do not seek treatment. Since many causes of dyspnea tend to increase with age, it is important to keep a wide differential diagnosis, investigate likely underlying causes, and treat accordingly.

ASSESSMENT OF DYSPNEA

In dying patients, dyspnea originates from five primary causes, which may be discerned by a focused history and physical:

- Existing disease, i.e., COPD, asthma, CHF
- Acute superimposed illness, i.e., atelectasis, pneumonia, pulmonary embolus
- Cancer-induced complications, i.e., bronchial obstruction, pleural effusion, lymphangitis carcinomatosa, superior vena cava syndrome, replacement of normal lung tissue with tumor
- Effects of cancer or other therapy, i.e., radiation fibrosis, pneumothorax, chemotherapy such as bleomycin or amiodarone
- Miscellaneous: anemia, uremia, ascites, anxiety, depression

A useful approach is to assess the symptom in a systematic way (Table 17–1). The OPQRST assessment method has been used to assess pain but can also be applied to other symptoms, such as dyspnea. It is also important to ask the patients about other related symptoms that may exacerbate dyspnea, such as fatigue, pain, cough, nausea/vomiting, and anxiety or depression. In elderly populations, including those with chronic, incurable illness, dypsnea may also be a side effect of medical treatments, including medications (e.g., amiodarone, bleomycin) and radiation.

Furthermore, in speaking with the patient, it is important to determine the emotional status, particularly whether the person speaks of his or her own death or suicidal ideations. The dyspnea assessment includes questions related to the various dimensions of dyspnea:

- Temporal dimension
- Sensory dimension
- Mental/cognitive dimension
- Affective/emotional dimension
- Behavioral dimension
- Physiologic dimension

Physical examination includes the following assessment parameters:

- Vital signs to determine if fever, low blood pressure, or irregular pulse may be contributing to fatigue and dyspnea

Table 17–1. The OPQRST Assessment of Symptoms

O: Onset	When did it begin? Was it over days or within a few hours? Acute vs. chronic.
P: Palliating factors, provocating factors	What makes it better? What makes it worse?
Q: Quality	What does it feel like? Get descriptions
R: Radiation or related factors	Does it spread anywhere? Is it related or associated with cough, fever, hemoptysis, chest tightness, palpitations, nausea, lightheadedness, etc?
S: Severity	How severe is it? How much does it affect your life? How much does it affect your function? Is this degree of dyspnea tolerable or acceptable to you? (Usually assessed with a scale from 0 to 10; none, mild, moderate, severe)
T: Temporal factors	When does it come, or when is it most severe? Is it there all the time, or does it come and go? Is it worse at any particular time of the day or night?

- General appearance, including affect (anxious, depressed, agitated, tearful, angry, or flat), self-care behaviors, speech patterns, intonation, and general responsiveness
- Assessment of cardiac, respiratory, renal, musculoskeletal, and skin status to identify physiological conditions, including signs of infection or dehydration/nutrition that may be associated with fatigue and other comorbid conditions
- Appropriate laboratory testing, such as complete blood count and other laboratory studies (electrolytes, blood gases, thyroid function tests), which may confirm diseases suspected

CAUSES OF DYSPNEA

The causes of dyspnea are as numerous and diverse as the causes of pain, and in good palliative care, it is important for the clinician to be familiar with these since therapeutic interventions are frequently best selected on the basis of etiology. Table 17–2 lists a differential diagnosis list for dyspnea, categorized by organ systems or anatomical–pathological correlations. In addition to the physiological processes, it is important to remember that anxiety and angst can be brought up by family, financial, legal, spiritual, and practical issues.

Dyspnea and Quality of Life

Regardless of age, dyspnea has a profound effect on a person's quality of life. Inability to carry out role performance tasks can result in decreased self-esteem, social isolation, depression, increased health-care utilization and costs, and increased anxiety.

MEASURING DYSPNEA

It is important to develop valid and reliable measures of symptoms so that response to treatment in individuals as well as to therapeutic strategies in group studies can be scientifically assessed. Although there are a number of ways to measure dyspnea, there is no gold standard.

Different symptom scoring measures can be used, depending on the reason for measuring dyspnea. If the objective is to evaluate purely subjective symptom relief, then a simple symptom scoring method will be sufficient. If the objective is to assess functional capacity, then objective markers such as exercise testing should be added. If the objective is to measure ventilatory abnormalities, such as in asthma or tumor related airflow obstruction, then tests of pulmonary function need to be carried out. To assess the psychosocial consequences of dyspnea on the patient and family, we need to ask about physical and role functioning as well as about mood and social restrictions.

Table 17–2. Differential Diagnoses of Dyspnea

1. Obstructive airway process	Tracheal obstruction: intrinsic/extrinsic asthma, COPD, aspiration
2. Parenchymal/pleural disease	Diffuse primary or metastatic cancer, lymphangitic metastases, pneumonia/infection, pleural effusion (malignant/other), pulmonary drug reaction, radiation pneumonitis, cystic fibrosis, pulmonary fibrosis, thick secretions, radiation, medications: bleomycin, combined mitomycin and vinca alkaloid chemotherapy,[16] amiodarone
3. Vascular disease	Pulmonary embolus, superior vena cava obstruction, pulmonary vascular tumor emboli
4. Cardiac disease	Congestive heart failure, ischemic heart disease, pericardial effusion (malignant/other)
5. Chest wall/respiratory muscles	Primary neurologic disease (e.g., ALS, malnutrition)
6. Systemic or metabolic	Anemia, liver failure, ascites, renal failure
7. Other	Anxiety, panic attacks, fatigue, pain

COPD, chronic obstructive pulmonary disease; ALS, amyotrophic lateral sclerosis.

At the level of simple scoring of physical symptoms, there are various scales used to grade the severity of dyspnea. Scaling of symptoms can be accomplished by the verbal categorical scales (e.g., none, mild, moderate, severe), numeric rating scales (1 = no dyspnea to 10 = severe dyspnea), and linear visual analogue scale (VAS, usually a 10 cm line anchored with "no dyspnea" at one end and "extreme dyspnea" at the other). In describing patient groups, it often makes more clinical sense to talk of the proportion of patients with none, mild, moderate, or severe dyspnea, rather than of mean values from 0 to 10 points or 0 to 100 mm.

In any verbal rating system it is important for users to be familiar with the meaning of the categories used. Thus, standardized and validated scales, such as the European Organization for Research and Treatment of Cancer Quality of Life Core Questionnaire (EORTC QL-30)[17,18] together with its Lung Module (QLQ-LC13),[19] are useful. The EORTC questionnaires were designed as self-rating instruments, to be completed by patients, but they can also be completed as part of a structured interview.

Palliative care patients vary in their symptoms and capabilities from day to day and over longer periods of time, but most study methods are not sensitive to these background variations. It is often useful to ask about physical functioning by asking the patient about the best and worst levels achieved.[20]

Exercise Tests

Exercise tests assess patient function in addition to patient self-reports. Obviously, these tests are more relevant for a patient population that is mobile and trying to remain functionally active. They include walking or bicycle ergometer tests[21,22] as well as shorter walking tests (up to 100 m).[23,24] However, clinicians must bear in mind that evidence of exercise capacity, at least in patients with COPD, is more strongly related to inspiratory muscle strength and lung function than to dyspnea and quality of life,

which are useful parameters in palliative care.[21]

Lastly, key biological parameters of dyspnea are lacking. Dyspnea does not correlate with respiratory rate, oxygen saturation percentage, spirometer readings,[25] or pulmonary function testing.

Certain factors can be associated with the intensity of dyspnea. Bruera et al.[26] prospectively assessed 135 consecutive ambulatory, terminally ill cancer patients for respiratory function (vital capacity, peak flow, maximal inspiratory pressure, and oxygen saturation), as well as ratings of dyspnea, anxiety, and fatigue/tiredness using VASs. Lung involvement by the tumor (primary or metastatic) was determined from the patient's chart. Multivariate analysis demonstrated that lung involvement ($p = 0.0016$) and anxiety ($p = 0.0027$) were independently correlated with the intensity of dyspnea. In the subgroup of patients with moderate to severe dyspnea, multivariate analysis found anxiety ($p = 0.0318$) and maximal inspiratory pressure ($p = 0.0187$) to be independent correlates of the intensity of dyspnea. The presence of cancer in the lungs, anxiety, and maximal inspiratory pressure were correlates of the intensity of dyspnea in this patient population.[26]

Thus, dyspnea is a multidimensional experience and needs to be assessed and measured in a multidimensional manner.

MANAGEMENT OF DYSPNEA

In managing dyspnea in the older adult palliative care patient, the goal is to achieve the best quality of life possible given the specific circumstance. Educating the patient and family about the disease process and reasons why they might feel dyspneic can be reassuring. Teaching and supporting patients and family ways of managing dyspnea is critical.

For therapeutic purposes, it is most helpful to think of dyspnea as a mechanical mismatch between afferent information from receptors in respiratory muscles, airways, and the thoracic cage and their corresponding motor activity. If an individual does not have the ventilatory capacity to meet demand, dyspnea results. The sections below examine three approaches to decreasing dyspnea: *(1)* increasing ventilatory capacity, *(2)* decreasing ventilatory demand, and *(3)* altering the central perception of dyspnea. Subsequent sections will address the pharmacological, nonpharmacological, and surgical approaches to managing dyspnea, highlighting differences in the management of dyspnea among patients with cancer versus those with nonmalignant conditions. Last, the psychological burden of dyspnea will be described.

Pharmacological Approach I: Increase Ventilatory Capacity

Bronchodilator therapy

Inhaled β_2 agonists (e.g., albuterol, metaproterenol) and the anticholinergic ipratropium bromide (Atrovent) are the most important agents in the pharmacological management of dyspnea in patients with COPD. They reduce the work of breathing by reducing airway resistance and associated hyperinflation, which compromises diaphragmatic function.[27] Bronchodilators offer improvement in dyspnea, exercise tolerance, and overall health status but do not alter the progressive decline in lung function that is the hallmark of COPD.[28] Their efficacy in patients with interstitial lung disease or respiratory compromise from lung cancer is anecdotal at best.

Ipratropium bromide is generally preferred to the short-acting β_2 agonists as a first-line agent due to its longer duration of action and absence of sympathomimetic side effects.[29] Some studies have suggested that ipratropium achieves superior bronchodilation in COPD patients.[30] Short-acting β_2 agonists are less expensive than ipratropium and have a more rapid onset of action, commonly leading to greater patient satisfaction. Use of both short-acting β_2 agonists and ipratropium at submaximal doses leads to improved bronchodilation compared to either agent alone, but the combination does not further reduce dyspnea.[31–33] Long-acting β_2 agonists (e.g., formoterol, salmeterol) and anticholinergics (tiotropium) appear to achieve equivalent or superior bronchodilation to ipratropium in addition to similar improvements in dyspnea and overall health status.[34–36] Both short- and long-acting bronchodilators have been reported to reduce dyspnea in advanced lung disease independent of their effects on forced expiratory volume in 1 second (FEV_1).[25,37]

Patients with dyspnea and COPD should receive a clinical trial of bronchodilator medications, even in the absence of documented reversal of airflow obstruction. Patients with interstitial lung disease or lung cancer in the absence of COPD do not generally benefit from bronchodilators, but a clinical trial may be appropriate. In all cases, bronchodilators should be discontinued in patients who do not experience a clear symptomatic benefit. Long-acting bronchodilators simplify dosing, improve compliance, and may offer improved symptom control. Medications can be delivered through metered-dose inhalers (MDIs), dry powder inhalers, and updraft nebulizers. Nebulizer and MDI delivery appear to offer similar efficacy, although nebulizers may be more convenient and effective in patients who are immobile and/or have difficulty mastering inhaler technique.[38]

Theophylline

Theophylline has fallen out of favor because of its narrow toxic–therapeutic window, significant drug interactions, and the availability of more potent and better-tolerated bronchodilators. Nonetheless, theophylline has been shown to improve respiratory muscle function,[39,40] increase minute ventilation,[41] reduce pulmonary vascular resistance, improve cardiac output and myocardial perfusion,[42] improve mucociliary clearance,[43,44] and reduce airway inflammation,[45,46] in addition to its beneficial effects on bronchomotor tone.[47] There is also a well-recognized propensity for stable COPD patients maintained on theophylline to decompensate when theophylline is withdrawn.[48]

Mahler and colleagues,[49] in a double-blind, placebo-controlled study of 12 patients with "nonreversible" COPD given sustained-release theophylline to maintain levels at 10–20 mcg/ml over 4 weeks, reported significant improvement in dyspnea without a change in exercise tolerance.[49] Martin and colleagues[50] found that nocturnal administration of sustained-release theophylline reduced sleep-related decline in FEV_1 and morning symptoms. Despite these beneficial effects, theophylline has not been shown consistently to improve the course of COPD when used as monotherapy. Recent data from a randomized controlled trial of 943 patients with COPD showed significantly greater improvement in dyspnea, pulmonary function, and exacerbation frequency in patients receiving both inhaled salmeterol and theophylline (200 mg/day) than either agent alone.[51] Similar reductions in dyspnea with the combination of theophylline and short-acting β_2 agonists have previously been documented.[52] Overall, it appears that some patients with COPD may receive additional dyspnea relief and improved exercise tolerance from the addition of theophylline to their bronchodilator regimen. In appropriate patients, the authors recommend a short-term (2–4 weeks) trial of long-acting theophylline preparations in doses that achieve a serum drug level of 10–12 mcg/ml. As always with symptomatic therapy, the drug should be discontinued in nonresponders.

Corticosteroids

The use of oral steroids in exacerbations of COPD is well supported[53] despite the variety of doses and durations of treatment studied and the increased rates of steroid-related side effects reported, particularly hyperglycemia.[54] The role of oral steroids in stable COPD is less clear. Only 10% of stable outpatients with COPD given oral corticosteroids have a 20% increase in FEV_1 compared to patients receiving placebo.[55] Recent studies challenge even these limited data.[56,57] Side effects of systemic corticosteroid therapy are significant; therefore, any spirometric gain must be weighed against steroid-related complications, such as diabetes, cataracts, osteoporosis, and others.[58] There are observational data that suggest an association between corticosteroid use and increased mortality.[58] Finally, the effect of oral steroids on dyspnea and functional status has not been well characterized.

An evidence-based approach to corticosteroid therapy in stable outpatients is very limited. Empirical trials of oral corticosteroids should be guided by the following principles: the baseline FEV_1 should be stable, i.e., not measured during an exacerbation, and taken on maximal bronchodilator therapy; the postbronchodilator value is considered the appropriate baseline. Corticosteroid therapy equivalent to 0.5 mg/kg qd of prednisone is given for 14–21 days. The drug should be discontinued unless there is a 20% increase in FEV_1. Patients with subjective benefit without spirometric improvement or a clear change in functional status are considered nonresponders and should be continued on treatment only if no other measures offer symptom relief. In patients who require maintenance therapy, the lowest dose and/or alternate-day dosing should be used in conjunction with measures to reduce the risk of osteoporosis.[59] Responders are often switched to inhaled corticosteroids, but there are few data to guide this practice (see below). Patients with COPD should not be treated with inhaled corticosteroids simply because these agents lack the full toxicity of oral preparations.

Inhaled corticosteroids have beneficial effects on health status and exacerbation rate in some stable COPD patients, although they do not affect the decline of lung function over time. Recent data from a multicenter randomized, placebo-controlled trial of over 1100 patients with COPD found no effect of chronic inhaled triamcinolone (600 mcg bid) on the rate of FEV_1 decline over a mean 40-month period.[60] However, there were significant reductions in dyspnea, other respiratory symptoms, and hospitalizations. These gains were accompanied by a significant loss of bone density in the treatment group. In another study, more severe, non-asthmatic COPD patients randomized to inhaled fluticasone (500 mcg bid) showed no significant improvement in FEV_1 over 36 months compared to those receiving placebo. However, fluticasone was associated with a significant reduction in COPD exacerbations and an improved standardized measurement of health status found to correlate with dyspnea intensity.[61]

Oral steroids have been used to treat many types of interstitial lung disease (ILD, also termed *diffuse parenchymal lung disease*). No randomized trial has demonstrated that any proposed therapy improves survival or quality of life compared with no treatment. Some forms of ILD appear to be prednisone-responsive, e.g., acute sarcoidosis, bronchiolitis obliterans organizing pneumonia (BOOP), and some forms with histological patterns of nonspecific interstitial pneumonitis or desquamative interstitial pneumonitis. Treatment of such patients is appropriate if not based on good outcome data. However, the most common clinical presentation of ILD in geriatric patients is idiopathic pulmonary fibrosis (IPF) and the histological subtype of usual interstitial pneumonitis (UIP), which typically presents in patients in their sixth and seventh decades. It is marked by progressive fibrosis of the basal and peripheral lung parenchyma. The associated scarring reduces pulmonary compliance, leading to pulmonary restriction and increased work of breathing manifesting as progressive dyspnea. Median survival with IPF/UIP is less than 3 years from diagnosis.

Traditionally IPF/UIP has been treated with corticosteroids and cytotoxic agents such as cyclophosphamide and azathioprine. However, no investigation has demonstrated a mortality benefit or superiority of any of these agents over no treatment at all.[62-66] Furthermore, a recent prospective study of 41 UIP patients treated with prednisone at doses of 40–100 mg/day for 3 months found a 100% incidence of steroid-related side effects.[67] The pulmonary community has shifted away from treatment of UIP with corticosteroids because of the absence of mortality benefit

and the high incidence of treatment-related side effects. Unfortunately, there are few therapeutic options for these patients who frequently suffer from disabling dyspnea. Some practitioners will use cytotoxic agents despite the absence of evidence for their efficacy because of their more favorable side-effect profile. There are preliminary data in a small number of patients with mixed subtypes of ILD suggesting that interferon-γ may prevent progression or even reverse fibrosis.[68] A large, randomized clinical trial is currently in progress to assess its potential efficacy in UIP patients.

How should steroids be used in patients with dyspnea?

Given the heterogeneity of patients studied, there is no way to predict which COPD patients will respond to inhaled versus oral corticosteroids. Therefore, short-term trials (e.g., 2 weeks) are appropriate in patients who are dyspneic despite optimal bronchodilation. The inhaled route may be preferable to systemic use because of a lower incidence of side effects. However, inhaled corticosteroids, especially newer, high-potency agents, are systemically absorbed and do have the potential for significant adverse effects.[69-72]

Corticosteroids are a ubiquitous group of drugs in palliative care and are indicated in the palliation of a number of respiratory symptoms: airways obstruction (asthma, COPD), tracheal tumor causing stridor, superior vena cava obstruction, lymphangitis carcinomatosa, and pneumonitis (e.g., after radiotherapy). Intravenous or oral dexamethasone or oral prednisolone is generally used, in doses high enough to work quickly without causing undue gastric toxicity or fluid retention (e.g., prednisolone 30–60 mg daily or dexamethasone 4–8 mg daily). Prednisone is only available orally.

The milligram equivalents in Table 17–3 facilitate changing to dexamethasone from other glucocorticoids.

Other miscellaneous therapies

Progesterone compounds have been shown to increase ventilation, probably by in-

Table 17–3. Dexamethasone Compared to Other Glucocorticoids

Dexamethasone	Methylprednisolone and triamcinolone	Prednisolone and prednisone	Hydrocortisone	Cortisone
0.75 mg	4 mg	5 mg	20 mg	25 mg

creasing the central sensitivity to CO_2, although they may also work at the peripheral chemoreceptors.[73] Studies of patients with COPD using medroxyprogesterone acetate at 60–100 mg/day have confirmed this action, but despite small improvements in arterial blood gases, symptomatic benefit has not been shown.[74,75] The progesterone group of drugs is extensively used in the management of breast and other hormone-responsive cancers. Paradoxically, one of their recognized adverse effects at high doses is the causation of dyspnea, which may be mediated by fluid retention, leading to pulmonary congestion, and by increased risk of venous thrombosis, leading to pulmonary embolism. Fortunately, the stimulation of ventilation by progesterones can be achieved at lower doses.[76]

Other classes of drugs that stimulate ventilation include nebulized local anesthetics,[77,78] almitrine (a peripheral chemoreceptor stimulant),[74] doxapram (stimulates carotid chemoreceptors at low doses but at higher doses stimulates medullary respiratory centers), and inhaled cannabis and the synthetic cannbinoid nabilone.[79,80] Nabilone may be helpful in sedating an anxious, dyspneic patient in borderline respiratory failure without aggravating CO_2 retention.[5] However, none of the other drugs has found significant use in palliative care due to significant toxic side effects.

Pharmacological Approach II: Decrease Ventilatory Demand

Oxygen therapy

Supplemental oxygen is one of the few life-prolonging therapies available for patients with advanced lung disease (ALD), specifically for patients with advanced COPD complicated by resting hypoxemia. In the Nocturnal Oxygen Therapy Trial (NOTT), 203 patients with severe COPD and hypoxemia at rest were randomized to 12 or 24 hours of oxygen therapy. After 26

months, mortality in the 24-hour treatment group was half that of the 12-hour group.[81] A subsequent randomized controlled trial by the British Medical Research Council reported a 5-year reduction in mortality from 66% to 45% in the group given oxygen for at least 15 hours a day.[81] However, these studies did not assess the effect of supplemental oxygen on dyspnea.

Supplemental oxygen therapy has multiple physiological effects. It variably depresses carotid body output and respiratory drive, improves respiratory muscle function, decreases respiratory system impedance, decreases pulmonary artery pressures, and improves oxygen delivery and cardiac function. Supplemental oxygen usually causes an increase in arterial partial pressure of CO_2 (PCO_2) by reducing the ventilatory response to CO_2.[38] Rarely, it may cause a significant increase in PCO_2 by altering ventilation–perfusion relationships or reducing respiratory drive.[82] This effect is almost exclusively seen in patients with resting hypercapnia. The effects of supplemental oxygen on arterial PCO_2 levels should be monitored on initiation of therapy in patients with ALD, particularly in those with significant hypercapnia.

The physiological effects of supplemental oxygen predictably improve exercise capacity in patients with ALD, but this change is generally modest.[83–85] The effect of supplemental oxygen on dyspnea is less consistent. In a randomized, double-blind, crossover trial of severely disabled hypoxemic patients with COPD and ILD, Swinburn and colleagues[86] reported significant reductions in rest dyspnea using 28% oxygen versus compressed air. This was not corroborated in a single-blind trial of eight patients with moderate to severe COPD and rest dyspnea.[87] Similarly, in patients with terminal cancer and rest dyspnea, some investigators have found that supplemental oxygen reduces rest dyspnea,[88] while others have found no difference between oxygen and compressed air delivered by nasal cannula.[89] This latter finding may reflect the presence of extrathoracic receptors on the face and in the nasal passages that mitigate the sensation of breathlessness.[90] Open windows and a fan to circulate air across the face frequently improve breathlessness. Oxygen may also act synergistically with opioids to relieve exertional dyspnea, as demonstrated by a reduced dyspnea score among 12 moderate to severe COPD patients during exercise compared to opioid therapy alone.[91]

Medicare reimbursement for home oxygen therapy is based on the enrollment criteria of the NOTT and not on symptomatic dyspnea:

1. Continuous therapy, either of the following:
   a. Partial pressure of arterial O_2 (PaO_2) 55 mm Hg or O_2 saturation by pulse oximetry (oxygen) (SpO_2) 88% taken at rest, while awake and breathing room air
   b. PaO_2 59 mm Hg or SpO_2 89% taken at rest, while awake and breathing room air, if there is evidence of any one or more of the following:
      i. Dependent edema suggesting CHF
      ii. Pulmonale on electrocardiogram
      iii. Hematocrit >56%
2. Prescription for nocturnal oxygen use only
3. Prescription for use only during exercise

However, the Medicare Hospice Benefit will pay for home oxygen therapy for treatment of dyspnea. Also, pulse oximetry has not been found to correlate with degree of dyspnea or the relief thereof.

Independent of the important issue of reimbursement, patients who do not meet Medicare criteria for home oxygen but who suffer from dyspnea refractory to standard therapy should be offered a trial of supplemental oxygen therapy. A letter to insurance companies documenting improved symptoms (some authors recommend a blinded trial of oxygen as evidence) and failure of other therapies to control dyspnea may result in reimbursement of long-term

oxygen therapy for this purpose. Although no optimal flow rate of oxygen has been defined, it seems reasonable to titrate flow rate to achieve effective palliation of dyspnea and/or improved exercise capacity while avoiding symptomatic hypercapnia.

Most patients receive supplemental oxygen through a nasal cannula. Face masks can be used but tend to interfere with speaking and eating and may contribute to a sense of suffocation. Transtracheal delivery through a percutaneous catheter may improve comfort, reduce nasal mucosal desiccation, and produce superior oxygen saturations at lower flow rates than nasal delivery. Direct flow into the trachea may also reduce inspired minute ventilation.[92] In a single-blind, randomized trial of 10 COPD patients receiving low- versus high-flow oxygen delivered through nasal and transtracheal routes, Bloom and colleagues[93] reported improved morale, depression, and exercise capacity with transtracheal oxygen compared to nasal administration. This was not supported in a study by Dewan and Bell.[85] Conflicting data along with the increased maintenance requirement and risk of infection or dislodgement with a transtracheal catheter probably account for its lack of widespread use despite the potential advantages.

Pharmacological Approach III: Alter Central Perception

When improving ventilatory capacity or reducing ventilatory drive cannot be achieved in the setting of ALD, another alternative way to palliate dyspnea is to interfere with neural pathways that give rise to the sensation of breathlessness. Several classes of drugs have been used for this purpose, including opioids, benzodiazepines, and neuroleptics.

Opioid therapy

How do opioids reduce dyspnea? Opioids are potent analgesics and mild sedatives with powerful effects on respiration to decrease ventilatory drive while facilitating higher tolerance to resultant hypoxemia and hypercapnia.[94] Morphine, the prototypical opioid, has a vasodilator action which reduces cardiac preload and is helpful for patients with heart failure. Opioids also have important cortical sedative ("narcotic") actions with measurable effects on cognitive function, as well as euphoric and anxiolytic effects. Thus, opioids can reduce the perception of dyspnea. Furthermore, opioids are unique in that they are the only sedative agents to have natural endogenous equivalents (endorphins), which may be responsible for mediating or modulating the normal responses to stimuli that induce dyspnea. This combination of physiological and higher cortical effects makes opioids attractive therapeutic agents for dyspnea.

Clinical studies of opioids for dyspnea. Clinical trials have yielded inconsistent results. In severe COPD, multiple trials suggest improvement in refractory dyspnea in patients given dihydrocodeine (15–60 mg tid),[91,95,96] morphine sulfate (0.8 mg/kg qd),[97] and hydromorphone (3 mg qid rectally).[98] In general, opioid use was associated with decreased minute ventilation, but hypercapnia and hypoxemia were well-tolerated. One of these trials reported a significant incidence of opioid-related side effects such as nausea, constipation, and drowsiness, which resulted in a 30% discontinuation rate in one study.[91]

Multiple well-designed studies have come to the opposite conclusion. One randomized, placebo-controlled trial of codeine (30 mg qid) failed to demonstrate improved dyspnea or exercise tolerance among 11 patients with severe COPD while reporting significant drowsiness.[99] A randomized, double-blind, placebo-controlled study using diamorphine at two doses (2.5 or 5 mg q6h for 2 weeks) in the setting of severe emphysema failed to show significant dyspnea reduction or improvement in exercise tolerance.[100] In a more recent randomized, double-blind, placebo-controlled crossover study of sustained-release morphine in severe COPD patients, a mean dose of 25 mg daily over 6 weeks did not improve measurements of quality of life, exercise tolerance, dyspnea, or oxygen saturation with a trend toward increased opioid side effects.[101]

In addition to subcutaneous, oral, and rectal administration of opioids to dyspneic COPD patients, nebulized delivery has been studied. In a double-blind, placebo-controlled trial, Young and colleagues[102] reported that nebulized morphine (mean dose 1.7 mg) significantly improved dyspnea-limited exercise times without untoward side effects in nine patients with severe COPD. In contrast, four subsequent trials of similar design in patients with multiple forms of ALD failed to demonstrate significant improvement in rest or exertional dyspnea despite nebulized doses ranging from low (1–2 mg) to high (10–25 mg).[103–106]

The literature shows more consistent improvements in dyspnea in terminally ill cancer patients. Bruera and colleagues[107] reported favorable effects of subcutaneous morphine in 19 of 20 terminally ill cancer patients without significant respiratory or hemodynamic changes. This finding was reproduced in a placebo-controlled trial by the same author of 10 terminally ill patients with dyspnea already receiving daily morphine with reported "good" control of pain. Patients receiving a 50% increase in their subcutaneous morphine dose reported an average 50% reduction in their dyspnea. They did not suffer significant effects on respiration or hemodynamics.[108] Cohen and colleagues[109] studied terminal lung cancer patients who lacked adequate pain control despite oxygen and intermittent dosing of opioids. Employing continuous intravenous morphine after 5- to 10-minute bolusing to achieve complete pain relief, six of eight patients reported complete relief of dyspnea within a period of 16–87 hours. Sedation was a significant side effect but was tempered by reducing the hourly amount without loss of effective analgesia or relief of dyspnea.

In summary, opioids are effective agents to treat dyspnea but have a significant incidence of side effects, particularly constipation and sedation. Tolerance of these side effects tends to be poor among ambulatory outpatients. For patients who have pain in addition to dyspnea and in those with refractory dyspnea in the setting of terminal cancer, a trial of opioids is clearly indicated.

For patients with nonmalignant ALD and dyspnea, the evidence is less clear. The current literature does not support the routine use of oral or inhaled opioid therapy in ambulatory outpatients with nonmalignant ALD and dyspnea. Nonetheless, therapeutic options are limited and clinical experience suggests that there are some patients who may benefit from opioid therapy. Therefore, a trial of opioids may be worthwhile in an attempt to reduce ventilatory drive when supplemental oxygen and pharmacological therapies fail to palliate dyspnea. When using opioids to provide effective dyspnea relief, the lowest dose should be employed, to minimize side effects.

Practically, how should opioids be used for dyspnea management? In many patients with cancer-related dyspnea, the dyspnea occurs intermittently, usually in relation to exertion, blockage of airways with mucus, or psychological factors. Therefore, it may be more prudent to use opioids on an as-needed basis rather than a standing basis, to maximize the effect but minimize side effects. Obviously, in patients with chronic dyspnea (such as COPD or lymphangitis carcinomatosa), regular respiratory sedation should be prescribed. Dose depends on current/prior use of opioids. For opioid-naive patients with severe dyspnea, start with 2–5 mg intravenous or subcutaneous morphine sulfate, every 5 minutes until symptoms improve. Morphine sulfate is the medication of choice (although all opioids are effective) and can be administered by any route: oral, subcutaneous, intravenous, or nebulized (nebs are contraindicated in patients with asthma). However, there is no clear evidence of benefit for nebulized morphine at doses below those that produce a systemic effect. Codeine has not been studied as an agent for dyspnea and is not considered effective as treatment for such.

Anxiolytics, neuroleptics, and antidepressants

Benzodiazepines are generally ineffective at relieving dyspnea in ALD. In a double-blind, placebo-controlled crossover trial of 18 "pink-puffer" COPD patients receiving 25 mg of diazepam daily, there was no change in dyspnea and diazepam significantly reduced exercise tolerance.[110] In 24 patients with COPD, alprazolam (0.5 mg bid) failed to relieve dyspnea or improve exercise tolerance compared to placebo, and investigators found a fall in PO_2 and increased $PaCO_2$ in patients given alprazolam.[111] A similar lack of effect on dyspnea or exercise tolerance along with an increased incidence of sedation has been documented with clorazepate compared to placebo in five severe COPD patients.[112]

Buspirone is an anxiolytic structurally and pharmacologically distinct from the benzodiazepines. It is associated with little sedation and may have mild respiratory stimulant activity. In a randomized, double-blind, placebo-controlled trial, Argyropoulou and colleagues[113] studied 16 patients with COPD and found that buspirone (20 mg qd) significantly reduced dyspnea and anxiety and improved exercise tolerance without changes in blood gases. This finding was not reproduced in a randomized, placebo-controlled trial of 11 COPD patients given 6 weeks of therapy at a dose of 10–20 mg/day.[114]

There is conflicting evidence for the use of neuroleptic medications to relieve dyspnea in ALD. Woodcock and colleagues[110] reported that promethazine, a phenothiazine derivative with potent H1 blocking activity and sedative properties, at a total dose of 125 mg/day had a modest effect on dyspnea while producing less sedation than valium. Rice and colleagues[99] failed to confirm a promethazine benefit at a dose of 25 mg qid. One uncontrolled study of 20 terminally ill cancer patients reported that chlorpromazine, given intravenously or rectally at a dose of 12.5–25 mg q 4–12 h, reduced restlessness and dyspnea in 18 of 20 patients.[115] Trials in ALD patients who are not actively dying are needed to corroborate this finding. There may be a synergistic role of neuroleptics when used with opioids. Light and colleagues[116] report improved dyspnea and exercise tolerance in seven stable patients with COPD taking 30 mg morphine combined with either promethazine (Phenergan) or prochlorperazine (Compazine) but not with morphine alone.

Overall, there are scant and conflicting data among a relatively small number of patients in trials to suggest that monotherapy with benzodiazepines or neuroleptics provide predictable relief of dyspnea or improved functional capacity in the setting of ALD. These agents are not recommended for relief of dyspnea in these patients, although specific symptoms such as restlessness, anxiety, or insomnia may merit a clinical trial in individual patients. A trial of buspirone may be more prudent than one of benzodiazepines. When used in conjunction with opioids, promethazine may act synergistically to palliate refractory dyspnea in ALD.

Practically, how should anxiolytics and other sedatives be used for dyspnea management? Various anxiolytics are available, such as diazepam (Valium), lorazepam (Ativan), and midazolam (Versed). These are available in oral, intravenous, subcutaneous, and rectal routes. For severe dyspnea, Valium 2–5 mg or Ativan 1 mg intravenously is generally used every 5–10 minutes until symptoms improve. Because these medications are sedating, it is probably best to use them on an as-needed basis. If patients suffer from anxiety as well, a standing dose (2–4 times qd) can be prescribed. Buspirone (Buspar) is available only orally, with a recommended initial dosage of 15 mg qd (7.5 mg bid or 5 mg tid). To achieve an optimal therapeutic response, at intervals of 2–3 days the dosage may be increased 5 mg qd, as needed. The maximum daily dosage should not exceed 60 mg qd. Buspirone should not be used in patients with renal or hepatic impairment.

Major tranquilizers/neuroleptics (chlorpromazine, promethazine, prochlorperazine) or barbiturates (pentobarbital, phenobarbital) may be needed to control terminal dyspnea/anxiety that is not manageable with opioids and benzodiazepines. Chlorpromazine (Thorazine) is available as oral, parenteral, and rectal preparations, 12.5–25 mg

q4–12h. Elderly and debilitated patients should start with initial doses at the lowest end of the dosage range (e.g., 12.5 mg qd). Such patients are more susceptible to hypotension and central nervous system effects and need to be monitored carefully. Promethazine (Phenergan) is available at 12.5–25 mg doses, which may be repeated, as necessary, at 4- to 6-hour intervals. It is available in oral (tablet, syrup), intravenous, and rectal preparations. Prochlorperazine (Compazine) is available as oral (regular or sustained-release capsules, syrup), intravenous, intramuscular, and rectal suppository formulations. Subcutaneous administration is not advisable due to local irritation. Dosage is 5 or 10 mg tablet tid or qid.

Other Pharmacological Interventions

Cough-suppressants can and should be used when cough exacerbates dyspnea. Treatment options include oral cough medicine, dextromethorphan, opiates, steroids, and/or inhaled lidocaine. Local anesthetics such as inhaled lidocaine may help manage cough, although this is controversial.

Nonpharmacological Approaches to Dyspnea in Advanced Lung Disease

Pulmonary rehabilitation

Integrated programs for patients with ALD include exercise training, breathing strategies, disease-specific education, and psychosocial support. In stable ALD patients with compensated comorbidities, such programs have been shown to improve dyspnea, exercise tolerance, and quality of life, independent of effects on pulmonary function.[117–119] As little as 3 hours a week for 6 weeks was recently found to increase quality of life on standardized measurement in 65 COPD patients for at least as long as the 6-month study period.[120] Pulmonary rehabilitation incorporating exercise and specific inspiratory muscle training may provide synergistic improvement in dyspnea and exercise capacity superior to long-acting bronchodilator therapy alone in the setting of moderate to severe COPD.[121] These programs are individualized to patient needs, environment, and level of function. Although most studies have been reported in COPD patients, the principles seem applicable to other groups of ambulatory ALD patients who might benefit. The goal of rehabilitation is to restore individuals with ALD to the highest level of independent function possible, but this may not be indicated for patients with decompensated lung disease or comorbidities which may cause an undue burden of symptoms without restoration of function. Nonetheless, most ambulatory ALD patients should be considered for pulmonary rehabilitation.

Progressive muscle relaxation

In a 4-week randomized controlled trial, 20 patients, mean age 61 (range 20–84) years were randomized to weekly sessions of 45 minutes of progressive muscle relaxation (PMR) plus daily home practice with taped instructions or to relaxation in lounge chairs for the same duration. Patients performing PMR were instructed to tense each muscle group for 5–10 seconds while inhaling, to hold their breath, then to relax while exhaling completely. Patients had reduced dyspnea, anxiety, respiratory rate, and heart rate during each weekly session. The beneficial effect was limited to the relaxation session, except for respiratory rate, which significantly decreased over the 4-week period.[122]

Inspiratory muscle training

In a randomized controlled trial, 19 COPD patients with dyspnea on exertion, mean age 61.1 years, were randomized to targeted inspiratory muscle training or sham training. All patients exercised with a PFLEX muscle trainer modified to give visual feedback on training intensity. The PFLEX consisted of a mouthpiece, a variable resistor, and a one-way expiratory valve. They trained for 15 minutes twice each day using nose clips, and the resistance was increased every 7–10 days. The control group used the same device but only trained at minimal resistance because of removal of the one-way valve. After 8 weeks of training, both groups showed an improvement in inspiratory muscle strength measured as maximal inspiratory pressure; however, the mean change in the treatment group (15.03 cm H_2O) was statistically significant, while the increase in the control group (5.2 cm H_2O) was not. There was also a significant improvement in dyspnea indices ($p = 0.003$) in the experimental group compared with controls.[123]

Exercise training

In a controlled trial of exercise retraining in patients with severe chronic bronchitis, 33 subjects were followed for a mean period of 10.3 months. The exercise program was supervised once a week, and daily training comprised a 12-minute walk and simple stair climbing exercises. Exercise training was assigned based on place of residence. Those living near the hospital were assigned to the experimental group. The intervention consisted of 2 minutes twice daily stepping up and down on two 24 cm steps. At the end of 6 months, the mean 12-minute walking distance increased was 518 feet compared to a decline for the control group of 39 feet ($p < 0.001$). Dyspnea improved significantly in the exercise group compared to the control group ($p < 0.02$).[124]

Noninvasive positive pressure ventilation

Data from multiple prospective, randomized trials convincingly support the use of noninvasive positive pressure ventilation (NPPV) in patients with acute exacerbations of COPD. It has been shown to reduce intubation rates, length of intensive care unit and hospital stays, nosocomial infection rates, and in-hospital mortality rates.[125–128] The benefits of NPPV in patients with advanced, stable COPD are more unclear. Randomized trials comparing oxygen plus NPPV to oxygen therapy alone in stable COPD patients have shown conflicting results. Meecham Jones and colleagues[129] studied 14 COPD patients using nocturnal NPPV in a 3-month crossover trial and demonstrated significant improvements in sleep, daytime and nocturnal gas exchange, and quality-of-life scores. Nonetheless, Strumpf and colleagues[130] failed to confirm these benefits in a similarly designed 3-month crossover trial of 23 patients with less severe COPD. They noted a high noncompliance rate as only seven patients completed the 3-month trial. Considering additional, unfavorable results of smaller, controlled trials of NPPV in stable COPD patients over shorter treatment periods, there are scant data to support its use in ALD outside of COPD patients with marked hypercapnia. Even in this subset of patients, no trial has convincingly demonstrated a survival advantage over long term-oxygen therapy. Practically, use of NPPV is tempered by the high financial cost and apparent high noncompliance rate associated with the home setting.

Noninvasive positive pressure ventilation has become an accepted therapy for chronic respiratory failure secondary to neuromuscular disease, thoracic deformity, and idiopathic hypoventilation. Uncontrolled cohort studies have shown that NPPV improves gas exchange, nocturnal hypoventilation, and daytime symptoms (cognitive dysfunction, morning headache, daytime hypersomnolence, and sleep difficulties) and reduces the need for tracheotomy in these patients. Despite the lack of prospective controlled trials addressing the use of NPPV in other forms of ALD, consensus opinion favors initiating NPPV in symptomatic patients, when $PaCO_2$ is >45 mm Hg, or when there is significant nocturnal desaturation.[131]

Miscellaneous/other interventions
- *Positioning:* sitting up and leaning forward helps relieve the sense of breathlessness
- *Increased air movement:* such as opening the window and having a bedside fan blowing across, not directly on, the face, which can help stimulate mechanoreceptors on the face and in the nostrils
- *Humidified air:* for patients with distressing cough

Surgical Approaches to Advanced Lung Disease

As palliative care expands beyond brink-of-death or end-of-life care, palliative care professionals will increasingly care for patients who may live for years with chronic, progressive illnesses for which there are no cure. Thus, palliative care therapies will include aggressive surgical interventions to improve symptoms.

Bullectomy

Bullectomy, or the surgical removal of lung bulla(e), is distinct from lung volume reduction surgery (described below). A minority of COPD patients have relatively normal pulmonary parenchyma apart from their bullae, which cause airflow obstruction through compression of normal bronchi and the mechanical disadvantages of hyperinflation. In these patients, removal of bulla(e) and re-expansion of normal lung may improve both pulmonary function and symptoms. There are no controlled trials, but multiple case series of COPD patients support subjective and objective improvements in lung function, with the magnitude of improvement (FEV_1 increases of 50%–200%) greatest in those whose bullae occupy up to 50% of the hemithorax.[132] Results are less favorable in those whose bullae occupy less than 30% of the hemithorax and in those with diffuse emphysema. In one of the largest case series to date, operative mortality was 2.1% while improvement in pulmonary function persisted up to 20 years.[133] Thus, bullectomy is an option for COPD patients with large bullae not associated with wide-spread emphysema, although these are by far the minority of COPD patients.

Lung volume reduction surgery

Lung volume reduction surgery (LVRS) is a surgical approach to patients dyspneic from advanced emphysema and hyperinflation. It involves removal of 20%–30% of apical emphysematous lung tissue to allow re-expansion of more normal lung, leading to improved expiratory airflow and respiratory mechanics.[134,135] In a case series of 89 patients with severe emphysema who underwent LVRS and were followed prospectively for 3 years, there were improvements in dyspnea and 6-minute walk distance, while surgical mortality varied from 4% to 15%.[136] Based on conflicting clinical trial data, the National Heart, Lung, and Blood Institute and the Center for Medicare and Medicaid Services recently sponsored the National Emphysema Treatment Trial (NETT),[137] a multicenter, randomized clinical trial in patients with advanced emphysema randomized to LVRS versus medical management. Patients must be nonsmoking for a minimum of 4 months and complete 6–10 weeks of pulmonary rehabilitation, following which they must be able to walk more than 140 meters in 6 minutes. Additional entry criteria include clinical and radiographic evidence of bilateral emphysema, FEV_1 <45% predicted, PO_2 >45 mm Hg, and PCO_2 <60 mm Hg. The primary outcome measure is survival over a 2-year minimum follow-up. Secondary outcome measures include exercise capacity measured by distance walked in 6 minutes, pulmonary function, oxygen requirement, quality of life, respiratory symptoms, and health-care utilization and costs. The trial is still enrolling patients. However, the safety monitoring board stopped enrollment in one group of patients with an unacceptably high mortality. In patients with FEV_1 <20% predicted and either homogeneous distribution of emphysema or a single breath-diffusing capacity of less than 20% predicted, 30-day mortality was 16% versus 0% in the medically treated group, with an overall 3-year relative risk of death of 3.9 (95% confidence interval 1.9–9).[138] Despite relatively small but significant gains in pulmonary function and exercise capacity in LVRS survivors, there were no differences in standardized measurements of health-related quality of life compared to medical patients. Until a particular subtype of COPD patient is identified for whom LVRS is predictably safe and effective at improving pulmonary function and symptoms, this operation cannot be recommended outside the ongoing research trial.

Lung transplant

Lung transplant remains an option for patients with chronic ALD for whom medical and surgical therapies fail and who are expected to die soon enough that transplant offers a potential survival advantage. Survival following lung transplantation at 1, 3, and 5 years is 70%, 55%, and 42%, respectively, with median survival approximately 3.8 years.[139] Transplants are typically limited to patients under age 65 (single lung) or age 60 (double lung). Therefore, they are not currently a realistic therapeutic option for the geriatric patient.

Other surgical options in chronic obstructive pulmonary disease

Surgical procedures aimed at palliating refractory dyspnea include vagal nerve transection or carotid body resection, with the goal of decreasing ventilatory drive by reducing chemoreceptor stimulus in the setting of hypoxemia. Bradley et al.[140] described five COPD patients with intractable dyspnea undergoing unilateral right vagotomy under local anesthesia. Two patients markedly improved, while three patients died within a year of the operation, two of whom developed respiratory infections possibly related to depressed cough reflex dampened by the operation. In another uncontrolled case series, three COPD patients underwent bilateral carotid body resection resulting in long-lasting, subjective dyspnea relief associated with decreased minute ventilation, oxygen consumption, and CO_2 production. However, all died within 2 years of the procedure, with two patients dying from severe respiratory insufficiency thought secondary to decreased hypoxemic ventilatory drive.[141] The potential role of these therapies in palliative care has not been pursued in larger, controlled trials due to poor outcomes in small case series.

Interventional approaches to dyspnea in lung cancer patients

Some causes of dyspnea are either exclusively seen in cancer patients or are more common in this population. Approximately 40% of all pleural effusions result from cancer, and lung cancer accounts for almost one-third of all malignant pleural effusions.[142] Pleural disease represents a significant cause of dyspnea in patients with cancer. *Thoracentesis* is the percutaneous drainage of pleural fluid. This can be done safely at the bedside with local anesthesia only and is effective at relieving dyspnea in the short term. Recurrence of pleural fluid is common. *Pleurodesis* is a technique of draining an effusion, then instilling a sclerosing agent into the pleural space with the goal of adhering the parietal and visceral pleural surfaces, to prevent accumulation of fluid in the pleural space.[143,144] Fever and pain are the most common side effects of pleurodesis and can be treated with antipyretics, analgesics, and the instillation of local anesthetic. Talc is superior to other sclerosing agents used in chemical pleurodesis, with a reported success rate (non-recurrence after initial drainage) of 93% compared to 72%, 67%, and 54% with doxycycline, tetracycline, and bleomycin, respectively.[145] Sterile, asbestos-free talc may not be readily available, however.

Pleurodesis is not usually performed following thoracentesis because success depends on draining the pleural space completely. Pleurodesis usually involves a chest tube and a 3- to 7-day inpatient hospitalization. An alternative to pleurodesis is the outpatient placement of a small-bore, biocompatible pleural catheter, which may be left in place for months.[146] This approach avoids hospitalization, facilitates repeated drainage at home through a special collection bottle, has a low rate of complications, and is at least as effective at causing pleural sclerosis as standard pleurodesis.[147]

Medical thoracoscopy, which employs local or conscious sedation in the ambulatory setting, may be used to manage pleural effusions refractory to chest tube drainage and pleurodesis. Unlike standard thoracoscopy and open thoracotomy, medical thoracoscopy does not require general anesthesia and can be performed in the outpatient setting. As such, it may be particularly useful for palliation of symptomatic cancer patients who are poor operative candidates.[148]

Interventional pulmonology employs several effective bronchoscopic and pleuro-scopic techniques as alternatives to surgery for the management of dyspnea, lung collapse, and/or pneumonia secondary to tumors causing endobronchial obstruction. Laser therapy, cryotherapy, electrocautery, brachytherapy, and photodynamic therapy are bronchoscopic treatments of airway lesions causing significant obstruction. Endobronchial stents yield effective, short-term palliation of symptomatic airway narrowing caused by extrinsic compression from tumors.[149] Referral to specialized centers is appropriate when these techniques promise effective palliation, even in advanced disease.

Both chemotherapy and radiation therapy offer opportunities for effective palliative therapy in patients with advanced lung cancer. An extensive literature exists on the role of chemotherapy in inoperable non-small cell lung cancer. A meta-analysis published in 1995 reported that in patients with stage IIIB and IV disease and good performance status (WHO performance status 0–1, <5% weight loss in the past 6 months), multidrug, platinum-based chemotherapy led to improved survival equivalent to a mean gain of 6 weeks at 1 year.[150] There was no survival benefit in patients with poor performance status. Older trials using alkylating agents (cyclophosphamide) were associated with decreased survival. More recent clinical trials have addressed the issue of quality of life as well as survival. Some show improved survival without any change in quality of life,[151–153] some show improved quality of life without any change in survival,[154] and others show variable effects on quality of life, with improvement in some areas but impairment in others related to medication effects.[155] These benefits are seen in all age groups.[156,157] It is difficult to make an unequivocal recommendation in a field under such intensive investigation. It seems safe to say that all patients, including the elderly, with inoperable non-small cell lung cancer and good performance status should be offered palliative chemotherapy. It remains to be seen which patients benefit most from what combination of agents. Patients with poor performance status should not routinely be given chemotherapy but may be appropriate candidates in individual circumstances. Accurate and complete information is essential to informed consent to proceed.[158]

Radiotherapy is an effective tool for palliation of symptoms, though it may be more effective for pain and hemoptysis than for dyspnea.[159] There is no strong evidence that any regimen gives greater palliation, although higher dose regimens are associated with more acute toxicity. There is evidence for a modest increase in survival (6% at 1 year and 3% at 2 years) in patients with better performance status given higher-dose radiotherapy.[160] A recent report used the technique of quality-adjusted life days (QALDs) to quantify the impact of targeted, high-dose radiotherapy for symptomatic non-small cell lung cancer.[161] The authors calculated that patients receiving palliative radiotherapy gained one-third of their QALDs from radiotherapy. There is retrospective evidence to suggest that patients age 75 and older have responses similar to younger patients.[162]

Complementary/Alternative Therapies for Dyspnea

There are also complementary or alternative interventions that can help patients with dyspnea. In a single-blind (patient) randomized, controlled trial of 24 patients with COPD and disabling breathlessness, acupuncture improved breathlessness and 6-minute walking distance compared to sham acupuncture at the end of 3 weeks.[163] In a single-blind, cross-over, randomized, controlled trial of 31 patients with severe COPD (mean age 67 years) enrolled in a 12-week pulmonary rehabilitation program, patients were taught acupressure to be practiced daily at home for 6 weeks, alternating with sham acupressure for 6 weeks. Dyspnea as measured by VAS was significantly less during the weeks of real acupressure ($p = 0.009$). Dyspnea scores (out of 100) were 58.5 at baseline, 49 after sham acupressure, and 43.4 after real acupressure.[164]

In a case series of cancer patients, VAS scores for dyspnea, relaxation, and anxiety were reduced for a minimum of 6 hours postacupuncture in patients with cancer-related dyspnea.[165]

Ethical Considerations

The fear of using opioid and other sedative drugs with the potential for respiratory depression to ease the distress of terminal dyspnea often leads to inadequate symptom control. Health professionals and the public often mistakenly equate use of medications to ease terminal dyspnea with euthanasia or assisted suicide. Ethically, the use of these medications is appropriate and essential as long as the intent is to relieve symptom distress, rather than shorten life. Medications will invariably have undesirable side effects, such as sedation or respiratory depression, but the primary intention is relief of suffering and symptoms. This is known as the rule of double effect.[166,167] There is no ethical or professional justification for withholding symptomatic treatment to a dying patient out of fear of potential respiratory depression. Understanding the patient's wishes for end-of-life symptom control and good communication with both family and other caregivers (e.g., nursing staff) regarding how and why drugs to relieve distressing dyspnea are administered is essential to avoid misunderstanding. Furthermore, doses required to relieve respiratory distress are usually well below respiratory depressant doses; transient sedation may occur in opiate-naive patients when agents are begun, but this generally clears over several days. Psychostimulants and/or steroids may be useful if sedation does not resolve on opiate doses required to relieve dyspnea.

Psychological Burden of Advanced Lung Disease

Depression and Anxiety

Psychiatric symptoms are common in patients with ALD. An estimated 42%–45% of patients with moderate to severe COPD suffer from depression, a rate higher than that reported in other populations of chronically ill patients[168,169] or the estimated

10% among age-matched controls.[170] Anxiety has been reported in up to 34% of hospitalized COPD patients.[171] One-third of patients with inoperable lung cancer self-reported depression in a recent study; the most important risk factor was the patient's degree of functional impairment.[172] When associated with ALD, depression and anxiety may amplify somatic symptoms, threaten quality of life, and increase disability.[173] Left untreated, psychological comorbidity may interfere with effective patient interaction with loved ones or threaten the integrity of established relationships. The urgency of treating depression and anxiety is proportional to the degree it causes functional and emotional impairment. Emotional and physical withdrawal may lead to isolation, which may be complicated by substance abuse and suicide. Pharmacotherapy and supportive counseling, specifically cognitive-behavioral therapy, are available treatments.

Pharmacological approaches

Multiple classes of drugs are available to treat depression, panic, and anxiety. Among antidepressant drug classes, the selective serotonin reuptake inhibitors (SSRIs) have the fewest side effects, despite drug interactions with tricyclic antidepressants (TCAs) and cardiac medications such as β-blockers, calcium channel blockers, and antiarrythmics frequently taken by older ALD patients whose course is complicated by cardiac illness. Among the SSRIs, sertraline, paroxetine, and the phenylpiperazine nefazodone have fewer side effects and drug interactions and may be better tolerated in elderly populations. Nefazodone and trazodone, when administered at bedtime, may improve sleep in ALD patients who suffer concomitant insomnia. If these agents fail to improve symptoms after time-limited trials of 1–2 months, other drug classes may be of benefit as monotherapy or as adjunctive medication. Use of TCAs (amitriptyline) is complicated in the geriatric population by anticholinergic side effects, typically confusion, dry mouth, constipation, or urinary retention (in male patients), which may be less

with second-generation formulations such as nortriptyline. Benzodiazepines may prove useful for panic and anxiety, though they carry the risk of causing respiratory depression, dependence, and withdrawal. Nonetheless, moderate doses under appropriate monitoring can be effective in patients with anxiety complicating ALD.[174] Buspirone, a novel anxiolytic, may be of benefit in that, unlike benzodiazepines, it does not depress ventilation and may actually have a respiratory stimulant effect (see Chapter 20).

Cognitive-behavioral therapy

In some patients with ALD, fearful cognitions such as suffocation related to disease-specific symptoms of dyspnea may lead to panic, which can cause increased autonomic arousal and variable amounts of hyperventilation. The result is dynamic hyperinflation and an increase in the work of breathing, creating a positive feedback cycle which intensifies dyspnea.[174] Cognitive-behavioral therapy, a time-limited form of psychotherapy including disease-specific education, thought restructuring, relaxation techniques, and guided therapy, may reduce panic sensations comparable to drug therapy in ALD patients.[175] With or without pharmacotherapy, it may help to reduce stimulus severity and provide enough mental desensitization to break a potentially deleterious cycle of fearful cognitions driving dyspnea intensification. Referral to a behavioral therapist is appropriate when a patient's cognition about the disease amplifies, drives somatic symptoms, and results in functional decline.

CONCLUSION

To the health-care professional, dyspnea signifies illness, a treatment side effect, depression, or anxiety. To patients and families, dyspnea is a symptom that keeps them from moving forward fully with life in addition to all of the above. Health professionals can be supportive by acknowledging dyspnea as real and taking it and its frustrations seriously. Understanding the possible etiology of dyspnea and the meaning of the symptom to the patient are important in determining its management. Assisting patients and families to live as fully as possible as they move along the illness trajectory may require consideration of nonpharmacological as well as pharmacological therapies to comprehensively and effectively treat dyspnea. Learning how to prevent and manage dyspnea is important to improving patient function, ability to socialize, and ultimately adjustment to a "new normal" baseline as they live with chronic or life-limiting illness.

REFERENCES

1. American Thoracic Society. Dyspnea. Mechanisms, assessment, and management: a consensus statement. Am J Respir Crit Care Med 159:321–340, 1999.
2. Education for Physicians on End-of-Life Care. Common Physical Symptoms. Module 10. The EPEC Project. 2002.
3. Ahmedzai S. Palliation of respiratory symptoms: dyspnoea. In: Doyle D, Hanks G, MacDonald N (Eds.). Oxford Textbook of Palliative Medicine. Oxford, Oxford University Press, pp. 586–603, 1998.
4. Crofton J, Douglas A. The structures and function of the respiratory tract. In: Respiratory Diseases. Crofton J, Douglas A, Eds. Oxford, Blackwell, p. 1–79, 1981.
5. Ahmedzai S. Respiratory distress in the terminally ill patient. Respir Dis Pract 5: 20–29, 1988.
6. Nejjari C, Tessier JF, Dartigues JF, et al. The relationship between dyspnoea and main lifetime occupation in the elderly. Int J Epidemiol 22:848–854, 1993.
7. Landahl S, Steen B, Svanborg A. Dyspnea in 70-year-old people. Acta Med Scand 207:225–230, 1980.
8. Hansen-Flaschen J. Advanced lung disease. Palliation and terminal care. Clin Chest Med 18:645–655, 1997.
9. Rousseau P. Nonpain symptom management in terminal care. Clin Geriatr Med 12:313–327, 1996.
10. SUPPORT Principal Investigators. A controlled trial to improve care for seriously ill hospitalized patients. The Study to Understand Prognoses and Preferences for Outcomes and Risks of Treatments (SUPPORT). JAMA 274:1591–1598, 1995.
11. Claessens MT, Lynn J, Zhong Z, et al. Dying with lung cancer or chronic obstructive pulmonary disease: insights from SUP-

PORT. Study to Understand Prognoses and Preferences for Outcomes and Risks of Treatments. J Am Geriatr Soc 48(Suppl 5):S146–S153, 2000.
12. Reuben DB, Mor V. Dyspnea in terminally ill cancer patients. Chest 89:234–236, 1986.
13. Vainio A, Auvinen A. Prevalence of symptoms among patients with advanced cancer: an international collaborative study. Symptom Prevalence Group. J Pain Symptom Manage 12:3–10, 1996.
14. Seale C, Cartwright A. The Year Before Death. Brookfield, VT, Ashgale, 1994.
15. Levenson JW, McCarthy EP, Lynn J, et al. The last six months of life for patients with congestive heart failure. J Am Geriatr Soc 48(Suppl 5):S101–S109, 2000.
16. Rivera MP, Kris MG, Gralla RJ, White DA. Syndrome of acute dyspnea related to combined mitomycin plus vinca alkaloid chemotherapy. Am J Clin Oncol 18: 245–250, 1995.
17. Aaronson NK, Ahmedzai S, Bergman B, et al. The European Organization for Research and Treatment of Cancer QLQ-C30: a quality-of-life instrument for use in international clinical trials in oncology. J Natl Cancer Inst 85:365–376, 1993.
18. Aaronson NK, Bullinger M, Ahmedzai S. A modular approach to quality-of-life assessment in cancer clinical trials. Recent Results Cancer Res 111:231–249, 1988.
19. Bergman B, Aaronson NK, Ahmedzai S, et al. The EORTC QLQ-LC13: a modular supplement to the EORTC Core Quality of Life Questionnaire (QLQ-C30) for use in lung cancer clinical trials. EORTC Study Group on Quality of Life. Eur J Cancer 5:635–642, 1994.
20. Peel ET, Soutar CA, Seaton A. Assessment of variability of exercise tolerance limited by breathlessness. Thorax 43:960–964, 1988.
21. Wijkstra P, et al. Relation of lung function, maximal inspiratory pressure, dyspnoea, and quality of life with exercise capacity in patients with chronic obstructive pulmonary disease. Thorax 49:468–472, 1994.
22. Morgan AD. Simple exercise testing. Respir Med 83:383–387, 1989.
23. Morice A, Smithies T. The 100 m walk: a simple and reproducible exercise test. Br J Dis Chest 78:392–394, 1984.
24. Morice A, Smithies T. Two-, six-, and 12-minute walking test in respiratory disease. BMJ 285:295, 1982.
25. Wolkove N, Dajczman E, Colacone A, Kreisman H. The relationship between pulmonary function and dyspnea in ob-

structive lung disease. Chest 96:1247–1251, 1989.

26. Bruera E, Schmitz B, Pither J, et al. The frequency and correlates of dyspnea in patients with advanced cancer. J Pain Symptom Manage 19:357–362, 2000.

27. Belman MJ, Botnick WC, Shin JW. Inhaled bronchodilators reduce dynamic hyperinflation during exercise in patients with chronic obstructive pulmonary disease. Am J Respir Crit Care Med 153:967–975, 1996.

28. Anthonisen NR, Connett JE, Kiley JP, et al. Effects of smoking intervention and the use of an inhaled anticholinergic bronchodilator on the rate of decline of FEV$_1$. The Lung Health Study. JAMA 272:1497–1505, 1994.

29. Colice GL. Nebulized bronchodilators for outpatient management of stable chronic obstructive pulmonary disease. Am J Med 100:11S–18S, 1996.

30. Tashkin DP, Ashutosh K, Bleecker ER, et al. Comparison of the anticholinergic bronchodilator ipratropium bromide with metaproterenol in chronic obstructive pulmonary disease. A 90-day multi-center study. Am J Med 81:81–90, 1986.

31. Campbell S. For COPD a combination of ipratropium bromide and albuterol sulfate is more effective than albuterol base. Arch Intern Med 159:156–160, 1999.

32. COMBIVENT Inhalation Aerosol Study Group. In chronic obstructive pulmonary disease, a combination of ipratropium and albuterol is more effective than either agent alone. An 85-day multicenter trial. Chest 105:1411–1419, 1994.

33. Dorinsky PM, Reisner C, Ferguson GT, et al. The combination of ipratropium and albuterol optimizes pulmonary function reversibility testing in patients with COPD. Chest 115:966–971, 1999.

34. Vincken W, van Noord JA, Greefhorst AP, et al. Improved health outcomes in patients with COPD during 1 yr's treatment with tiotropium. Eur Respir J 19:209–216, 2002.

35. Rennard SI, Anderson W, ZuWallach R, et al. Use of a long-acting inhaled beta2-adrenergic agonist, salmeterol xinafoate, in patients with chronic obstructive pulmonary disease. Am J Respir Crit Care Med 163:1087–1092, 2001.

36. Cazzola M, Donner CF. Long-acting beta2 agonists in the management of stable chronic obstructive pulmonary disease. Drugs 60:307–320, 2000.

37. Hay J, Stone P, Carter J, et al. Bronchodilator reversibility, exercise performance and breathlessness in stable chronic obstructive pulmonary disease. Eur Respir J 5:659–664, 1992.

38. Berry RB, Shinto RA, Wong FH, et al. Nebulizer vs spacer for bronchodilator delivery in patients hospitalized for acute exacerbations of COPD. Chest 96:1241–1246, 1989.

39. Grazzini M, Stendardi L, Rosi E, Scano G. Pharmacological treatment of exercise dyspnoea. Monaldi Arch Chest Dis 56:43–47, 2001.

40. Murciano D, Auclair MH, Pariente R, Aubier M. A randomized, controlled trial of theophylline in patients with severe chronic obstructive pulmonary disease. N Engl J Med 320:1521–1525, 1989.

41. Sherman MS, Lang DM, Matityahu A, Campbell D. Theophylline improves measurements of respiratory muscle efficiency. Chest 110:1437–1442, 1996.

42. Matthay RA. Favorable cardiovascular effects of theophylline in COPD. Chest 92(Suppl 1):22S–26S, 1987.

43. Ziment I. Theophylline and mucociliary clearance. Chest 92(Suppl 1):38S–43S, 1987.

44. Wanner A. Effects of methylxanthines on airway mucociliary function. Am J Med 79:16–21, 1985.

45. Rabe KF, Dent G. Theophylline and airway inflammation. Clin Exp Allergy 28(Suppl 3):35–41, 1998.

46. Minoguchi K, Kohno Y, Oda N, et al. Effect of theophylline withdrawal on airway inflammation in asthma. Clin Exp Allergy 28(Suppl 3):57–63, 1998.

47. Wolfe JD, Tashkin DP, Calvarese B, Simmons M. Bronchodilator effects of terbutaline and aminophylline alone and in combination in asthmatic patients. N Engl J Med 298:363–367, 1978.

48. Kirsten DK, Wegner RE, Jorres RA, Magnussen H. Effects of theophylline withdrawal in severe chronic obstructive pulmonary disease. Chest 104:1101–1107, 1993.

49. Mahler DA, Matthay RA, Snyder PE, et al. Sustained-release theophylline reduces dyspnea in nonreversible obstructive airway disease. Am Rev Respir Dis 131:22–25, 1985.

50. Martin RJ, Pak J. Overnight theophylline concentrations and effects on sleep and lung function in chronic obstructive pulmonary disease. Am Rev Respir Dis 145:540–544, 1992.

51. ZuWallack RL, Mahler DA, Reilly D, et al. Salmeterol plus theophylline combination therapy in the treatment of COPD. Chest 119:1661–1670, 2001.

52. Guyatt GH, Townsend M, Pugsley SO, et

al. Bronchodilators in chronic air-flow limitation. Effects on airway function, exercise capacity, and quality of life. Am Rev Respir Dis 135:1069–1074, 1987.

53. Niewoehner DE, Erbland ML, Deupree RH, et al. Effect of systemic glucocorticoids on exacerbations of chronic obstructive pulmonary disease. Department of Veterans Affairs Cooperative Study Group. N Engl J Med 340:1941–1947, 1999.

54. Snow V, Lascher S, Mottur-Pilson C. Evidence base for management of acute exacerbations of chronic obstructive pulmonary disease. Ann Intern Med 134: 595–599, 2001.

55. Callahan CM, Dittus RS, Katz BP. Oral corticosteroid therapy for patients with stable chronic obstructive pulmonary disease. A meta-analysis. Ann Intern Med 114:216–223, 1991.

56. Weiner P, Weiner M, Rabner M, et al. The response to inhaled and oral steroids in patients with stable chronic obstructive pulmonary disease. J Intern Med 245:83–89, 1999.

57. Rice KL, Rubins JB, Lebahn F, et al. Withdrawal of chronic systemic corticosteroids in patients with COPD: a randomized trial. Am J Respir Crit Care Med 162:174–178, 2000.

58. Schols AM, Wesseling G, Kester AD, et al. Dose dependent increased mortality risk in COPD patients treated with oral glucocorticoids. Eur Respir J 17:337–342, 2001.

59. Libanati CR, Baylink DJ. Prevention and treatment of glucocorticoid-induced osteoporosis. A pathogenetic perspective. Chest 102:1426–1435, 1992.

60. The Living Health Study Research Group. Effect of inhaled triamcinolone on the decline in pulmonary function in chronic obstructive pulmonary disease. N Engl J Med 343:1902–1909, 2000.

61. Burge PS, Calverley PM, Jones PW, et al. Randomised, double blind, placebo controlled study of fluticasone propionate in patients with moderate to severe chronic obstructive pulmonary disease: the ISOLDE trial. BMJ 320:1297–1303, 2000.

62. Baughman RP, Alabi FO. Nonsteroidal therapy for idiopathic pulmonary fibrosis. Curr Opin Pulm Med 7:309–313, 2001.

63. Kolb M, Kirschner J, Riedel W, et al. Cyclophosphamide pulse therapy in idiopathic pulmonary fibrosis. Eur Respir J 12:1409–1414, 1998.

64. Lynch JP 3rd, White E, Flaherty K. Corticosteroids in idiopathic pulmonary fibrosis. Curr Opin Pulm Med 7:298–308, 2001.

65. Douglas WW, Ryu JH, Schroeder DR. Idiopathic pulmonary fibrosis: impact of oxygen and colchicine, prednisone, or no therapy on survival. Am J Respir Crit Care Med 161:1172–1178, 2000.

66. Zisman DA, Lynch JP 3rd, Toews G-B, et al. Cyclophosphamide in the treatment of idiopathic pulmonary fibrosis: a prospective study in patients who failed to respond to corticosteroids. Chest 117:1619–1626, 2000.

67. Flaherty KR, Toews G-B, Lynch JP 3rd, et al. Steroids in idiopathic pulmonary fibrosis: a prospective assessment of adverse reactions, response to therapy, and survival. Am J Med 110:278–282, 2001.

68. Ziesche R, Hofbauer F, Wittmann K, et al. A preliminary study of long-term treatment with interferon gamma-1b and low-dose prednisolone in patients with idiopathic pulmonary fibrosis. N Engl J Med 341:1264–1269, 1999.

69. Toogood JH. Side effects of inhaled corticosteroids. J Allergy Clin Immunol 102: 705–713, 1998.

70. Boulet LP, Cockcroft DW, Toogood J, et al. Comparative assessment of safety and efficacy of inhaled corticosteroids: report of a committee of the Canadian Thoracic Society. Eur Respir J 11:1194–1210, 1998.

71. Meibohm B, Hochhaus G, Mollmann H, et al. A pharmacokinetic/pharmacodynamic approach to predict the cumulative cortisol suppression of inhaled corticosteroids. J Pharmacokinet Biopharm 27: 127–147, 1999.

72. Nielsen LP, Dahl R. Therapeutic ratio of inhaled corticosteroids in adult asthma. A dose-range comparison between fluticasone propionate and budesonide, measuring their effect on bronchial hyperresponsiveness and adrenal cortex function. Am J Respir Crit Care Med 162:2053–2057, 2000.

73. Patrick J. Studies of respiratory control in man. In: Pallot D (Ed.). Control of Respiration. London, Croom Helm, pp. 203–220, 1983.

74. Daskalopoulou E, Patakas D, Tsara V, et al. Comparison of almitrine bismesylate and medroxyprogesterone acetate on oxygenation during wakefulness and sleep in patients with chronic obstructive lung disease. Thorax 45:666–669, 1990.

75. Al-Damluji S. The effect of ventilatory stimulation with medroxyprogesterone on exercise performance and the sensation of dyspnoea in hypercapnic chronic bronchitis. Br J Dis Chest 80:273–279, 1986.

76. Mikami M, Tatsumi K, Kimura H, et al. Respiration effect of synthetic progestin in

small doses in normal men. Chest 96: 1073–1075, 1989.

77. Winning AJ, Hamilton RD, Shea SA, et al. The effect of airway anaesthesia on the control of breathing and the sensation of breathlessness in man. Clin Sci (Colch) 68:215–225, 1985.

78. Labaille T, Clergue F, Samii K, et al. Ventilatory response to CO_2 following intravenous and epidural lidocaine. Anesthesiology 63:179–183, 1985.

79. Ahmedzai S, Carter R, Mills RJ, Moran F. Effects of nabilone on pulmonary function. In: Marihuana '84. Proceedings of the Oxford Symposium on Cannabis. Oxford, IRL Press, pp. 371–378, 1984.

80. Vachon L, Fitzgerald MX, Solliday NH, et al. Single-dose effects of marihuana smoke. Bronchial dynamics and respiratory-center sensitivity in normal subjects. N Engl J Med 288:985–989, 1973.

81. Noxturnal Oxygen Therapy Trial Group. Continuous or nocturnal oxygen therapy in hypoxemic chronic obstructive lung disease: a clinical trial. Ann Intern Med 93: 391–398, 1980.

82. Robinson TD, Freiberg DB, Regnis JA, Young IH. The role of hypoventilation and ventilation-perfusion redistribution in oxygen-induced hypercapnia during acute exacerbations of chronic obstructive pulmonary disease. Am J Respir Crit Care Med 161:1524–1529, 2000.

83. McDonald CF, Blyth CM, Lazarus MD, et al. Exertional oxygen of limited benefit in patients with chronic obstructive pulmonary disease and mild hypoxemia. Am J Respir Crit Care Med 152:1616–1619, 1995.

84. Garrod R, Paul EA, Wedzicha JA. Supplemental oxygen during pulmonary rehabilitation in patients with COPD with exercise hypoxaemia. Thorax 55:539–543, 2000.

85. Dewan NA, Bell CW. Effect of low flow and high flow oxygen delivery on exercise tolerance and sensation of dyspnea. A study comparing the transtracheal catheter and nasal prongs. Chest 105:1061–1065, 1994.

86. Swinburn CR, Mould H, Stone TN, et al. Symptomatic benefit of supplemental oxygen in hypoxemic patients with chronic lung disease. Am Rev Respir Dis 143: 913–915, 1991.

87. Liss H, Grant B. The effect of nasal flow on breathlessness in patients with chronic obstructive pulmonary disease. Am Rev Respir Dis 137:1285–1288, 1988.

88. Bruera E, Schoeller T, MacEachern T. Symptomatic benefit of supplemental oxygen in hypoxemic patients with terminal cancer: the use of the N of 1 randomized controlled trial. J Pain Symptom Manage 7:365–368, 1992.

89. Booth S, Kelly MJ, Cox NP, et al. Does oxygen help dyspnea in patients with cancer? Am J Respir Crit Care Med 153: 1515–1518, 1996.

90. Schwartzstein RM, Lahive K, Pope A, et al. Cold facial stimulation reduces breathlessness induced in normal subjects. Am Rev Respir Dis 136:58–61, 1987.

91. Woodcock AA, Gross ER, Gellert A, et al. Effects of dihydrocodeine, alcohol, and caffeine on breathlessness and exercise tolerance in patients with chronic obstructive lung disease and normal blood gases. N Engl J Med 305:1611–1616, 1981.

92. Couser JI Jr, Make BJ. Transtracheal oxygen decreases inspired minute ventilation. Am Rev Respir Dis 139:627–631, 1989.

93. Bloom BS, Daniel JM, Wiseman M, et al. Transtracheal oxygen delivery and patients with chronic obstructive pulmonary disease. Respir Med 83:281–288, 1989.

94. Weil JV, McCullough RE, Kline JS, Sodal IE. Diminished ventilatory response to hypoxia and hypercapnia after morphine in normal man. N Engl J Med 292:1103–1106, 1975.

95. Johnson M, Woodcock AA, Geddes DM. Dihydrocodeine for breathlessness in "pink puffers." BMJ 286:675–677, 1983.

96. Bar-Or D, Marx JA, Good J. Breathlessness, alcohol, and opiates. N Engl J Med 306:1363–1364, 1982.

97. Light R, Muro JR, Sato RI, et al. Effects of oral morphine on breathlessness and exercise tolerance in patients with chronic obstructive pulmonary disease. Am Rev Respir Dis 139:126–133, 1989.

98. Robin E, Burke C. Single-patient randomized clinical trial. Opiates for intractable dyspnea. Chest 90:888–892, 1986.

99. Rice KL, Kronenberg RS, Hedemark LL, Niewoehner DE. Effects of chronic administration of codeine and promethazine on breathlessness and exercise tolerance in patients with chronic airflow obstruction. Br J Dis Chest 81:287–292, 1987.

100. Eiser N, Denman WT, West C, Luce P. Oral diamorphine: lack of effect on dyspnoea and exercise tolerance in the "pink puffer" syndrome. Eur Respir J 4:926–931, 1991.

101. Poole PJ, Veale AG, Black PN. The effect of sustained-release morphine on breathlessness and quality of life in severe chronic obstructive pulmonary disease. Am J Respir Crit Care Med 157:1877–1880, 1998.

102. Young IH, Daviskas E, Keena VA. Effect of low dose nebulised morphine on exercise endurance in patients with chronic lung disease. Thorax 44:387–390, 1989.

103. Beauford W, Saylor TT, Stansbury DW, et al. Effects of nebulized morphine sulfate on the exercise tolerance of the ventilatory limited COPD patient. Chest 104:175–178, 1993.

104. Leung R, Hill P, Burdon J. Effect of inhaled morphine on the development of breathlessness during exercise in patients with chronic lung disease. Thorax 51:596–600, 1996.

105. Masood AR, Reed JW, Thomas SH. Lack of effect of inhaled morphine on exercise-induced breathlessness in chronic obstructive pulmonary disease. Thorax 50:629–634, 1995.

106. Noseda A, Carpiaux JP, Markstein C, et al. Disabling dyspnoea in patients with advanced disease: lack of effect of nebulized morphine. Eur Respir J 10:1079–1083, 1997.

107. Bruera E, Macmillan K, Pither J, MacDonald RN. Effects of morphine on the dyspnea of terminal cancer patients. J Pain Symptom Manage 5:341–344, 1990.

108. Bruera E, MacEachern T, Ripamonli C, Hanson J. Subcutaneous morphine for dyspnea in cancer patients. Ann Intern Med 119:906–907, 1993.

109. Cohen MH, Anderson AJ, Krasnow SH, et al. Continuous intravenous infusion of morphine for severe dyspnea. South Med J 84:229–234, 1991.

110. Woodcock AA, Gross ER, Geddes DM. Drug treatment of breathlessness: contrasting effects of diazepam and promethazine in pink puffers. BMJ 283:343–346, 1981.

111. Man G, Hsu K, Sproule B. Effect of alprazolam on exercise and dyspnea in patients with chronic obstructive pulmonary disease. Chest 90:832–836, 1986.

112. Eimer M, Cable T, Gal P, et al. Effects of clorazepate on breathlessness and exercise tolerance in patients with chronic airflow obstruction. J Fam Pract 21:359–362, 1985.

113. Argyropoulou P, Patakas D, Koukou A, et al. Buspirone effect on breathlessness and exercise performance in patients with chronic obstructive pulmonary disease. Respiration 60:216–220, 1993.

114. Singh NP, Despars JA, Stansbury DW, et al. Effects of buspirone on anxiety levels and exercise tolerance in patients with chronic airflow obstruction and mild anxiety. Chest 103:800–804, 1993.

115. McIver B, Walsh D, Nelson K. The use of chlorpromazine for symptom control in dying cancer patients. J Pain Symptom Manage 9:341–345, 1994.

116. Light RW, Stansbury DW, Webster JS. Effect of 30 mg of morphine alone or with promethazine or prochlorperazine on the exercise capacity of patients with COPD. Chest 109:975–981, 1996.

117. Griffiths TL, Burr ML, Campbell IA, et al. Results at 1 year of outpatient multidisciplinary pulmonary rehabilitation: a randomised controlled trial. Lancet 355:362–368, 2000.

118. Ries AL, Kaplan RM, Limberg TM, Prewitt LM. Effects of pulmonary rehabilitation on physiologic and psychosocial outcomes in patients with chronic obstructive pulmonary disease. Ann Intern Med 122:823–832, 1995.

119. Lacasse Y, Wong E, Guyatt GH, et al. Meta-analysis of respiratory rehabilitation in chronic obstructive pulmonary disease. Lancet 348:1115–1119, 1996.

120. Finnerty JP, Keeping I, Bullough I, Jones J. The effectiveness of outpatient pulmonary rehabilitation in chronic lung disease: a randomized controlled trial. Chest 119:1705–1710, 2001.

121. Weiner P, Magadle R, Berar-Yanay N, et al. The cumulative effect of long-acting bronchodilators, exercise, and inspiratory muscle training on the perception of dyspnea in patients with advanced COPD. Chest 118:672–678, 2000.

122. Renfroe KL. Effect of progressive relaxation on dyspnea and state anxiety in patients with chronic obstructive pulmonary disease. Heart Lung 17:408–413, 1988.

123. Harver A, Mahler DA, Daubenspeck JA. Targeted inspiratory muscle training improves respiratory muscle function and reduces dyspnea in patients with chronic obstructive pulmonary disease. Ann Intern Med 111:117–124, 1989.

124. Sinclair DJ, Ingram CG. Controlled trial of supervised exercise training in chronic bronchitis. BMJ 280:519–521, 1980.

125. Celikel T, Sungur M, Ceyhan B, Karakurt S. Comparison of noninvasive positive pressure ventilation with standard medical therapy in hypercapnic acute respiratory failure. Chest 114:1636–1642, 1998.

126. Antonelli M, Conti G, Rocco M, et al. A comparison of noninvasive positive-pressure ventilation and conventional mechanical ventilation in patients with acute respiratory failure. N Engl J Med 339:429–435, 1998.

127. Brochard L, Mancebo J, Wysocki M, et al. Noninvasive ventilation for acute exacerbations of chronic obstructive pulmonary disease. N Engl J Med 333:817–822, 1995.

128. Kramer N, Meyer TJ, Meharg J, et al. Randomized, prospective trial of noninvasive positive pressure ventilation in acute respiratory failure. Am J Respir Crit Care Med 151:1799–1806, 1995.

129. Meecham Jones DJ, Paul EA, Jones PW, Wedzicha JA, et al. Nasal pressure support ventilation plus oxygen compared with oxygen therapy alone in hypercapnic COPD. Am J Respir Crit Care Med 152:538–544, 1995.

130. Strumpf DA, Millman RP, Carlisle CC, et al. Nocturnal positive-pressure ventilation via nasal mask in patients with severe chronic obstructive pulmonary disease. Am Rev Respir Dis 144:1234–1239, 1991.

131. Robert D, Willig TN, Leger P. Long-term nasal ventilation in neuromuscular disorders: report of a consensus conference. Eur Respir J 6:599–606, 1993.

132. Sung DT, Payne WS, Black LF. Surgical management of giant bullae associated with obstructive airway disease. Surg Clin North Am 53:913–920, 1973.

133. Benditt JO, Albert RK. Surgical options for patients with advanced emphysema. Clin Chest Med 18:577–593, 1997.

134. Stirling GR, Babidge WJ, Peacock MJ, et al. Lung volume reduction surgery in emphysema: a systematic review. Ann Thorac Surg 72:641–648, 2001.

135. Flaherty KR, Martinez FJ. Lung volume reduction surgery for emphysema. Clin Chest Med 21:819–848, 2000.

136. Flaherty KR, Kazerooni EA, Curtis JL, et al. Short-term and long-term outcomes after bilateral lung volume reduction surgery: prediction by quantitative CT. Chest 119:1337–1346, 2001.

137. The National Emphysema Treatment Trial Research Group. Rationale and design of the National Emphysema Treatment Trial: a prospective randomized trial of lung volume reduction surgery. Chest 116:1750–1761, 1999.

138. National Emphysema Treatment Trial Research Group. Patients at high risk of death after lung-volume-reduction surgery. N Engl J Med 345:1075–1083, 2001.

139. Hosenpud JD, Bennett LE, Keck BM, et al. The Registry of the International Society for Heart and Lung Transplantation: eighteenth official report–2001. J Heart Lung Transplant 20:805–815, 2001.

140. Bradley GW, Hale T, Pimble J, et al. Effect of vagotomy on the breathing pattern and exercise ability in emphysematous patients. Clin Sci (Colch) 62:311–319, 1982.

141. Stulbarg MS, Winn WR, Kellett LE. Bilateral carotid body resection for the relief of dyspnea in severe chronic obstructive pulmonary disease. Physiologic and clinical observations in three patients. Chest 95:1123–1128, 1989.

142. American Thoracic Society. Management of malignant pleural effusions. Am J Respir Crit Care Med 162:1987–2001, 2000.

143. Sahn SA. Malignancy metastatic to the pleura. Clin Chest Med 19:351–361, 1998.

144. Rodriguez-Panadero F, Antony VB. Pleurodesis: state of the art. Eur Respir J 10:1648–1654, 1997.

145. Walker-Renard PB, Vaughan LM, Sahn SA. Chemical pleurodesis for malignant pleural effusions. Ann Intern Med 120:56–64, 1994.

146. Putnam JB Jr, Walsh GL, Swisher SG, et al. Outpatient management of malignant pleural effusion by a chronic indwelling pleural catheter. Ann Thorac Surg 69:369–375, 2000.

147. Putnam JB Jr, Light RW, Rodriguez RM, et al. A randomized comparison of indwelling pleural catheter and doxycycline pleurodesis in the management of malignant pleural effusions. Cancer 86:1992–1999, 1999.

148. Seijo LM, Sterman DH. Interventional pulmonology. N Engl J Med 344:740–749, 2001.

149. Vonk-Noordegraaf A, Postmus PE, Sutedja TG. Tracheobronchial stenting in the terminal care of cancer patients with central airways obstruction. Chest 120:1811–1814, 2001.

150. Non-small Cell Lung Cancer Collaborative Group. Chemotherapy in non-small cell lung cancer: a meta-analysis using updated data on individual patients from 52 randomised clinical trials. BMJ 311:899–909, 1995.

151. Ranson M, Davidson N, Nicolson M, et al. Randomized trial of paclitaxel plus supportive care versus supportive care for patients with advanced non-small-cell lung cancer. J Natl Cancer Inst 92:1074–1080, 2000.

152. Cullen MH, Billingham LJ, Woodroffe CM, et al. Mitomycin, ifosfamide, and cisplatin in unresectable non-small-cell lung cancer: effects on survival and quality of life. J Clin Oncol 17:3188–3194, 1999.

153. Roszkowski K, Pluzanska A, Krzakowski M, et al. A multicenter, randomized, phase III study of docetaxel plus best supportive care versus best supportive care in chemotherapy-naive patients with metastatic or non-resectable localized non-small cell lung cancer (NSCLC). Lung Cancer 27:145–157, 2000.

154. Anderson H, Hopwood P, Stephens RJ, et al. Gemcitabine plus best supportive care

(BSC) vs BSC in inoperable non-small cell lung cancer—a randomized trial with quality of life as the primary outcome. UK NSCLC Gemcitabine Group. Non-Small Cell Lung Cancer. Br J Cancer 83:447–453, 2000.

155. Gridelli C, The ELVIS trial: a phase III study of single-agent vinorelbine as first-line treatment in elderly patients with advanced non-small cell lung cancer. Elderly Lung Cancer Vinorelbine Italian Study. Oncologist 6(Suppl 1):4–7, 2001.

156. Earle CC, Tsai JS, Gelber RD, et al. Effectiveness of chemotherapy for advanced lung cancer in the elderly: instrumental variable and propensity analysis. J Clin Oncol 19:1064–1070, 2001.

157. Hickish TF, Smith IE, O'Brien ME, et al. Clinical benefit from palliative chemotherapy in non-small-cell lung cancer extends to the elderly and those with poor prognostic factors. Br J Cancer 78:28–33, 1998.

158. Silvestri G, Pritchard R, Welch HG. Preferences for chemotherapy in patients with advanced non-small cell lung cancer: descriptive study based on scripted interviews. BMJ 317:771–775, 1998.

159. Langendijk JA, ten Velde GP, Aaronson NK, et al. Quality of life after palliative radiotherapy in non-small cell lung cancer: a prospective study. Int J Radiat Oncol Biol Phys 47:149–155, 2000.

160. Macbeth F, Toy E, Coles B, et al. Palliative radiotherapy regimens for non-small cell lung cancer. Cochrane Database Syst Rev 2001. CD002143

161. Schaafsma J, Coy P. Response of global quality of life to high-dose palliative radiotherapy for non-small-cell lung cancer. Int J Radiat Oncol Biol Phys 47:691–701, 2000.

162. Patterson CJ, Hocking M, Bond M, Teale C. Retrospective study of radiotherapy for lung cancer in patients aged 75 years and over. Age Ageing 27:515–518, 1998.

163. Jobst K, Chen JH, McPherson K, et al. Controlled trial of acupuncture for disabling breathlessness. Lancet 2:1416–1419, 1986.

164. Maa SH, Gauthier D, Turner M. Acupressure as an adjunct to a pulmonary rehabilitation program. J Cardiopulm Rehabil 17:268–276, 1997.

165. Filshie J, Penn K, Ashley S, Davis CL. Acupuncture for the relief of cancer-related breathlessness. Palliat Med 10:145–150, 1996.

166. Quill TE, Dresser R, Brock DW. The rule of double effect—a critique of its role in end-of-life decision making [see comments in N Engl J Med 338:1389–1390, 1998]. N Engl J Med 337:1768–1771, 1997.

167. Manfredi PL, Morrison RS, Meier DE. The rule of double effect. N Engl J Med 338:1390, 1998.

168. Katon W. The epidemiology of depression in medical care. Int J Psychiatry Med 17:93–112, 1987.

169. Light RW, Merrill EJ, Despars JA, et al. Prevalence of depression and anxiety in patients with COPD. Relationship to functional capacity. Chest 87:35–38, 1985.

170. McSweeney AJ, Heaton RK, Grant I, et al. Chronic obstructive pulmonary disease; socioemotional adjustment and life quality. Chest 77(Suppl 2):309–311, 1980.

171. Yellowlees PM, Alpers JH, Bowden JJ, et al. Psychiatric morbidity in patients with chronic airflow obstruction. Med J Aust 146:305–307, 1987.

172. Hopwood P, Stephens RJ. Depression in patients with lung cancer: prevalence and risk factors derived from quality-of-life data. J Clin Oncol 18:893–903, 2000.

173. Greenberg GD, Ryan JJ, Bourlier PF. Psychological and neuropsychological aspects of COPD. Psychosomatics 26:29–33, 1985.

174. Smoller JW, Pollack MH, Otto MW, et al. Panic, anxiety, dyspnea, and respiratory disease. Theoretical and clinical considerations. Am J Respir Crit Care Med 154:6–17, 1996.

175. Corner J, Plant H, A'Hern R, Bailey C. Non-pharmacological intervention for breathlessness in lung cancer. Palliat Med 10:299–305, 1996.

18

Gastrointestinal Symptoms

NIGEL P. SYKES

The gastrointestinal tract produces a large number of symptoms, many of which become more common with increasing age. Some gastrointestinal symptoms are also among the most distressing in palliative care, particularly when associated with advanced cancer but also, to a lesser degree, in neurological and other types of progressive disease. The care of a person who has the combination of old age and a condition requiring palliative care therefore requires knowledge of the management of several key gastrointestinal symptoms, one or more of which is most likely present.

This chapter briefly reviews symptoms selected for their high occurrence and troublesomeness, starting at the mouth and working downward.

MOUTH PROBLEMS

Mouth problems are extremely common in any palliative care population;[1] and if inadequately treated, they can multiply. For instance, a dry mouth more easily becomes infected, increases the risk of dental caries,

and interferes with communication. Taste distortion exacerbates anorexia.

Dry Mouth

There is no clear evidence that aging diminishes salivary flow, although there are certainly age-related changes in salivary gland structure. Neither is it always apparent that a complaint of dry mouth is associated with impaired salivation. Dry mouth is common in terminally ill patients and appears to occur more frequently as disease progresses. Factors in the later stages of illness include the following:

- Increasing use of medication, some with anticholinergic actions
- Reduction in food intake and decreased firmness of the food that is still taken, both of which reduce the masticatory stimulus to salivation
- Possibly an increase in mouth breathing

Management

- Ensure that the mouth is clean. In weak and debilitated patients, mouth care may be needed every 2 hours. Relatives can help.

- Encourage frequent drinks when they can be tolerated.
- Identify and, if possible, stop contributing medications.
- Salivary flow is stimulated by astringent tastes such as citrus fruits and acid drops, but these will increase the discomfort of a sore mouth.
- Certain fruits are said to improve mucosal coating because of the enzymes they contain, e.g., ananase in the case of pineapple and papain in papaya.
- Several proprietary artificial salivas are available, based on either methylcellulose or mucin. Both types of preparation form a moisture-retaining gel, and different flavorings are available. However, it is worth recalling when treating Jewish or Moslem patients that the mucin preparations are derived from by-products of the bacon industry.
- Pilocarpine 5 mg tid[2] increases salivary flow except in those who have suffered severe radiotherapy damage to the salivary glands. The effect is not always immediate and may be accompanied by runny eyes and rhinorrhea.

Infections

Candida has been found in 83% of patients with advanced cancer,[3] although around half of the candidal infections were asymptomatic. Infection may be the result, rather than the cause, of mouth problems; and general oral hygiene, particularly of dentures, in the terminally ill may be more important than antifungals. *Candida albicans* is the commonest oral fungal infection; but others, such as *C. glabrata*, can also be found and vary in their sensitivity to antifungal drugs. The elderly are particularly susceptible to oral *Candida*, especially if they are diabetic or exposed to antibiotics or steroids.

Classically, *Candida* presents as white plaques, which are easily scraped off, leaving an erythematous surface beneath; but it can also produce simply a red smooth mucosa. Either appearance may be accompanied by angular cheilitis. *Candida* can also affect the esophagus to give painful swallowing and hence dysphagia. Endoscopy will show the characteristic mucosal signs, but it is generally more practical to have a high index of suspicion and give a trial of antifungal therapy.

Management

- Nystatin suspension is cheap and still often effective for oral candidiasis, although its activity is reduced by chlorhexidine, which is a constituent of many mouthwashes.[3] As nystatin is essentially a topical agent, it requires careful application, which if the patient is unable, takes significant nursing time and is inappropriate for esophageal or systemic candidiasis.
- The good bioavailability of fluconazole makes it a suitable alternative for these problems. Itraconazole is a further alternative, although drug interactions and hepatotoxicity may be important. Ketoconazole can be hepatotoxic, is impaired by low gastric acid (e.g., H_2-blockers), and interacts with many medications.

The vesicles of herpes infections are extremely painful, especially if they extend to the esophagus, and often make the person systemically unwell. Prompt initiation of acyclovir probably hastens the clearance of lesions and symptoms.

Mouth dryness in an immunosuppressed patient can also lead to bacterial infections, particularly with coliforms and staphylococci. Appropriate antibiotics and careful oral hygiene are indicated.

Other Oral Problems

Mucositis can be due to chemotherapy, notably with 5-fluorouracil or methotrexate, or to radiotherapy to the head and neck. It will eventually clear spontaneously but can be reduced by benzydamine oral rinse[4] or sucralfate.[5]

Taste alterations are present in 25% of cancer patients at presentation and affect around half of those with advanced malignancy. The problem is worsened by factors such as dry mouth, chemotherapy, and infection. Certain medications can also distort taste; e.g., dexamethasone can induce a metallic taste in the mouth, and ramipril can make food and drink taste salty. Reversible factors should be dealt with, but beyond this, steroids may help, if only by enhancing appetite sufficiently to overcome the aversive effect of the taste changes. It may also be helpful to introduce compensations into the diet, such as spices to overcome a dulled palate or white instead of red meat if there is an increased sensitivity to bitterness and, hence, to foods containing urea.

DYSPHAGIA

In one series of 800 palliative care patients, dysphagia affected 12% of individuals.[6] Of these, about 30% were not confirmed on objective assessment, and it was suggested that these cases represented the results of anxiety or poor appetite rather than physical impairment of swallowing. Dry mouth or insufficient mastication in edentulous patients can also cause dysphagia where no actual obstruction or neurological derangement of swallowing exists.

Assessment

Neurogenic dysphagia involves liquids initially and only later solids, whereas mechanical obstruction affects solids first. The oropharyngeal phase of swallowing is most affected by a neurological abnormality, with an inability to make food leave the mouth; however, mechanical obstruction often involves the esophageal phase so that food leaves the mouth but becomes stuck in the esophagus. In addition, swallowing may be painful, and there may be complaints of coughing during eating (suggestive of aspiration), drooling, nasal regurgitation, or late regurgitation of undigested food. The latter should be distinguished from vomiting.

Investigation

Investigation by barium swallow, endoscopy for structural disorders, and manometric and video studies for neuromuscular disorders may be appropriate. A speech and language therapy assessment can both elucidate pathology and suggest therapy.

Esophageal cancers are the most likely to cause obstruction, giving rise to 30% of cases of malignant dysphagia, followed by gastric and oropharyngeal cancers. Dysphagia associated with neural infiltration by tumor has been seen, particularly in squamous cancers of the head and neck, and sometimes responds to steroids.[7]

Nearly 60% of dysphagia cases in advanced cancer can be ameliorated by conservative management.[6] The principal measures are as follows:

- Provision of a diet of the correct consistency for each patient's needs, attuned to the individual's tastes, and presented as attractively as possible.
- Attention to the temperature of food and drink. Some patients after surgery or radiotherapy to the head and neck have a temporary loss of sensation in the mouth, resulting in uncoordinated swallowing. Very cold or warm food may help re-educate the swallowing mechanism. A similar effect of cold has been found in amyotrophic lateral sclerosis patients with bulbar involvement, in whom application of a source of cold beneath the chin prior to eating can assist swallowing.
- In neurogenic dysphagia, very watery liquids may be more difficult to swallow than substances of thicker consistency, and the addition of thickeners can help.
- Careful attention to oral hygiene, including clearance of infection where necessary.
- Good general symptom control, with particular attention to pain and nausea.
- Use of steroids if a cytotoxic effect may be expected, esophageal compression from mediastinal nodal deposits is likely, or in head and neck cancer, where symptoms may result from neural infiltration.
- Allow adequate time for eating, and help the patient to find the most satisfactory position of the head to aid swallowing, especially if the oropharyngeal phase of swallowing is impaired.

External beam radiotherapy relieves dysphagia due to low esophageal obstruction in 50% of patients but may require a treatment schedule too onerous for the frail. Intracavitary irradiation has shown a 65% success rate in a similar group of patients after a single treatment, with little morbidity.[8]

Palliation of esophageal tumors can also be achieved by endoscopic use of lasers. Typically, response rates of at least 75% are reported, with repeat treatments being needed up to every 4 weeks or so and low morbidity in the hands of experienced operators.[9]

A malignant esophageal stricture may be dilated by bouginage, but multiple procedures may be needed to restore luminal patency and dilation may have to be repeated later. Alternatively, the dilation can be maintained by endoscopic insertion of an indwelling flexible esophageal tube, which preserves the ability to eat a soft diet and drink fluids. Patient education regarding diet and regular flushing of the tube with carbonated drinks is important if blockage is to be avoided. Although the quality of swallowing with this technique is reported to be slightly less than after laser, it has the benefit of not usually requiring repetition and is therefore probably the approach of choice for those who are elderly and unwell.

Nasogastric intubation, parenteral nutrition, and formation of a gastrostomy are inappropriate in the management of dysphagia caused by incurable malignant obstruction. The first two of these procedures are restrictive, and none facilitates the swallowing of saliva. Hence, aspiration is likely to ensue, resulting in prolongation of an uncomfortable death rather than of a worthwhile life.

ANOREXIA

Anorexia, loss of appetite, becomes virtually universal by the last stages of progressive illness. Because it accompanies physical deterioration, anorexia can be a focus of anxiety for the patient and, particularly, the family. Anorexia is a contributor to the weight loss of the cachexia syndrome seen in some cancers and in cardiac failure, but cachexia reflects widespread and very profound changes in the body's metabolism and is not simply due to inadequate food intake. Weight loss commences prior to reduction in appetite and can be reversed effectively only by cure of the underlying disease, probably reflecting the role of cytokine release in its mediation.

Management

Appetite can fail for many reasons, and a therapeutic approach to anorexia must be multifaceted. To a significant extent, anorexia is a sign of diminishing health and unlikely to be fully reversible, certainly not permanently reversible. It is therefore a problem only if it is so defined by the patient, and family and friends need to be told gently that the reason the patient is so ill is not because he or she is not eating enough. Rather, the lack of appetite is a reflection of the severity of the disease, and their life should not be made miserable by being browbeaten into eating more than they want or can handle.

Nevertheless, potentially reversible factors need to be assessed and dealt with if present:

- Further treatment for the underlying disease.
- Relief of nausea.
- Attention to oral hygiene and, in particular, clearance of candidal infection.
- Relief of dysphagia, e.g., by placement of an esophageal stent.
- Dietary advice and assurance that the menu being offered is actually to the person's taste (there is no evidence that parenteral nutrition has benefit in this group of anorexic patients).[10]
- Identification and management of depression or anxiety.

Only after this is it appropriate to consider pharmacological treatments for appetite:

- Corticosteroids are the principal category of drugs used to stimulate appetite. Dexamethasone 3–6 mg and prednisolone 20–40 mg daily are effective at stimulating appetite and providing a sense of well-being.[11] However, there is no weight gain or increase in survival. The effect has been reported to last only a few weeks, but whether this reflects a development of tolerance or an increasing resistance to the drug's effects because of advancing disease is often unclear in practice. Around 80% of cancer patients gain appetite and well-being benefits from steroids if they are started more than 2 weeks before death, but only 25% benefit if commencement was within the last fortnight of life.[12] This benefit has to be weighed against the often serious adverse effects of steroid use. Steroids should therefore be tried for a week and, if not clearly helping, stopped. Tailing off is not necessary after this duration and magnitude of dose. If there is benefit, the patient should be left on the lowest effective dose, to be withdrawn once it is no longer effective.

- Progestogens have fewer adverse effects than corticosteroids but are considerably more expensive. Megestrol acetate is better than placebo at increasing appetite, weight, and well-being.[11] The weight gain is dose-related and due to an increase in fat rather than either muscle or fluid. An appropriate starting dose is 160 mg daily, but doses up to 1600 mg per day have been used. Medroxyprogesterone 1 g per day has similar effects.[13]
- Various other drugs, including cannabinoids, have been tried in anorexia and cachexia but require more extensive studies before they can be accepted for routine use.

NAUSEA AND VOMITING

About 60% of palliative care patients experience nausea and 30% vomiting. Effective therapy results from careful assessment of the physiological and anatomical origins of the symptoms in an individual and a choice of an antiemetic made in light of this and of the drug's profile of neurotransmitter actions. Although the attempt is worth making, many instances of nausea and vomiting are probably multifactorial, while increasing knowledge of the mechanisms underlying nausea and vomiting currently does more to add appreciation of their complexity than to facilitate effective therapy.

Clinical Assessment

The first question is whether the patient is really vomiting: regurgitation is often mistaken for vomiting. Clues in the history are the site of any cancer (notably esophageal tumor), the absence of preliminary nausea, a temporal association with eating, and the presence of undigested and recently eaten food in the "vomit."

Similar enquiry can help elucidate other causes of vomiting:

- Gastric outlet obstruction characteristically produces large-volume vomits, free of bile if the obstruction is complete. Episodes occur suddenly without preceding nausea, producing undigested food in the vomit from meals taken several hours previously. Hiccups and heartburn may be present.
- Morning vomiting associated with neurological or intellectual abnormalities suggests cerebral metastases, classically in the posterior fossa.
- An alternative and more common explanation of nausea and vomiting accompanied by drowsiness or confusion is hypercalcemia. Think of it especially in patients with myeloma or breast or squamous lung carcinoma, particularly if they also have bone metastases. Uremia can cause the same picture.
- Constipation appears to precipitate nausea in some people but may itself be a symptom of intestinal obstruction, which is discussed separately (see below, Intestinal Obstruction).
- Recent administration of chemotherapy or radiotherapy should be determined. Anticipatory nausea and vomiting can be a problem in patients who have experienced multiple courses of cytotoxics,

where learned responses mean that even encountering hospital staff associated with administration of treatment can bring on an episode.

- A detailed drug and alcohol history is essential. Drugs frequently associated with nausea and vomiting include opioids, cytotoxics, antibiotics, anticonvulsants, digoxin, NSAIDs and theophylline. Also check that previous unsuccessful antiemetic therapy is not being repeated.
- Anxiety can induce nausea and vomiting via corticomedullary connections.
- Aversive smells or tastes or movement may, in the presence of other emetic stimuli, be enough to precipitate vomiting.

Management

The cause of the vomiting should be diagnosed, to be able to choose an appropriate antiemetic and to identify and deal with reversible factors:

- Biochemical screening for urea, corrected calcium, glucose, and, if appropriate, digoxin and anticonvulsant levels is worthwhile. Uremia in the elderly terminally ill is all too often irreversible, but knowing about it will assist selection of an appropriate antiemetic (see Antiemetics, below).
- The symptoms of hypercalcemia are poorly correlated with the degree of excess calcium. Regardless of the severity of hypercalcemia, the good side effect profile of the bisphosphonates has established them as the treatment of choice. Good hydration should be ensured using a saline infusion if necessary as renal excretion of calcium requires both good perfusion volume and the availability of sodium ions. Diuretics should normally be stopped as they worsen dehydration and exacerbate renal damage from calcium.
- In anxiety, the first need is for calm listening and explanation, with the timely availability of support. Phenothiazines can be helpful through their dual role as anxiolytics and established antiemetics, but benzodiazepines may also be effective.

Antiemetics

Antiemetic drugs are neurotransmitter blocking agents. Where they function depends on where their target receptors are found, and what types of vomiting they control depends on the function of the nuclei with those receptors.

During vomiting, a complex and coordinated series of events takes place:

- Autonomic activity to produce sweating and hypersalivation
- Coordinated contractions of abdominal and diaphragmatic muscle
- Relaxation of the gastroesophageal sphincter
- Closure of the epiglottis and nasopharynx as the vomit is expelled

These actions require the orchestrated involvement of multiple closely sited nuclei in the medulla. The functional bringing together of these nuclei has been called the *integrative vomiting center* or the *emetic pattern generator*, but these entities have no clear neuroanatomical basis.

The important practical points are that the relevant medullary nuclei form a sort of final common pathway for nausea and vomiting and are well supplied principally, although not exclusively, with muscarinic cholinergic and H_1 histamine receptors (Fig. 18–1). By implication, agents that block these receptors should act in this area and be capable of acting across a range of different causes of vomiting. From Table 18–1 it can be seen that cyclizine, scopolamine, and the phenothiazines are particularly relevant. Among these, levomepromazine (methotrimeprazine) has a very broad spectrum of neurotransmitter blocking activity and has proved a highly effective antiemetic in palliative care and during chemotherapy. Doses can be much lower (6.25–25 mg orally or half of these doses subcutaneously) than previously used, avoiding the potential side effects of sedation and hypotension.[14] Unfortunately, levomepromazine is no longer available in the United States.

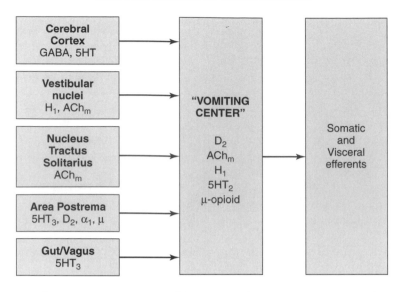

Figure 18–1. Schematic representation of the principal neurotransmitter distributions in central nervous system areas involved with control of nausea and emesis. GABA, γ-aminobutyric acid; 5-HT, 5-hydroxytryptamine; H_1, histamine 1; ACh_m, muscarinic cholinergic receptor; D_2, dopamine type 2.

Chemical stimuli to nausea and vomiting, such as uremia and hypercalcemia, are detected by the chemoreceptor trigger zone in the area postrema, which lies outside the blood–brain barrier in the floor of the fourth ventricle, together with the closely associated nucleus tractus solitarius. These areas also appear to mediate radiotherapy-induced sickness. They are rich in dopamine (D_2) and muscarinic receptors but also carry relays of 5-hydroxytryptamine$_3$ (5-HT$_3$) serotonergic fibers from the upper gut via the vagus. Inputs from the gut are important in cytotoxic-related vomiting

and in gastric distension. Suitable antiemetics here are the phenothiazines, the butyrophenones, and ondansetron and related drugs (Table 18–1).

Metoclopramide and domperidone are less potent D_2 antagonists. However, metoclopramide is useful in gastric stasis or functional bowel obstructions because of its upper intestinal prokinetic effects mediated through agonism at local 5-HT$_4$ receptors. Domperidone is often viewed as equivalent to metoclopramide but appears to act solely at dopamine receptors outside the blood–brain barrier. It therefore should be less

Table 18–1. Receptor Activities of Selected Antiemetic Drugs

	D_2	ACh_m	H_1	5-HT$_3$	5-HT$_4$
Hyoscine	−	+++	−	−	−
Cyclizine	−	+	+++	−	−
Haloperidol	+++	−	−	−	−
Chlorpromazine	++	+	++	−	−
Metoclopramide	++	−	−	+	++
Domperidone	++	−	−	−	−
Ondansetron	−	−	−	+++	+
Levomepromazine	++	+	+	+	−

D_2, dopamine type 2 receptors; ACh_m, muscarinic cholinergic receptors; H_1, histamine type 1 receptors; 5-HT$_3$, 5-hydroxytryptamine type 3 receptors; 5-HT$_4$, 5-hydroxytryptamine type 4 receptors.

likely than haloperidol or metoclopramide to precipitate parkinsonian adverse effects in the elderly, but its more limited potency and range of effects together with a poor oral bioavailability (15%)[15] diminish its effectiveness. The 5-HT$_4$ activity of metoclopramide is shared by cisapride, which may be useful alongside other antiemetics that lack a prokinetic action as it will not add to dopaminergic system adverse effects. Currently, cisapride is unavailable in the United Kingdom, and access is restricted (because of life-threatening arrythmias) in the United States.

Cannabinoid receptors exist in the brain stem, and cannabis users are said to experience less vomiting after chemotherapy. However, the available cannabinoids such as nabilone cause psychomimetic side effects, which the elderly seem to find particularly unpleasant. Although addition of a phenothiazine can help, these effects and the drowsiness that can ensue if they are used alongside opioids currently limit the palliative care use of these drugs.

About 10% of patients with nausea and vomiting are said to require a combination of antiemetics for the control of their symptoms. Appreciation of the modes of action of different drugs allows the prescription of rational combinations of drugs which complement rather than duplicate each other. With the partial exception of cyclizine, which is prone to precipitate when the concentration of other drugs in a solution rises, the agents mentioned appear to combine satisfactorily with each other when paired in a syringe for subcutaneous infusion.

INTESTINAL OBSTRUCTION

The prevalence of bowel obstruction in advanced cancer varies hugely according to the characteristics of the patient group studied. In an unselected group of hospice inpatients, 3% had malignant intestinal obstruction,[16] but 16% of those with colonic carcinoma present with obstruction,[17] and at death 51% of women with ovarian cancer are found to have bowel obstruction.[18]

In advanced cancer, bowel obstruction is frequently multifactorial and, especially in ovarian cancer, can occur at more than one level of the intestine. The principal categories of cause are as follows:[19]

- Intraluminal: tumor originating in the bowel itself
- Extramural: compression or kinking of the bowel by external tumor masses or adhesions
- Motility disorders: gut motility can be impaired by tumor infiltration of the intestinal muscle or its controlling neural networks, particularly common in ovarian cancer but lung carcinoma has been associated with a paraneoplastic syndrome which gives rise to a similar pseudo-obstructive picture
- Other factors, such as severe constipation precipitated by opioid analgesia, causing fecal impaction

Clinical Assessment

The complete picture of bowel obstruction is of a patient with the following:

- Colicky abdominal pain
- Nausea and feculent vomiting
- Abdominal distension
- Absolute constipation

However, the onset of malignant obstruction is often gradual, and bowel function may initially fluctuate between normal and obstructed patterns of function, with episodes of diarrhea occurring during periods of partial obstruction. Abdominal distension will be absent if the bowel is tethered at several sites. The presence of extensive intra-abdominal disease frequently gives rise to a constant pain as a background to the intermittent colic.

Management

Surgery is the only curative treatment and should always be considered as an option. However, the overall mortality rate for surgery in acute bowel obstruction is 69% in patients aged over 70.[20] Also, by the time of presentation of obstruction, many patients, regardless of age, are too unwell for surgery or have evidence of multiple sites of obstruction which render them inoperable. Perhaps paradoxically, abdominal distension in the context of obstruction is a good prognostic sign for operability as it indicates that the bowel is not widely tethered.

Intravenous fluids and nasogastric intubation are appropriate preparations for surgery but not as symptom control. Figures of 0%–14% have been reported for sustained symptom relief.[19] More effective and less burdensome for patients is medical management using drug combinations delivered parenterally to avoid the uncertainties of oral absorption in this situation. This is usually done by continuous subcutaneous infusion from a portable syringe driver.[16] The rectal route is an alternative if a syringe driver is unavailable, but there is no evidence for any advantage to the intravenous route.

- Continuous background pain is controlled with an opioid such as morphine.
- Colic is managed by an antispasmodic, of which the most often used is scopolamine butylbromide. This is started at 60 mg qd, and the dose is titrated against response to a reported maximum of 380 mg qd.[21] Scopolamine butylbromide may also lessen secretions in intestinal obstruction.[22]
- It is not easy to make a completely rational choice of antiemetic. The aim is to reduce nausea and then the frequency of vomits. Haloperidol 5–15 mg qd, metoclopramide 40–80 mg qd, diphenhydramine 100–200 mg qd, cyclizine 100–150 mg qd, or levomepromazine 6.25–25 mg qd are the most commonly used drugs and doses in practice. Metoclopramide has the potential to exacerbate colic in complete obstruction because of its prokinetic action, but it may have a particular therapeutic role in incomplete obstructions, where it may aid resolution. Doses of 30–240 mg qd have been used, but the higher ranges cause volume difficulties in conventional portable syringe drivers. Patients with malignant intestinal obstruction have high circulating levels of serotonin, which suggests a theoretical role for 5-HT$_3$ antagonists in obstruction-related vomiting.[23]
- As an adjunct in the management of both vomiting and colic, octreotide, a long-acting analogue of somatostatin, antagonizes both intestinal secretion and motility. It has been shown to reduce the volume of nasogastric aspirate and the occurrence of nausea and vomiting in malignant bowel obstruction.[22] On clinical grounds, a dose range of 100–900 mcg qd has been proposed;[24] but for other indications, octreotide is used in far higher doses,[25] and it may be appropriate to do so here as well, providing additional response is obtained with each titration increment.
- Steroids are commonly used to reduce obstruction through their anti-inflammatory effect of reducing tumor bulk. However, the innate variability of intestinal obstruction makes any response difficult to attribute with certainty, and a meta-analysis of the small studies to date yielded only a suggestion of improvement.[26]
- It is appropriate to give stool softeners to ease the passage of stool through any gut constriction, but bowel stimulants (e.g., senna, bisacodyl) are avoided as they can worsen colic. Occasionally, antidiarrheal drugs are needed instead.
- No restrictions are placed on diet, but patients tend to choose small meals of low-residue foods. Fluid replacement is a psychologically appropriate response to a complaint of thirst that cannot be satisfied orally, but the evidence is that it may actually make matters worse rather than better.[22] Extra fluids are given most unobtrusively by subcutaneous infusion.[27]
- The symptoms of high obstructions are much more difficult to control than those arising more distally. Percutaneous venting gastrostomies have been used for this indication, although results have not been good enough to prompt their widespread adoption.

Around 70%–90% of patients can be pain-free with this approach. Nausea should usually be controllable, but vomiting may be reduced to once or twice a day,[16] rather than totally abolished, to limit adverse effects. Most patients in this situation live only a few weeks, but a few have been reported to survive up to 7 months.[16]

CONSTIPATION

Background

Constipation is common in those requiring palliative care and increases in prevalence with advancing years. Sixty-three percent of elderly people in hospital have been found to be constipated compared with 22% of the same age group living at home.[28] This is not widely removed from the 60% found in cancer palliative care patients who are not taking opioid analgesia.[29] The importance of the condition lies in the distress it causes as a symptom, which in some surveys has been more troublesome than pain.

Objective criteria have been suggested, in particular an average of fewer than three stools per week or the existence of straining during at least 25% of defecations; but many people who would not meet these criteria nevertheless consider themselves to be constipated. The range of normal bowel function is very wide, and what matters is the deviation from what the individual considers normal for himself or herself rather than a deviation from a population average.

The reasons why chronic illness produces constipation are multiple. Most activity in the large bowel consists of mixing movements, and peristaltic activity to move colonic contents distally occurs only a few times a day, triggered by gastric emptying of meals and by general physical activity. As meals become smaller and less frequent and mobility is reduced, both triggers will become less effective. There is often reduced intake of fluid as well as food, which results in more complete water absorption from the bowel and consequently a drier, harder stool.

Among drugs, morphine and other opioids are probably the most important single constipating factor that can be isolated; but they operate against a background of widespread constipation arising from debility. Opioids reduce gut peristalsis and rectal sensitivity, increase sphincter tone throughout the bowel, and may increase net water absorption from the gut contents. In addition, any drug with anticholinergic effects has constipating potential, as, in particular, do anticonvulsants and iron.

Assessment

History taking should include an enquiry about constipation and, if it is present, details about the patient's current bowel frequency, need to strain at stool, and how these differ from what has normally been experienced in the past. If there has been a change, a rectal examination is needed unless there is a clear report of a satisfactory evacuation within the past day or so. The purpose of the examination is to assess the consistency of the stool and, particularly, to uncover the existence of fecal impaction in the rectum, which might need local intervention to remove it.

Impaction that produces overflow of liquid stool past the fecal mass, leading the patient to complain of diarrhea, is a major pitfall in the clinical assessment of bowel function. Any diarrhea that occurs following a period of constipation, is frequent but of small volume, or produces fecal incontinence should prompt a rectal examination. Up to 98% of impactions are said to occur in the rectum and, therefore, should be picked up by adequate clinical assessment.

Bowel distension from constipation can cause nausea or urinary incontinence in the elderly or debilitated, so the onset of either of these symptoms ought to stimulate enquiry about bowel function.

Occasionally, there is doubt as to whether a patient has severe constipation or an intestinal obstruction. Erect and supine abdominal radiographs are then indicated to help make the distinction; but in general, investigations are not required in the routine assessment of constipation.

Management

The pathophysiology of constipation suggests several prophylactic measures, although in practice the possibility of making significant changes in these areas diminishes as the disease progresses and disability increases:

- Increasing dietary fiber. Specialist dietary advice can help in maximizing dietary fiber intake when appetite is declining or dysphagia is increasing.
- Encouraging oral fluids. Adequate fluid intake is very important as dehydration will result in a dry stool that is difficult to expel.
- Improving mobility. Good control of symptoms, physiotherapy, and the provision of appropriate mobility aids will help avoid constipation through facilitating activity.
- Constipating drugs should be avoided or a laxative made available at the time of first prescription, without waiting until constipation is established.

Most people undergoing palliative care who are constipated will require laxative therapy. The basic division of laxatives is between stimulants and softeners. This division seems useful in clinical practice, although in fact any drug that stimulates peristalsis will accelerate transit, allow less time for water absorption, and thus produce a softer stool. Similarly, softening the stool involves increasing its bulk, which will result in increased distension of the intestinal wall and a consequent stimulation of reflex enteric muscle contraction.

The results of laxative drug trials do not allow a clear recommendation of one agent over another because of the small size of the studies, the number of different preparations, and the various end points and conditions involved. However:

- Systematic review evidence of studies in elderly people suggests that any kind of laxative can increase stool frequency by about 1.4 bowel actions per week compared with placebo.[30]

- There is limited experimental evidence that the optimal combination of effectiveness with few adverse effects and low dose is achieved using a combination of stimulant and softening laxatives rather than either alone.[31]
- Laxative preparations vary significantly in price and physical characteristics. Ready-made combinations tend to be expensive. Given the lack of major differences in efficacy, both cost and individual patient acceptability should be strong influences in prescribing choice.

The aim of laxative therapy is comfortable defecation, not any particular frequency of evacuation. No single laxative dose is adequate for everyone, and many patients are subjected to both rectal interventions and an inadequate oral dose of laxative. The dose needs to be titrated against the response and the advent of adverse effects and should be increased prophylactically if, say, opioids are introduced or their dose is substantially increased.

Oral laxatives

Stimulant laxatives. Examples of stimulant laxatives include senna, bisacodyl, sodium picosulfate, danthron (only available in combination preparations).

- Starting doses: senna 15 mg daily, bisacodyl 10 mg daily, sodium picosulfate 5 mg daily, danthron 50 mg daily
- Act directly on the myenteric nerves to evoke gut muscle contraction
- Reduce gut water absorption
- Evidence for intestinal damage from these agents is poor
- Can produce marked colic, particularly if not combined with a softening agent
- Onset of action 6–12 hours
- Danthron causes red urinary discoloration and perianal rashes

Softening laxatives, osmotic laxatives. Examples of softening laxatives include magnesium sulfate, magnesium hydroxide, lactulose, and polyethylene glycol (PEG).

- Starting doses: magnesium hydroxide or sulfate 2–4 g daily, lactulose 15 ml bid, PEG one sachet in 125 ml water daily (fecal impaction eight sachets in 1 l of water over 6 hours)
- Magnesium sulfate and hydroxide have stimulant as well as osmotic actions at higher doses. The sulfate is the more potent. They are cheap.
- Magnesium sulfate used alone can be useful for resistant constipation. There is a risk of hypermagnesemia with chronic use.
- Lactulose is expensive, needed in large volumes if used alone in marked constipation, and a cause of flatulence in around 20% of users.
- Polyethyleneglycol (Go-lytely, Miralax) has been reported to be effective as an oral treatment for fecal impaction.[32]

Surfactant laxatives. Examples of surfactant laxatives include docusate sodium, poloxamer (available only in combination with danthron).

- Starting dose: docusate sodium 300 mg daily
- Increase water penetration of the stool
- Evidence for laxative efficacy limited

Lubricant laxative: liquid paraffin.

- Starting dose: 10 ml daily
- Chronic paraffin use can cause fat-soluble vitamin deficiencies, has been associated with anal fecal leakage, and has been reported to cause a bezoar. None of these adverse effects has been linked with the emulsion of liquid paraffin with magnesium hydroxide, which is currently the most common form in which it is used in Britain.
- Cheap

Bulking agents
Examples of bulking agents include bran, methylcellulose, and ispaghula.

- Starting doses: bran 8 g daily, others 3–4 g daily

- Bulking agents are "normalizers" rather than true laxatives: they will soften a hard stool but make firmer a loose one.
- Increase stool bulk partly by providing material that resists bacterial breakdown and, hence, remains in the gut and partly by providing a substrate for bacterial growth and gas production
- Effective in mild constipation but probably not in severe constipation
- Need to be taken with ample water (at least 200–300 ml); this and their consistency are unacceptable to many ill patients.
- If taken with inadequate water, a viscous mass may result, which can cause intestinal tract obstruction.

Rectal laxatives
Most patients prefer oral laxatives to rectal, whose use should accordingly be minimized by optimizing laxative treatment by mouth. There is, however, a particular role for enemas and suppositories in the relief of fecal impaction and in bowel management in patients where neurological damage, e.g., from spinal cord compression, results in fecal incontinence. Evidence to guide their use is scantier even than that for oral laxatives. Anything introduced into the rectum can stimulate defecation via the anocolonic reflex, but among rectal laxatives only bisacodyl suppositories have a pharmacological stimulant action. Glycerine suppositories and arachis or olive oil enemas soften and lubricate the stool, as do proprietary mini-enemas, which contain mixtures of surfactants.

DIARRHEA

Diarrhea is much less common than constipation in cancer care, occurring in around 10% of admissions for palliative care.[33]

The bowel receives about 9 l of fluid daily, 2 l from oral intake and the remainder from gastric, biliary, pancreatic, and intestinal secretions. All but some 150 ml of this total is reabsorbed. The difference between constipation and diarrhea amounts to 100 ml or so of water per day, indicating a remarkably fine control of fluid balance across the gut wall. This control is exercised via the myenteric neural plexus but is also subject to influence by luminal factors such as fatty acids, bile salts, and drugs such as opioids and some cytotoxic chemotherapy agents.[34]

Clinical Findings

Although diarrhea is frequent evacuation of loose stool, patients may use the word to describe other situations, such as an increase in frequency of any kind of stool, a single relatively loose bowel action per day, or fecal leakage or incontinence, any of which might represent constipation rather than true diarrhea. Therefore, a complaint of diarrhea must be elucidated by a careful history, including an account of drugs such as laxatives and elixir preparations, which might contain osmotically active sugars, and recent chemotherapy or radiotherapy. Abdominal and rectal examinations should also be performed, to exclude fecal impaction or loss of sphincter tone.

Investigations

In this patient group, investigations of diarrhea are not usually warranted because the cause emerges through history or examination or because any infective cause is likely to be short-lived and self-limiting. However, if the patient is toxic or the diarrhea continues beyond about 3 days, stool samples should be taken and cultured for pathogens such as *Clostridium difficile*, *Escherischia coli*, *Salmonella* or *Shigella*. Prolonged diarrhea should also prompt monitoring and correction of fluid and electrolyte balance.

Management

The most common cause of diarrhea in palliative medicine is an excessive laxative dose.[35] However, an unduly long suspension of laxative therapy results in a pattern of alternating constipation and diarrhea; it is usually adequate to suspend the laxatives for 24 hours and then resume a dose step down.

Specific therapies exist for certain causes of diarrhea:

- Fat malabsorption, pancreatic enzyme replacement
- Chologenic diarrhea, cholestyramine 4–12 g tid, calcium carbonate
- Radiation-induced diarrhea, cholestyramine 4–12 g tid, aspirin
- Carcinoid syndrome, cyproheptadine initially 12 mg qd (also consider octreotide, see below)
- Ulcerative colitis, mesalazine 1.2–2.4 g qd, steroids
- Pseudomembranous colitis, vancomycin 125 mg qid, metronidazole 400 mg tid

Most treatment for diarrhea is symptomatic. Available drugs are either absorbent or adsorbent, taking up water and toxins into or onto their structures, or are motility- and secretion-modifying agents.

- Absorbent agents: bulk-forming agents, e.g., methylcellulose, pectin
- Adsorbent agents (limited evidence for efficacy in acute diarrhea): kaolin, attapulgite
- Motility- and secretion-modifying agents

Opioids
- Codeine: 10–60 mg q4h (morphine usually if already in use for pain)
- Diphenoxylate (combined with atropine): 10 mg stat, then 5 mg 6qh
- Loperamide: 4 mg stat, then 2 mg after each loose stool up to 16 mg qd

Somatostatin Analogues
- Octreotide: 300 mcg qd subcutaneous titrated up to 2400 mcg qd if necessary

The most effective general antidiarrheals are the opioids, of which loperamide is the most specific since in adults it has an oral bioavailability close to 1% and its effects are therefore limited almost exclusively to the gut.[36]

REFERENCES

1. Jobbins J, Bagg J, Finlay IG, Addy M, Newcombe RG. Oral and dental disease in ter-

minally ill cancer patients. BMJ 304:1612, 1992.

2. Davies AN, Daniels C, Pugh R, Sharma K. A comparison of artificial saliva and pilocarpine in the management of xerostomia in patients with advanced cancer. Palliat Med 12:105–111, 1998.

3. Finlay I. Oral fungal infections. Eur J Palliat Care 2(Suppl 1):4–7, 1995.

4. Epstein EB, Stevenson-Moore P, Jackson S, Mohamed JH, Spinelli JJ. Prevention of oral mucositis in radiation therapy: a controlled study with benzydamine hydrochloride rinse. Int J Radiat Oncol Biol Phys 16:1571–1575, 1989.

5. Solomon MA. Oral sucralfate suspension for mucositis. N Engl J Med 315:459–460, 1986.

6. Sykes NP, Baines M, Carter RL. Clinical and pathological study of dysphagia conservatively managed in patients with advanced malignant disease. Lancet ii:726–728, 1988.

7. Carter RL, Pittam MR, Tanner NSB. Pain and dysphagia in patients with squamous carcinomas of the head and neck: the role of perineural spread. J R Soc Med 75: 598–606, 1982.

8. Rowland CG, Pagliero KM. Intracavitary irradiation in palliation of carcinoma of oesophagus and cardia. Lancet 2:981–983, 1985.

9. Loizou LA, Grigg D, Atkinson M, Robertson C, Bown SG. A prospective comparison of laser therapy and intubation in endoscopic palliation for malignant dysphagia. Gastroenterology 100:1303–1310, 1991.

10. Fainsinger R. The modern management of cancer related cachexia in palliative care. Prog Palliat Care 5:191–195, 1997.

11. Fainsinger R. Pharmacological approach to cancer anorexia and cachexia. In: Bruera E, Higginson I (Eds.). Cachexia–Anorexia in Cancer Patients. Oxford, Oxford University Press, 1996.

12. Farr WC. The use of corticosteroids for symptom management in terminally ill patients. Am J Hosp Care 7:41–46, 1990.

13. Simons JP, Schols AM, Hoefnagels JM, Westerterp KR, ten Velde GP, Wouters EF. Effects of medroxyprogesterone acetate on food intake, body composition, and resting energy expenditure in patients with advanced, nonhormone-sensitive cancer: a randomised, placebo-controlled trial. Cancer 82:553–560, 1998.

14. Twycross RG, Barkby GD, Hallwood PM. The use of low dose levomepromazine (methotrimeprazine) in the management of nausea and vomiting. Prog Palliat Care 5: 49–53, 1997.

15. Brunton LL. Agents affecting gastrointestinal water flux and motility; emesis and antiemetics; bile acids and pancreatic enzymes. In: Hardman JG, Limbird LE, Molinoff PB, Ruddon RW, Gilman AG (Eds.). Goodman and Gilman's The Pharmacological Basis of Therapeutics, 9th ed. New York, McGraw-Hill, pp. 917–936, 1996.

16. Baines MJ, Oliver DJ, Carter RL. Medical management of intestinal obstruction in patients with advanced malignant disease: a clinical and pathological study. Lancet ii:990–993, 1985.

17. Philips RKS, Hittinger R, Fry JS, Fielding LP. Malignant large bowel obstruction. Br J Surg 72:296–302, 1985.

18. Dvoretsky PM, Richards KA, Angel C, Rabinowitz L, Beecham JB, Bonfiglio TA. Survival time, causes of death, and tumor/treatment-related morbidity in 100 women with ovarian cancer. Hum Pathol 19: 1273–1279, 1988.

19. Baines MJ. The pathophysiology and management of malignant intestinal obstruction. In: Doyle D, Hanks GW, MacDonald N (Eds.). Oxford Textbook of Palliative Medicine, (2nd ed.). Oxford, Oxford University Press, pp. 526–534, 1998.

20. Parker MC, Baines MJ. Intestinal obstruction in patients with advanced cancer. Br J Surg 83:1–2, 1996.

21. Ventafridda V, Ripamonti C, Caraceni A, Spoldi E, Messina L, De Conno F. The management of inoperable intestinal obstruction in terminal cancer patients. Tumori 76:389–393, 1990.

22. Ripamonti C, Mercadante S, Groff L, Zecca E, De Conno F, Casuccio A. Role of octreotide, scopolamine butylbromide, and hydration in symptom control of patients with inoperable bowel obstruction and nasogastric tubes: a prospective randomized trial. J Pain Symptom Manage 19:23–34, 2000.

23. Hutchison SMW, Beattie G, Shearing CH. Increased serotonin excretion in patients with ovarian carcinoma and intestinal obstruction. Palliat Med 9:67–68, 1995.

24. Riley J, Fallon MT. Octreotide in terminal malignant obstruction of the gastrointestinal tract. Eur J Palliat Care 1:23–25, 1994.

25. Harris AG, O'Dorisio TM, Woltering EA, Anthony LB, Burton FR, Geller RB, Grendell JH, Levin B, Redfern JS. Consensus statement: octreotide dose titration in secretory diarrhea. Diarrhea Consensus Development Panel. Dig Dis Sci 40:1464–1473, 1995.

26. Feuer DJ, Broadley KE. Systematic review and meta-analysis of corticosteroids for the resolution of malignant bowel obstruction in advanced gynaecological cancers. Ann Oncol 10:1–7, 1999.

27. Fainsinger RL, MacEachern T, Miller MJ, Bruera E, Spachynski K, Kuehn N, Hanson J. The use of hypodermoclysis for rehydration in terminally ill cancer patients. J Pain Symptom Manage 9:298–302, 1994.

28. Wigzell FW. The health of nonagenarians. Gerontol Clin 11:137–144, 1969.

29. Sykes NP. The relationship between opioid use and laxative use in terminally ill cancer patients. Palliat Med 12:375–382, 1998.

30. Petticrew M, Watt I, Sheldon T. Systematic review of the effectiveness of laxatives in the elderly. Health Technol Assess 1:1–52, 1997.

31. Sykes NP. A volunteer model for the comparison of laxatives in opioid-induced constipation. J Pain Symptom Manage 11: 363–369, 1997.

32. Culbert P, Gillett H, Ferguson A. Highly effective new oral therapy for faecal impaction. Br J Gen Practice 48:1599–1600, 1998.

33. Sykes NP. Constipation and diarrhoea. In: Doyle D, Hanks GW, MacDonald N (Eds.). Oxford Textbook of Palliative Medicine, (2nd ed.) Oxford, Oxford University Press, pp. 513–526, 1998.

34. Ippoliti C. Antidiarrheal agents for the management of treatment-related diarrhea in cancer patients. Am J Health Syst Pharm 55:1573–1580, 1998.

35. Twycross RG, Lack SA. Diarrhoea. In: Control of Alimentary Symptoms in Far Advanced Cancer. London, Churchill Livingstone, pp. 208–209, 1986.

36. Ruppin H. Review: loperamide—a potent antidiarrhoeal drug with actions along the alimentary tract. Aliment Pharmacol Ther 1:179–190, 1987.

19

Fatigue

DEBORAH WITT SHERMAN AND MARIANNE LAPORTE MATZO

On the palliative care unit, Ms. Garcia, a 72-year-old woman diagnosed with metastatic breast cancer, reports "feeling constantly tired." Mr. Ling, an 80-year-old man diagnosed with end-stage chronic obstructive pulmonary disease (COPD), complains of being "extremely weak," while Mr. Tuck, a 66-year-old man diagnosed with advanced acquired immunodeficiency syndrome (AIDS), states "I am exhausted." Their distress is associated with their inability to carry on with their activities of daily living and to experience prior pleasures, such as walks with their family or even talking with one another. Their chief complaint was translated by the clinician and documented as fatigue. Fatigue is one of the most common symptoms experienced by patients with cancer and other incurable, progressive illnesses, which negatively influences the quality of their lives.[1,2] Fatigue affects patients' relationships with others, self-perception, ability to function, and sense of hope, thereby compounding the suffering associated with life-threatening illness. Like pain, fatigue is what the patient says it is, since it is a subjective experience. In palliative care, it is of value to understand the experience of fatigue within various patient populations, including the older adult, and its relevance to various disease states and associated therapies.[3]

PREVALENCE OF FATIGUE

Given that the symptom of fatigue has been poorly defined clinically, it is difficult to find valid surveys regarding the prevalence of fatigue in patients with progressive disease. However, in a study conducted by the World Health Organization, which included 1840 palliative care patients, half (51%) of the patients reported fatigue.[4] The overall prevalence of *fatigue*, defined as diminished energy, for patients with metastatic cancer has been reported in multiple surveys to exceed 75%.[5] In a study of the dimensions of symptom distress in women with advanced lung cancer, fatigue was among the most prevalent.[6] Prevalence rates have been reported to be as high as 95% for patients receiving chemotherapy, radiation therapy, and immunotherapy.[7] Fatigue has also been documented in patients with end-stage renal disease, coronary artery disease, and all gradations of rheumatoid arthritis, diseases that commonly afflict older adults.[8] In the palliative care patient population, fatigue, poor appetite, and diminished sense of well-being were the most intense symptoms reported.[9]

FATIGUE IN THE OLDER ADULT

When treating the older adult in palliative care, the potential for confounding comorbidities secondary to the patient's age cannot be ignored. It is often difficult to discern if the fatigue is secondary to treatment modalities, depression, congestive heart failure, constipation, infection, anemia, hypothyroidism, diabetes, or fibromyalgia, to name but a few conditions in the differential. The conventional wisdom is that fatigue is a normal consequence of aging, and both patients and professionals erroneously believe that fatigue is inevitable and untreatable. In fact, older adults may not even report symptoms of weakness and fatigue to their primary care provider. Therefore, the health-care provider should include a careful and routine assessment of fatigue for all older adult patients. Many causes of fatigue can be treated, even for the geriatric palliative care patient. The goal for the health-care provider related to fatigue is to improve the patient's quality of life by treating the symptom and teaching the older adult coping mechanisms and lifestyle changes.

THE CONCEPT OF FATIGUE

Fatigue has been characterized by patients by such descriptors as *worn out, weary, exhausted, sleepiness, low energy, tired, worn down, bone-tired,* and *rubber knees.* Practitioners also use terms such as *listlessness, lassitude, lethargy,* and *malaise.* The historical development of the concept of fatigue indicates the following identifying criteria: *(1)* a subjective perception, *(2)* an alteration in neuromuscular and metabolic processes, *(3)* a decrease in physical performance, and *(4)* a deterioration in mental and physical activities.[8] To date, there has been no clear consensus regarding the definition of fatigue or a description of it. However, there is an appreciation of the differentiation between "normal" fatigue, experienced by the majority of the population, and clinical fatigue, associated with disease or its treatments.[5] The assessment of etiology, severity, duration, or impact of clinical fatigue is important in developing a conceptual and operational definition.

Currently, there are various definitions of fatigue documented in the literature. Piper et al.[10] defined fatigue as "a subjective feeling of tiredness that is influenced by circadian rhythm; it can vary in unpleasantness, duration, and intensity; when acute it serves a protective function and when prolonged, excessive or chronic, it may lead to an aversion to activity." The North American Nursing Diagnosis Association defined fatigue as "an overwhelming, sustained sense of exhaustion and decreased capacity for physical or emotional work."[11] One of the most comprehensive definitions, relevant to palliative care, is "the awareness of a decreased capacity for physical and/or mental activity due to an imbalance in the availability, utilization, and/or restoration of resources needed to perform activity."[12]

Some practitioners differentiate fatigue from weakness, while others believe that they accompany each other and comprise a syndrome known as asthenia.[8] Asthenia is an unpleasant sensation experienced when an individual's physiological resources are exceeded, particularly within the context of several clinical conditions, including chronic fatigue syndrome, depression, acute or chronic infection, chronic heart failure, chronic pulmonary disease, AIDS, cancers, and endocrine diseases such as diabetes.[13]

At various points in the illness trajectory, patients interpret fatigue differently. For many patients newly diagnosed with a life-threatening illness, fatigue has been an indication or warning symptom of the diagnosis. As treatment ensues, it may be understood as a side effect of treatment, while for patients with recurrence or exacerbation of illness, fatigue is interpreted as physical decline.[8]

MULTIDIMENSIONAL ASPECTS OF FATIGUE

Fatigue, like pain, is a multidimensional, subjective experience of diverse etiologies.[5] As a complex phenomenon, fatigue has physical, emotional, cognitive, and behavioral dimensions.[2]

The possible physical etiologies of fatigue in the medically ill include medical and physical conditions, specifically the underlying disease itself, associated treatments (chemotherapy, radiation, surgery, biological response modifiers), intercurrent systemic disorders (anemia, infection, pulmonary disorders, hepatic failure, heart failure, renal failure, malnutrition, neuromuscular disorders), sleep disorders, chronic pain, use of centrally acting drugs, as well as lack of mobility and exercise.[14] From a physiological perspective, fatigue has been attributed to excessive energy consumption and the depletion of hormones, neurotransmitters, or other essential substrates.[12]

The mechanism or pathophysiology of fatigue/asthenia differs from one clinical condition to another. Within a physiological context, fatigue can be classified according to two types: central or peripheral. In *central fatigue*, the motor pathways in the central nervous system (CNS) fail to sustain recruitment and/or frequency of motor units or the generation of descending volleys in the motor cortex due to neurotransmitter depletion. Pharmacologically altered brain 5-hydroxytryptamine activity may influence dopamine concentration in the brain, altering the perception of fatigue. In *peripheral fatigue*, there is failure in the propagation of muscle action potential, resulting in impaired excitation–contraction.[13] The question is whether a person's failure to exert effort is caused by a failure in the neural drive, such as fatigue in the CNS, or a failure of neurotransmission in the muscles.

In the case of cancer-related fatigue/asthenia, there are three associated physiological mechanisms that may effect the CNS or muscles:

1. Direct tumor effects (i.e., mechanical destruction, such as metastasis, or metabolically by lipolytic factors or tumor degradation products)
2. Tumor-induced humoral mediators (i.e., tumor necrosis factors [asthenin/cachectin] and other cytokines such as interleukin-1 [IL-1], interferon, or IL-6)
3. Tumor-accompanying factors (i.e., cachexia, infection, anemia, hypoxia, neurological disorders, pharmacological side effects, dehydration, or paraneoplastic or metabolic factors)[13]

In cancer populations, there has been a documented relationship between asthenia and cachexia, although one may exist without the other. However, in patients with advanced cancer, both are usually present, with asthenia as an epiphenomenon of the cachexia syndrome. In malignancy, changes in carbohydrate, fat, and protein metabolism as well as direct tumor factors and cytokines, previously mentioned, lead to cachexia and loss of muscle mass. This partially explains cachexia-related asthenia.

The concept of fatigue also encompasses emotional, cognitive, and behavioral dimensions. Psychosocial etiological factors in the medically ill include anxiety or depressive disorders, stress, and related environmental reinforcers.[15] In healthy individuals, overexertion may produce ordinary fatigue, which is relieved relatively quickly by rest. Fatigue may also be interpreted as satisfaction given the accomplishment of hard work. However, fatigue associated with illness is perceived as more severe and comes on after a shorter period of time and less exertion than ordinary fatigue. It is often described as a general feeling of tiredness or "sapped" energy that occurs on a daily basis and is present intermittently throughout the day or during the evening after a day of normal activities. Fatigue also leads to a decline in mental or intellectual activities, as well as diminished motivation or capacity to attend.[5] It is often associated with decreased ability to concentrate, which impedes engagement in a variety of activities.[3]

For many individuals, fatigue is interpreted as an exacerbation of their condition. For example, in a study by Small and Lamb,[3] patients with COPD expressed an increase in fatigue as their breathing became more labored. They believed that the cause of their fatigue was their inability to obtain sufficient oxygen and that labored breathing was a central feature of their fatigue. With restrictions of their activities imposed by fatigue, patients with COPD also expressed a loss of strength. The less they were able to do, the more tired they became with effort. Fatigue was also exacerbated by interrupted sleep, which led to prolonged and extreme feelings of exhaustion, and by psychological stress, which increased their fatigue through its effect on their breathing. These patients also described the impact of fatigue on activities of daily living. As a result of fatigue, they were unable to do heavy chores around the house or spur-of-the-moment activities. For many, fatigue limited self-care abilities. For example, even showering resulted in feelings of exhaustion. Lack of energy also resulted in changes in mood, such as irritability and frustration. Patients explained that "what bothers me most is not being able to get up and do what I want to do." The psychosocial impact of fatigue also resulted in changes in family roles and interfered with family and social relationships given that patients were too tired to participate fully in related events. Furthermore, patients frequently avoided social situations that they believed would trigger or exacerbate their fatigue.

A qualitative study which explored fatigue in cancer patients illustrated it as a process involving experience, consequences, and actions. The experience of fatigue related to issues of loss, psychological stress, abnormal weakness, and difficulty taking initiative. The consequences of fatigue were social limitation and changes in self-esteem and quality of life, while action related to each participant's ways of coping. With knowledge of the different expressions of fatigue and recognition of the consequences, interventions can be developed to facilitate effective coping.[16]

CLASSIFICATION OF FATIGUE AS ACUTE OR CHRONIC

Fatigue has been classified as either acute or chronic. According to Piper,[17] acute fatigue is a protective state, identifiably linked to a single cause, in usually healthy individuals. Acute fatigue has a rapid onset and short direction and is viewed as normal when alleviated by restorative techniques, such as rest, diet, exercise, and stress management. Acute fatigue has minor effects on activities of daily living and quality of life. In contrast, chronic fatigue has an unknown purpose and cause and may be experienced without any relationship to exertion or activity. Chronic fatigue is frequently experienced by patients with life-threatening illness, having an insidious onset and persisting over time. Chronic fatigue is viewed as abnormal or pathological and generally not relieved by restorative techniques. In contrast to acute fatigue, chronic fatigue has a significant negative effect on activities of living and quality of life.

CAUSES OF FATIGUE

A biological mechanism in a healthy individual, known as the *conservation withdrawal system*, is controlled by the parasympathetic nervous system to safeguard against the exhaustion of reserves. This system gives the body the signal that it is fatigued and that it needs to rest. When the body is experiencing the stress and pathology of chronic disease or cancer, its reserves can become totally depleted and ultimately unable to counterbalance physiological insults. The older adult with cancer may experience fatigue in relation to the advanced stage of the disease and concurrent anemia and cachexia. Coexisting symptoms, such as nausea and vomiting, anorexia/cachexia, pain, immobility, shortness of breath, possible gastric obstruction, and anxiety or depression, also are associated with the elder's experience of fatigue.[18] Medication and drugs can cause fatigue, such as analgesics, psychotropics, β-blockers, and alcohol.[5]

Treatment for cancer (surgery, radiation, chemotherapy, biotherapeutic therapy) can also cause feelings of fatigue. With surgery, there is the anxiety resulting from preoperative regimens and the postoperative fatigue that can result from pain, direct tissue damage, anesthesia, sedatives, analgesics, and immobility. Fatigue may continue for as long as six-months after a surgical intervention.[19] Nearly 100% of patients treated with radiotherapy will experience fatigue, which tends to peak toward the end of the cycle. The fatigue experienced is dose-dependent. Approximately 95% of patients who receive chemotherapy feel that fatigue is one of the worst symptoms experienced within the first 2 weeks after treatment. Bio-therapeutic agents (interferon, interleukins) cause dose-related fatigue in 50%–70% of patients.[5]

Patients with chronic conditions, such as fibromyalgia, may manifest progressive symptoms of psychogenic fatigue, physiological fatigue, and pain. Given the unknown etiology of fibromyalgia, there are limited treatment options for it, with relief primarily achieved by the palliation of symptoms. Older adults who have lived with conditions like fibromyalgia, rheumatoid arthritis, or chronic fatigue syndrome are at higher risk for suicide, particularly when comorbid depression occurs. In such situations, interventions such as medication management should be initiated.[20]

CORRELATES OF FATIGUE IN VARIOUS PATIENT POPULATIONS

Fatigue has been associated anecdotally with many factors, such as sleep disorders, anemia, systemic infection, depression, or the use of centrally acting drugs such as opioids.[5] Fatigue has also been associated with older age, advanced disease, and combined therapies.[21]

Fatigue was the most commonly reported symptom for patients with heart failure and increased significantly over time.[22] Given that fatigue is integral to the experience of heart failure, interventions are needed to assist patients to cope with the experience of fatigue, such as pacing of activities, relaxation, and restful sleep. Exercise may reduce fatigue in patients with heart failure. However, caution is needed regarding the safety and benefits of exercise training for patients with mild to moderate heart failure, given a lack of empirical data regarding the risk/benefit ratio.

In another study, 40% of stroke patients described fatigue as one of their worst symptoms.[23] This symptom was not related to time post-stroke, severity, or the location of the lesion, suggesting that fatigue can contribute to functional impairment.

In older populations, fatigue is a common symptom, particularly evident in the older adult in long-term care facilities, where it is associated with pain, multiple medications, depression, and functional impairment.[24] Depression may be the causal factor if fatigue is worse in the morning, particularly if accompanied by unexplained weight loss.[25] The American Psychiatric Association has identified fatigue as a symptom of depression, but often it is difficult to determine if chronic fatigue is etiologically unrelated to an affective disorder or if the symptoms of chronic fatigue precipitated the depression.[26] Depression has been cited as a correlate of fatigue in patients with primary biliary cirrhosis,[27] COPD,[28] human immunodeficiency (HIV) disease,[29] and various forms of cancer.[30–35]

In addition to depression as a correlate of fatigue in patients with breast cancer, fatigue has been associated with significantly higher levels of pain, sleep disturbance, and dyspnea.[36,37] Patients with advanced lung cancer experienced dyspnea on walking, depression, as well as appetite loss.[38]

FATIGUE AND QUALITY OF LIFE

Regardless of the age of the patient, fatigue has a profound effect on quality of life. Incapacity to carry out role tasks can result in decreased self-esteem, social isolation, depression, increased health-care utilization and costs, and increased morbidity.[39] In one study, 71% of cancer patients reported that fatigue affected their activities of daily living, and 61% reported that fatigue affected their daily lives more than pain.[40] The aspects of life that were affected "very much" or "somewhat" by fatigue were ability to work, physical well-being, ability to enjoy life in the moment, emotional well-being, intimacy with partner, ability to take care of the family, relationships with family and friends, and concerns about mortality and survival. As a goal of care and an outcome variable in palliative care, quality of life is a priority of patients, families, and health professionals. To promote quality of life, fatigue, as a symptom, must be appropriately assessed and effectively treated.

ASSESSMENT OF FATIGUE

As a subjective symptom, practitioners most often rely on a patient's self-report of fatigue to evaluate its severity. However, the assessment of fatigue also includes observable characteristics, as well as impact on quality of life. A comprehensive assessment of fatigue obtained through a health history, review of systems including fatigue assessment, physical examination, and laboratory data can assist the practitioner in discriminating between physiological and psychogenic fatigue, depression, and the presence of correctable causes of fatigue.

Health history should include a medical, psychiatric, family, social, and medication history, which may reveal associated conditions, such as diabetes, hypothyroidism, sleep apnea, anxiety or depressive disorders, inherited metabolic disorders, a history of alcohol or illegal drug use, and the possibility of infection often associated with fatigue.

Review of systems regarding fatigue focuses on changes in other body systems that may indicate potential health problems associated with fatigue, such as respiratory disorders (e.g., dyspnea), cardiac problems, anemia, cancer, depression, or electrolyte disorders. In elderly populations, including those with chronic, incurable illness, fatigue may be a side effect of medical treatments, including both prescription and over-the-counter medications. In speaking with the patient, it is important to determine the emotional status, particularly whether the person speaks of his or her own death or suicidal ideations or has other signs and symptoms of anxiety or depression.

The fatigue assessment includes questions related to the six dimensions of fatigue.[41]

1. Temporal dimension, which includes assessment of the timing of fatigue (when it occurs), onset (from hours to years), duration (chronic for more than 6 months), and pattern (wake up fatigued, evening fatigue, or transient fatigue), as well as changes in this dimension over time
2. Sensory dimension, which focuses on how the fatigue feels, e.g., is the fatigue localized (tired eyes, arms, legs) or generalized (e.g., whole-body tiredness, weariness, weakness, lethargy), and what is its intensity or severity (using a 0–10 scale); additional assessment questions include what exacerbates the fatigue (e.g., pain, nausea, vomiting, environmental heat, or noise), what helps the patient feel better or alleviates the symptoms (e.g., rest, food, or listening to music)
3. Mental/cognitive dimension, which assesses attention span, recall, ability to concentrate and focus, and if the patient reports being "mentally tired"
4. Affective/emotional dimension, which assesses irritability, impatience, mood changes, depression, and the significance of the fatigue
5. Behavioral dimension, which considers the effect that fatigue has on the patient's ability to perform activities of daily living (e.g., bathing, dressing, cooking, socializing, or sexual activity), including observations by family or practitioners regarding the patient's posture, gait, appearance (e.g., drooping shoulders), or lack of energy; acute behavioral manifestations can include a

change in alertness, while chronic manifestations may not be obvious to the practitioner because of the ability of many patients to adapt to their fatigue; if the patient also has a dementing illness, the behavioral dimension may be the only clue that the practitioner has regarding the presence of fatigue

6. Physiologic dimension, which includes a complete physical examination and laboratory tests

Physical examination includes the following assessment parameters:

- Vital signs to determine if fever, low blood pressure, or irregular pulse may contributors
- General appearance, including affect (anxious, depressed, agitated, tearful, angry, or flat), self-care behaviors, speech patterns, intonation, and general responsiveness
- Assessment of cardiac, respiratory, renal, musculoskeletal, and skin status to identify physiological conditions, including signs of infection or dehydration/nutrition that may be associated with fatigue and other comorbid conditions
- Appropriate laboratory testing, such as complete blood count and other laboratory studies (electrolytes, blood gases, thyroid function tests), which may identify underlying causes of fatigue

Table 19–1 also provides questions related to the assessment of the pattern of sleep and rest, patient's perceptions/expression of fatigue, and the impact on quality of life.[20]

MEASURING FATIGUE

Given its subjectivity and the general lack of consensus in the literature regarding a definition of fatigue, measurement remains a challenge. Early attempts at developing an instrument to measure fatigue focused on healthy populations. However, these instruments were less than satisfactory in elderly and chronically ill populations.[12] More recently, self-assessments and self-reports have been developed to measure fatigue. However, construct validity of an instrument is difficult to establish since there are various aspects of fatigue, such as its character, precursors or causes, or effects, and each aspect can be addressed from a physiological, psychosocial, or behavioral perspective. Aaronson and colleagues[12] identified salient characteristics to assess when measuring fatigue: (1) subjective quantification, (2) subjective distress, (3) subjective assessment of the impact on activities of daily living, (4) correlates, and (5) key biological parameters. Researchers must consider the aspect of fatigue that they are interested in examining when selecting a specific measure. It is recommended, how-

Table 19–1. Assessment of Patterns of Sleep/Rest, Perceptions/Expressions of Fatigue, and Impact on Quality of Life

Sleep/rest patterns	Perceptions/expressions of fatigue	Impact on quality of life
Do you nap?	What do you believe is the cause of your fatigue?	Do you feel the quality of your life has changed because of fatigue?
Do you feel rested after a nap?	Are you distressed by fatigue?	Can you work?
Do you have difficulty falling asleep at night or staying asleep?	What do you think is the meaning of this symptom?	Do you socialize?
Has the quality of your sleep at night changed?	Do you feel hopeful?	Has fatigue affected your relationship with others?
How do you feel when you awaken?	Has your appetite changed?	Are you able to enjoy life?
Has your sleeping environment changed?	Do you have other symptoms, such as pain?	Has fatigue affected your outlook?

ever, that researchers use the same multidimensional set of measures across clinical populations to limit discrepant findings among studies and enhance generalizability.

Several instruments are being used[12] to assess the salient characteristics of fatigue in research studies, including the Visual Analog Scale of Fatigue,[42] the Multidimensional Assessment of Fatigue,[43] the Symptom Distress Scale,[44] the Sleep Scale,[45] and the Profile of Mood States.[46] For the clinician, a simple verbal numeric scale is the most efficient assessment tool. Clinicians should consistently use the same scale and give the same instructions each time. The patient should be asked to rate the fatigue at the time of assessment and in the last 24 hours. The same scale, using 0 (no fatigue) to 10 (worst fatigue imaginable), can be used for assessment of all symptoms and gives the patient and clinician a consistent mode of communication.

Lastly, key biological parameters have been based on common blood tests to identify pathological states commonly associated with fatigue, such as hypothyroidism, renal failure, and anemia. However, specific biological measures should be selected based on the clinical population under study.

MANAGEMENT OF FATIGUE

In managing fatigue in the older adult palliative care patient, the goal is to achieve the best quality of life possible given the specific circumstance. Having the energy to do what is important to the patient so that he or she may finalize specific tasks or interact in special relationships is a valuable outcome of treatment. Within the context of palliative care, the management of fatigue must be considered in relation to the age and developmental stage of patients, their wishes and preferences, and the extent of disease and coexisting symptoms.[8] Interventions may focus on treating symptoms that exacerbate fatigue or on preventing fatigue by balancing rest with activity and identifying those activities that increase fatigue or restore energy. Portenoy[47] pro-

posed guidelines for the evaluation and management of fatigue, suggesting modification in drug regimens; correction of metabolic abnormalities; pharmacological treatment for anemia, depression, and insomnia; and symptomatic interventions including cognitive therapies, exercise, modification of activity and rest, sleep hygiene approaches, and nutritional support. Interventions for fatigue will be discussed under nonpharmacological and pharmacological approaches and are selected in accordance with the underlying cause of the fatigue. Review of the literature indicates that data on outcomes of nonpharmacological and pharmacological interventions for fatigue remain limited. Nonpharmacological interventions for fatigue include education/cognitive interventions, coping strategies, exercise, energy balance and conservation, and nutritional considerations.

Education/cognitive interventions include preparatory information and anticipatory guidance regarding the likelihood of fatigue as a side effect of many treatment options, the disease itself, or the emotional reaction to the disease. Older adults are often comforted to know that fatigue may be an expected outcome and not a sign of disease progression. An analogy that can be helpful is to conceptualize fatigue as a depletion of a "bank account" of energy. Within the context of a person's lifestyle and expectations, strategies can be employed that "increase deposits" and "minimize withdrawals."[48] Patients may be encouraged to keep a daily fatigue journal to identify the factors and activities associated with the depletion and restoration of energy (Fig. 19–1). Such a journal will also help the older adult to communicate with the health-care practitioner regarding various concerns, which may be alleviated by effective symptom management, and to plan a schedule to optimize peak energy times. The journal also provides the practitioner with objective evidence of how the patient is doing on a day-to-day basis.

Coping strategies, such as emotion-focused and problem-focused coping, were identified as valuable approaches to fatigue.

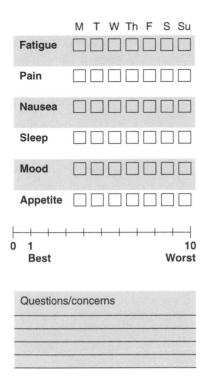

Figure 19–1. Fatigue journal example.

In one study,[3] patients with COPD considered their fatigue as a natural consequence of their condition and identified a number of emotion-focused and problem-focused strategies to enhance their sense of coping. Emotion-focused strategies included being positive with an upbeat look on life, accepting the physical limitations by living within the limits imposed, use of distraction by not dwelling on fatigue, taking things one day at a time, listening to music, and normalizing the condition by attempting to live life normally and fully while maintaining independence. Problem-focused coping strategies included energy conservation, to avoid any unnecessary or excessive use of energy, and energy restoration, in which they used their energy to avoid further deconditioning and deterioration in physical functioning through muscle-strengthening exercises, asking for help when necessary, and through relaxation strategies such as "sitting down and resting," "putting your feet up with a cup of tea," or "taking relaxing baths."

Energy balance and conservation involves finding a balance between rest and exercise that will give patients the most energy to do the things that they would like to do. Given that daytime inactivity and nighttime restlessness have been associated with cancer-related fatigue, interventions to promote daytime activity and nighttime rest are key to managing fatigue and preventing loss of biological rhythmicity.[3] It is suggested that the older person sleep no longer than necessary, which establishes a more solid, less fragmented sleep pattern. Waking up and going to sleep at the same time each day strengthens the circadian cycles and assists in establishing and maintaining a regular sleep cycle, as does exposure to light daily.[8] Encourage patients to establish a specific bedtime and wake time, as well as bedtime routines. A light bedtime snack and something warm to drink often promote sleep. Bedtime routines can help the reticular activating system in the brain shut down in preparation for sleep. Strategies to promote restful sleep also include reduction of environmental stimuli (e.g., noise, light), diversional activities (e.g., music, aromatherapy, massage), and avoidance of alcohol and stimulants (e.g., caffeine, nicotine, steroids). Adjusting the room temperature and humidity, as well as using pillows, may also be helpful in providing support and comfort. If the patient is unable to fall asleep in 20 minutes, suggest getting out of bed, going into another room to read with a dim light, and returning to bed when sleepy.

It helps patients adjust to and accept fatigue if the clinician acknowledges that it is not a sequestered symptom but one that will affect all aspects of the older adult's life. As such, patients will need explicit encouragement to save their energy and plan for activities that are very important to them. They should be asked what activities they enjoy most and encouraged to schedule those activities for the time of day that they have the most energy. Breaks should be scheduled during activities to help restore energy levels, as well as to take short naps (15–20 minutes), which tend to be more restorative than long ones. Energy-conservation techniques should be reinforced with the older adult, such as doing activities while sitting down, using a power scooter for grocery shopping, storing frequently used items at chest level to avoid bending and stretching, putting a terry robe on after the shower instead of using energy to dry off, or wearing slip-on shoes. Recommending devices such as a raised toilet seat, reaching device, and walker can also help conserve energy for patients with progressive fatigue.

Patients should also be encouraged to ask for help with specific chores. Some older adults will see this type of interdependence as very threatening. However, practitioners may help them to see their energy as something to be "budgeted" and used for something that they enjoy or that is very important for them to do. Older adults should always feel that they have the option to "spend" their energy on anything that they wish, being mindful of their energy as a limited resource. Often, reframing their fatigue in this way gives provides a sense of control and creates a willingness to accept help when needed. Spending time with family and friends is also very important in promoting a sense of well-being, which may lessen the perception of fatigue. Prioritizing who they would like to visit with can be helpful, as well as planning such visits at a time of day when the patient has the most energy to avoid excessive fatigue. Health professionals may also assist in addressing the negative impact of psychological and social stressors and how to avoid or modify them.[49]

Exercise, as a problem-focused coping strategy, is another effective intervention for patients who are fatigued. Exercise can take place in a structured rehabilitation/physical therapy department, particularly for those with neuromusculoskeletal deficits or who are fatigued due to cardiac or respiratory problems and would benefit from related rehabilitation therapy. For others, there may be simply a personal commitment to walk outdoors on a regular basis. Whichever is chosen, the exercise program should be individualized with consideration for the patient's physical condition and other medical problems. Patients should be instructed not to exercise to exhaustion, but the activity should be done regularly during the week to be beneficial. Movement can prevent loss of muscle tone, which is difficult to regain, and helps reduce the incidence of falls. Endorphins are liberated with physical activity, resulting in improvement in mood and sense of well-being. Exercise that utilizes the entire body, such as walking, swimming, gardening, or golf, will help maintain tone, strength, and flexibility. Older patients are encouraged to exercise at least 6 hours before their typical bedtime so that they will not have difficulty falling asleep. In several studies of patients with cancer-related fatigue, exercise and rest were the most commonly used and effective strategies for managing the symptom.[34,50,51]

Nutritional status is also an important consideration in explaining the development of fatigue. Deficiences in various B vitamins, vitamin C, magnesium, sodium, zinc, L-tryptophan, L-carnitine, coenzyme Q_{10}, and essential fatty acids may contribute to the experience of fatigue yet are primarily due to illness rather than inadequate diet.[52] Furthermore, low-fat foods and small meals may be easier to digest in the older adult, resulting in less energy used for digestion. Given that nutrition and hydration are important in preventing fatigue, increasing fluids may be of benefit, unless contraindicated by other medical problems. Protein intake and supplements can also be encouraged if the older person is having trouble with a regular diet. Recent data suggest that for patients with advanced cancer, foods rich in ω-3 polyunsaturated fatty acids, such as flaxseed oil and fish oil, may decrease cytokines such as tumor necrosis factor and IL-1β, increase weight and appetite, and decrease fatigue.[53] Megesterol acetate may also stimulate appetite and provide energy, thereby lessening fatigue.[48]

PHARMACOLOGICAL MANAGEMENT OF FATIGUE

The pharmacological management of fatigue is different from the management typically provided for other symptoms when there are often medications available to treat the underlying cause. In the case of fatigue, the cause may not be treatable, and medications may not be the primary intervention. Each medication that the patient receives should be reviewed for its potential to produce sedation and fatigue. Distressing symptoms should be optimally treated as their relief often decreases associated fatigue. Patients should be made aware that the fatigue experienced with opioid therapy will cease as tolerance to opioids develops. Optimizing the use of nonopioid and adjuvant analgesics may also reduce fatigue associated with pain management. Even modest improvements in fatigue can improve the older adult's quality of life.[48]

Corticosteroids, stimulants, and antidepressants have also been of benefit in the treatment of fatigue (Table 19–2). There is empirical support for the use of low-dose corticosteroids for patients with multiple symptoms and advanced disease who experience fatigue;[54] however, there are insufficient data on optimal type and dosage. Corticosteroids can also improve appetite, elevate mood, and serve as adjuvant analgesics, resulting in an improved sense of well-being, although the duration of effect may be limited. Most commonly, dexamethasone 2–8 mg twice daily or prednisone 10–40 mg twice daily is prescribed. However, to date, there have been no comparative studies.[15] The predictable side effects of corticosteroids (i.e., diabetes, hypertension, peptic ulcer, and delirium) must be balanced against their potential benefit in the context of a limited prognosis.

Although the use of psychostimulants to treat cancer-related fatigue has not been empirically tested, anecdotal evidence indicates that the use of psychostimulants is worth considering with older adults whose clinical profile would not contraindicate a trial.[15,55] There is also clinical experience in using psychostimulants to treat depression in the older adult population.[56] Although there have been no controlled comparisons of dextroamphetamine and pemoline, pemoline is reported to have fewer sympathomimetic effects.[15] Pemoline is available in a chewable formulation that will absorb through the buccal mucosa for those who are no longer able to swallow. However, given the risk of hepatotoxicity from pemoline, not seen with other psychostimulants, methylphenidate is suggested for initial treatment.[5] The initial dose of methylphenidate is usually 2.5–5 mg given in the morning and early afternoon. The dose can be gradually increased until favorable effects occur or until toxicities, such as anorexia, insomnia, anxiety, confusion, tremor, or tachycardia, supervene. To limit toxicity in the medically ill, dose escalation should be undertaken with caution and over longer intervals.[15]

When fatigue is associated with clinical depression, a trial of an antidepressant drug is appropriate. Antidepressants, such as the selective serotonin reuptake inhibitors, are preferred because of their side-effect profile and the fact that they are more likely to be activating.[15] A sedating antidepressant, such as trazodone or mirtazapine, may be beneficial when given at bedtime for patients who have difficulty sleeping.[57]

If fatigue is the result of anemia, treatment with recombinant erythropoietin has been shown in randomized studies to increase the hemoglobin level and improve energy levels as well as quality of life.[58] Anemia can also be treated with blood transfusions, but this intervention is not without risks, which may include systemic infections such as HIV or hepatitis B or C, acute hemolytic reactions, bacterial contamination, and allergic reactions (e.g., urticaria, anaphylaxis).[59]

It is important to evaluate the efficacy of both pharmacological and nonpharmacological fatigue interventions on a regular basis through formal assessment and reassessment of symptom severity.

Table 19–2. Pharmacological Therapies for the Treatment of Fatigue

Class of drug	Examples	Mechanism of action	Comments
Corticosteroids	Dexamethasone (2–8 mg bid)	Unclear	May mask signs of acute infection, side effects include diabetes, hypertension, peptic ulcer, and delirium
	Prednisone (10–40 mg bid)	Duration and benefits limited to months	
Stimulants	Methylphenidate (2.5–5 mg qd or bid)	Stimulates central nervous system and respiratory centers, increases appetite and energy levels, improves mood, reduces sedation[60]	Titrate to effect, rapid onset of action, fewer side effects than many antidepressants, may cause agitation, risk of toxicity increases with dose[57]
	Dextroamphetamine (2.5–5 mg qd or bid) Pemoline (18.75 mg qd or bid)		No controlled comparisons between efficacy of each of these drugs, response to one does not predict response to others, sequential trials to determine the most useful drug suggested[5]
Antidepressants	Trazodone (25–50 mg at bedtime, increase as tolerated to a maximum of 300 mg qd)[57]	Reduces depressive symptoms associated with fatigue, can improve sleep, primary choice for treatment of depression in cancer patients	
	Paroxetine (10 mg) Fluoxetine (10 mg)		
Selective serotonin reuptake inhibitors (SSRIs)	Sertraline (25 mg)	Inhibits serotonin reuptake	Give once daily in the morning, fluoxetine has a have long half-life and should be used cautiously in the terminally ill older adult
Tricyclic antidepressants	Nortriptyliine (25 mg tid, qid)	Blocks reuptake of various neurotransmitters at the neuronal membrane, can improve sleep	Other tricyclics, such as amitriptyline, should not be used in the older adult, particularly in patients with cardiovascular disease as adverse reactions include arrythmias or anticholinergic toxicity, including constipation, dry mouth, tachycardia, and orthostasis
Erythropoietin	150 U/kg subcutaneously 3 times a week	Increases hemoglobin with effects on energy, activity and overall quality of life while decreasing transfusion requirements[61]	Monitor hematocrit and reduce dose if it approaches 36% or increases by >points in 2 weeks

FATIGUE IN FAMILY CAREGIVERS

Family caregivers are often profoundly fatigued by the stressors inherent in caregiving. Caregivers bear the physical and emotional burdens of assisting patients with activities of daily living and treatments. They often must assume new roles and responsibilities and deal with additional financial distress.[48] As a result, family caregivers may also develop anxiety or depressive disorders associated with fatigue. Severe family fatigue is commonly experienced in four situations: *(1)* inadequate relief of patient's pain and suffering, *(2)* inadequate resources to cope with home care, *(3)* unrealistic expectations of family caregivers of themselves or health professionals and *(4)* emotional distress that persists even when there is adequate relief of patient suffering.[62]

Palliative care recognizes patient and family as the unit of care; therefore, assessment and interventions to relieve caregiver burden are essential. Validating the needs and concerns of family caregivers is important. Helping family caregivers to set priorities with regard to competing demands, optimizing stress and coping strategies, encouraging relaxation and rest, and the treatment of depression while assisting with respite care is important in preventing or alleviating caregiver fatigue.[48]

CONCLUSION

To the health-care professional, fatigue signifies illness, a treatment side effect, depression, or the emotional strain of illness or caregiving. To patients and families, fatigue is a symptom that keeps them from moving forward fully with life.[63] Health professionals can be supportive by acknowledging fatigue as real and taking it and its frustrations seriously. Understanding the possible etiology of fatigue and the meaning of the symptom to the patient are important in determining its management. Assisting patients and families to live as fully as possible as they move along the illness trajectory may require consideration of nonpharmacological as well as pharmacological therapies to comprehensively and effectively treat fatigue. Learning how to prevent fatigue and/or restore energy is important to improving patient function, ability to socialize, and ultimately adjustment to a "new normal" baseline as they live with chronic or life-limiting illness.[64]

REFERENCES

1. Ferrell BR, Grant M, Dean GE, et al. Bone tired: the experience of fatigue and its impact on quality of life. Oncol Nurs Forum 23:1539–1547, 1996.

2. Richardson A, Ream E. Research and development: fatigue in patients receiving chemotherapy for advanced cancer. Int J Palliat Nurs 2:199–204, 1996.

3. Small S, Lamb M. Fatigue in chronic illness: the experience of individuals with chronic obstructive pulmonary disease and with asthma. J Adv Nurs 30:469–478, 1999.

4. Vainio A, Auvinen A. Prevalence of symptoms among patients with advanced cancer: an international study. J Pain Symptom Manage 12:3–10, 1996.

5. Breitbart W, Esch JF, Portenoy RK. Fatigue in Cancer and AIDS. The Network Project. Memorial Sloan-Kettering Cancer Center, New York, 1997.

6. Sarna L, Brecht M. Dimensions of symptom distress in women with advanced lung cancer: a factor analysis. Heart Lung 26:23–30, 1997.

7. Irvine DM, Vincent L, Bubela N, et al. A critical appraisal of the research literature investigating fatigue in the individual with cancer. Cancer Nurs 14:188–199, 1991.

8. Dean GE, Anderson PR. Fatigue. In: Ferrel BR, Coyle N (Eds.). The Textbook of Palliative Nursing. New York, Oxford University Press, pp. 91–100, 2001.

9. Jenkins CA, Schulz M, Hanson J, et al. Demographic, symptom, medication profiles of cancer patients seen by a palliative care consult team in a tertiary referral hospital. J Pain Symptom Manage 19:174–184, 2000.

10. Piper BF, Lindsey AM, Dodd MJ, et al. The development of an instrument to measure the subjective dimension of fatigue. In: Funk SG, Funk EM, Champagne MT, et al. (Eds.). Key Aspects of Comfort. New York, Springer, pp. 199–208, 1989.

11. Tiesinga, LJ, Dassen TWN, Halfens RJG. Fatigue: a summary of the definitions, dimensions and indicators. Nurs Diagn 7: 51–62, 1996.

12. Aaronson LS, Teel CS, Cassmeyer V, et al. Defining and measuring fatigue. Image J Nurs Sch 31:45–50, 1999.

13. Neuenschwander H, Bruera E. Pathophysiology of cancer asthenia. In: Bruera E, Portenoy RK (Eds.). Topics in Palliative Care, vol 2. New York: Oxford University Press, pp. 171–181, 1998.

14. Chochinov H, Breitbart W. Handbook of Psychiatry in Palliative Medicine. New York, Oxford University Press, 2000.

15. Portenoy R. Physical symptom management in the terminally ill. In: Chochinov HM, Breitbart W (Eds.). Handbook of Psychiatry in Palliative Medicine. New York, Oxford University Press, pp. 116–119, 2000.

16. Magnusson K, Moller A, Ekman T, Wallgreen A. A qualitative study to explore the experience of fatigue in cancer patients. Eur J Cancer Care 8:224–232, 1999.

17. Piper BF. Fatigue: current bases for practice. In: Funk SG, Funk EM, Champagne MT, et al. (Eds.). Key Aspects of Comfort. New York, Springer, pp. 187–198, 1989.

18. Atkinson A, Barsevick A, Cella D, Cimprich B, Cleeland C, Donnelly J, Eisenberger M, Escalanted C, Hinds P, Jacobsen PB, Kaldor P, Knight SJ, Perteman A, Piper BF, Rugo H, Sabbatini P, Stahl C. NCCN Practice Guidelines for cancer-related fatigue. Oncology 14:151–161, 2000.

19. Groenwald SL, Frogge MH, Goodman M, et al. (Eds.). Cancer Nursing Principles and Practice. Sudbury, MA, Jones and Bartlett, 1993.

20. Cahill C. Differential diagnosis of fatigue in women. J Obstet Gynecol Neonatal Nurs 28:81–86, 1999.

21. Fobair P, Hoppe RT, Bloom J, et al. Psychosocial problems among survivors of Hodgkin's disease. J Clin Oncol 4:805–814, 1986.

22. Friedman M, King K. Correlates of fatigue in older women with heart failure. Heart Lung 24:512–518, 1995.

23. Ingles JL, Eskes GA, Phillips SJ. Fatigue after stroke. Arch Phys Med Rehabil 80:173–178, 1999.

24. Liao S, Ferrell BA. Fatigue in an older population. J Am Geriatr Soc 48:426–430, 2000.

25. Frazer DW, Leicht ML, Baker MD. Psychological manifestations of physical disease in the elderly. In: Carstensen LL, Edelstein BA, Dornbrand L (Eds.). The Practical Handbook of Clinical Gerontology. Thousand Oaks, CA, Sage, pp. 217–235, 1996.

26. Aaronson LS, Teel CS, Cassmeyer V, et al. Defining and measuring fatigue. Image J Nurs Sch 31:45–50, 1999.

27. Cauch-Dudek K, Abbey S, Stewart DE, et al. Fatigue in primary biliary cirrhosis. Gut 43:705–710, 1998.

28. Breslin E, vander Schans S, Breukink S, et al. Perception of fatigue and quality of life in patients with COPD. Chest 114:958–964, 1998.

29. Ferrando S, Evans S, Goggin K, et al. Fatigue in HIV illness: relationship to depression, physical limitations, and disability. Psychosom Med 60:759–764, 1998.

30. Berger AM, Farr L. The influence of daytime inactivity and nighttime restlessness on cancer-related fatigue. Oncol Nurs Forum 26:1663–1671, 1999.

31. Loge JH, Abrahamsen AF, Ekeberg O, et al. Fatigue and psychiatric morbidity among Hodgkin's disease. J Pain Symptom Manage 19:91–99, 2000.

32. Mast M. Correlates of fatigue in survivors of breast cancer. Cancer Nurs 21:136–142, 1998.

33. Miaskowski C, Lee KA. Pain, fatigue, and sleep disturbances in oncology outpatients receiving radiation therapy for bone metastasis: a pilot study. J Pain Symptom Manage 17:320–322, 1999.

34. Schwartz AL. Patterns of exercise and fatigue in physically active cancer survivors. Oncol Nurs Forum 25:485–491, 1998.

35. Woo B, Dibble SL, Piper BF, et al. Differences in fatigue by treatment methods in women with breast cancer. Oncol Nurs Forum 25:915–920, 1998.

36. Bower JE, Ganz PA, Desmond KA, Rowland JH, Meyerowitz BE, Belin TR. Fatigue in breast cancer survivors: occurrence, correlates, and impact on quality of life. J Clin Oncol 18:743–753, 2000.

37. Okuyama T, Akechi T, Kugaya A, Okamura H, Imoto S, Nakano T, Mikami I, Hosaka T, Uchitomi Y. Factors correlated with fatigue in disease-free breast cancer patients: application of the Cancer Fatigue Scale. Support Care Cancer 8:215–222, 2000.

38. Okuyama T, Tanaka K, Akechi T, Kugaya A, Okamura H, Nishiwaki Y, Hosaka T, Uchitomi Y. Fatigue in ambulatory patients with advanced lung cancer: prevalence, correlated factors, and screening. J Pain Symptom Manage 22:554–564, 2001.

39. Ferrell BR, Grant M, Dean GE, et al. Bone tired: the experience of fatigue and its impact on quality of life. Oncol Nurs Forum 23:1539–1547, 1996.

40. Vogelzang NJ, Breitbart W, Cella D, et al. Patient, caregiver, and oncologist perceptions of cancer-related fatigue: results of a tripart assessment survey. Semin Hematol 34:4–12, 1997.

41. Piper BF. Measurements of fatigue. In: Stromberg M, Olsen K (Eds.). Instruments for Clinical Research, 2nd ed. Boston, Jones and Bartlett, 1995.

42. Lee KA, Hicks G, Nino-Murcia G. Validity and reliability of a scale to assess fatigue. Psychiatry Res 36:291–298, 1991.

43. Tack B. Dimensions and Correlates of Fatigue in Older Adults with Rheumatoid Arthritis. San Francisco, University of California, 1991, Dissertation.

44. McCorkle R, Young K. Development of a symptom distress scale. Cancer Nurs 3:248–256, 1978.

45. Snyder-Halpern R, Verran JA. Instrumentation to describe subjective sleep characteristics in healthy subjects. Res Nurs Health 10:155–163, 1987.

46. McNair DM, Lorr M, Dropplemann LF. EdITS Manual for the Profile of Mood States. San Diego, EdITS/Educational Testing Service, 1992.

47. Portenoy R. Cancer-related fatigue: guidelines for evaluation and management. Oncologist 4:1–10, 1999.

48. Abbey S. Psychiatric aspects of fatigue in the terminally ill. In: Chochinov HM, Breitbart W (Eds.). Handbook of Psychiatry in Palliative Medicine. New York, Oxford University Press, pp. 175–185, 2000.

49. Winningham ML, Nail LM, Burke MB, et al. Fatigue and the cancer experience: the state of the knowledge. Oncol Nurs Forum 21:23–36, 1994.

50. Dimeo FC, Stieglitz RD, Novelli-Fischer U, Kuel J. Effects of physical activity on the fatigue and psychologic status of cancer patients during chemotherapy. Cancer 85: 2273–2277, 1999.

51. Schwartz AL. Daily fatigue patterns and effect of exercise in women with breast cancer. Cancer Pract 8:16–24, 2000.

52. Werbach MR. Nutritional strategies for treating chronic fatigue syndrome. Altern Med Rev 5:93–198, 2000.

53. Kalman D, Villani LJ. Nutritional aspects of cancer-related fatigue. J Am Diet Assoc 97:650–654, 1997.

54. Tannock I, Gospodarowicz M, Meakin W, et al. Treatment of metastatic prostatic cancer with low-dose prednisone: evaluation of pain and quality of life as pragmatic indices of response. J Clin Oncol 7:590–597, 1989.

55. Sarhill N, Walsh D, Nelson KA, Homsi J, LeGrand S, Davis MP. Methylphenidate for fatigue in advanced cancer: a prospective open-label pilot study. Am J Hosp Palliat Care 18:187–192, 2001.

56. Breitbart W, Mermelsltein MV. An alternative psychostimulant for the management of depressive disorders in cancer patients. Psychosomatics 33:352–356, 1992.

57. Beers MH, Berkow R. Care of the dying patient. In: The Merck Manual of Geriatrics, 3rd ed. Whitehouse Station, NY, Merck, pp. 115–127, 2000.

58. Glaspy J, Bukowski R, Steinber D, et al. Impact of therapy with epoetin alfa on clinical outcomes in patients with nonmyeloid malignancies during cancer chemotherapy in community oncology practice. J Clin Oncol 15:1218–1234, 1997.

59. Labovich TM. Transfusion therapy: nursing implications. Clin J Oncol Nurs 1:61, 1997.

60. Bruera E, Chadwick S, Brenneis C. Methylphenidate associated with narcotic treatment of cancer pain. Cancer Treat Rep 70: 295–297, 1985.

61. Krammer L, Muir C, Gooding-Gellar N, et al. Palliative care and oncology: opportunities for nursing. Oncol Nurs Update 6:1–12, 1999.

62. Cherny NI. The treatment of suffering in patients with advanced cancer. In: Chochinov HM, Breitbart W (Eds.). Handbook of Psychiatry in Palliative Medicine. New York, Oxford University Press, pp. 375–396, 2000.

63. Greenberg D. Fatigue. In: Holland J (Ed.). Psycho-oncology. New York, Oxford University Press, pp. 485–493, 1998.

64. Harpham W. Resolving the frustration of fatigue. CA Cancer J Clin 49:178–189, 1999.

20

Delirium, Anxiety, and Depression

ELIZABETH GOY AND LINDA GANZINI

Although the final chapter of a person's life can be psychologically and socially rich, mental disorders often supervene, worsening quality of life for patients and distressing their caregivers. Emotional difficulties develop into mental disorders when psychological or behavioral disturbances become pervasive, cause distress, and impair a person's ability to function. Although epidemiological studies of the prevalence of mental disorders among geriatric patients in palliative care settings are not available, the most common and troublesome syndromes include delirium, anxiety, mood disorders, and behavioral difficulties in end-stage dementia.

DELIRIUM

Delirium is a disorder characterized by impairments in attention, concentration, and cognition resulting from insults such as medical illnesses and medications.[1] Delirium's clinical importance in palliative care is as a marker of worsening illness and harbinger of death and in its association with declining function, worsening behavioral difficulties, caregiver burden, and need for higher levels of care.[2] Delirium can be a source of suffering for patients and their families because it results in fear, anxiety, and dysphoria in patients; and it curtails remaining opportunities to communicate and to direct one's care.[3] Like other geriatric syndromes, delirium may represent the first or only symptom of a new illness. Management of delirium in palliative care can be clinically challenging, and there are few clinical trials to support potentially beneficial interventions.

Clinical discourse and research on delirium has been impeded by the many terms used to refer to this syndrome, including acute confusional state, encephalopathy, organic brain syndrome, acute brain failure, and intensive care unit psychosis.[4,5] In hospice, delirium is sometimes referred to as terminal restlessness or terminal agitation.[6] In recent years, experts have advocated for use of the term *delirium* exclusively. Delirium is defined in both the *International Classification of Diseases*,

Table 20–1. *Diagnostic and Statistical Manual*, Volume IV[1] (DSM-IV) and *International Classification of Diseases, 9th Revision, Clinical Modification*[7] (ICD-9-CM) Criteria for Delirium

DSM-IV

A. Disturbance of consciousness (i.e., reduced clarity of awareness of the environment) with reduced ability to focus, sustain, or shift attention

B. A change in cognition (e.g., memory deficit, disorientation, language disturbance) or the development of a perceptual disturbance that is not better accounted for by a pre-existing, established, or evolving dementia

C. The disturbance develops over a short period of time (usually hours to days) and tends to fluctuate during the course of the day

D. There is evidence from the history, physical examination, or laboratory findings that the disturbance is caused by the direct physiological consequences of a general medical condition

ICD-9-CM

Delirium: Transient organic psychotic conditions with a short course in which there is a rapidly developing onset of disorganization of higher mental processes manifested by some degree of impairment of information processing, impaired or abnormal attention, perception, memory, and thinking. Clouded consciousness, confusion, disorientation, delusions, illusions, and often vivid hallucinations predominate in the clinical picture.

9th revision (ICD-9)[7] and the *Diagnostic and Statistical Manual* of the American Psychiatric Association (DSM-IV)[1] (Table 20–1).

Clinical Features of Delirium

Delirium develops over hours to days, and symptoms characteristically fluctuate throughout the course of the day, sometimes quite rapidly. Although clinicians often observe that delirium worsens in the evening and night, one study of over 300 patients older than 75 years in a variety of settings reported that almost half of patients had delirium predominantly in the morning.[8]

Delirious patients struggle to focus, sustain, and shift attention appropriately. In conversation, they are easily distracted by irrelevant stimuli, have difficulty staying on track, and may shift from one subject to another. Because of disorganized thinking and incoherent speech, delirious patients are often unreliable historians. Although delirium often renders patients sleepy or lethargic, at other times they appear alert even when attention and concentration are severely impaired. Tests of attention on cognitive examination include the ability to repeat a list of random numbers (unimpaired elderly should be able to repeat at least five), ability to say the days of the week backward (unimpaired elderly should have no errors), or serial subtractions.[3,9] Other evidence of cognitive impairment includes problems with memory, especially short-term memory and disorientation; language; abstraction; and visuoperceptual ability.[10]

Delirium has been subtyped on the basis of the patient's psychomotor state. Hypomotoric patients, sometimes described as "quietly delirious," are typically lethargic, listless, and apathetic, with decreased motor activity. Hyperactive patients are hypervigilant; restless; wandering; at times loud, angry, or irritable; and often agitated.[11] In studies of elderly patients in a variety of settings, approximately one-quarter have hypoactivity, one-quarter have hyperactivity, and about half have a mixed motor presentation.[8,12,13] Among elderly patients, hypoactive delirium is often misdiagnosed as depression or not recognized.[14] Hypoactive delirium is associated with more severe medical illness, longer hospital stays, and development of decubitus ulcers and has a worse prognosis.[12] In contrast, agitated/hyperactive patients are younger and more likely to have drug/alcohol withdrawal; have a better prognosis, shorter length of hospital stay, and more falls; and are more likely to receive psychoactive medications, including neuroleptics and benzodiazepines.[11,12] The sleep/wake cycle is disturbed in both the hyperactive and hypoactive presentations, with nighttime agitation and impaired sleep continuity.[10]

Psychotic and emotional symptoms are common in delirious patients. For example, 77% of over 300 patients older than 75 years had emotional symptoms, including dysphoria, irritability, emotional lability, and anxiety.[8] Among patients in a medical surgical setting who became tearful, 76% were found to have a cognitive disorder, most often delirium.[15] Perceptual disturbances including misinterpretations, illusions, and true hallucinations (particularly visual but also auditory and tactile) are especially common in hyperactive delirium. Delusions are usually simple and of the paranoid type, and they wax and wane in severity with the disorder.

Diagnosis of Delirium

Several instruments have been developed to aid clinicians in diagnosing delirium and determining its severity. The Confusion Assessment Method allows clinicians to make reliable diagnoses and has been used in a variety of settings; however, this instrument was not designed to allow severity ratings.[16] Instruments measuring the severity of delirium include the Memorial Delirium Assessment Scale, which was developed for patients with advanced cancer.[17] The Delirium Rating Scale rates both presence and absence of the diagnosis as well as severity.[18] One of the most popular instruments for measuring cognition in geriatric populations is the Folstein Mini-Mental State Examination (MMSE).[19] Although scores in the impaired range do not specifically indicate delirium (patients with dementia typically score in the impaired range), sudden precipitous declines in MMSE score warrant further examination for delirium.

Epidemiology of Delirium

The prevalence of delirium ranges from 1.1% in community-dwelling persons over the age of 55 to 10%–40% in elderly patients in medical inpatient units to 25%–40% in hospitalized cancer patients

to 9%–44% in elderly patients following surgical interventions and to 60% of persons age 75 years or older in nursing homes.[20,21] In studies of palliative care inpatients, approximately 20% were delirious on admission; the point prevalence in this setting was 20%–61%, and the incidence was 33%–85%. Eighty to ninety percent of terminally ill patients approaching death will develop delirium.[22–26] The disorder is overlooked by health-care practitioners even in settings where it is prevalent;[10,23] however, families may notice restlessness, irritability, mood changes, sleep problems, and distractibility.[10]

Risk factors for delirium include older age, especially age over 80 years; multiple severe or unstable medical problems; dementia or cognitive impairment; polypharmacy; dehydration/azotemia; infection; fractures; visual impairment; fever or hypothermia; psychoactive drug use; male gender; and alcohol abuse.[2,20,27] Inouye[2] points out that some of these factors predispose patients to the development of delirium in that they result in increased vulnerability to this syndrome. Other factors precipitate delirium; that is, they are the noxious insults that ultimately result in a patient becoming delirious. The elderly in palliative care may be at risk of developing delirium because they have more predisposing factors and precipitating factors. Old age is a predisposing factor, perhaps because of age-related brain changes, such as reduced cholinergic activity, or because other risk factors, such as dementia or polypharmacotherapy, are more prevalent in old age.[27]

When delirium develops, clinicians retrospectively examine the chain of events leading up to it and may find many possible precipitating or predisposing factors. For example, Francis et al.[28] reported that among 2219 elderly patients admitted to medical inpatient service, a definitive or probable cause was found in 31%, whereas a possible cause was found in 69%. Similarly, Brauer et al.,[21] examining elderly patients with a hip fracture, reported that in only 6% of cases could a definite cause be found, and in 26% the cause was rated as probable. In the majority of patients, the "cause" was one of several possible comorbid conditions.[5,21] As the number of risk factors increases, the relative risk of developing delirium increases in a multiplicative manner.[29] For example, Lawlor et al.,[5] in a study of advanced cancer patients, found a median of three precipitating factors per episode of delirium.

The most common precipitants of delirium in palliative care are drugs, infections, metabolic disorders, and end-organ disease.[30] Among the drug causes of delirium, medications with anticholinergic effects are the most consistently identified, including tricyclic antidepressants, which may be used to treat pain; antipsychotics, including the older low-potency medications such as thorazine and thioridazine and the newer atypicals such as olanzapine; H_2-blockers such as cimetidine; and antisecretory agents such as scopolamine.[31] Over 600 marketed drugs have anticholinergic effects, and these medications are disproportionately prescribed for the elderly.[31] In palliative care settings, opioids, especially if used for more than several days, are frequently implicated. The effects of opioids range from mild alterations in alertness and attention to frank delirium. Morphine and meperidine are anecdotally associated with delirium more frequently than other opioids, though there are no controlled trials; delirium may be more common in the context of repeated doses, renal impairment, and old age.[3] Alcohol, sedatives/hypnotics, and drugs of abuse can be direct causes of delirium; or delirium may result from withdrawal in drug-dependent patients.

Other common causes of delirium include dehydration with or without hypo- and hypernatremia; progressive end-organ failure resulting in uremia, hepatic failure, hypercarbia, and pulmonary edema; and any systemic infection or sepsis. Many brain injuries result in global confusion along with focal neurological deficits.[5,30] In older patients, delirium can be the first and most prominent manifestation of any of these illnesses.

Complications of Delirium

Complications of delirium include behavioral and affective disturbances, worsening pain syndromes, falls, and self-injury.[20] Pain is more difficult to control in delirious patients.[22,32-34] Among nonterminally ill, elderly, hospitalized patients, delirium is associated with three times the risk of functional decline and three times the risk of nursing home placement.[35] Delirious patients experience fear, anxiety, and depressive symptoms. Misdiagnosed depression or anxiety may lead to ineffective or harmful pharmacological or psychotherapeutic interventions.

Outcome of Delirium

In medical inpatients, delirium is an important independent determinant of death even after adjustment for age, illnesses severity, dementia, and functional status.[28,35] In advanced cancer patients referred to palliative care programs, delirium independently predicts mortality, even when functional status, other symptoms (such as anorexia, weight loss, and dyspnea), and clinical prediction of survival are taken into account.[5,23,36-38] Despite this association, between one-half and two-thirds of patients with advanced cancer in palliative care settings who develop delirium will improve significantly before death, many without intervention.[5,22,23] Among advanced cancer patients, reversible causes of delirium include psychoactive medications and dehydration; hypoxia and metabolic abnormalities are associated with nonreversibility.[5]

Assessment and Treatment of Delirium

The most important approach to the treatment of delirium is to reverse underlying precipitants and to address underlying vulnerabilities. Within palliative care, the goals of finding and treating the causes are balanced against emphasis on comfort, quality of life, and avoidance of burdensome diagnostic interventions.[3] Achieving this balance will depend on the patients' and families' goals and the patients' setting. Palliative care patients with hyperactive delirium often require treatment because they are a danger to themselves; the delirium is frightening and distressing to the patient and increases family members' emotional distress, burden, and exhaustion.[6,32] Treatment of hypoactive delirium in palliative care is more controversial as many hospice professionals consider quiet delirium to be part of the dying process and consistent with a peaceful, unanxious death. Hallucinations in the final days of life, especially those of a spiritual nature, are considered normative and part of the "letting go" process by some.[39] For many, however, hallucinations are frightening and may require treatment.[30] Care providers should be educated as to the nature of the delirium and its cause. Attention should be given to safety issues, including risks of falls, self-harm, and wandering. Restraints should be avoided whenever possible as they may worsen agitation. Patients may be less behaviorally disturbed with a familiar environment and familiar care providers.[10]

Inouye and coinvestigators[29] implemented a standardized protocol for the management of six risk factors for delirium among geriatric medical inpatients, including cognitive impairment, sleep deprivation, immobility, visual impairment, hearing impairment, and dehydration. This intervention was associated with a reduced incidence, total number of days, and total number of episodes of delirium.[29] However, Brauer et al.,[21] in a study of delirium in elderly hip fracture patients, reported that 74% improved markedly or completely by the time of discharge, without interventions aimed at healing the delirium.

Among patients with advanced disease or who are in palliative care settings, randomized protocols are lacking, but several helpful interventions have been suggested by experts. Palliative care specialists report that hydration by hypodermoclysis and *opioid rotation* (changing to a different opioid at an equianalgesic dose) reduced the incidence of agitated delirium from one in four to one in ten.[40]

Neuroleptic medications offer the most effective symptomatic relief in delirium ex-

cept if due to alcohol/sedative hypnotic withdrawal or in the context of recurrent seizures in which benzodiazepines are recommended. Neuroleptics are indicated for patients with agitation, fearfulness, hallucinations, paranoia, or aggression. They may be less helpful for confused behavior, wandering, restlessness, or calling out and at times can worsen these latter behaviors if the patient develops *akathisia*, a syndrome of subjective motor restlessness. Breitbart et al.[41] reported in a randomized trial of delirious acquired immunodeficiency virus (AIDS) patients that those receiving neuroleptics (haloperidol or chlorpromazine) had improvement in symptoms of delirium compared to those treated with lorazepam: improvement was noted both in patients with hyperactive and in those with hypoactive symptoms. Haloperidol is most often recommended as it rarely causes orthostatic hypotension or cardiovascular adverse effects; can be given orally, subcutaneously, intramuscularly, and intravenously; and has a wide therapeutic window.[6] The most common adverse effects, in addition to akathisia, include drug-induced parkinsonism and acute dystonia, though the overall incidence is low.[41,42] There are no clear advantages to the newer atypical antipsychotics unless patients have known intolerance to haloperidol secondary to extrapyramidal symptoms. Atypical neuroleptics are recommended for long-term treatment in the elderly because of less liability for development of extrapyramidal syndromes such as tardive dyskinesia. However, development of tardive dyskinesia is not of concern in the short-term treatment of delirium. In addition, the newer atypicals are comparatively expensive, may cause more orthostatic hypotension (e.g., risperidone), and have more anticholinergic effects that may worsen confusion (e.g., olanzapine).

Investigators have reported the degree to which other forms of sedation, such as midazolam, diazepam, lorazepam, propofol, or methotrimepazine, are indicated for agitated delirium in the final days of life.[30] Sedation can be considered when more conservative treatments have not been effective. Midazolam and propofol are administered only by constant intravenous infusion, which is not appropriate for many palliative settings.[43] These interventions may further rob the patient of awareness and opportunities to communicate but may improve patient comfort. The goals and risks of sedation should be discussed with the patient if he or she has decision-making capacity or with a caregiver if the patient lacks decision-making capacity. Sedation is used in 4%–36% of patients near the end of life, with substantial variation across treatment settings but delirium being the most common indication.[22,44,45] Further studies are needed to confirm that careful prospective assessment and management will decrease the need for sedation for agitated delirium at the end of life.

ANXIETY

Clinical Features and Diagnosis of Anxiety

Anxiety is characterized by apprehensive anticipation of future danger or misfortune accompanied by psychological symptoms such as worrying, vigilance, and rumination as well as by physical feelings such as tension, jitters, palpitations, dyspnea, chest discomfort, or abdominal distress.[1] Mild anxiety is a ubiquitous symptom and, although uncomfortable, rarely represents a psychiatric disorder. Anxiety can be a common and understandable response to the uncertainties of living with a life-limiting disorder, concerns about the dying process, and worries about the looming time limits for attending to unresolved problems. When severe and resulting in impaired functioning, anxiety may be the primary manifestation of a true anxiety disorder or a symptom of another psychiatric disorder, such as a mood disorder or delirium. Anxiety may also be a specific conditioned response to radiation or chemotherapy.[46]

Certain anxiety disorders may precede development of life-limiting illness but complicate the course. For example, posttraumatic stress disorder in combat veterans, marked by worsening nightmares, recollections of the traumatic event, and symptoms of hyperarousal such as irritability, startle, and hypervigilance, may symptomatically worsen during episodes of illness and cognitive decline.[47] Generalized anxiety disorder and obsessive-compulsive disorder, which generally have their onset in young adults, may interfere with the ability to tolerate medical regimens.[1]

Other anxiety disorders may have their onset after diagnosis of a life-limiting illness. New anxiety can be a manifestation of a medical illness (e.g., worsening pulmonary or cardiac disease), pain, medications such as steroids or β-adrenergic stimulants, withdrawal from alcohol or benzodiazepines, or akathisia resulting from neuroleptics. There is a moderate correlation between dyspnea in cancer patients and anxiety.[48] Specific phobias may result from noxious treatments, and more generalized posttraumatic stress disorder has been reported in cancer survivors.[49] Anxiety in elderly palliative care patients often results from another psychiatric disorder, most commonly delirium, depression, or dementia.

Epidemiology of Anxiety

The prevalence of anxiety disorder among the seriously ill is not well studied, but several large studies have examined it as a symptom. For example, Kutner et al.[50] received nurses' reports on 348 clients from 16 hospices: nurses reported that 43% of clients endorsed nervousness. Donnelly and Walsh[51] reported anxiety in 23% of 1000 advanced cancer patients who received palliative care consultations. Hopwood and Stephens[52] reported that 34% of 987 inoperable lung cancer patients had anxiety and 21% had anxiety with depression. Women appear to have more anxiety symptoms than men, but there is no evidence that age influences prevalence.[51,52]

Assessment and Treatment of Anxiety

The approach to new-onset anxiety should include assessment of its intensity, context, and pervasiveness; exploration of history of previous anxiety and its treatment; consideration of a new underlying medical illness; and exclusion of delirium and depression. For anxiety related to difficulties in adjusting, worries and fears are best addressed by exploration of the sources of the fears, practical discussion, and active support of the patient and family. Panic disorder, symptoms of posttraumatic stress disorder, obsessive-compulsive disorder, and anxiety in the context of depression can be treated with medications in the selective serotonin uptake inhibitor (SSRI) class. Buspirone, a nonbenzodiazepine anxiolytic, is useful in the treatment of chronic anxiety and causes minimal psychomotor or cognitive impairment, but there is little evidence of efficacy for patients in palliative care.[53] Benzodiazepines are primarily used for brief treatment of adjustment disorders and generalized anxiety disorder and, in general, represent second-line treatment of other anxiety disorders. As with other treatments for elderly patients in palliative care, the evaluation of anxiety reflects a balance between setting the goals of the patient and the length of remaining life. For example, the evaluation and treatment of anxiety secondary to a suspected pulmonary embolus may be different for a patient receiving active treatment in a hospital setting and for a patient in home hospice. The SSRIs have an onset of action of several weeks and can briefly worsen anxiety. Therefore, in patients with less than 1–2 months of life, especially if they are minimally ambulatory, benzodiazepines should be considered for rapid relief of symptoms. The most common adverse effects to benzodiazepines, especially in ill elderly patients, include ataxia, cognitive impairment, and excessive sleepiness.[54] Opioids are indicated for treatment of anxiety secondary to dyspnea in terminally ill patients. Anxiety in the course of delirium is best addressed with neuroleptics.[46]

DEPRESSIVE DISORDERS

Major *depression* is a disabling mental disorder marked by low mood or loss of pleasure or interest in usually preferred activi-

ties for at least 2 weeks, accompanied by change in appetite, sleep disruption, restlessness and/or lack of energy, impaired concentration, amplified feelings of guilt or worthlessness, and preoccupation with death or suicide.[1] Although psychiatric nosology includes other types of depressive disorder, major depression is the most pernicious and relevant to geriatric patients in palliative care.

The overlap of physical illness symptoms with signs and symptoms of depression complicates reliable diagnosis of depression during illness.[55] In ill patients, somatic complaints attributable to physical disease, such as loss of appetite, sleep problems, loss of energy, and difficulty concentrating, can inflate scores on scales used to measure depression, such as the Beck Depression Inventory (BDI)[56] and the Geriatric Depression Scale (GDS),[57] even though they may be unrelated to depression.[58] Conversely, if a depressed individual reports primarily somatic symptoms, the clinician might focus disproportionately on physical etiologies and neglect the mood state. Overall, studies of terminally ill populations comparing inclusion and exclusion of somatic symptoms in determining prevalence rates of depression indicate that somatic items contribute less to diagnostic variance than expected when the psychological symptoms are of at least moderate severity.[59,60]

Epidemiology of Depression

Among healthy community-based adults over age 65, the prevalence of depression is lower than for any other adult age category.[61] The prevalence of depression in older, medically compromised adults varies across settings. Among hospitalized geriatric patients, the prevalence of major depression is between 10% and 20% and as many as 30% meet criteria for minor depression (those with depressed mood or loss of pleasure with one to three other symptoms of depression lasting at least 2 weeks).[62] Prevalence rates of depression range from 1% to 15% in elderly community samples[63,64] to 10% to 20% of Alzheimer's patients,[65] 23% of elderly emergency room patients,[66] 9% to 25% of cancer patients,[60,67] 33% of older adults with Lewy body dementia,[68] 36% of older adults in rehabilitation facilities,[69] up to 45% of patients with coronary artery disease[70] and vascular dementia,[65] and up to 60% of nursing home residents.[71,72]

Among medically ill older adults who are depressed, only a small portion are treated for depression,[64,73,74] suggesting that the risk of overlooking a correct depression diagnosis in medically ill older adults is far greater than that of overdiagnosing depression.[73,75] The roots of underdetection and undertreatment of depression in seriously ill older adults are manifold but include under-reporting by the older adult patient and observational biases on the part of health-care practitioners. Older patients, possibly concerned about the stigma of a mental health diagnosis and not acculturated to talk about emotions or focused more on their physical symptoms, may minimize their distress or present it in the form of physical ailments.[58] There may also be a greater tendency to ignore distress; such denial allows the patient to cope with the challenges of chronic or terminal illness but limits insight about mood state. Physicians or caregivers might incorrectly assume the depressive symptoms are a feature of normal aging, reflect appropriate sadness from facing a terminal illness,[73,76] or are directly caused by the medical condition.[77] Uncapher and Arean[78] reported that physicians were able to correctly recognize depression as well as risk of suicide from case vignettes, regardless of the age of the patient in the vignette. However, physicians were less willing to treat depression, less likely to use therapeutic interventions, and more likely to consider suicidal ideation as normative in the older patient compared to the younger patient.

Risk Factors and Complications of Depression

Medical illness and functional impairment appear to be risk factors for depression, though studies vary regarding their contribution. Geriatric subjects with functional limitations at baseline were also found to be more vulnerable to depression when they were acutely ill or in pain;[79] however, those in rehabilitation units were more likely to be depressed (35.9% of the sampled population) than those in acute-care settings (20%–30%).[80] Conversely, other published research indicates that poor health contributes more to depression than physical disability; for example, in one study of older adults, medical conditions, but not functional difficulties, contributed to later development of depressive symptoms.[81] A variety of medical conditions have been associated with development of depression in older patients, including cancer, chronic obstructive pulmonary disease, neurological disorders, cardiac disorders, and endocrine disorders. This vulnerability to depression may be correlated more strongly with the severity of illness than the specific type of illness.[62] The interpretation of the contributions of functional status and medical illness to depression is further complicated when the patient has pain.[82] For example, pain, functional disability, and depression are interrelated in many cancer studies.[83] Overall, these findings suggest that health-care providers should proceed with raised suspicion of depression in older patients who present with functional impairment, pain, or chronic or multiple medical conditions.

There is broad evidence supporting an association between depression and cognitive impairment in older patients.[84–86] Inconsistent evidence regarding the direction of causality[87] suggests that depression and cognitive ability may have interactive, reciprocal influences. Many neurological disorders affect the basal ganglia, including Parkinson's disease, the Lewy body variant dementia, and vascular dementia. Executive dysfunction, reflecting cerebral frontal lobe impairment, has been cited as a predictor of relapse and recurrence of depression in older adults[88,89] and is associated with slower response to psychopharmacological treatment and greater levels of functional impairment.[90] Patients with vascular dementia have a higher 1-month prevalence of depression than those with Alzheimer's dementia.[65]

Other reported risk factors for late-life depression in medically ill adults include bereavement, major life stress events,[79] loss of autonomy (including nursing home placement),[71] diminished sense of purpose or meaning in life,[91] and previous history of depression.[62] Supportive social and family bonds offer some protection against the development of depression,[92] while older adults who suffered abuse or neglect were significantly more likely to meet clinical criteria for depression.[93] Major depression and alcohol abuse commonly co-occur in elderly patients, with comorbidity rates ranging from 11% to 36%;[94] and in one prospective study, heavy alcohol consumption predicted later development of depression in elderly men.[95]

Depression also complicates the course of many medical illnesses. Many, though not all, studies[96] demonstrate that depression is associated with longer hospitalization and shortened survival (from suicide as well as general medical causes) in geriatric medical inpatients and community-dwelling elders.[97–104] Mortality after mild depression in the geriatric population appears more likely for men than women, but both genders are more vulnerable when diagnosed with major depression.[105] The effect of depression on survival in palliative care settings is not known. One of the more interesting questions stimulated by these findings is whether treatment of depression affects mortality or disability outcomes as there are no controlled trials demonstrating improved survival. Ganzini and colleagues[101] reported that depressed, medically ill, older inpatients were at greater risk for death 30 months after diagnosis than their non-depressed counterparts, regardless of whether they had been given prescriptions for antidepressant medication. However, medication compliance within the sample was not known.

Assessment of Depression

Routine inquiry about mood state should be an essential part of the health evaluation of older and seriously ill patients. Experts have recommended replacing somatic items with questions or scale items addressing depressed appearance, social withdrawal, brooding, self-pity, guilt, worthlessness/hopelessness, inability to be cheered up,[106] perception of the illness as punishment, unrealistic worries about being a burden, persistent suicidal ideation, complicating panic attacks, and treatment-resistant chronic pain.[77] Follow-up validations of this modified assessment demonstrated that once psychological symptoms are at least of moderate severity, assessments with and without somatic items identify essentially the same group of patients.[60]

Exploration of hopelessness, defined as negative expectancies toward the future, may be particularly valuable.[107] While some hopelessness may be expected in those who have learned of a terminal diagnosis, a more detailed conversation allows exploration of the impact and pervasiveness of hopelessness on the individual's life.[108] In studies of patients with amyotrophic lateral sclerosis, hopelessness contributed more to overall suffering than depression.[109] Chochinov et al.,[110] in a study of terminally ill cancer patients, demonstrated that hopelessness accounted for more variation in suicidal ideation than did depression. Breitbart et al.[108] reported that among 92 terminally ill cancer patients, depression and hopelessness were independent predictors of desire for hastened death.

A number of assessment methods are available for depression, some of them modified to minimize the impact of medical illness on diagnosis. Structured clinical interviews that guide the evaluator through the diagnostic criteria specified by the DSM-IV serve as the gold standard for accuracy of diagnosis. Because they can be time-consuming, they typically require administration by a trained clinician; and as their length can be especially challenging for medically ill older patients, they are more often used for research studies. A number of shorter self-report scales provide valid data while placing a lesser burden on frail respondents. Devised especially for older adults, the GDS[57] is a 30-item scale answered with yes/no judgments. The GDS incorporates fewer somatic symptom-based items than the BDI[55] and has had broad use in geriatric clinical and research settings.[77] The Hospital Anxiety and Depression Scale (HADS)[111] also minimizes the influence of somatic complaints, although it is not specifically tailored to older adults.[112] Designed to evaluate for depression and anxiety among patients in medical settings, the HADS is a 14-item scale allotting seven items to each construct. It takes approximately 5 minutes to administer and provides a reliable, sensitive measure of even mild mood disturbance.[112]

Several brief screening instruments for depression in palliative care groups have been developed. Chochinov et al.,[113] in a study of cancer patients with a mean age of 71.0 years, reported that simply asking "Are you depressed?" provided sensitive and specific screening, which corresponded well with results of more in-depth diagnostic interviewing. Lees and Lloyd-Williams[114] demonstrated that asking hospice-enrolled patients to mark their mood on a 10-centimeter line with happy and sad at either end correlated well with the longer HADS. Both approaches represent quick screening tools on which a depressive response clearly indicates the need for follow-up comprehensive mood assessment.

Treatment of Depression

Nonpharmacological interventions for depression in the terminally ill have not been examined extensively in controlled studies, but emerging evidence from studies of cancer patients suggests that psychotherapy can improve depressive symptoms, increase well-being,[115–121] and even prolong life.[122] Typically, counseling and therapy are coupled with psychotropic medication, though in mild depression psychotherapy alone can provide adequate relief.[123] The debilitation of depression coupled with terminal illness places severe limitations on the scope and duration of psychotherapy. Lengthy analysis of life events and influences is inappropriate in this context. Table 20–2 lists key components of psychotherapy.[67,76,123,124]

Although some geriatric palliative care patients with mild depression may benefit from psychotherapy alone, hesitation to prescribe an antidepressant may deprive patients of the opportunity to live out the final period of life without depression. The choice of antidepressant is influenced by life expectancy. For patients with an expected life of >2 months, SSRIs, such as citalopram, sertraline, or paroxetine, are recommended because of their benign side-effect profile. Less is known about newer antidepressants in severely ill, geriatric patients, though a study of mirtazapine for pain in cancer patients found that it was well tolerated with minimal analgesia but substantial improvement in depressive symptoms, sleep, and appetite (S. Passik, unpublished data).

Patients with short life expectancy may not have an opportunity to respond to an SSRI if intolerance occurs and/or response takes several weeks. The importance of considering life expectancy was demonstrated in a study by Lloyd-Williams et al.[67] of over 1000 patients admitted to a palliative care unit. Physicians prescribed antidepressants for 10%; 96% were prescribed a tricyclic antidepressant or SSRI, but 76% received these agents in the final 2 weeks

Table 20–2. Components of Palliative Psychotherapy

1. Listening to expressions of emotion and provision of sympathy and validation
2. Addressing fears about dying or distressing loved ones
3. Engaging in life review
4. Provision of cognitive-behavioral work focused on identifying and challenging negative thoughts as well as identifying past successful coping strategies and strengths
5. Training in coping skills and problem solving to enhance adjustment and improve the fighting spirit
6. Provision of social support, including group therapy shared by others with comparable medical situations
7. Provision of supportive family interventions as warranted

of life, a time period in which these agents are rarely therapeutic. Many experts recommend psychostimulants, such as amphetamine, methylphenidate, or pemoline, in palliative care patients. Response often occurs within 2 days, and side effects resulting in discontinuation occur in 10%.[125] Noncontrolled studies in cancer patients demonstrate response rates of 69%.[126] In addition, psychostimulants both augment opioid analgesia and diminish opioid sedation. Abuse is rare, though dependence may occur after several months of treatment. Randomized trials of psychostimulants are needed to verify their effectiveness in this population.

MOOD AND BEHAVIORAL DISTURBANCES IN END-STAGE DEMENTIA

Dementia is a heterogeneous disorder chiefly characterized by progressive memory loss, cognitive disturbance, and functional disability. While the variable presentation of dementia does not always lend itself readily to fixed staging criteria, the Functional Assessment Staging (FAST) scale proposed by Reisberg[127] provides an organizational reference point for professional communication and is used to predict longevity and define the point at which hospice care becomes appropriate. End-stage dementia corresponds to FAST stage 7. At this terminal stage, patients are unable to complete basic functional skills, such as walking, grooming, and dressing; unable to speak or communicate meaningfully; and incontinent of bowel and bladder.[128] While the range of behavior problems in mild to moderate dementia is extensive, the progressive debilitation and immobility associated with end-stage dementia lead most commonly to restlessness, repetitive moaning, combativeness, and resistance to care before culminating in lethargy and coma.[128]

Assessment and Treatment of Psychiatric Disturbances in End-Stage Dementia

Treatment of agitation begins with thorough assessment of the specific behaviors in question, their severity, and the surrounding environmental precipitants and consequences of the behaviors.[129] Agitation in terminal dementia may result from the disease itself or new medical illness (including constipation or urinary retention), medication, fever, pain,[130] delirium, or other psychiatric disorders. Environmental factors, such as room temperature, noise level, or change in surroundings, and psychosocial factors, such as social isolation, are also possible precipitants. Palliative interventions for agitation in end-stage dementia are intended to comfort rather than cure taking into account the burdens of the assessment and treatment relative to the goals of comfort care. Typical interventions include initial evaluation for illness, treatment to minimize pain or possible discomfort of infection (i.e., fever), calm reassurance, and caregiver support and education. Slow-stroke massage, which has been used effectively in moderately demented populations, may be a calming technique for resistance and combativeness in end-stage dementia.[131]

Recent guidelines based on expert consensus[132] offer diagnostic and management considerations for mild and severe agitation (Table 20–3). Care providers are encouraged to evaluate for possible environmental contributions to agitation and adjust accordingly. For example, a demented patient who becomes agitated during bathing may benefit from a modified bathing procedure that allows the patient to remain in bed covered with warmed towels while being cleansed soothingly.[133] This example represents a first-line treatment strategy for mild to moderate agitation. When agitation is severe, particularly when the potential for harm to self or others arises, immediate intervention with medication is warranted, with environmental adjustments following as appropriate. The range of pharmacological options includes conventional high-potency antipsychotics, atypical antipsychotics, SSRIs, other antidepressants such as trazodone, and less often sedatives. No protocol for choosing an agent has been validated by empirical trials. Expert opinion, however, suggests that the psycho-

Table 20–3. Overview: Assessment and Treatment of Agitation in Terminal Dementia

Differential diagnosis
1. Onset or exacerbation of illness? Related pain or discomfort?
2. Contribution of medication or substance abuse?
3. Environmental/psychosocial problems?
4. Psychiatric disturbance?

| | Level of agitation | |
	Mild	Severe
Typical presentation	Moaning, crying, repetitive movements	Screaming, aggression, combativeness, self-injury
First-line treatment	Environmental intervention plus medication	Medication plus environmental intervention
Second-line treatment	Environmental intervention alone	Medication alone

Source: Alexopoulos et al.[132]

tropic should match the domain of treatment. For example, as outlined by Tariot and coauthors,[134] a patient with prominent suspiciousness and paranoia should receive a trial of an antipsychotic first. A patient with prominent tearfulness and poor motivation should receive an SSRI first. Further considerations include choosing agents to minimize side effects, giving an adequate dose, and discontinuing the agent if it is not clearly helping.[134]

Family and caregiver education should address the common causes of agitation in dementia and provide suggestions for evaluating and managing it. Educated caregivers play a decisive role in observing situations that trigger agitation and in identifying creative and acceptable changes to the environment that result in improved behavior. Management suggestions most relevant to the terminal stage of dementia include use of a calming voice and soothing activities such as massage and gentle grooming if tolerated; provision of comforting social contact; minimization of noise in the environment; and use of redirection and distraction techniques rather than arguing or scolding.[135]

Depression has been cited as a predictor of physical and verbal aggression in dementia.[136] The identification of depression in end-stage dementia is complicated by the patient's loss of language and communication skills since self-report is a critical source of diagnostic information; however,

tearfulness or anguished facial expression can be indicators of depression in terminal dementia.[135] Psychosocial contributions to low mood should also be considered as the dementia patient has lost most resources for meaningful interaction with others. Gentle touch and soothing social presence are possible interventions that caregivers can provide. Continuation of a previously prescribed antidepressant or new trial of an antidepressant should be readily considered for the agitated patient.[128]

CAREGIVER ISSUES FOR DEPRESSED AND/OR DEMENTED, MEDICALLY ILL ELDERLY

Caregivers face emotional, physical, social, financial, and spiritual challenges during their sojourn with seriously ill, depressed older adults. Caregivers, who are often family members,[137] rate their own health worse as their stress scores increase.[138,139] The negative affective characteristics of depression, such as withdrawal, brooding, complaining, and pessimism, often culminate in poor-quality social relationships[140] and worsening morale and mood of the caregiver.[138,141] Depression is one of two patient characteristics associated with the most significant levels of stress for their caregivers.[138] Caregivers report having greatest difficulty with the neurovegetative symptoms of depression, such as impaired concentration, loss of energy, and reduced interest and pleasure.[142]

Behavioral disturbance associated with dementia is a marked source of caregiver distress.[139] After a period of particular vulnerability to stress during the last month of the patient's life, the death of the patient often produces a sense of relief but compounded by guilt and sorrow.[143] The mental health of the caregiver is yet further threatened when both depression and dementia are present in the patient. The burden and stress associated with caregiving in this "double whammy" scenario leave the caregiver at significant risk for depression.[144]

Caregiver beliefs about the causes of difficulties with their charges turn out to be a very important predictor of the nature of the caregiving relationship as well as the course of the patient's recovery from depression. Caregivers were more sympathetic to their charges and reported less distress when they were educated about their patients' illness and coached to attribute symptoms to the disease rather than the personal failings of the patient.[145] Caregiver beliefs that depressive symptoms were under the control of the patient were associated with greater likelihood of the patient's depressive relapse.[71] Overall, these findings indicate that patient adjustment and care might be positively influenced by education of the caregiver about depression and its effects and helping caregivers recognize that observed symptoms are part of the disease rather than willful misbehavior by the patient.

The needs of caregivers for older, terminally ill patients with psychiatric complications are complex, yet they fall generally into two domains: education and support. Education should reflect the individual cultural preferences of the caregiver and recipient.[146,147] Caregivers may also benefit from learning to analyze problem behaviors in terms of their antecedents (possible triggers) and consequences (possible rewards) that maintain the behavior.[147] Caregivers need guidance and support to remember their self-care as their own health plays an important role in the welfare of both giver and recipient of care.

Caregiver distress can be moderated by support of various forms. Health-care providers, family members, and various affiliations and organizations relevant to the caregiver are important potential sources of support. Individual counseling and support groups offer more structured sources of information and understanding and serve as a place for caregivers to discuss their feelings. Other forms of instrumental support include specialty organizations, such as the Alzheimer's Association; respite care; employee assistance programs; and hospice organizations.[137]

REFERENCES

1. American Psychiatric Association. Diagnostic and Statistical Manual of Mental Disorders, vol IV. Washington DC, American Psychiatric Press, 1994.
2. Inouye SK. Predisposing and precipitating factors for delirium in hospitalized older patients. Dement Geriatr Cogn Disord 10:393–400, 1999.
3. Casarett DJ, Inouye SK. Diagnosis and management of delirium near the end of life. Ann Intern Med 135:32–40, 2001.
4. Lipowski ZJ. Delirium: Acute Confusional States. New York, Oxford University Press, pp. 38–46, 1990.
5. Lawlor PG, Gagnon B, Mancini IL, et al. Occurrence, causes, and outcome of delirium in patients with advanced cancer: a prospective study. Arch Intern Med 160: 786–794, 2000.
6. Breitbart W, Chochinov HM, Passik S. Psychiatric aspects of palliative care. In: Doyle D, Hanks GWC, MacDonald N (Eds.). Oxford Textbook of Palliative Medicine, 2nd ed. New York, Oxford University Press, pp. 933–954, 1998.
7. International Classification of Diseases, 9th rev, Clinical Modification 5th ed. Los Angeles, Practice Management Information Corporation, 1997.
8. Sandberg O, Gustafson Y, Brannstrom B, Bucht G. Clinical profile of delirium in older patients. J Am Geriatr Soc 47: 1300–1306, 1999.
9. Pompei P, Foreman M, Cassel CK, Alessi C, Cox D. Detecting delirium among hospitalized older patients. Arch Intern Med 155:301–307, 1995.
10. American Psychiatric Association. Practice guideline for the treatment of patients with delirium. Am J Psychiatry 156(5 Suppl): 1–20, 1999.
11. Liptzin B, Levkoff SE. An empirical study

of delirium subtypes. Br J Psychiatry 161: 843–845, 1992.

12. O'Keeffe ST, Lavan JN. Clinical significance of delirium subtypes in older people. Age Ageing 28:115–119, 1999.

13. Meagher DJ, O'Hanlon D, O'Mahony E, Casey PR, Trzepacz PT. Relationship between symptoms and motoric subtype of delirium. J Neuropsychiatry Clin Neurosci 12:51–56, 2000.

14. Farrell K, Ganzini L. Misdiagnosing delirium as depression in medically ill elderly patients. Arch Intern Med 155:2459–2464, 1995.

15. Green RL, McAllister TW, Bernat JL. A study of crying in medically and surgically hospitalized patients. Am J Psychiatry 144:442–447, 1987.

16. Inouye SK, van Dyck CH, Alessi CA, Balkin S, Siegal AP, Horwitz RI. Clarifying confusion: the confusion assessment method. A new method for detection of delirium. Ann Internal Med 113:941–948, 1990.

17. Breitbart W, Rosenfeld B, Roth A, Smith MJ, Cohen K, Passik S. The Memorial Delirium Assessment Scale. J Pain Symptom Manage 13:128–137, 1997.

18. Trzepacz PT, Baker RW, Greenhouse J. A symptom rating scale for delirium. Psychiatry Res 23:89–97, 1988.

19. Folstein MF, Folstein SE, McHugh PR. "Mini-mental state." A practical method for grading the cognitive state of patients for the clinician. J Psychiatr Res 12:189–198, 1975.

20. Fann JR. The epidemiology of delirium: a review of studies and methodological issues. Semin Clin Neuropsychiatry 5:64–74, 2000.

21. Brauer C, Morrison RS, Silberzweig SB, Siu AL. The cause of delirium in patients with hip fracture. Arch Intern Med 160:1856–1860, 2000.

22. Gagnon P, Allard P, Masse B, DeSerres M. Delirium in terminal cancer: a prospective study using daily screening, early diagnosis and continuous monitoring. J Pain Symptom Manage 19:412–426, 2000.

23. Bruera E, Miller L, McCallion J, Macmillan K, Krefting L, Hanson J. Cognitive failure in patients with terminal cancer: a prospective study. J Pain Symptom Manage 7:192–195, 1992.

24. Pereira J, Hanson J, Bruera E. The frequency and clinical course of cognitive impairment in patients with terminal cancer. Cancer 79:835–842, 1997.

25. Massie MJ, Holland J, Glass E. Delirium in terminally ill cancer patients. Am J Psychiatry 140:1048–1050, 1983.

26. Minagawa H, Uchitomi Y, Yamawaki S, Ishitani K. Psychiatric morbidity in terminally ill cancer patients. A prospective study. Cancer 78:1131–1137, 1996.

27. Trzepacz PT. Delirium. Advances in diagnosis, pathophysiology, and treatment. Psychiatr Clin North Am 19:429–448, 1996.

28. Francis J, Martin D, Kapoor WN. A prospective study of delirium in hospitalized elderly. JAMA 263:1097–1101, 1990.

29. Inouye SK, Bogardus ST Jr, Charpentier PA, et al. A multicomponent intervention to prevent delirium in hospitalized older patients. N Engl J Med 340:669–676, 1999.

30. Breitbart W, Strout D. Delirium in the terminally ill. Clin Geriatr Med 16:357–372, 2000.

31. Tune LE. Serum anticholinergic activity levels and delirium in the elderly. Semin Clin Neuropsychiatry 5:149–153, 2000.

32. Fainsinger RL, Tapper M, Bruera E. A perspective on the management of delirium in terminally ill patients on a palliative care unit. J Palliat Care 9:4–8, 1993.

33. Lynch EP, Lazor MA, Gellis JE, Orav J, Goldman L, Marcantonio ER. The impact of postoperative pain on the development of postoperative delirium. Anesth Analg 86:781–785, 1998.

34. Bruera E, Fainsinger RL, Miller MJ, Kuehn N. The assessment of pain intensity in patients with cognitive failure: a preliminary report. J Pain Symptom Manage 7:267–270, 1992.

35. Inouye SK, Rushing JT, Foreman MD, Palmer RM, Pompei P. Does delirium contribute to poor hospital outcomes? A three-site epidemiologic study. J Gen Intern Med 13:234–242, 1998.

36. Caraceni A, Nanni O, Maltoni M, et al. Impact of delirium on the short term prognosis of advanced cancer patients. Italian Multicenter Study Group on Palliative Care. Cancer 89:1145–1149, 2000.

37. Morita T, Tsunoda J, Inoue S, Chihara S. The Palliative Prognostic Index: a scoring system for survival prediction of terminally ill cancer patients. Support Care Cancer 7:128–133, 1999.

38. Metitieri T, Bianchetti A, Trabucchi M. Delirium as a predictor of survival in older patients with advanced cancer. Arch Intern Med 160:2866–2868, 2000.

39. Farber S, Egnew TR, Stempel J, Vleck J. End-of-Life Care: AAFP Home Study Self-Assessment, Monograph 250/251. American Academy of Family Physicians, 2000.

40. Bruera E, Franco JJ, Maltoni M, Wantanabe S, Suarez-Almozor M. Changing pattern of agitated impaired metal status in patients with advanced cancer: association

with cognitive monitoring, hydration and, opioid rotation. J Pain Symptom Manage 10:287–291, 1995.

41. Breitbart W, Marotta R, Platt MM, et al. A double-blind trial of haloperidol, chlorpromazine, and lorazepam in the treatment of delirium in hospitalized AIDS patients. Am J Psychiatry 153:231–237, 1996.

42. Mazzocato C, Stiefel F, Buclin T, Berney A. Psychopharmacology in supportive care of cancer: a review for the clinician: II. Neuroleptics. Support Care Cancer 8:89–97, 2000.

43. Krakauer EL, Penson RT, Truog RD, King LA, Chabner BA, Lynch TJ Jr. Sedation for intractable distress of a dying patient: acute palliative care and the principle of double effect. Oncologist 5:53–62, 2000.

44. Fainsinger RL, De Moissac D, Mancini I, Oneschuk D. Sedation for delirium and other symptoms in terminally ill patients in Edmonton. J Palliat Care 16:5–10, 2000.

45. Fainsinger RL, Waller A, Bercovici M, et al. A multicentre international study of sedation for uncontrolled symptoms in terminally ill patients. Palliat Med 14:257–265, 2000.

46. Payne DK, Massie MJ. Anxiety in palliative care. In: Chochinov HM, Breitbart W (Eds.). Handbook of Psychiatry in Palliative Medicine. New York, Oxford University Press, pp. 63–74, 2000.

47. Weintraub D, Ruskin P. Posttraumatic stress disorder in the elderly: a review. Harv Rev Psychiatry 7:144–152, 1999.

48. Bruera E, Schmitz B, Pither J, Neumann CM, Hanson J. The frequency and correlates of dyspnea in patients with advanced cancer. J Pain Symptom Manage 19:357–362, 2000.

49. Alter CL, Pelcovitz D, Axelrod A, et al. The identification of PTSD in cancer survivors. Psychosomatics 37:137–143, 1996.

50. Kutner JS, Kassner CT, Nowels DE. Symptom burden at the end of life: hospice providers' perceptions. J Pain Symptom Manage 21:473–480, 2001.

51. Donnelly S, Walsh D. The symptoms of advanced cancer. Semin Oncol 22(Suppl 3):67–72, 1995.

52. Hopwood P, Stephens RJ. Symptoms at presentation for treatment in patients with lung cancer: implication for the evaluation of palliative treatment. The Medical Research Council (MCR) Lung Cancer Working Party. Br J Cancer 71:633–636, 1995.

53. Massie MJ, Lesko LM. Psychopharmacological management. In: Holland JC, Rowland JH (Eds.). Handbook of Psychoon-cology. New York, Oxford University Press, pp. 470–491, 1990.

54. Atkinson RM, Ganzini L. Substance abuse in old age. In: Cummings J, Coffey E (Eds.). Textbook of Geriatric Neuropsychiatry. Washington DC, American Psychiatric Press, pp. 297–322, 1994.

55. Mulsant BH, Pollock BG. Treatment-resistant depression in late life. J Geriatr Psychiatry Neurol 11:186–193, 1998.

56. Beck A. Depression Inventory. Philadelphia, Center for Cognitive Therapy, 1978.

57. Yesavage JA, Brink TL, Rose TL, et al. Development and validation of a geriatric depression screening scale: a preliminary report. J Psychiatr Res 17:37–49, 1982–1983.

58. Whall AL, Hoes-Gurevich ML. Missed depression in elderly individuals. Why is this a problem? J Gerontol Nurs 25:44–46, 1999.

59. Chochinov HM. Psychiatry and terminal illness. Can J Psychiatry 45:143–150, 2000.

60. Chochinov HM, Wilson KG, Enns M, Lander S. Prevalence of depression in the terminally ill: effects of diagnostic criteria and symptom threshold judgments. Am J Psychiatry 151:537–540, 1994.

61. Fisher JE, Zeiss AM, Carstensen LL. Psychopathology in the aged. In: Sutker PB, Adams HE (Eds.). Comprehensive Handbook of Psychopathology, 2nd ed. New York, Plenum, pp. 815–842, 1993.

62. Koenig HG. Differences in psychosocial and health correlates of major and minor depression in medically ill older adults. J Am Geriatr Soc 45:1487–1495, 1997.

63. Katona C, Livingston G. Impact of screening old people with physical illness for depression. Lancet 356:91–92, 2000.

64. Unützer J, Simon G, Belin TR, Datt M, Katon W, Patrick D. Care for depression in HMO patients aged 65 and older. J Am Geriatr Soc 48:871–878, 2000.

65. Ballard C, Neill D, O'Brien J, McKeith IG, Ince P, Perry R. Anxiety, depression and psychosis in vascular dementia: prevalence and associations. J Affect Disord 59:97–106, 2000.

66. Meldon SW, Emerman CL, Moffa DA, Schubert DS. Utility of clinical characteristics in identifying depression in geriatric ED patients. Am J Emerg Med 17:522–525, 1999.

67. Lloyd-Williams M, Friedman T, Rudd N. A survey of antidepressant prescribing in the terminally ill. Palliat Med 13:243–248, 1999.

68. Ballard C, Holmes C, McKeith I, et al. Psychiatric morbidity in dementia with Lewy bodies: a prospective clinical and neuro-

pathological comparative study with Alzheimer's disease. Am J Psychiatry 156: 1039–1045, 1999.

69. Shah A, Hoxey K, Mayadunne V. Suicidal ideation in acutely medically ill elderly inpatients: prevalence, correlates and longitudinal stability. Int J Geriatr Psychiatry 15:162–169, 2000.

70. Spertus JA, McDonell M, Woodman CL, Fihn SD. Association between depression and worse disease-specific functional status in outpatients with coronary artery disease. Am Heart J 140:105–110, 2000.

71. Bell M, Goss AJ. Recognition, assessment and treatment of depression in geriatric nursing home residents. Clin Excell Nurse Pract 5:26–36, 2001.

72. Casten RJ, Rovner BW, Shmuely-Dulitzki Y, Pasternak RE, Pelchat R, Ranen N. Predictors of recovery from major depression among geriatric psychiatry inpatients: the importance of caregivers' beliefs. Int Psychogeriatr 11:149–157, 1999.

73. Koenig HG, George LK. Depression and physical disability outcomes in depressed medically ill hospitalized older adults. Am J Geriatr Psychiatry 6:230–247, 1998.

74. Rapp SR, Parisi SA, Walsh DA, Wallace CE. Detecting depression in elderly medical inpatients. J Consult Clin Psychol 56: 509–513, 1988.

75. Kitchell MA, Barnes RF, Veith RC, Okimoto JT, Raskind MA. Screening for depression in hospitalized geriatric medical patients. J Am Geriatr Soc 30:174–177, 1982.

76. Block SD. Assessing and managing depression in the terminally ill patient. ACP-ASIM End-of-Life Care Consensus Panel. Ann Intern Med 132:209–218, 2000.

77. Kurlowicz LH, Streim, JE. Measuring depression in hospitalized, medically ill, older adults. Arch Psychiatr Nurs 12:209–218, 1998.

78. Uncapher H, Arean PA. Physicians are less willing to treat suicidal ideation in older patients. J Am Geriatr Soc 48:188–192, 2000.

79. Livingston G, Watkin V, Milne B, Manela MY, Katona C. Who becomes depressed? The Islington Community Study of Older People. J Affect Disord 58:125–133, 2000.

80. Fenton FR, Cole MG, Engelsman N, Mansouri L. Depression in older medical inpatients. Int Clin Psychopharmacol 8: 333–336, 1993.

81. Meeks S, Murrell SA, Mehl RC. Longitudinal relationships between depressive symptoms and health in normal older and middle-aged adults. Psychol Aging 15: 100–109, 2000.

82. Spiegel D, Bloom JR. Group therapy and hypnosis reduce metastatic breast carcinoma pain. Psychosom Med 45:333–339, 1983.

83. Wilson KG, Chochinov HM, de Faye BJ, Breitbart W. Diagnosis and management of depression in palliative care. In: Chochinov H, Breitbart W (Eds.). Handbook of Psychiatry in Palliative Medicine. New York, Oxford University Press, pp. 25–50, 2000.

84. Rovner BW, Broadhead J, Spencer M, Carson K, Folstein MF. Depression and Alzheimer's disease. Am J Psychiatry 146: 350–353, 1989.

85. Wragg RE, Jeste DV. Overview of depression and psychosis in Alzheimer's disease. Am J Psychiatry 146:577–587, 1989.

86. Li Y, Meyer JS, Thornby J. Depressive symptoms among cognitively normal versus cognitively impaired elderly subjects. Int J Geriatr Psychiatry 16:455–461, 2001.

87. Payne JL, Lyketsos CG, Steele C, et al. Relationship of cognitive and functional impairment to depressive features in Alzheimer's disease and other dementias. J Neuropsychiatry Clin Neurosci 10:440–447, 1998.

88. Alexopoulos GS, Meyers BS, Young RC, et al. Executive dysfunction and long-term outcomes of geriatric depression. Arch Gen Psychiatry 57:285–290, 2000.

89. Lesser IM, Boone KB, Mehringer CM, Wohl MA, Miller BL, Berman NG. Cognition and white matter hyperintensities in older depressed patients. Am J Psychiatry 153:1280–1287, 1996.

90. Kiosses DN, Alexopoulos GS, Murphy C. Symptoms of striatofrontal dysfunction contribute to disability in geriatric depression. Int J Geriatr Psychiatry 15:992–999, 2000.

91. Reker GT. Personal meaning, optimism, and choice: existential predictors of depression in community and institutional elderly. Gerontologist 37:709–716, 1997.

92. George LK. Social structure, social processes, and social-psychological states. In: Binstock RH, George LK (Eds.). Handbook of Aging and the Social Sciences, 3rd ed. San Diego, Academic Press, pp. 186–204, 1990.

93. Dyer CB, Pavlik VN, Murphy KP, Hyman DJ. The high prevalence of depression and dementia in elder abuse or neglect. J Am Geriatr Soc 48:205–208, 2000.

94. Oslin DW, Katz IR, Edell WS, Ten Have TR. Effects of alcohol consumption on the treatment of depression among elderly patients. Am J Geriatr Psychiatry 8:215–220, 2000.

95. Saunders PA, Copeland JR, Dewey ME, et al. Heavy drinking as a risk factor for depression and dementia in elderly males. Findings from the Liverpool Longitudinal Community Study. Br J Psychiatry 159: 213–216, 1991.

96. Teno JM, Harrell FE Jr, Knaus W, et al. Prediction of survival for older hospitalized patients: the HELP survival model. Hospitalized Elderly Longitudinal Project. J Am Geriatr Soc 48:S16–S24, 2000.

97. Bruce ML, Leaf PJ. Psychiatric disorders and 15-month mortality in a community sample of older adults. Am J Public Health 79:727–730, 1989.

98. Sharma VK, Copeland JR, Dewey ME, Lowe D, Davidson I. Outcome of the depressed elderly living in the community in Liverpool: a 5-year follow-up. Psychol Med 28:1329–1337, 1998.

99. Murphy E, Smith R, Lindesay J, Slattery J. Increased mortality rates in late-life depression. Br J Psychiatry 152:347–353, 1988.

100. Rovner BW, German PS, Brant LJ, Clark R, Burton L, Folstein MF. Depression and mortality in nursing homes. JAMA 265: 993–996, 1991.

101. Ganzini L, Smith DM, Fenn DS, Lee MA. Depression and mortality in medically ill older adults. J Am Geriatr Soc 45:307–312, 1997.

102. Koenig HG, Shelp F, Goli V, Cohen HJ, Blazer DG. Survival and health care utilization in elderly medical inpatients with major depression. J Am Geriatr Soc 37: 599–606, 1989.

103. Shah DC, Evans M, King D. Prevalence of mental illness in a rehabilitation unit for older adults. Postgrad Med J 76:153–156, 2000.

104. Silverstone PH. Depression increases mortality and morbidity in acute life-threatening medical illness. J Psychosom Res 34: 651–657, 1990.

105. Schoevers RA, Geerlings MI, Beekman AT, et al. Association of depression and gender with mortality in old age. Results from the Amsterdam Study of the Elderly (AMSTEL). Br J Psychiatry 177:336–342, 2000.

106. Endicott J. Measurement of depression in patients with cancer. Cancer 53:2243–2249, 1984.

107. Beck AT, Weissman A, Lester D, Trexler L. The measurement of pessimism: the Hopelessness Scale. J Consult Clin Psychol 42:861–865, 1974.

108. Breitbart W, Rosenfeld B, Pessin H, et al. Depression, hopelessness, and desire for hastened death in terminally ill patients with cancer. JAMA 284:2907–2911, 2000.

109. Ganzini L, Johnston WS, Hoffman WF. Correlates of suffering in amyotrophic lateral sclerosis. Neurology 52:1434–1440, 1999.

110. Chochinov HM, Wilson KG, Enns M, Lander S. Depression, hopelessness and suicidal ideation in the terminally ill. Psychosomatics 39:366–370, 1998.

111. Zigmond AS, Snaith RP. The Hospital Anxiety and Depression Scale. Acta Psychiatr Scand 67:361–370, 1983.

112. Herrmann C. International experiences with the Hospital Anxiety and Depression Scale: a review of validation data and clinical results. J Psychosom Res 42:17–41, 1997.

113. Chochinov HM, Wilson KG, Enns M, Lander S. "Are you depressed?" Screening for depression in the terminally ill. Am J Psychiatry 154:674–676, 1997.

114. Lees N, Lloyd-Williams M. Assessing depression in palliative care patients using the visual analogue scale: a pilot study. Eur J Cancer Care (Engl) 8:220–223, 1999.

115. Linn MW, Linn BS, Harris R. Effects of counseling for late-stage cancer patients. Cancer 49:1048–1055, 1982.

116. Massie MJ, Holland JC. Diagnosis and treatment of depression in the cancer patient. J Clin Psychiatry 45:25–28, 1984.

117. Greer S, Moorey S, Baruch JD, et al. Adjuvant psychological therapy for patients with cancer: a prospective randomised trial. BMJ 304:675–680, 1992.

118. Spiegel D, Bloom JR, Yalom I. Group support for patients with metastatic cancer. A randomized outcome study. Arch Gen Psychiatry 38:527–533, 1981.

119. Fallowfield LJ, Hall A, Maguire GP, Baum M. Psychological outcomes of different treatment policies in women with early breast cancer outside a clinical trial. BMJ 301:575–580, 1990.

120. Fawzy FI, Cousins N, Fawzy NW, Kemeny ME, Elashoff R, Morton D. A structured psychiatric intervention for cancer patients. I. Changes over time in methods of coping and affective disturbance. Arch Gen Psychiatry 47:720–725, 1990.

121. Fawzy FI, Kemeny ME, Fawzy NW, et al. A structured psychiatric intervention for cancer patients. II. Changes over time in immunolgical measures. Arch Gen Psychiatry 47:729–735, 1990.

122. Spiegel D, Bloom JR, Kraemer HC, Gottheil E. Effect of psychosocial treatment on survival of patients with metastatic breast cancer. Lancet 2:888–891, 1989.

123. Koenig HG. Late life depression: how to

treat patients with comorbid chronic illness. Interview by Alice V. Luddington. Geriatrics 54:56–62, 1999.

124. Spiegel D. Cancer and depression. Br J Psychiatry 30:109–116, 1996

125. Olin J, Masand P. Psychostimulants for depression in hospitalized cancer patients. Psychosomatics 37:57–62, 1996.

126. Macleod AD. Methylphenidate in terminal depression. J Pain Symptom Manage 16:193–198, 1998.

127. Reisberg B. Functional Assessment Staging (FAST). Psychopharmacol Bull 24:653–659, 1988.

128. Shuster JL Jr. Palliative care for advanced dementia. Clin Geriatr Med 16:373–386, 2000.

129. Ballard CG, O'Brien J, James I, Swann A. Identification and measurement of behavioural and psychological symptoms in dementia. In: Ballard CG, O'Brien J, James I, Swann A (Eds.). Dementia: Management of Behavioral and Psychological Symptoms. New York, Oxford University Press, pp. 3–15, 2001.

130. Geda YE, Rummans TA. Pain: cause of agitation in elderly individuals with dementia. Am J Psychiatry 156:1662–1663, 1999.

131. Rowe M, Alfred D. The effectiveness of slow-stroke massage in diffusing agitated behaviors in individuals with Alzheimer's disease. J Gerontol Nurs 25:22–34, 1999.

132. Alexopoulos GS, Silver JM, Kahn DA, Frances A, Carpenter D (Eds.). Treatment of agitation in older persons with dementia. Postgrad Med pp. 1–80, 1998. Available at http://www.psychguides.com/.

133. Sloane PD, Rader J, Barrick AL, et al. Bathing persons with dementia. Gerontologist 35:672–678, 1995.

134. Tariot PN, Ryan JM, Porsteinsson AP, Loy R, Schneider LS. Pharmacologic therapy for behavioral symptoms of Alzheimer's disease. Clin Geriatr Med 17:359–376, 2001.

135. Kahn D, Gwyther LP, Frances A. Agitation in older persons with dementia. A guide for families and caregivers. Postgrad Med 81–88, 1998. Available at http://www.psychguides.com/.

136. Menon AS, Gruber-Baldini AL, Hebel JR, et al. Relationship between aggressive behaviors and depression among nursing home residents with dementia. Int J Geriatr Psychiatry 16:139–146, 2001.

137. Query JL Jr, Flint LJ. The caregiving relationship. In: Vanzetti N, Duck S (Eds.). A Lifetime of Relationships. Pacific Grove, CA, Brooks/Cole, pp. 455–483, 1996.

138. Desbiens NA, Mueller-Rizner N, Virnig B, Lynn J. Stress in caregivers of hospitalized oldest-old patients. J Gerontol A Biol Sci Med Sci 56:M231–M235, 2001.

139. Miller B, Townsend A, Carpenter E, Montgomery RVJ, Stull D, Young RF. Social support and caregiver distress: a replication analysis. J Gerontol B Psychol Sci Soc Sci 56:S249–256, 2001.

140. Coyne JC. Toward an interactional description of depression. Psychiatry 39:28–40, 1976.

141. Parmalee P, Katz I. "Caregiving" to depressed older persons: a relevant concept? Gerontologist 32:436–437, 1992.

142. Hinrichsen GA, Hernandez NA, Pollack S. Difficulties and rewards in family care of the depressed older adult. Gerontologist 32:486–492, 1992.

143. Jones PS, Martinson IM. The experience of bereavement in caregivers of family members with Alzheimer's disease. Image J Nurs Sch 24:172–176, 1992.

144. Cohen D, Eisdorfer C. Depression in family members caring for a relative with Alzheimer's disease. J Am Geriatr Soc 36:885–889, 1988.

145. Wadley VG, Haley WE. Diagnostic attributions versus labeling: impact of Alzheimer's disease and major depression diagnoses on emotions, beliefs, and helping intentions of family members. J Gerontol B Psychol Sci Soc Sci 56:P244–P252, 2001.

146. Harper BC, Lartigue M, Doka KJ. Cultural differences: sensitivities required for effective caring. In: Doka KJ, Davidson JD (Eds.). Caregiving and Loss. Washington DC, Hospice Foundation of America, pp. 139–151, 2001.

147. Zarit SH. Interventions with family caregivers. In: Zarit SH, Knight BG (Eds.). A Guide to Psychotherapy and Aging. Washington DC, American Psychiatric Association Press, pp. 139–159, 1996.

IV

COMMUNICATION

21

Advance Care Planning for Frail, Older Persons

JOAN M. TENO

Nearly four decades ago, Luis Kuntner proposed the living will in response to a tragic case of son shooting his mother who was dying of cancer and in pain and on a ventilator. A living will was proposed so that people could state, in advance, their preferences for life-sustaining treatment if physically or physiologically, irreversibly ill. Since 1969, the use of a written advance directive, such as the living will or durable power of attorney, for health care has been widely promoted and codified in both state and federal law with the passage of the Patient Self-Determination Act.

Despite this widespread enthusiasm for advance directives, their role has been questioned in both normative and empirical research. Concerns have been voiced over the difficulty of interpreting terms such as *irreversibly ill* or *hopelessly ill* to the clinical situation that an individual patient faces, the validity and stability of patient preferences stated in advance of an uncertain future, and the degree of leeway that a proxy should have in following a patients' written preferences.

Empirical research has identified important concerns with the process of completing and invoking advance directives. For example, Morrison and colleagues[1] noted that written advance directives were rarely transferred with the patient from the nursing home to the acute-care hospital. Schneiderman and colleagues[2] found, in a randomized controlled trial, that offering advance directive did not impact on healthcare costs, the use of life-sustaining treatment, and several other outcomes. The Study to Understand Prognoses and Preferences for Outcomes and Risks of Treatments (SUPPORT) revealed that physicians rarely counseled patients about advance directives; rather, attorneys were most likely to be involved in completing written advance directives. Of even more concern, seriously ill patients and physicians rarely talked about an advance directive. Physicians were often unaware that the patient had an advance directive even when it was placed in the medical record, and persons with advance directives and a stated preference to forgo cardiopulmonary resuscitation (CPR) often did not have a do-not-resuscitate (DNR) order.[3] While such concerns may be interpreted as suggesting that written advance directives have little role in medical decision making, an alternate interpretation is that there is a need to incorporate a much broader notion of advance directives into advance care planning (ACP).

HOW DOES ADVANCE CARE PLANNING DIFFER FROM ADVANCE DIRECTIVES?

Advance directives were formulated mainly as legal documents to allow a competent person to state preferences in advance of a period of decision incapacity. The focus of advance directives is usually on when the patient is "hopelessly ill." At the time the living will is created, the ethical and legal debate was over the morality of withholding and withdrawing life-sustaining treatment. Now DNR orders, stopping mechanical ventilation, and forgoing a feeding tube are common medical practices. We are now faced with a much greater challenge: the timing of such decisions, or at what point in the disease trajectory does one stop? For some progressive, chronic illnesses, such as cancer, the stopping point is when treatment is futile, while for many older persons with multiple chronic illnesses, "when" is a much more difficult question. For many persons, "when" is a time period in which the patient's quality of life is diminished to a point that death is the preferable alternative. Such prognostic uncertainty calls for a process of communication that occurs over time and not merely the one-time completion of a written, legal document. Advance care planning involves a much broader vision, which encompasses ongoing communication and negotiation regarding treatment preferences as well as formulation of contingency plans.

Advance care planning (ACP) is an outgrowth of patient-centered medical care that promotes shared decision making such that medical care will meet the patient's needs and expectations. Unlike advance di-

Table 21–1. Key Steps of Advance Care Planning

Step 1: Actively listen to the patient about his or her understanding and current quality of life.
Step 2: Work with the patient to create goals of care that are based on mutual understanding of where the patient is in the disease trajectory.
Step 3: Formulate contingency plans to honor those goals.

rectives, ACP is integrated into patient care from the first clinic encounter to the deathbed. The specificity and content of ACP differ throughout the patient's disease trajectory. There are two overarching goals of ACP. First, ACP is the process of communication that facilitates the patient's desired involvement in formulating preferences for current and future medical decisions. An outcome of this communication and negotiation is a set of treatment goals for present and future outcome states that can be anticipated. A second goal of ACP is the formulation of contingency plans that facilitate the patient in achieving desired treatment goals. For example, a 78-year-old with advanced chronic obstructive pulmonary disease tells his physician that he desires no further hospitalizations. Documentation of those preferences in the medical record and even in an advance directive accomplishes only the first goal of ACP. The second goal is accomplished only when a plan is formulated for amelioration of the terminal dyspnea that the majority of such patients will encounter.[4]

Advance care planning focuses on the process of communication, negotiation, and formulation of contingency plans (Table 21–1). A written advance directive is a tool that allows a patient preference to be honored. Thus, a written advance directive is a potential outcome of ACP.

INCORPORATING ADVANCE CARE PLANNING INTO CARE OF THE OLDER PATIENT

Early on, ACP can focus on the naming of a surrogate and preferences unique to that person's religious beliefs or values (e.g., a preference to forgo the use of blood products based on religious beliefs; Table 21–2). As the disease progresses, health-care providers work with the patient and family to recognize any critical turning point in the disease trajectory. A critical turning point is when there is transition in the focus of goals of care. Early in the disease trajectory, the majority of patients want medical care to extend life. As the disease progresses, some change these treatment preferences due to increasing burdens of treatment and diminishing quality of life. This change in focus of care from life-extending treatment to comfort, even if life is shortened, is gradual and ought to be patient-directed to the extent that the patient desires such involvement in decision making.

Important to the vision outlined is the notion of disease trajectory. While some have defined *disease trajectory* based on functional parameters, a much broader definition incorporates a patient's preferences and will to live. For simplicity, four sentinel time periods for ACP are when the person is *(1)* without a serious illness; *(2)* living with one or more chronic progressive illnesses *(3)* at a critical turning point in which the treatment goals start to change, and *(4)* actively dying. For older persons dying of multiple chronic illnesses, the critical turning point is not typically based on physiological futility of treatment but on patient preferences and self-perceived quality of life. Many decisions are based on a sense of "weariness" with the life that confronts them. Simply stated, the "bad days" far outnumber the "good days," and death may become the preferable option to living with an undesirable quality of life. The challenge to the health-care provider is to ensure that this weariness is not confounded by depression or other mood disorders.

For the person without a serious illness, the focus of ACP is on naming a proxy or surrogate and elicitation of atypical preferences (e.g., not wanting blood transfusions because of religious beliefs). Unless the patient wants to be specific, the focus of ACP is on general preferences and naming a proxy decision maker in a way that would allow flexibility to respond to unpredictable future circumstances. Once a patient is diagnosed with a serious illnesses, ACP should take on increasing specificity if the patient desires this level of involvement in future medical decision making. Health-care providers should work with the patient and family to make patient-directed transitions in the goals of care. Factors that inform these transitions are the disease, its response to treatment, whether there are further treatment options, patients' values, and their perceptions of quality of life that inform their own treatment preferences.

To illustrate the importance of disease trajectory and ACP, two cases will be presented. The first focuses on ACP for an older person with chronic, progressive illness that has resulted in only a minimal impact on patient functioning, while the second examines the role of ACP in a dying person.

ADVANCE CARE PLANNING EARLY IN THE DISEASE TRAJECTORY

Mr. Perkins, a new 87-year-old white patient, arrives in your office with his completed advance directive, which proclaims **No CPR, No Feeding Tubes, NO VENTS!!** What do you do? File the directive and apply a red dot to his chart that signifies that he is not to be resuscitated? Make sure that the directive is on the state-required form? Tell him that he needs to state preferences for hospitalizations, dialysis, and the use of vasopressors? Or none of the above? The correct answer is none of above. You should acknowledge that you are glad that he has brought his advance directive but that your next step is to complete a history and physical exam. A first key step to ACP in this patient is determining where he is in his disease trajectory. Simply stated, how does he feel about his quality of life while living with several progressive, chronic illnesses?

Mr. Perkins has hypertension, benign prostatic hypertrophy, lumbar stenosis, and congestive heart failure that requires an angiotensin-converting enzyme inhibitor and diuretic. His wife recently died, and he entered an assisted-care facility to avoid being a burden on his son and daughter-in-law. While he has some difficulty walking, secondary to his lumbar stenosis, he is able to perform all other basic activities of daily living. His physical exam is unremarkable. Understanding his values and goals is an important part of this patient's history and physical exam. One should not accept his advance directive at face value. Research has shown that the majority of advance directives are completed without counseling by a physician or other health-care provider, as was the case with Mr. Perkins. He had seen a TV program that prompted him to complete his advance directive. Based on that program, he believed that all mechanical ventilators did was lead to suffering and prolonged dying.

An important part of the new office visit for Mr. Perkins is ACP, a three-step process which ensures that valid patient preferences are formulated, if desired, and that a plan is put in place to ensure those preferences will be honored (Table 21–2). While Mr. Perkins is doing well now, it would not be unexpected for him to die in the next several years. The most important threat to his longevity is his congestive heart failure, a disease which is difficult to prognosticate given that patients often appear the same on the day before death as they did several months or years before.[5] The first step in ACP is actively listening to how Mr. Perkins is living with his disease and life trajectory. Despite the recent death of his wife, he is making a good adaptation to his new home and notes that he has wonderful relationships with his grandsons via e-mail. He considers every day a gift to be treasured. His previous doctor has told him that his congestive heart failure can be controlled with medicines. Mr. Perkins has researched congestive heart failure on the worldwide web.

Listening to the patient is important.

1. How does the patient understand his disease?

2. What mental framework does he use to communicate his understanding of his prognosis?
3. How is the illness influencing the patients' quality of life?

In Mr. Perkins' case, you have learned important information to guide ACP based on a brief conversation. Mr. Perkins is doing well. From his viewpoint, his quality of life is satisfactory. Additionally, you have learned that he is among a growing minority of older Americans using the worldwide web as a source of medical information. Your style of communication with him should take into account that he is a sophisticated consumer and that he will use the web to educate himself.

The second step of ACP is to formulate goals and preferences, to the extent desired by the patient. Here, Mr. Perkins has already stated some very clear goals. However, they were not formulated with a health-care provider, and those preferences are based on a misunderstanding of the use of mechanical ventilators, which could be life-saving for a person with congestive heart failure. Your obligation as Mr. Perkins' physician is to educate him about the availability of time-limited trials of therapy: often, patients with congestive heart failure can be on a ventilator briefly, with the potential to return to their previous level of functioning. In a patient with a good quality of life, physicians should discuss time-limited trials that could allow a chance to see whether the patient can be restored to his or her previous level of functioning. Based on this conversation, some patients will change their preferences. Others will not want to change their preferences. It is important that Mr. Perkins understands his options and makes an informed choice consistent with his underlying values and preferences. If he did not want to change his advance directive, you should try to ensure that this choice is not based on grief or depression.

Once the health-care provider and patient have formulated a set of preferences and future treatment goals, the health-care

Table 21–2. Adapting Advance Care Planning to Patient Circumstances: Possible Issues and Actions

Health status	Issues for discussion	Actions	Persons to lead action
Healthy	Surrogate decision maker	Suggest completion of durable power of attorney	C
	Health concerns	Discuss possibilities in a medical emergency	C, P
	Preferences or beliefs	Discuss values and preferences with surrogate, document	P
		strong preferences in patient record	C
Diagnosis of serious illness	Surrogate decision decision maker	Complete durable power of attorney	P
	Prognosis and options	Discuss possible and likely outcome states in relation to care options	C, P, F
	Preferences or beliefs	Discuss values and preferences in the event of an emergency,	P
		document preferences in patient record	C
Diagnosis of life-threatening illness	Surrogate decision maker	Determine status and location of durable power-of-attorney documents	C, P, F
	Preferences	Discuss and document preferences for end-of-life care and make arrangements as appropriate	C, P, F
	Goals	Discuss hopes and expectations for the last stage of life	C, P
	Contingency plans	Make specific plans for likely complications and urgent situations	C, P, F
Advanced age	Surrogate decision maker	Determine status and location of durable power-of-attorney documents	C, P, F
	Preferences	Discuss and document preferences for end-of-life care and make arrangements as appropriate	C, P, F
	Goals	Discuss hopes and expectations for the last stage of life	C, P
	Contingency plans	Make specific plans for likely complications and urgent situations	C, F

C, caregiver; P, patient; F, family.
Sources: Field and Cassel[6] and Teno and Lynn.[7]

provider must take on the most important step of ACP, formulating a plan of care that honors those preferences and goals. Without such plans, a patient could end up in the emergency room at 3:00 AM, being cared for by physicians who are unaware of his treatment preferences. This can be prevented by formulating a contingency plan in ACP that will ensure that the patient's preferences are honored. In this sense, ACP can prevent a serious medical error: an informed patient's preferences not being honored.

ADVANCE CARE PLANNING IN THE DYING PATIENT

Advance care planning plays a pivotal role in the care of dying persons. First, previously formulated preferences for outcomes where death is preferred to life may inform decisions to either forgo or withdraw life-sustaining treatment. Second, health-care providers should work with the patient and family to arrive at a patient-directed transition in goals of care. Such transitions may be forced when there are no further treatment options or the toxicities of treatment outweigh any potential benefits of treatment. Other times, transitions occur when the patient is seriously ill and weary of living with illness. In such cases, patients' voice preferences to forgo treatment, such as hospitalization for future events. As an example, consider the following case.

Grace* was a 65-year-old college professor, an adoptive mother of a 15-year-old son, and victim of colon cancer. She battled with this illness for 5 years, becoming an authority on how to find out about, and gain access to, the latest treatment protocols on a compassionate-use basis. She endured multiple surgeries with the ultimate goal of surviving and to see her son grow up. After a final surgery complicated by fungemia, she returned to an inpatient hospice to die. Her first action was to rearrange the furniture in her room to have her bed face the window. She took control of her surroundings.

My first visit with Grace and her husband was preceded by the nurse's comment that "I had to do something with the morphine drip." Her medical record from her oncologist noted that she had a written advance directive stating that she was a DNR and the focus of her care should be on her comfort.

Despite severe cachexia and dyspnea at rest, Grace does not want her morphine increased. The inpatient hospice staff is concerned that she is unnecessarily suffering and that her current actions are contrary to her previously stated preferences to focus on her comfort. Her score on the Folstein Mini-Mental Status Exam is 30/30, yet she feels not at her usual cognitive level. A discussion with her reveals that she is fully aware of her medical illness and prognosis, and she states her wish to maintain her

alertness to allow maximal amount of time to spend with her son.

Preferences stated in an advance directive are not applicable to this patient. These preferences would apply only if the patient had impaired decision-making capacity. Grace's decision-making capacity does not appear to be impaired. Fluids are given, and the morphine dose is decreased. Subjectively, she states that her mental status improves. She lives another 6 weeks in the inpatient unit, becoming increasingly fatigued, weak, edematous, and experiencing worsening dyspnea. The patient now states that she believes that her death is near.

The first step of ACP is to listen to the patient and her perceptions of her current quality of life. In later conversations with Grace, she has reached a critical turning point. Every day is now a struggle that, despite her determination, she finds difficult to endure. Next, you must communicate and negotiate with the patient regarding her current goals of care. The patient's quality of life has reached a point where it is becoming unacceptable to her. There are no treatment options, including experimental ones, for this patient. Communication is not about resuscitation preferences. Indeed, under this circumstance, consideration should be given to banning questions like "Do you want to be a full-code?" Rather, your conversation with this patient is very clear. She views her quality of life as suboptimal. A potential means of opening a dialogue is to ask her "Grace, tell me, what are your concerns now?" Future conversations should follow the lead of those concerns. For example:

GRACE: My breathing . . . it is a struggle just to take each breath.

DOCTOR: As we have discussed in the past, we can give medicines such as morphine or lorazepam to help, but they may make you sleepy and not as able to interact with your son.

GRACE: I love my son. He knows that. The times that we have spent these last weeks were invaluable. But my breathing, the weakness, it is just too much . . .

DOCTOR: I understand. We are going to increase the rate of the morphine drip and work with

---

*This is a composite case and does not represent the care of an actual patient.

you to find a point where you feel comfortable. You may feel groggy, but what I am hearing you tell me is that you want me to focus on your comfort, even if you are sedated. This is important. Am I correct that if you do become sedated from the medications you don't want me to reduce them to maintain your alertness?

GRACE: Yes.

The drip was increased and lorazepam was used. Grace died, sedated but comfortable. Although the conversation was brief, the foundation for it was laid in discussions over the prior 6 weeks. Based on the physician's understanding that the patient had reached a critical turning point, the focus was on her preference for sedation. This was not the first time her preference for sedation was discussed. Throughout the inpatient stay, this was discussed, given her initial desire to maintain alertness. The staff worked with Grace to arrive at a patient-directed use of medications to treat her symptoms yet maintain her alertness.

Dying is unlike any other period in a person's life. The person dying from a chronic, progressive, and eventually fatal illness, such as Grace, is quite different. Many people with Grace's prognosis and symptom burden would not have wanted intravenous hydration, further lab work, or careful titration of opiates to maintain mental clarity. However, this patient's preference was clear. Closure with her son was important. The goals of care for a dying person cannot be reasonably anticipated. In this chapter, a three-step approach to ACP has been outlined, with the ultimate goal of promoting patient autonomy. Unlike completing a written advance directive, advance care planning is a dynamic process that changes over the patient's disease trajectory. Early on, the content of ACP should focus on naming a proxy and stating unusual preferences. As the patient is diagnosed with a chronic, progressive illness, the focus is on understanding patient preferences regarding potential adverse out-

come states. Finally, death nears, the health-care provider works with the patient and family to achieve the patient's changing goals of care. Understanding where patients are on their disease trajectory is key to ACP. Based on that understanding, health-care providers must work with patients and families to arrive at treatment goals for the present and any future events that can be anticipated. Finally, health-care providers present patients and families with contingency plans that will ensure that those preferences are honored.

REFERENCES

1. Morrison RS, Olson E, Mertz KR, Meier DE. The inaccessibility of advance directives on transfer from ambulatory to acute care settings [see comments]. JAMA 274:478–482, 1995.
2. Schneiderman LJ, Kronick R, Kaplan RM, Anderson JP, Langer RD. Effects of offering advance directives on medical treatments and costs. Ann Intern Med 117:599–606, 1992.
3. Teno JM, Lynn J, Wenger N, et al. Advance directives for seriously ill hospitalized patients: effectiveness with the patient self-determination act and the SUPPORT intervention. SUPPORT Investigators. Study to Understand Prognoses and Preferences for Outcomes and Risks of Treatment [see comments]. J Am Geriatr Soc 45:500–507, 1997.
4. Lynn J, Teno JM, Phillips RS, et al. Perceptions by family members of the dying experience of older and seriously ill patients. Ann Intern Med 126:97–106, 1997.
5. Fox E, Landrum McNiff K, Zhong Z, Dawson NV, Wu AW, Lynn J. Evaluation of prognostic criteria for determining hospice eligibility in patients with advanced lung, heart, or liver disease. SUPPORT Investigators. Study to Understand Prognoses and Preferences for Outcomes and Risks of Treatments [see comments]. JAMA 282:1638–1645, 1999.
6. Field MJ, Cassel CK (Eds.). Approaching Death: Improving Care at the End of Life. Washington DC, National Academy Press, 1997.
7. Teno JM, Lynn J. Putting advance-care planning into action. J Clin Ethics 7:205–213, 1996.

22

Doctor–Patient Communication

JAMES A. TULSKY

Palliative care aims to meet the disparate needs of patients and families during a time of life-limiting illness. Good communication is indispensable to uncovering patient and family needs and individually negotiating the goals of care. Everyone defines good care differently,[1] and whether patient suffering is caused by pain, nausea, unwanted medical intervention, or spiritual crisis, the common pathway to treatment is through a provider able to elicit these concerns and equipped to help the patient and family address them.

Good communication brings real and tangible benefits. In patients with cancer, the number and severity of unresolved concerns predict high levels of emotional distress and future anxiety and depression.[2–4] Conversely, considerable evidence suggests that improved physician–patient communication correlates with improved health outcomes, patient satisfaction, and emotional well-being.[5–9] For example, primary-care patients exhibit decreased anxiety and are more satisfied with their physicians if they discuss advance care planning.[10] The mech-

anisms for this impact are likely twofold. First, improved communication increases the likelihood that the patient's needs will be recognized and addressed. Second, the communication itself may be therapeutic. Simply telling one's story may improve objective health outcomes.[11]

This chapter reviews recent literature concerning health-care provider communication at the end of life, surveys principles of communication relevant to palliative care with particular emphasis on the role of affect, and provides practical advice regarding some of the common topics that arise when caring for older patients with life-limiting illness.

WHAT IS THE PRESENT STATE OF COMMUNICATION DURING ADVANCED ILLNESS?

Unfortunately, the quality of communication between health-care providers and patients with life-limiting disease is generally poor. Studies show that the discussion of bad news frequently does not meet patient needs or falls short of expert recommendations.[2,12–18] Both physicians and nurses tend to underestimate cancer patients' concerns[19] and commonly do not elicit the full range of patients' concerns or attend to patients' affect.[20] Rather than using facilitative communication techniques, such as open-ended questions or empathic responses, when inquiring about psychosocial issues, they often block discussion of these issues by changing the subject or ignoring patients' emotional states.[14,21] Even in a hospice setting, one study revealed that only 40% of patients' concerns were elicited.[22] As a result, cancer patients tend to disclose fewer than 50% of their concerns,[21,22] which leads further to physicians' inaccurate assessments of patient distress.[15] One large audiotape study of oncology visits with terminally ill patients found that physicians dedicated only 23% of their time to health-related quality-of-life issues and frequently missed opportunities to address issues that seemed to be most important to patients.[23] Finally, physicians rarely talk with seriously ill patients about their goals, values, or treatment decisions.[24–31] A significant gap exists between the idealized model of provider–patient communication at the end of life and the reality of practice.

ETIOLOGY OF POOR COMMUNICATION

Why is the "state of the art" so abysmal? First, health-care providers are not selected for their communication skills. Cognitive aptitude does not always correlate positively with empathy. Second, until recently there has been little training regarding communication skills generally and less so with regard to these difficult topics.[32] For example, in a survey of over 3200 oncologists, few had any formal training in palliative care or communication skills. Oncology programs are not alone in devoting little attention to this subject. At both the medical school and residency levels, inadequate attention is given to care of the seriously ill.[33] Among graduating students at two medical schools, only 48% said they had adequate role models for how to discuss end-of-life issues. At another school, 41% of students on a medicine rotation and 73% on a surgery rotation had never observed a staff physician talk with a dying patient. Finally, physicians have difficulty inquiring directly about the emotional status of dying patients because of their feelings about the patient or about their own mortality.

Considerable evidence suggests physicians' personal feelings toward their patients are important to the doctor–patient relationship,[34–36] and many have suggested that physicians' emotional responses to their patients may interfere with their care.[37–41] For example, a study of surrogate decision–making found that physicians' predictions of their patients' wishes regarding life-sustaining treatment were closer to their own choices than to the choices expressed by their patients.[42]

Caring for those with advanced illness may elicit significant stress in physicians and a variety of reactions, including guilt ("If only I'd convinced him to get that screening colonoscopy"), impotence ("There's nothing I can do for her"), failure ("I messed up. I'm a bad doctor"), loss ("I'm really going to miss this person"), resentment ("This patient is going to keep me in the hospital all night"), and fear ("I know they're going to sue me").[43] Physicians may have unconscious feelings of omnipotence and troublesome responses stem from physicians' needs to preserve their image as "powerful healers" who can master any situation.[39] Feeling they have failed the patient, physicians may respond by acting defensively, wishing the patient would die to avoid dealing with them, or treating too aggressively to ensure that "everything has been done to save the patient."

Empathizing with seriously ill patients often evokes anxiety about physicians' own mortality. They respond by withdrawing from patients,[44] avoiding threatening topics,[16,21,45] employing blocking behaviors that distance them from addressing affective concerns,[46] or falsely reassuring patients that "everything is OK."[39]

Empirical data support these claims about physicians' anxieties regarding death. Physicians score higher on death anxiety scales than other professional groups.[47] They also find caring for terminally ill patients stressful. In a survey of 598 oncologists, 56% reported being burned out and 53% attributed these feelings to continuous exposure to fatal illness.[48] When caring for dying patients, physicians often report sadness, helplessness, failure, disappointment, and loneliness.[49] These feelings, particularly if unrecognized, may affect patient care.[50,51]

Such feelings are normal and common. However, they can affect one's ability to interact successfully with the patient. For example, feelings of failure may motivate one to avoid the patient, while feelings of loss may make discussions about dying too difficult. The first step toward managing such feelings is to acknowledge that they exist. The next step is to discuss them with colleagues or confidants. In most cases, however, patients do not benefit from hearing such thoughts. When considering sharing such feelings with a patient, a good rule is to ask oneself "Am I doing this for me or for the patient?" If the answer is truly the latter, then it may be appropriate to share.

GENERAL PRINCIPLES OF GOOD COMMUNICATION

A considerable body of evidence supports certain general communication skills. More accurate assessment of anxiety and depression is associated with good eye contact, clarifying of disclosures, responsiveness to cues of emotional distress, supportive comments, and asking explicitly about psychological content (Table 22–1).[52] Disclosure of concerns is promoted by open-ended questions, focusing on psychological aspects of illness, summarizing, educated guesses, and demonstrations of empathy. Likewise, disclosure is inhibited by closed-ended or leading questions, focusing on physical as-

Table 22–1. General Communication Skills to Enhance Disclosure of Concerns

Maintain good eye contact
Ask open-ended rather than closed-ended questions
Focus on the patient's concerns as well as your agenda for the visit
Observe and respond to the patient's affect
Ask about the patient's life outside of medicine and attend to psychosocial issues
Ensure your nonverbal behavior signifies attentiveness

Source: Tulsky and Arnold.[100]

pects of illness and offering advice and premature reassurance.[20] Furthermore, short demonstrations of empathy can reduce patient anxiety.[53] Training programs that emphasize these sorts of skills have been, for the most part, successful.[9,54–57]

The following sections identify and elaborate on general skills that are useful in all encounters with elderly patients. These are followed by practical advice for specific situations that arise in palliative care.

Advance Preparation

Whenever possible, important medical information, particularly bad or sad news, should be delivered during a scheduled meeting. This allows patients to prepare themselves for the type of information they will hear and to make sure that appropriate family members or friends are present. It also allows the physician to allocate the necessary time to the encounter.

Communication best occurs face-to-face. Telephones accentuate physical communication difficulties, such as hearing loss and speech problems, and there is no opportunity to employ the benefits of nonverbal communication. If the topic is emotionally threatening, it is more difficult to assess and ensure the patient's safety at the other end of the telephone. If one is anticipating an emotionally charged conversation with a patient, as when expecting results of a biopsy of a suspicious lesion, it is best to schedule an office visit. Frequently, the physician is caught off guard and discovers unexpectedly a bad result. In such cases, it is still best to schedule a time to discuss the results face-to-face. For example, one can call the patient and say "I have received the results of your blood tests, and I would like to discuss these results with you in person. Can you come in tomorrow at lunchtime?" Most patients will understand that all is not well, however; will not ask further questions; and will come in for the visit, when everything can be discussed. In effect, they have received a "warning shot" about the bad news and have begun to prepare themselves. Some patients, however, will respond by requesting to know the facts: "Is it cancer?" Even though it may seem evasive, it is worth trying to avoid delivering the news, even at this point, with a statement such as "I can imagine that you are concerned about the results, and I will answer all of your questions. There are a number of things we need to talk about, and I think I can help you better if we speak face-to-face." If the patient continues to insist on hearing the information, then one is obliged to answer directly, employing all of the appropriate skills for delivering bad news. In such a case, it is valuable to inquire directly about the patient's support at home and immediate plan of action.

One also needs to approach all such conversations prepared with basic medical information and anticipating the most likely questions regarding treatment options, prognosis, and resources for support and guidance.

Sensory Issues and Control of the Environment

When speaking with older adults, choosing a quiet, private room with good lighting enhances the patient's ability to comprehend. The physician should sit at eye level and within reach of the patient. If possible, one's pager or cellular phone should be turned off, or at least on quiet mode, and one should avoid interruptions. As presbycusis first affects higher sound frequencies, it is helpful to speak slowly in a clear, loud, low voice.[58] If patients wear hearing-assistive devices, they should be in place.

Increasingly, we encounter non-English-speaking patients. One must absolutely employ the assistance of an interpreter in such settings. However, it is equally important to avoid using family members as interpreters. Not only does this run the risk of faulty translation or reinterpretation of the physician's statements, it also places family members in the uncomfortable position of being the physician's and patient's spokesperson. The common practice of using bilingual young children as translators is particularly problematic. Many health-care facilities now employ professional translators or maintain lists of language skills among facility staff members.

WHAT IS EFFECTIVE COMMUNICATION IN ADVANCED ILLNESS?

According to patients, family members, and health-care providers, goals for communication include talking with patients in an honest and straightforward way, being willing to talk about dying, giving bad news in a sensitive way, listening to patients, encouraging questions from patients, and being responsive to patients' readiness to talk about death.[18] Patients want physicians to achieve a balance between being honest and straightforward and not discouraging hope. For some, this requires leaving open the possibility that unexpected "miracles" might happen, discussing outcomes other than a cure that can offer patients hope and meaning, and helping patients prepare for the losses they may experience. Because patients must receive adequate information to make informed choices, they wish to receive that information in an emotionally supportive way.[59] Patients want to discuss emotional concerns but frequently are unwilling to bring them up spontaneously and may need to be prompted.[60] Therefore, communication with seriously ill patients should be informative, be patient-centered rather than physician-centered,[61] and attend to patients' emotional needs. Many models have been proposed;[62–66] this chapter focuses on the role of emotions in such discussions.

Role of Affect in Communication

Most difficulties in communication are the result of inattention to affect. *Affect* refers to the feelings and emotions associated with the content of the conversation. Feelings such as anger, guilt, frustration, sadness, and fear modify our ability to hear, to communicate, and to make decisions. For example, after hearing bad news, most patients are so overwhelmed emotionally that they are unable to comprehend very much about the details of the illness or a treatment plan.[13,67] Conversations between doctors and patients often transpire only in the cognitive realm. Emotion is frequently not acknowledged or handled directly, and physicians miss opportunities to do so.[68,69] Consider the following conversations observed in a study of empathic communication and missed opportunities:[70]

DOCTOR: Does anybody in your family have breast cancer?

PATIENT: No.

DOCTOR: No?

PATIENT: After I had my hysterectomy. I was taking estrogen, right?

DOCTOR: Yeah?

PATIENT: You know how your breasts get real hard and everything? You know how you get sorta scared?

DOCTOR: How long were you on the estrogen?

PATIENT: Oh, maybe about 6 months.

DOCTOR: Yeah, what, how, when were you, when did you have the, uh, hysterectomy?

In this exchange, the doctor ignores the patient's fears and proceeds with factual questions. Not only is this patient unlikely to feel supported, she may also fail to give detailed information about her symptoms and hinder treatment. In contrast, in the following conversation, the physician recognizes the patient's expression of affect and delivers an empathic response. This is likely to continue the conversation in the realm of the emotions and leave the patient feeling supported.

DOCTOR: How do you feel about the cancer—about the possibility of it coming back?

PATIENT: Well, it bothers me sometimes, but I don't dwell on it. But I'm not as cheerful about it as I was when I first had it. I just had very good feelings that everything was going to be all right, you know. But now I dread another operation.

DOCTOR: You seem a little upset; you seem a little teary-eyed talking about it.

Emotion-Handling Skills

One barrier to eliciting patient affect is the fear of being unable to manage the emotional response. This section describes an approach to handling emotions that is also likely to further elicit the sorts of concerns described earlier. The primary goal of emotion handling is to convey a sense of empathy. *Empathy* is the sense that "I could be you" and is what patients are usually feeling when they comment about a physician that really cared for them.[71] Robert Smith has created a useful mnemonic to recall four basic techniques to use when confronted by patient emotions, *NURS* (Name, Understand, Respect, and Support).[72] This discussion adds a final *E* for Explore (Table 22–2).

Naming the emotion acknowledges the feeling and demonstrates that it is a legitimate area for discussion. Statements such as "That seems sad for you" can serve this purpose well, although one needs to be careful not to inappropriately label the patient. Therefore, naming is often best done in a quizzical fashion that does not presuppose the emotion (e.g., "Many people would feel angry if that happened to them. I wonder if you ever feel that way?").

Expressing a sense of understanding normalizes the patient's emotion and conveys empathy. However, expressing understanding must be done cautiously to prevent a response such as "How can you possibly

Table 22–2. NURSE-ing an Emotion

Name the emotion
Understand the emotion
Respect or praise the patient
Support the patient
Explore what underlies the emotion

Source: Fischer et al.[81]

understand what I'm going through; have you ever had a stroke?" A typical statement might be "Although I've never shared your experience, I do understand that this has been a really hard time for you."

Respect reminds us to praise patients and families for what they are doing and how they are managing with a difficult situation. Offering respect defuses defensiveness and makes people feel good about themselves and more capable of handling the future. A useful statement might be "I am so impressed with how you've continued to provide excellent care for your mother as her dementia has progressed."

Support is essential to helping people in distress not feel alone. Simple statements such as "I will be there with you throughout this illness" can be tremendously comforting. Health-care providers ought not to feel the entire support burden on their shoulders; support can include other members of a team. For example, "We will send a nurse to your home to check in on you in a couple of days, and if you'd like, I could ask the chaplain to pay you a visit."

Finally, patients will frequently make statements that deserve further exploration. For example, a patient may say "After you gave me the results of the test, I thought that this is going to be it." A simple response such as "Tell me more" may help reveal the patient's fears and concerns about cancer, which will be helpful in planning future treatment.

HOPE IN THE CONTEXT OF PALLIATIVE CARE

Physicians struggle to promote hope in the patient with advanced disease and to support a positive outlook, fearing that discussing death may decrease patient hopefulness.[18,73–76] As a result, they frequently convey prognosis with an optimistic bias or do not give this information at all.[77] This is relevant to treatment choices; patients with more optimistic assessments of their own prognosis are more likely to choose aggressive therapies at the end of life.[78,79] In turn, fearing the loss of hope, patients frequently cope by expressing denial and may be unwilling to hear what is said.[80]

It is not clear that health-care providers can either steal or instill hope. However, they can provide an empathic, reflective presence that will help patients draw strength from their existing resources. Physicians should recognize that it is not their job to "correct" the patient's hope for a miracle. The key question is whether the hope is interfering with appropriate planning and behavior. A patient who has completed his will and said his good-byes but is still hoping for a miracle is different from a patient who is making long-term investments and does not plan for custody of a minor child despite a 3-month prognosis.

Physicians can respond in several ways (after demonstrating empathy, as discussed above). Acknowledging hope may allow the physician and patient to "hope for the best but prepare for the worst." They can also recognize that people hope for many different things and leave space for patients to hope for outcomes and futures that are more likely to occur. One might say "I know you are hoping that your disease will be cured. Are there other things that you want to focus on?" Or "If we cannot make that happen, what other shorter-term goals might we focus on?" Finally, one can ask about what tasks are left undone as a way to get patients to begin to think in a shorter time course.

PRACTICAL SUGGESTIONS FOR SPECIFIC SITUATIONS

Communicating Bad News

Communicating bad news draws upon the skills discussed previously. Many protocols exist for the delivery of bad news, grouping behaviors into several key domains: preparation, content of message, dealing with patient responses, and ending the encounter (Table 22–3).[17,81] The primary el-

Table 22–3. Key Elements of Delivering
Bad News
_____

Preparation
   Find out what patient knows and believes
   Find out what patient wants to know
   Suggest that a supportive person accompany the
      patient
   Learn about the patient's condition
   Arrange the encounter in a private place with
      enough time

Content
   Get to the point quickly
   Fire "warning shot" (e.g., "I have bad news")
   State the news clearly, simply, and sensitively
   Avoid false reassurance
   Make truthful, hopeful statements
   Provide information in small chunks

Handle patient's reactions
   Inquire about meaning of the condition for the
      patient
   NURSE expressed emotions
   Assure continued support

Wrap-up
   Set up a meeting within next few days
   Offer to talk to relatives/friends
   Suggest that patients write down questions
   Provide a way to be reached in emergencies
   Assess suicidality
_____
Source: Fischer et al.[81]

ements of preparation have been addressed
above.

Content of message

Uncovering what the patient already knows
or believes is extremely valuable prior to
revealing bad news.[81] This allows physicians to begin their explanation from the
patient's perspective, aligning themselves
with patients and making communication
more efficient and effective. When a test is
ordered is a good time to assess this. One
might ask "Is there anything that you are
particularly concerned about?" If the patient mentions a serious illness that might
be present, the physician can follow-up by
asking about the patient's specific fears and
concerns. Consider, for example, an elderly
woman with a breast mass. Her doctor is
concerned that it might be breast cancer.
Here is how the physician might approach
the patient:[81]

DOCTOR: Is there anything that you are particularly worried that this might be?

PATIENT: I guess anyone would be scared that it's
cancer.

DOCTOR: I'm afraid that it might be cancer.
There are other things that it might be too, however. That's why we are going to do the biopsy—
to find out. What worries you most about
cancer?

PATIENT: My mother died of colon cancer. She
suffered terribly with it. In the end, she was so
weak and thin . . . she had to "do her business"
in a bag, you know? And she always seemed to
be in pain.

At the end of this exchange, note how
the physician begins to find out what the
patient's fears are in an effort to anticipate
the patient's reactions to the news if the test
result does turn out to be bad.

When prepared to deliver the message
content, the physician should begin by fir-
ing a brief "warning shot" and then stating the news in clear and direct terms. One
should avoid spending time "beating
around the bush" prior to sharing the news.
For example:

DOCTOR: We have the test results back, and I'm
afraid they don't look good.

PATIENT: Oh no, what is it?

DOCTOR: The biopsy shows you have cancer.

Perhaps most important is what follows
this exchange. The clinician should remain
silent and allow the patient an opportunity
to absorb the news. One can strike an empathic stance, maintain comfortable eye
contact, and perhaps use a nonverbal ges-
ture such as reaching out and touching the
patient's hand. However, silence is imperative to allow patients an opportunity to
process the information, formulate a response, and experience their emotions. The
clinician who feels uncomfortable during
this silent phase needs to appreciate that the
discomfort is rarely shared by the patient,
who is engrossed in thoughts about the
meaning of the news and the future. Furthermore, very little that is said by the
physician at this time will be remembered
by the patient, so it is best not to say it at

all. If the patient makes no verbal response after, perhaps, two minutes, it can be useful to check in: "I just told you some pretty serious news. Do you feel comfortable sharing your thoughts about this?"

Dealing with the response
The remainder of the conversation should be spent primarily handling the patient's response. This includes using the NURSE skills to empathize with the patient's experience. It is also important to explore the meaning the news has for the patient and to achieve a shared understanding of the disease and its implications. For example:

DOCTOR: What is most troubling to you about having cancer?

PATIENT: It's a death sentence—my mother died from cancer, my brother died from cancer. I guess it's my turn now.

DOCTOR: Given your experience, I can see how this is really scary for you. And cancer can be very serious. However, in your case, there are a lot of treatment options, and you have a good chance of surviving with this disease.

PATIENT: So this won't kill me?

DOCTOR: I certainly hope not. And, I'll be there with you every step of the way, fighting this illness.

The preponderance of literature stresses the importance of maintaining hope while remaining truthful.[17] As discussed above, hopeful messages need to be tailored to patients' specific concerns, particularly addressing misconceptions and fears. Once patients' concerns have been explored, patients can be reassured more effectively. When effective treatment is available, this fact should be explained. When the treatment options are poor, hope may be found by alleviating patients' worst fears. Doctors may reassure patients that they will not be abandoned during their illness, that the doctor will remain available if things get worse, that everything will be done to maintain the patient's comfort, and that they will continue to watch for new treatment developments.[82] Often, people find hope and strength from their religious or spiritual beliefs, from having their individ-

uality respected, from meaningful relationships with others, and from finding meaning in their lives.[75] Exploring these with the patient over time may help to foster realistic hope. Although physicians may have a desire to make an overly reassuring statement to the patient right after revealing the diagnosis, hopeful statements that are truthful and made after taking the time to explore the patient's concerns are more likely to be accepted by the patient.[83] One can offer a realistic sense of hope, whether biomedical ("We'll keep our eyes open for new treatments and discuss them as they become available") or psychosocial ("I look forward to talking with you more about how we can help you live every day as fully as possible, despite this illness").

Patients may have specific questions about further tests, treatment options, and prognosis. It is important to respond to these seriously. However, many patients will suffer comprehension difficulties in such emotionally challenging situations. Give simple, focused bits of information, use nonvague language that patients can understand, carefully observe the patient's verbal and nonverbal reactions to what you say, and most importantly, avoid information-packed speeches.

Ending the encounter
The clinician must end the encounter in a way that leaves the patient feeling supported and with some sense of hope. Support can be provided through meeting patients' immediate health needs and risks. One must treat pain and palliate other symptoms. Patients should be asked how they plan to cope with the news; and if their response raises any concerns about suicide, these should be directly addressed. One should minimize aloneness through statements of nonabandonment and referral to other resources such as support groups, counselors, or pastoral care.

Lastly, one should provide a specific follow-up plan: "I'd like you to keep a list of questions so I can answer them for you on our next visit this Tuesday. We'll talk about all your options again at that time. Okay? And please feel free to call me." The physician needs to remember that the goal of this conversation is not to leave a happy patient. That is rarely possible (or even desirable) after delivering bad news. Instead, one hopes to leave a patient who feels supported and cared for and can look forward to a specific plan of action.

Advance Care Planning

Discussions about advance care planning encompass many goals: preparing for death and dying, exercising control, relieving burdens placed on loved ones, helping patients make decisions consistent with their values, and leaving patients feeling supported and understood.[84] Unfortunately, these goals are frequently not met. Audiotape studies of actual discussions about advance care planning demonstrate that information is frequently presented in ways that may be misunderstood by patients, uncertainty is addressed insufficiently, empathic opportunities are missed, and scenarios and treatments discussed do not reflect the most challenging situations confronted in real life.[28,29] These data are not surprising. Patients struggle with hypothetical future treatment decisions while confronting the emotional impact of discussing their own mortality. Clinicians must respond to patients' cognitive and affective demands, yet few providers receive formal training in such communication.[33,85]

The first step in preparing to discuss advance care plans is deciding on the appropriate goals for the discussion.[86] What one hopes to accomplish will vary depending on the clinical situation.[87] Advance care planning includes many different tasks: informing the patient, eliciting preferences, identifying a surrogate decision maker, and providing emotional support. Frequently, one cannot accomplish all of these in one conversation, and focusing on the goals of the discussion allows the physician to tailor the encounter. Advance care planning is a process completed over time, which allows patients and providers an opportunity for thoughtful reflection and interaction.

For a healthy, older patient, physicians might establish who the patient would like to appoint as a health-care surrogate. They might ask whether the patient already has a written advance directive and explore the patients' thoughts about dying and life-sustaining treatments in general. For an elderly patient with a serious chronic illness, the doctor might also discuss the patient's attitudes about specific interventions that are likely to occur. For example, the physician might ask about attitudes toward mechanical ventilation in a patient with severe chronic obstructive pulmonary disease (COPD). Finally, if the illness has progressed to the point where it seems that the patient will soon die, the doctor will shift the focus from future treatment in hypothetical scenarios to establishing what the goals should be for care provided in the present. In all cases, advance care planning can help patients prepare for death, discuss their values with their loved ones, and achieve a sense of control.[84] It can help build trust between doctors and their patients so that when difficult treatment decisions arise, doctors, patients, and their loved ones can communicate openly and achieve resolution.

Initiating the conversation

There are a number of ways to begin the discussion.[86] Often, physicians can relate the topic to a recent serious illness. For example, if the patient had been previously hospitalized for COPD, the doctor may begin an advance directive discussion this way:

DOCTOR: How have you been doing since you were discharged from the hospital?

PATIENT: Pretty well. The breathing is pretty much back to normal . . . you know.

DOCTOR: Good. You know, I was pretty worried about you when the medics brought you to the ER.

PATIENT: So was I. I was never that bad before. I really felt like I was suffocating.

DOCTOR: That sounds like it must have been awful.

PATIENT: Yeah.

DOCTOR: Well, I realized that you and I have never had a chance to talk about what we should do if you were sicker, say, so sick that you couldn't tell me what you wanted, and we had to do things like put you on a breathing machine . . .

Another way to begin is to ask about experiences with relatives or friends who have died. Elderly patients are no strangers to death. They have been to many funerals of family members and friends. They are likely to have observed serious illness closely and perhaps have had loved ones in some of the situations which the physician is describing. They are likely to have much information and misinformation about end-of-life care and to have thought about their own deaths. Opening a discussion in this manner can naturally lead to a discussion about how decisions were made and what the patient thought of that particular death. This will provide valuable insights into the patient's own values. Finally, when there is no such event to which to link the discussion, doctors can simply declare that they discuss the topic with all of their patients. One can reassure patients, when true, that one is not bringing the topic up because the patient's death is imminent or because the physician has information about the patient's condition that is not being shared.

Providing information

Patients must have adequate information to make informed decisions. It helps to start by asking patients what they understand about their medical illness. If the patient's condition is more serious than he or she realizes, then the physician will need to shift focus. The physician will want to put off discussing advance care plans, focusing the discussion instead on explaining the seriousness of the patient's condition.

Patients are more interested in what the expected health outcome will be than in details about the interventions themselves.[25,88] When elderly patients are provided with outcome data about the prognosis after cardiopulmonary resuscitation, they become less interested in receiving the intervention.[78,89] Patients consider withholding treatments primarily to avoid an outcome judged by them to be worse than death.[90]

They may also worry that the burden of treatment outweighs the potential benefit. Therefore, patients should understand the impact of common life-sustaining interventions on quality of life. In contrast, vivid descriptions of the nature of the treatments themselves (e.g., intubation, cardioversion, intensive care unit care) may alarm patients but be less helpful.

Eliciting preferences

Patients state preferences after learning about potential options and evaluating these in light of their personal values. *Values* refers to deeply held beliefs such as a desire for personal independence or the importance of a religious practice. By exploring patients' values and goals, clinicians can help them clarify their specific preferences. Sometimes one can ask explicitly about such values (e.g., "What makes life worth living for you?"). Alternatively, values may be elicited in the process of asking about specific treatment preferences. For example, after a patient makes a statement about end-of-life care (e.g., "I'd never want to be on one of those machines"), the clinician may respond by simply asking "Why?" The answer to this question (e.g., "Because I never want to be a burden on my family or society") may uncover a patient's core values, which will impact greatly on treatment decisions.

Identifying what conditions the patient would find unacceptable can also help to clarify preferences. A useful question is "Can you imagine any situations in which life would not be worth living?"[91] Typically, patients mention persistent vegetative state or similar dire scenarios. This question can be followed by asking what the patient would be willing to forgo to avoid such states.

For many patients, dealing with uncertainty comprises the most difficult aspect of decision making. When doctors ask patients if they would want a particular treatment, patients often state that the treatment should be provided "if it will help me, but if it won't help me, don't do it." Such statements ignore the reality that physicians are often uncertain about the outcome. Everyone responds to uncertainty differently, and the patient's approach to this issue should be discussed explicitly as well. For example, one may ask "What if we are not sure whether we will be able to get you off the breathing machine?" Depending on the patient's answer to this question, the doctor can explore what the chance of success needs to be to pursue aggressive treatment. Some patients will state that any possibility of recovery is worth pursuing, while others will refuse curative treatment when the likelihood of recovery drops below a particular threshhold.[79] Some patients are comfortable using numbers in talking about probabilities; others are less quantitatively facile.[92–94] The patient's preferences should dictate the extent to which numbers are used in this discussion. Offering a treatment trial is also a useful way to provide clarity in the face of uncertainty.

It is impossible to elicit meaningful preferences for every intervention in every possible situation. By focusing on a patient's values and goals, the physician can help the patient make decisions about future or current treatments that are consistent with those goals. Discussions should move back and forth, from preferences to reasons and values to information and back again, ensuring that the patient understands the implications of stated preferences and that the doctor understands the patient's values. In this way, when the physician is faced with an unanticipated clinical situation, the patient's stated values and goals can be used to help determine the appropriate course of action. It is also frequently worthwhile to inquire specifically about some controversial treatments, such as artificial nutrition and hydration. This is particularly true in states that require the patients' specific directive to withhold these treatments. Finally, many patients will be satisfied leaving decisions to the judgment of their physician and family members, with only general instructions, and this should be respected.

Choosing surrogate decision makers
Identifying who is to act as the patient's health-care proxy may be the most impor-

tant outcome of a conversation about advance care planning. Does the patient wish this to be a single individual or an entire family? Given the literature demonstrating poor concordance between patient preferences and surrogate perceptions of those preferences, the clinician would be wise to stress the need for the patient to communicate with the selected proxy decision maker.[95] Patients should also be asked how much leeway their proxies should have in decision making.[96] Should proxies adhere strictly to patients' stated preferences, or ought they have more flexibility when making actual decisions?

These discussions can be emotionally difficult, even when they are welcome. It is important to draw upon the emotion-handling skills described earlier; to acknowledge patient's feelings of sadness, fear, or anger when they come up; and to validate those feelings by stating your understanding of their reaction. The physician can admit that the discussion can be difficult and support the patient by stating how helpful he or she has been in helping to understand his or her preferences. Another way doctors can provide support to the patient is to assure the patient that they will do whatever they can to meet their goals (such as comfort) and to articulate what some of those things might be. In this way, doctors can assure patients that they will continue to care for them, even if they are in a condition in which they would not want life-sustaining treatment.

Communicating over the Transition
Physicians and patients may face the greatest communication challenges as they discuss progression of disease, the transition from curative therapy to palliation, and the referral for hospice care. Such times of transition involve the recognition of loss, redefinition of self-concept and social role, and great emotional stress. Patients are likely to feel sadness, anger, and denial. Physicians frequently have difficulty with such discussions because they feel a sense of failure and are worried that patients will feel abandoned or that they will be overcome in the conversation by anxiety or de-

spair.[81] Furthermore, they may have their own unresolved issues about mortality or fear the patient's anticipated emotional response.

Again, it is useful to identify the goals of these conversations. They include eliciting emotional, psychological, and spiritual concerns and providing empathic and practical support. Of course, it is also important to help patients acknowledge their illness and to make appropriate health-care decisions, such as enrolling in hospice. However, conversations should not be dominated by the physicians' agenda, and patients must be given ample space to make decisions according to their own timetables. According to a recent study, patients facing terminal illness desire a physician who will talk in an honest and straightforward way, be willing to talk about dying, give bad news in a sensitive way, listen, encourage questions, and be sensitive to when they are ready to talk about death.[18] They also wish for physicians to maintain hope while being truthful. Easier said than done. As a general rule, it is important for physicians to employ behaviors that promote the sharing of concerns by patients and to avoid behaviors, such as reassurance, that inhibit such sharing. Table 22–4 lists useful open-ended questions with which one can initiate such conversations.

As a patient responds to these questions, the physician should continue to focus on the psychosocial and spiritual aspects of their illness and not allow the biomedical issues to dominate. It is important to avoid false reassurance.[46] A particular form of response that can be extremely effective at these times is the "wish statement"[97] These are particularly effective in response to statements that appear to demonstrate significant denial of the severity of illness. For example:

PATIENT: I'm going to get better. I know that this new chemotherapy they're offering at the university will make the difference.

DOCTOR: I wish that there was a treatment that would make this cancer go away.

PATIENT: You mean that you don't think it will work.

DOCTOR: It's hard to come to terms with this, but unfortunately I don't believe it would help you overcome your cancer.

PATIENT: I was afraid you might say that. What do we do now?

DOCTOR: There's a lot that we can do. Let's talk about what goals are most important for you right now.

The wish statement allows the doctor to demonstrate empathy toward the patient and to align himself or herself with the patient's hopes. At the same time, it implicitly conveys the message that certain goals are unrealistic. In this way, the physician can address the patient's denial without losing the therapeutic alliance.

Dreaded Questions

Finally, it is useful to consider several of the questions that many physicians find most difficult to answer. Responding to such questions draws upon the many skills described in this chapter, and it is useful to keep several additional points in mind.[98] Check the reason for the question (e.g., "Why do you ask that now?"), show interest in the patient's ideas, and empathize with their concerns. One must also be prepared to admit that one does not know. The most important thing a physician can do is remain curious. One should not assume that one knows what the question is "really" about. A patient who is asking "How long do I have?" may be wondering if he or she is going to live until Christmas, whether reports that the disease is fatal are accurate, or whether he or she is going to get out of the hospital. Acknowledge the

Table 22–4. Open-Ended Questions to Initiate Conversations about Dying

What concerns you most about your illness?

How is treatment going for you (your family)?

As you think about your illness, what is the best and the worst that might happen?

What has been most difficult about this illness for you?

What are your hopes (your expectations, your fears) for the future?

As you think about the future, what is most important to you (what matters the most to you)?

Source: Lo et al.[64]

question, but make sure you understand it before trying to answer (e.g., "That is a really tough question. What are you concerned about?"). It is also important to recognize that it is not necessarily the physician's job to solve the problem. Physicians do not have the answers to questions such as "Why me?" and may not be able to diminish the feelings of sadness and loss. What one can do is to acknowledge and normalize the feelings. In allowing the patient to be heard, the physician may decrease the patient's sense of being alone in the disease and thus decrease suffering.

Having anticipated replies can be useful and several examples follow:[64]

PATIENT: How long do I have to live?

DOCTOR: I wonder if it is frightening not knowing what will happen next, or when.

This response acknowledges that underlying such a question is tremendous emotion, most likely fear. It will be important for the physician to give a factual response to this question. However, the patient will not be prepared to hear this response until the doctor has addressed his or her emotional concerns. The suggested answer above allows patients to speak about their fears and worries. When the physician needs to use a more factual response, the following is a way of being honest while maintaining hope: "On average, a person in your situation lives three to four months, but some people have much less time, and others may live over a year. I would take care of now any practical or family matters that you wish to have completed before you die, but continue to hope that you are one of the lucky people who gets a bit more time."

FAMILY: Does this mean you're giving up on him?

DOCTOR: Absolutely not. But tell me, what do you mean by giving up?

Suggesting that a patient receive palliative care risks conveying a sense of abandonment. Physicians must be emphatic that palliative care and hospice are active forms of care that can be employed at the same time as beneficial life-prolonging measures and that aim to meet patients' varying goals

at the end of life. However, further exploration of patients' or families concerns about abandonment are important to understanding their perceptions and attitudes toward care at the end of life.

PATIENT: Are you telling me that I am going to die?

DOCTOR: I wish that were not the case, but it is likely in the near future. I am also asking, how would want to spend the remaining time if it were limited?

This wish statement helps the physician identify with the patient's loss. The following sentence is an attempt by the physician to reframe the patient's understanding of the situation. He or she has acknowledged that the patient is dying but now seeks to understand what the patient's goals might be in light of this new information. Creating new goals in this way provides an outlet for the patient's hope.

Communication Issues with Cognitively Impaired Patients

Coexisting cognitive impairment associated with dementia, delirium, anxiety, or depression complicates the physician's efforts to communicate complex and emotion-laden information. As when obtaining informed consent, capacity to participate in such discussions is situation-specific. For example, a patient with mild to moderate dementia may be quite capable of indicating who he or she trusts to make decisions or to indicate what hurts and where, but he or she may not be able to come to terms with information about prognosis or the burdens and benefits of a range of treatment options. Clinicians must titrate the content of the information given according to their assessment of patients' capacity to integrate such information. Whenever possible, psychiatric comorbidities should be ameliorated to optimize patients' abilities to understand their situation and participate in treatment decisions. Further, if the disease process is likely to soon worsen cognition and decisional capacity, the clinician should rapidly prioritize the importance of communication about goals and preferences for care as well as identify trusted surrogates, lest the opportunity pass irrevocably.

When caring for older adults with impaired cognition, communication often occurs primarily between the physician and the patient's family. Although the law prioritizes identification of a single preferred decision maker, such as a health-care proxy or durable power of attorney for health care, in most families decisions are made collectively. The physician should determine explicitly how and which family surrogates prefer to receive information, make decisions, and communicate with the health-care team. Formally scheduled family meetings, including as many concerned and involved family members as possible, are often critically important to establishing a shared understanding of the medical situation, the treatment alternatives, and their priority in the context of what is known about the patient's preferences and best interests. In such communications, the physician's goal is not only to promote decision making that is concordant with the patient's previously expressed values and wishes but also to support family caregivers as they struggle to come to terms with the responsibility of their decision-making role and work to arrive at the best option on behalf of their loved one. The aim is to enable the family to look back on their care of the patient with pride and a sense of having done everything possible to assure excellent care in terms of not only life-prolonging efforts but also relief of suffering.

Once the decision makers are established, the same approach to conveying bad news, advance care planning, and discussing the transitions to palliative care described above for the individual patient may be employed. After many years of struggle with advanced chronic illness, family caregivers are as much a part of the unit of care as the patient him- or herself. Inquiries as to their health, well-being, and practical and psychosocial needs as well as a willingness to listen to these concerns are powerful indicators of the physician's respect for and appreciation of their role and have been shown to increase families' satisfaction with quality of care.

Bereavement

Caring for elderly patients means caring for bereaved patients. The loss of spouses, siblings, other family members, and close friends is extremely common among older persons. A full discussion of bereavement is beyond the scope of this chapter; however, it is useful to review several key elements of communication with patients after loss.[99] Patients ought to be encouraged to tell their stories of loss, including details of the days and weeks around the death of their loved one. Similarly, patients benefit by recalling earlier positive memories of the person. Physicians can explore how the patient has responded to the grief ("How have things been different for you since your husband died?") and identify the patient's social support and coping resources ("Has anyone been particularly helpful to you recently?" and "What helps you get through the day?"). Lastly, one should not overlook the frequently enormous practical ramifications of loss, such as financial difficulties, functional dependence, the need to leave a home, and transportation.

Good communication skills provide the pathway to excellent care for elderly persons. The fundamentals of such communication are listening, attending to patients' emotional needs, and achieving a shared understanding of the concerns at hand. Specific tasks such as delivering bad news, discussing advance care planning, helping patients through the transition to hospice care, and responding to bereavement require using these skills to ensure that patients' concerns are elicited and addressed and that patients are informed and feel supported.

ACKNOWLEDGMENTS

This chapter is adapted from Tulsky and Arnold[100] and Tulsky.[101]

REFERENCES

1. Steinhauser KE, Christakis NA, Clipp EC, McNeilly M, McIntyre L, Tulsky JA. Fac-

tors considered important at the end of life by patients, family, physicians, and other care providers. JAMA 284:2476–2482, 2000.

2. Butow PN, Kazemi JN, Beeney LJ, Griffin AM, Dunn SM, Tattersall MH. When the diagnosis is cancer: patient communication experiences and preferences. Cancer 77:2630–2637, 1996.

3. Heaven CM, Maguire P. The relationship between patients' concerns and psychological distress in a hospice setting. Psychooncology 7:502–507, 1998.

4. Parle M, Jones B, Maguire P. Maladaptive coping and affective disorders among cancer patients. Psychol Med 26:735–744, 1996.

5. Bertakis KD, Roter D, Putnam SM. The relationship of physician medical interview style to patient satisfaction. J Fam Pract 32:175–181, 1991.

6. Cohen SR, Mount BM, Tomas JJN, Mount LF. Existential well-being is an important determinant of quality of life: evidence from the McGill Quality of Life Questionnaire. Cancer 77:576–586, 1996.

7. Fakhoury W, McCarthy M, Addington-Hall J. Determinants of informal caregivers' satisfaction with services for dying cancer patients. Soc Sci Med 42:721, 1996.

8. Kaplan SH, Greenfield S, Ware JE Jr. Assessing the effects of physician–patient interaction on the outcomes of chronic disease. Med Care 27:S110–S127, 1989.

9. Roter DL, Hall JA, Kern DE, Barker LR, Cole KA, Rocxa RP. Improving physicians' interviewing skills and reducing patients' emotional distress: a randomized clinical trial. Arch Intern Med 155:1877, 1995.

10. Tierney WM, Dexter PR, Gramelspacher GP, Perkins AJ, Zhou XH, Wolinsky FD. The effect of discussions about advance directives on patients satisfaction with primary care. J Gen Intern Med 16:32–40, 2001.

11. Smyth JM, Stone AA, Hurewitz A, Kaell A. Effects of writing about stressful experiences on symptom reduction in patients with asthma or rheumatoid arthritis: a randomized trial. JAMA 281:1304–1309, 1999.

12. Clark RE, LaBeff EE. Death telling: managing the delivery of bad news. J Health Soc Behav 23:366–380, 1982.

13. Eden OB, Black I, MacKinlay GA, Emery AE. Communication with parents of children with cancer. Palliat Med 8:105–114, 1994.

14. Ford S, Fallowfield L, Lewis S. Can on-

cologists detect distress in their out-patients and how satisfied are they with their performance during bad news consultations? Br J Cancer 70:767–770, 1994.

15. Ford S, Fallowfield L, Lewis S. Doctor-patient interactions in oncology. Soc Sci Med 42:1511, 1996.

16. Friedrichsen MJ, Strang PM, Carlsson ME. Breaking bad news in the transition from curative to palliative cancer care—patient's view of the doctor giving the information. Support Care Cancer 8:472–478, 2000.

17. Ptacek JT, Eberhardt TL. Breaking bad news. A review of the literature. JAMA 276:496–502, 1996.

18. Wenrich MD, Curtis JR, Shannon SE, Carline JD, Ambrozy DM, Ramsey PG. Communicating with dying patients within the spectrum of medical care from terminal diagnosis to death. Arch Intern Med 161:868–874, 2001.

19. Goldberg R, Guadagnoli E, Silliman RA, Glicksman A. Cancer patients' concerns: congruence between patients and primary care physicians. J Cancer Educ 5:193–199, 1990.

20. Maguire P, Faulkner A, Booth K, Elliott C, Hillier V. Helping cancer patients disclose their concerns. Eur J Cancer 32A:78–81, 1996.

21. Maguire P. Improving communication with cancer patients. Eur J Cancer 35:1415–1422, 1999.

22. Heaven CM, Maguire P. Disclosure of concerns by hospice patients and their identification by nurses. Palliat Med 11:283–290, 1997.

23. Detmar SB, Muller MJ, Wever LD, Schornagel JH, Aaronson NK. The patient–physician relationship. Patient–physician communication during outpatient palliative treatment visits: an observational study. JAMA 285:1351–1357, 2001.

24. Emanuel LL, Barry MJ, Stoeckle JD, Ettelson LM, Emanuel EJ. Advance directives for medical care—a case for greater use. N Engl J Med 324:889–895, 1991.

25. Layson RT, Adelman HM, Wallach PM, Pfeifer MP, Johnston S, McNutt RA. Discussions about the use of life-sustaining treatments: a literature review of physicians' and patients' attitudes and practices. J Clin Ethics 5:195–203, 1994.

26. Miles SH, Bannick-Mohrland S, Lurie N. Advance-treatment planning discussions with nursing home residents: pilot experience with simulated interviews. J Clin Ethics 1:108–112, 1990.

27. Miller DK, Coe RM, Hyers TM. Achieving consensus on withdrawing or with-

holding care for critically ill patients. J Gen Intern Med 7:475–480, 1992.

28. Tulsky JA, Chesney MA, Lo B. How do medical residents discuss resuscitation with patients? J Gen Intern Med 10:436–442, 1995.

29. Tulsky JA, Fischer GS, Rose MR, Arnold RM. Opening the black box: how do physicians communicate about advance directives? Ann Intern Med 129:441–449, 1998.

30. Ventres W, Nichter M, Reed R, Frankel R. Do-not-resuscitate discussions: a qualitative analysis. Fam Pract Res J 12:157–169, 1992.

31. Ventres W, Nichter M, Reed R, Frankel R. Limitation of medical care: an ethnographic analysis. J Clin Ethics 4:134–145, 1993.

32. Novack DH, Volk G, Drossman DA, Lipkin M. Medical interviewing and interpersonal skills teaching in US medical schools. Progress, problems, and promise. JAMA 269:2101–2105, 1993.

33. Billings JA, Block S. Palliative care in undergraduate medical education. Status report and future directions. JAMA 278:733–738, 1997.

34. Smith RC. Teaching interviewing skills to medical students: the issue of "countertransference." J Med Educ 59:582–588, 1984.

35. Smith RC. Unrecognized responses and feelings of residents and fellows during interviews. J Med Educ 61:982–984, 1986.

36. Smith RC, Zimny GH. Physicians emotional reactions to patients. Psychosomatics 29:392–397, 1988.

37. Eissler KK. The Psychiatrist and the Dying Patient. New York, International Universities Press, 1955.

38. Konior GS, Levine AS. The fear of dying: how patients and their doctors behave. Semin Oncol 2:311–316, 1975.

39. Spikes J, Holland J. The physician's response to the dying patient. In: Strain JJ, Grossman (Eds.). Psychological Care of the Medically Ill: A Primer in Liaison Psychiatry. New York, Appleton-Century-Crofts, pp. 138–148, 1975.

40. Weissman AD. Misgivings and misconceptions in the psychiatric care of terminal patients. Psychiatry 33:67–81, 1970.

41. White LP. The self-image of the physician and the care of dying patients. Ann N Y Acad Sci 164:822–837, 1969.

42. Schneiderman LJ, Kaplan RM, Pearlman RA. Do physicians own preferences for life-sustaining treatment influence their perceptions of patients' preferences? J Clin Ethics 4:28–33, 1993.

43. Quill TE, Townsend P. Bad news: delivery, dialogue, and dilemmas. Arch Intern Med 151:463–468, 1991.

44. Benoliel JQ. Health care providers and dying patients: critical issues in terminal care. Omega 18:341–363, 1987–1988.

45. The AM, Hak T, Koeter G, van Der Wal G. Collusion in doctor–patient communication about imminent death: an ethnographic study. BMJ 321:1376–1381, 2000.

46. Maguire P. Barriers to psychological care of the dying. BMJ 291:1711–1713, 1985.

47. Benoliel JQ. Health care delivery: not conducive to teaching palliative care. J Palliat Care 4:41–42, 1988.

48. Whippen DA, Canellos GP. Burnout syndrome in the practice of oncology: results of a random survey of 1,000 oncologists. J Clin Oncol 9:1916–1920, 1991.

49. Schaerer R. Suffering of the doctor linked with death of patients. Palliat Med 7:27–37, 1993.

50. Cochrane JB, Levy MR, Fryer JE. Death anxiety, disclosure behaviors, and attitudes of oncologists toward terminal care. Omega 22:1–12, 1990–91.

51. Neimeyer GJ, Behnke M, Reiss J. Constructs and coping: physicians' response to patient death. Death Educ 7:245–264, 1983.

52. Marks JN, Goldberg DP, Hillier VF. Determinants of the ability of general practitioners to detect psychiatric illness. Psychol Med 9:337–353, 1979.

53. Fogarty LA, Curbow BA, Wingard JR, McDonnell K, Somerfield MR. Can 40 seconds of compassion reduce patient anxiety? J Clin Oncol 17:371–379, 1999.

54. Smith RC, Lyles JS, Mettler J, et al. The effectiveness of intensive training for residents in interviewing. Ann Intern Med 128:118–126, 1998.

55. Levinson W, Roter D. The effects of two continuing medical education programs on communication skills of practicing primary care physicians. J Gen Intern Med 8:318–324, 1993.

56. Fallowfield L, Jenkins V, Farewell V, Saul J, Duffy A, Eves R. Efficacy of a Cancer Research UK communication skills training model for oncologists: a randomised controlled trial. Lancet 359:650–656, 2000.

57. Jenkins V, Fallowfield L. Can communication skills training alter physicians' beliefs and behavior in clinics? J Clin Oncol 20:765–769, 2002.

58. Adelman RD, Greene MG, Ory MG. Communication between older patients and their physicians. Clin Geriatr Med 16:1–24, 2000.

59. Parker PA, Baile WF, de Moor C, Lenzi R, Kudelka AP, Cohen L. Breaking bad news about cancer: patients' preferences for communication. J Clin Oncol 19:2049–2056, 2001.

60. Detmar SB, Aaronson NK, Wever LD, Muller M, Schornagel JH. How are you feeling? Who wants to know? Patients' and oncologists' preferences for discussing health-related quality-of-life issues. J Clin Oncol 18:3295–3301, 2000.

61. Dowsett SM, Saul JL, Butow PN, et al. Communication styles in the cancer consultation: preferences for a patient-centred approach. Psychooncology 9:147–156, 2000.

62. Baile WF, Glober GA, Lenzi R, Beale EA, Kudelka AP. Discussing disease progression and end-of-life decisions. Oncology 13:1021–1031, 1999.

63. Larson DG, Tobin DR. End-of-life conversations: evolving practice and theory. JAMA 284:1573–1578, 2000.

64. Lo B, Quill T, Tulsky J. Discussing palliative care with patients. Ann Intern Med 130:744–749, 1999.

65. Parle M, Maguire P, Heaven C. The development of a training model to improve health professionals' skills, self-efficacy and outcome expectancies when communicating with cancer patients. Soc Sci Med 44:231–240, 1997.

66. von Gunten CF, Ferris FD, Emanuel LL. The patient–physician relationship. Ensuring competency in end-of-life care: communication and relational skills. JAMA 284:3051–3057, 2000.

67. Sell L, Devlin B, Bourke SJ, Munro NC, Corris PA, Gibson GJ. Communicating the diagnosis of lung cancer. Respir Med 87:61–63, 1993.

68. Levinson W, Gorawara-Bhat R, Lamb J. A study of patient clues and physician responses in primary care and surgical settings. JAMA 284:1021–1027, 2000.

69. Mishler EG. The Discourse of Medicine: Dialectics of Medical Interviews. Norwood, NJ, Aplex, 1984.

70. Suchman AL, Markakis K, Beckman HB, Frankel R. A model of empathic communication in the medical interview. JAMA 277:678–682, 1997.

71. Spiro HM. What is empathy and can it be taught? In: Spiro HM (Ed.). Empathy and Practice of Medicine: Beyond Pills and the Scalpel. New Haven, Yale University Press, pp. 7–14, 1993.

72. Smith RC, Hoppe RB. The patient's story: integrating the patient- and physician-centered approaches to interviewing. Ann Intern Med 115:470–477, 1991.

73. Christakis NA. Death Foretold: Prophecy and Prognosis in Medical Care. Chicago, University of Chicago Press, 2000.

74. Delvecchio MJ, Good BJ, Schaffer C, Lind SE. American oncology and the discourse on hope. Cult Med Psychiatry 14:59–79, 1990.

75. Herth K. Fostering hope in terminally-ill people. J Adv Nurs 15:1250–1259, 1990.

76. Koopmeiners L, Post-White J, Gutknecht S, et al. How healthcare professionals contribute to hope in patients with cancer. Oncol Nurs Forum 24:1507–1513, 1997.

77. Lamont EB, Christakis NA. Prognostic disclosure to patients with cancer near the end of life. Ann Intern Med 134:1096–1105, 2001.

78. Murphy DJ, Burrows D, Santilli S, et al. The influence of the probability of survival on patients' preferences regarding cardiopulmonary resuscitation. N Engl J Med 330:545–549, 1994.

79. Weeks JC, Cook EF, O'Day SJ, et al. Relationship between cancer patients' predictions of prognosis and their treatment preferences. JAMA 279:1709–1714, 1998.

80. Kreitler S. Denial in cancer patients. Cancer Invest 17:514–534, 1999.

81. Fischer GS, Tulsky JA, Arnold RM. Communicating a poor prognosis. In: Portenoy RK, Bruera E (Eds.). Topics in Palliative Care, vol 4. New York, Oxford University Press, 2000. pp. 75–91.

82. Carnes JW, Brownlee HJ Jr. The disclosure of the diagnosis of cancer. Med Clin North Am 80:145–151, 1996.

83. Buckman R. Breaking bad news: why is it still so difficult? BMJ 288:1597–1599, 1984.

84. Singer PA, Martin DK, Lavery JV, Thiel EC, Kelner M, Mendelssohn DC. Reconceptualizing advance care planning from the patient's perspective. Arch Intern Med 158:879–884, 1998.

85. Tulsky JA, Chesney MA, Bernard L. See one, do one, teach one?—House staff experience discussing do-not-resuscitate orders. Arch Intern Med 156:1285–1289, 1996.

86. Fischer GS, Arnold RM, Tulsky JA. Talking to the older adult about advance directives. Clin Geriatr Med 16:239–254, 2000.

87. Teno JM, Lynn J. Putting advance-care planning into action. J Clin Ethics 7:205–213, 1996.

88. Frankl D, Oye RK, Bellamy PE. Attitudes of hospitalized patient toward life support: a survey of 200 medical inpatients. Am J Med 86:645–648, 1989.

89. Schonwetter RS, Walker RM, Kramer DR,

Robinson BE. Resuscitation decision making in the elderly: the value of outcome data. J Gen Intern Med 8:295–300, 1993.

90. Patrick DL, Starks HE, Cain KC, Uhlmann RF, Pearlman RA. Measuring preferences for health states worse than death. Med Decis Making 14:9–18, 1994.

91. Pearlman RA, Cain KC, Patrick DL, et al. Insights pertaining to patient assessments of states worse than death. J Clin Ethics 4:33–41, 1993.

92. Mazur DJ, Hickam DH. Patients' interpretations of probability terms [see comments]. J Gen Intern Med 6:237–240, 1991.

93. O'Connor AM. Effects of framing and level of probability on patients' preferences for cancer chemotherapy. J Clin Epidemiol 42:119–126, 1989.

94. Woloshin KK, Ruffin MT, Gorenflo DW. Patients' interpretation of qualitative probability statements. Arch Fam Med 3:961–966, 1994.

95. Seckler AB, Meier DE, Mulvihill M, Paris BE. Substituted judgment: how accurate are proxy predictions? Ann Intern Med 115:92–98, 1991.

96. Sehgal A, Galbraith A, Chesney M, Schoenfeld P, Charles G, Lo B. How strictly do dialysis patients want their advance directives followed? JAMA 267:59–63, 1992.

97. Quill TE, Arnold RM, Platt F. "I wish things were different": expressing wishes in response to loss, futility, and unrealistic hopes. Ann Intern Med 135(7):551–555, 2001.

98. Faulkner A. ABC of palliative care. Communication with patients, families, and other professionals. BMJ 316:130–132, 1998.

99. Casarett D, Kutner JS, Abrahm J, for the End-of-Life Care Consensus Panel. Life after death: a practical approach to grief and bereavement. Ann Intern Med 134:208–215, 2001.

100. Tulsky JA, Arnold RM. Communication at end of life. In: Berger AM, Portenoy RK, Weissman DE (Eds.). Principles and Practice of Palliative Care and Supportive Oncology, 2nd ed. Philadelphia, Lipincott Williams & Wilkins, pp. 673–684, 2002.

101. Tulsky JA. Doctor–patient communication issues. In: Cassell C, Leipzig RM, Cohen HJ, Larson EB, Meier DE, Capello CF (Eds.). Geriatric Medicine, 4th ed. New York, Springer-Verlag (in press).

23

Decision Making for the Cognitively Impaired

TIMOTHY E. QUILL AND ROBERT McCANN

My (TQ) father-in-law's illness with Alzheimer's disease started slowly and subtly, as we didn't recognize the warning signs for several years. Once recognized, his condition continued for 4 years of progressive disability and dependence before he died of pneumonia at age 89 with less than optimal palliation of his symptoms. Had we known the course that his illness would take, we might not have treated several earlier infections. However, the illness progressed slowly, and no catastrophic event occurred where the invasive treatments that we knew he did not want could have been forgone. Although his former self would have been appalled by his deteriorated condition over the last 2 years of his life, he remained pleasant and cooperative even when he could no longer talk, manage any of his activities of daily living, or make decisions about his medical care. How should we make decisions for him, and what ethical and legal issues need to be considered?

Because of improvements in public health and increasing medical abilities to diagnose and treat many formerly fatal illnesses, women in the United States can now expect to live into their mid-80s and men into their late 70s. The hope of this progress was that healthy life would be prolonged considerably, the period of morbidity before death would be compressed and carefully palliated, and death would come in a timely and peaceful way.[1] Unfortunately, this is often not the case. Many patients with chronic illness experience extended periods of chronic illness and dependence as they near the end of their lives. To make matters even more complex, many patients lose the ability to speak for themselves as death approaches. Table 23–1 illustrates the percentage of patients with declining decision-making capacity as death approaches.[2] Patients with Alzheimer's disease have severely impaired mental capacity 1 year prior to death and show a sharp decline over their final year. It therefore behooves physicians to elicit patient values while they have mental capacity intact, knowing that a substantial number will lose that capacity prior to dying.

In the 20% of such incapacitated patients with advance directives (ADs), the documents often guide the most invasive of

Table 23–1. Intact Decision-Making Capacity Prior to Death in the Elderly (%)

Diseases other than Alzheimer's
   1 year = 87% (intact)
   1 month = 78%
   1 day = 51%
Alzheimer's disease
   1 year = 39% (Intact)
   1 month = 24%
   1 day = 8%

Source: Lentzer.[2]

treatments. However, ADs frequently provide little useful information about less invasive but commonly occurring treatments, such as artificial nutrition, hydration, or the use of antibiotics. In the setting of uncertainty about the patient's wishes, the default approach is often to provide all treatments that have not been explicitly refused. Unfortunately, there is always some uncertainty about what an incapacitated patient would want.

CAPACITY, COMPETENCE, AND SURROGATE DECISION MAKERS

My father-in-law lost his capacity to do things gradually in progressive steps over time rather than with an abrupt event. First to go was his ability to balance the checkbook, a distressing turn for this fastidious former banker and investor. He then started getting lost while driving his car, so we had the painful task of taking his keys away. Yet at that time he was still capable of participating in most medical decisions. When he became septic after an incontinence evaluation, he was willing to go to the hospital to receive antibiotics if that was needed to prolong his life. Once in the hospital, he became very confused and at times psychotic, and my wife as his health-care proxy asked that a do-not-resuscitate (DNR) order be issued based on his AD and on his clinical condition. He recovered in a more deteriorated condition than prior to admission, and we subsequently did not involve him in medical decision making as he showed no interest and it seemed cruel to have him struggle with issues that he could not adequately comprehend.

The definition of *capacity* to make medical decisions is narrow and clinical. It refers to

the ability to comprehend and participate in decision making about the particular medical question at hand. Thus, the inability to balance the checkbook or drive a car has no bearing on this question. My father-in-law's capacity to make the decision to go to the hospital was somewhat uncertain. He was clearly not prepared to stay home and risk dying from a potentially treatable illness; it was unclear whether he realized how difficult the hospitalization could be or that he might emerge from the hospitalization much more debilitated than he was when he went in. In circumstances where capacity is uncertain, decisions should usually be made jointly by the surrogate decision makers, the patient, and physician.

Capacity is assessed by the clinicians caring for the patient and is decision-specific, focused on understanding the particular clinical question and its implications. If there is uncertainty about the patient's ability to make a decision or if the decision seems inconsistent with past patient values, it may be useful to have a mental health professional assess the patient. This is particularly important if there is an associated mental illness or a potentially distorting role of depression, anxiety, or delirium. However, mental health consultation is not a legal or ethical requirement for less complex decisions. *Competence* is a legal determination made in the courts, particularly around the ability of a person to manage his or her funds. Thus, a person may be deemed incompetent to manage funds but have the capacity to make some medical decisions. However, many people who are not competent to manage their financial affairs also lack the capacity to make medical decisions. While the terms are often used interchangeably, we usually refer to capacity when deciding whether a person understands the pertinent issues around medical therapies. Assessing competence through the courts is usually too time-consuming to be helpful in immediate life-and-death medical crises, but it is occasionally necessary when conflicts are not resolvable through consensus building or with the help of mental health and ethics consultations.

Table 23–2. Decision-Making Hierarchy

Patient with capacity
Advance directive
Health-care proxy
Living will
Substituted judgment
Best interests

An agreed-upon hierarchy for surrogate decision making is outlined in Table 23–2.[3] The patient with full mental capacity clearly heads the list. His or her immediate wishes based on fully informed consent should guide treatment whenever possible. *Advance directives* are written or oral declarations made by the patient when he or she had capacity. They are invoked when the patient has lost the capacity to make medical decisions as determined by the physician. Health-care proxies and living wills are two types of written advance directives. In a health-care proxy form, a patient names a health-care agent who presumably understands the patient's values to make medical decisions for him or her should he or she lose capacity. The health-care agent's job is to represent the patient using the patient's values as much as possible. The living will may give guidance about the patient's overall philosophy but may or may not directly address the patient's specific dilemma. These documents are useful if they provide a clear idea of a patient's values and are specific enough to address the present situation and guide therapy. Unfortunately, many advance directives are not specific enough and, therefore of limited help.

If there is no advance directive, or the directive is not specific enough to guide therapy, then the persons closest to the patient must use substituted judgment to try to represent the patient by making decisions as they believe the patient would. Substituted judgment is an inexact science, for one can never know with certainty what a patient would want under particular circumstances. However, previous statements made by the patient illustrating his or her values along with prior experiences with se-rious illness and death can be helpful in judging whether he or she would want medical therapy aimed at life prolongation. If prior statements by the patient indicate that he or she conceived his or her quality of life to be poor, then a care plan aimed at palliation rather than life prolongation is most appropriate. However, if the quality of life prior to a sentinel event was very good, a trial of aggressive therapy aimed at life prolongation is what many people would choose. In substituted judgment, it is important that the person(s) speaking on the patient's behalf represents what the patient would want even though it may not be what he or she might want for him- or herself or for the patient. When choosing a health-care agent, a patient should convey the circumstances where life might not be worth living and make sure the proxy will be able to represent his or her wishes.

If nothing is known about the patient's wishes and values around a particular circumstance, then decision makers are left with trying to do what they believe is in the patient's "best interests." Here, the shift is away from the patient's personal values, which are unknown, and toward doing what those caring for the patient think is the best thing to do. In these instances, we are attempting to judge how the average person would balance the benefits and burdens of various treatment alternatives. There may be considerable difference of opinion about this question; the values of the caregivers may not be homogeneous, yet they must still struggle with the question.

Finally, there are three special circumstances where legal involvement may be necessary. First, incapacitated patients who have no family or friends to represent them and whose wishes and values are unknown should be assigned a court-appointed guardian to represent their best interests and ensure a dialogue with the health-care providers. Assigning a guardian can take several weeks to months, which makes this process challenging if immediate life-and-death decisions must be faced. In general, while the process is initiated, life-prolonging therapies should be continued unless they are near futile. Second, patients who have never had decision-making capacity should be represented by their families if they are actively involved in their care or by court-appointed guardians if there is no family to speak for them. Here, best interests must be used to guide therapeutic choices as the patients never had the capacity to complete an advance directive or to make statements allowing substituted judgment. Making judgments on the quality of life of such patients is very difficult. Their day-to-day caregivers can often give valuable insight into these judgments. Finally, where there is major concern about whether family members are representing the patient's best interests and this conflict of interest is unresolvable, the courts may be asked to intervene and name an independent guardian. With careful consensus building based on the patient's values, such referrals should be infrequent.

CHALLENGES OF SURROGATE DECISION MAKING

How would my father-in-law have viewed his quality of life as his condition deteriorated? The answer to that question would depend in no small measure on whether one was taking his perspective from before he was afflicted with Alzheimer's disease or after he was transformed by his illness. From the former perspective, there is little doubt in the mind of any family member that he would rather be dead than forced to live in diapers, incapable of speech, unable to get out of bed without two people assisting him, and unable to feed himself. Yet from the unknowable vantage point of the present, he did not appear uncomfortable or anguished most of the time, and he passively assented to each new potential indignity with equanimity and almost cheerfulness. There were rare moments when he would say how much he hated his current existence, but there was no sense that he was in any way prepared for, much less yearning for, death. In fact, other than completing an advance directive many years previously, my father-in-law preferred not to discuss end-of-life issues, and he seemed as afraid of death as he was afraid of suffering. It was in this context that we had to engage in substituted judgment decision making.

Quality of life and degree of suffering are difficult to define precisely, in part because they contain both objective and subjective elements.[4] The lack of evidence of outward physical suffering may not constitute a high quality of life for a given person. Activities of daily living can be measured and described, as can scales of performance and function; but again, how acceptable such losses of ability are to particular persons can only be understood by asking them. Circumstances that healthy individuals feel would make life not worth living (such as being quadriplegic or ventilator-dependent) may become acceptable when one is forced to live with such losses and the only alternative is death. However, we cannot abrogate the responsibility of addressing quality of life and suffering issues for incapacitated patients because of uncertainty about how they actually perceive their situation. The impact of such a strategy would be to discount the suffering of all incapacitated patients because it cannot be fully verified. This would violate a central norm of medicine, to do our best to understand and relieve human suffering.

Research about surrogate decision makers' ability to make decisions as the patient would based on hypothetical scenarios shows that there are inaccuracies.[5] In fact, some family members over-ride previous wishes of patients even though the family would not want the same therapies for themselves.[6] Informed about these discrepancies, most patients would still empower family members to make decisions on their behalf. The more wide-ranging discussions that surrogate decision makers and patients have had about end-of-life possibilities in advance, the more able they will be to make difficult decisions that are likely to reflect the patient's particular world view (before becoming incapacitated). Surrogates need to be reminded that it is the patient's values they are supposed to be representing and not their own. When conflict arises within a family trying to exercise substituted judgment, primary data about prior patient statements should be sought. When a patient's wishes are known, surrogate decision makers should articulate those wishes as if the patient were representing him- or herself. Unfortunately, most patients have not explicitly chosen a surrogate, nor have they explicitly articulated their end-of-life philosophy. Some states have enacted laws that empower family members closest to the patient to be formally named surrogate decision makers in the absence of such directives. Most patients expect this to occur as close family members are in the best position to represent the patient's values and to create an appropriate dialogue with health-care providers. Although there is growing ethical consensus that this is an appropriate way to proceed in these uncertain circumstances, laws in some states (e.g., New York and Missouri) suggest that certain end-of-life decisions (e.g., not starting or stopping a feeding tube) cannot be made without explicit knowledge of the patient's wishes.

The states' rights to determine the level of "clear and convincing evidence" in these types of medical decision has been affirmed by the Supreme Court.[7] It is useful to know the laws in your particular state and to know that the courts want health-care providers and families generally to make these decisions as best they can despite the associated uncertainty.[8]

A CONSENSUS-BASED APPROACH

Although it was clear from his advance directive that my father-in-law would not want cardiopulmonary resuscitation, intubation, dialysis, or a feeding tube, there were a number of smaller decisions that had a bearing on the quality as well as the length of his life. Although we all agreed that he would have been spared a lot of indignity and suffering if he had died with his initial episode of sepsis, neither he nor we as his surrogate decision makers were prepared to let him die at that point. Yet as he deteriorated further, a similar trip to the hospital would have been unacceptable from our point of view. Unlike the dying cancer patient, beyond a basic home DNR order, there was no clear contingency plan for such emergencies. My father-in-law developed an episode of celluli-

tis, which was treated with oral antibiotics and dressing changes, and an episode of bronchitis, which was also treated with oral antibiotics. Neither of these illnesses seemed severe enough to end his life, and both untreated would have been associated with considerable suffering. Although it seemed appropriate to treat, such simple treatments also probably prolonged his life and the associated suffering. We were not offered (nor did we consider) alternatives such as narcotics aimed primarily at palliation of symptoms. When he was incapable of speech, transfers, toileting, and feeding himself, we chose to discontinue all medicines not related to immediate comfort, though this too did not seem to alter the quality or length of his shrinking life. In making each of these decisions, we would speak together as a family about what seemed to be the best thing to do and then discuss it with his physician, who would generally concur. Unfortunately, there was not a template or guidelines for us to follow. It seemed as if we were operating in a vacuum.

In this setting, there was total agreement about trying to protect my father-in-law's quality of life, but there was considerable uncertainty about the proper course. When the patient's advance directives (both formal and informal) are not clarifying or nonexistent and medical and palliative care guidelines are unclear, a consensus-based approach among those who care for the patient is appropriate.[9] Close family members, professional and non-professional caregivers, as well as physicians and other members of the health-care team who know the patient should be consulted and involved. When there is conflict about how to proceed, a mediated session where everyone is allowed to express their views about the proper course and an effort to find common ground with a central focus on what is known about the patient's values and wishes is appropriate. The patient's previously expressed values, when known, should be the "template" for discussions using substituted judgment. When the patient's values are not known, we need to estimate an "average person's" values and how "most people might want to be treated" in the present situation (i.e., best interests).

Physicians have the potential to overpower or underpower their roles in these discussions. In particular, they need to actively use their knowledge about medical care and palliative care, as well as about the patient's wishes, to guide the process. Simply providing options to families without any direction is just as unacceptable as imposing an approach that does not have what is known about the particular patient's values and wishes at its center.[10] If decisions are very difficult for families to make despite reasonably clear evidence about the patient's wishes (e.g., stopping a ventilator or feeding tube that a patient clearly would not want), the physician should clearly recommend that course based on the patient's wishes and ask for the family to passively assent rather than forcing them to take full responsibility for the decision. An eye should always be kept on easing the grief and bereavement of family members when possible by facilitating a consensus discussion that keeps the patient's values and statements at its core. This can dramatically ease the perceived burden of the family and the pretense that family and physician have ultimate control over life and death.

Most advance directive documents address the major invasive treatments, such as cardiopulmonary resuscitation, dialysis, and other "extraordinary" treatments; but they do not address other potentially life-prolonging treatments, such as antibiotics or chronic disease-directed medications that have the potential to prolong life or prolong dying. It is impossible to anticipate all of the possible treatments that may be relevant in this regard, for one does not know in advance which treatments might meet a patient's goals at different points in the illness trajectory. Thus, early in a patient's illness, when quality of life is still relatively good, it may make sense to continue noninvasive chronic treatments and to add basic antibiotics for infections. Later, as debility and associated suffering increase, those same treatments might be stopped and a new infection might be treated with symptom palliation rather than antibiotics. Figure 23–1 schematically illustrates this trade-off and shows how palliation can become the predominant objective as death approaches and quality of life deteriorates.

The question of artificial hydration and nutrition deserves special consideration, in part because of the special societal meanings attached to *feeding* and *starvation* and in part because this treatment is considered separately by law in some states in comparison to other life-sustaining therapies. There are two main ways in which this treatment is used: *(1)* to temporarily sustain someone who is going through an acute illness but may regain the ability to

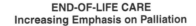

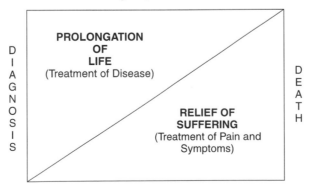

Figure 23–1. Balance of palliative care and disease-directed care.

eat and drink independently when he or she recovers and *(2)* to sustain someone who has permanently lost the ability to eat and drink from the progression of the underlying condition. Many times it is unclear whether a feeding tube will be of more benefit or burden to a patient after it is initiated, so the possibility of a time-limited clinical trial, which can be stopped if it becomes overly burdensome, is important. Feeding tubes are sometimes used to try to prevent aspiration pneumonia, though there are no data supporting the notion that feeding tubes prevent the aspiration of oral or gastric secretions.[11] There is controversy about how much suffering is associated with dying from not eating and drinking, though limited data derived from cancer patients suggest that associated symptoms can be relatively easily palliated with good mouth and skin care.[12] While the laws in New York and Missouri require a relatively high standard of knowledge about a patient's specific wishes with regard to stopping or not starting artificial hydration and nutrition, most states treat it like any other life-sustaining therapy that surrogate decision makers would have the right to consent to or refuse on the patient's behalf.[8] Because of this legal uncertainty and the potential clinical and psychological importance of the decision, many advance directive forms prompt patients to make their wishes known about this particular treatment.

In addition to making the patient's wishes known about particular treatments in advance, many nursing facilities and home care agencies are now asking patients and their families their wishes about where and how to be treated. Thus, in addition to the decision about attempting cardiopulmonary resuscitation, patients and their surrogate decision makers might be asked if the patient wants to go to the hospital for treatment of acute illnesses or to accept only those treatments that can be made available at home or in the nursing facility (e.g., antibiotics and intravenous fluids). For those who choose not to go to the hospital, decisions might be made in advance about whether they want treatment for

acute illnesses that can be relatively easily reversed (infections, temporary dehydration) at their current setting, if possible, or if they want a more purely comfort-oriented approach, where the primary treatment would be symptom palliation. It is desirable to document more detailed directives to guide therapy should the patient experience sentinel events. Table 23–3 represents such a document, which might be used by a nursing home to help guide therapy and keep track of patient wishes. Such documents are particularly useful in the off-hours and on weekends, when persons caring for a patient may have no knowledge of his or her wishes and values.

PALLIATIVE CARE AND HOSPICE FOR INCAPACITATED PATIENTS

As my father-in-law became more and more debilitated from the slow but relentless progression of his Alzheimer's disease, he and we as a family clearly could have benefited from an intensive palliative care program such as hospice. He did not meet the requirement of being likely to die within 6 months, even though in all other aspects he would have qualified and benefited from the program. Instead, we paid for aide services each day to supplement the care that his wife and daughter could provide since he required total care with all of his activities of daily living. Fortunately, we had resources to pay for such expensive care. He had no acute needs that Medicare would pay for, and there were no associated formal programs to help the

Table 23–3. Nursing Home Levels of Care

1. Hospitalize with no restrictions on care
2. Hospitalize with do-not-resuscitate order
3. Hospitalize only for readily reversible illnesses (i.e., fracture, infection)
4. Do not hospitalize but provide all available medical treatments available at nursing home
5. Do not hospitalize and direct all medical interventions toward providing comfort and not at life prolongation. Artificial Feeding is:
   a. Not to be used under any circumstance
   b. To be used short term or while prognosis is in doubt
   c. To be used indefinitely if unable to eat and drink

family cope with the loss of the man they knew and with the demands of his daily care. When it finally took two additional persons to do any transfers or toileting, we reluctantly admitted him to a skilled nursing facility for additional help. We all knew that, when competent, he would clearly say that he would rather be dead than in a nursing facility, but in his current condition, he couldn't say "no;" he seemed sad but not devastated by the transfer. As a family, we certainly felt we had let him down; but from a practical point of view, we had no choice.

Once in the nursing facility, he continued his slow decline. He would smile during my wife's daily visits and passively allow himself to be fed and cleaned up after soiling himself. On very rare occasions, he would have a moment of lucidity where he would let it be known how hard this all was, but most of the time his inner experience was totally unknown to us. All of his medicines were stopped, and we made a decision that he would not go back to the hospital and that we would pursue a purely comfort-oriented approach.

Several months later, he developed an acute respiratory infection. We discussed the situation with his doctor and agreed not to treat with antibiotics. He was fully alert at first and had a tremendous amount of secretions that he could not handle. Over the next week, he gradually got sicker, with increasing shortness of breath and hard-to-manage secretions. Many on the staff were uncomfortable with our nontreatment decision. His suffering from untreated infectious symptoms was increasing, and it was pathetic to see him dying in this way. After a sleepless night, my wife and I decided that it made sense to more aggressively palliate his shortness of breath and congestion with sedation (as we would have days before if he were dying with cancer but did not because the disease was Alzheimer's). We made plans to visit with his doctor that day to make a more humane plan but received a call before the appointment that my father-in-law had died. Once again, it felt as if we had let him down.

Once a person loses the ability to speak for him- or herself, palliative care should become a central element in the treatment plan. Since the patient can no longer represent her- or himself, we should always try to address and maximize quality-of-life issues on their behalf. Addressing pain and suffering and trying to represent the patient's values as much as possible based on past statements, documents, and behavior is at the core of treatment. Of course, as illustrated in Figure 23–1, this approach in no way precludes the provision of disease-directed, life-prolonging therapy, especially if the patient's quality of life remains good (given what is known of the patient's values) and the treatments do not entail considerable additional suffering. However, as death approaches and/or suffering increases, palliation becomes the predominant objective for most patients and families.

Unfortunately, most patients with Alzheimer's disease have too long and uncertain a prognosis to qualify for Medicare-certified hospice programs, but this should not preclude the provision of hospice-like care devoted to enhancing quality of life as a part of nursing facilities' and home-care agencies' plan of care. Model programs have been developed where symptoms are aggressively treated, quality-of-life issues are extensively discussed, planning is done about the appropriateness of hospitalization, and end-of-life issues are openly explored. The purpose of these programs is to enhance the patient's quality of life and to keep the patient's own values as our guide in balancing palliative care with care aimed at life prolongation. Preliminary data suggest better satisfaction, better symptom palliation, less hospitalization, and no change in length of life when such programs are compared with usual care.[13]

Finally, when incapacitated patients are near death and a decision is made not to treat infections or any other life-threatening illnesses, a clear plan of aggressive palliation must be made. Like any other medical care plan, it needs to be evaluated frequently and altered as required. It should make no difference if the patient is dying from Alzheimer's or advanced cancer, though in the former case, the family will almost always have to consent on the patient's behalf. Several last-resort treatments are available to incapacitated patients for severe terminal symptoms.[14,15] If the predominant symptom is pain, analgesic doses can be increased until the patient is out of pain or sedated and then maintained at that level. If the patient is on life-sustaining therapy, perhaps started at another time when quality of life was better, such treatment can be stopped if the consensus is that the patient would not want it under the circumstances. Finally, if symptoms become severe and cannot be relieved any other way (as was the case with my father-in-law), sedation can be provided, where the patient is sedated until he appears comfortable. Artificial hydration and nutrition do not enhance comfort at this stage and may actually cause discomfort by increasing oral secretions, leading to respiratory distress and the need for suctioning. The purpose of sedation is to relieve suffering, so it is fully consistent with the fundamental ethos of the medical profession (and with the doctrine of double effect); then, no life-prolonging therapies are initiated.[16]

CONCLUSION

Those who care for incapacitated patients have an important and difficult job. These patients are vulnerable and sick and cannot speak for themselves. The medical task is to enhance the quality and meaning of their lives and to try to give them a central voice in balancing disease-driven and palliative treatments by keeping what is known about their values and wishes at the center of clinical decision making. Alleviating discomfort and avoiding harm are imperative. It is a challenging and uncertain process, so every effort should be made to achieve a consensus among those who care about the patient on the proper course of action. The Quinlan court[17] perhaps put it best: "if [the patient] could wake up and fully comprehend [his or her] condition, and then had to return to it, what would [he or she] tell you to do?" Our severely ill, incapacitated patients are counting on us not to walk away from this challenge.

REFERENCES

1. Fries JF. Aging, natural death, and the compression of morbidity. N Engl J Med 303:130–135, 1980.
2. Lentzer HR, Pamuk ER, Rhodenhiser EP, et al. The quality of life in the year before death. Am J Public Health 82:1093–1098, 1992.
3. President's Commission for the Study of Ethical Problems in Medicine and Biomedical and Behavioral Research. Deciding to forego life-sustaining treatment: a report on the ethical, medical and legal issues in treatment decisions. Washington DC, United States Government Printing Office, 1983.
4. Morrison RS, Siu AL, Leipzig RM, Cassel CK, Meier DE. The hard task of improving quality of care at the end of life. Arch Intern Med 160:743–747, 2000.
5. Sulmasy DP, Terry PB, Weisman CS, Miller DJ, Stallings RY, Stallings RY. The accuracy of substituted judgments in patients with terminal diagnoses. Ann Intern Med 128:621–629, 1998.
6. Sonnenblick M, Friedlander Y, Steinberg A. Dissociation between wishes of terminally ill patients and decisions by their offspring. J Am Geriatr Soc 41:599–604, 1993.
7. Lovejoy F. Nancy Cruzan and the right to die. N Engl J Med 323:670–673, 1990.
8. Meisel A, Snyder L, Quill TE. Seven legal barriers to end-of-life care: myths, realities and grains of truth. JAMA 284:2495–2501, 2000.
9. Karlawish JH, Quill TE, Meier DE. A consensus-based approach to providing palliative care to patients who lack decision-making capacity. ACP-ASIM End-of-Life Care Consensus Panel. Ann Intern Med 130:835–840, 1999.
10. Quill TE, Brody H. Physician recommendations and patient autonomy: finding a balance between physician power and patient choice. Ann Intern Med 125:763–769, 1996.
11. Finucane TE, Bynum JP. Use of feeding tube to prevent aspiration pneumonia. Lancet 348:1421–1424, 1996.
12. McCann TM, Hall WJ, Groth-Juncker A. Comfort care for terminally ill patients: the appropriate use of nutrition and hydration. JAMA 272:1263–1266, 1994.
13. Ahronheim JC, Morrison RS, Morris J, Baskin-Lyons S, Meier DE. Palliative care in advanced dementia: a randomized controlled trial and descriptive analysis. J Palliat Med 3:265–273, 2000.
14. Quill TE, Lo B, Brock DW. Palliative options of last resort: a comparison of volun-

tarily stopping eating and drinking, terminal sedation, physician-assisted suicide, and voluntary active euthanasia. JAMA 278: 2099–2104, 1997.

15. Quill TE, Coombs-Lee B, Nunn S, for the University of Pennsylvania Center for Bioethics Assisted Suicide Consensus Panel. Palliative treatments of last resort: choosing the least harmful alternative. Ann Intern Med 132:488–493, 2000.

16. Quill TE, Byock I, for the ACP-ASIM End-of-Life Care Consensus Panel. Responding to terminal suffering: the role of terminal sedation and voluntary refusal of food and fluids. Ann Intern Med 132:408–414, 2000.

17. Quinlan, In re, 137 N.J. Super. 227, 348 A. 2d 801 (Ch. Div., 1975), rev'd, 70 N.J. 10, 355 A. 2d 647, cert. denied sub nom. Garger v. New Jersey, 429 U.S. 922, 50 L. Ed. 2d 289, 97 S. Ct. 319 (1976) overruled in part, In re Conroy, 98 N.J. 321, 486 A. 2d 1209 (1985). 2000.

V

STRUCTURES OF CARE FOR THE CHRONICALLY ILL WITH PALLIATIVE CARE NEEDS

24

Can We Make the Health-Care System Work?

JANICE LYNCH SCHUSTER, SARAH MYERS, SUSAN K. ROGERS,
SUSAN C. EMMER, AND JOANNE LYNN

Ordinary Americans are likely to have a healthy start in life and to be protected from occupational, reproductive, and infectious diseases that once cut many lives short. Indeed, most will grow old and will generally be healthy for most of their years. However, potential disaster awaits many Americans at the end of life: unrelieved pain and other symptoms, indignities and powerlessness, impoverishment and family burden, and quite simply a care system that repeatedly makes serious errors and abrogates the human experience of coming to the end of life. It is true that not all people have a very difficult course at the end of life, but many do; thus, all are scared, often more scared of the uncertainties of the "care" system than of dying itself, and many have no idea what to expect: the average American knows very little about the long course of living with a fatal, chronic disease, a very different death from the sudden, swift one that tends to be prominent in the American media.

One of the most urgent problems in this arena is that no one can count on good end-of-life care; the health-care system is, in fact, a jumble of services, programs, and providers connected primarily by an array of financial mechanisms, including Medicare, Medicaid, and private insurance plans. To individuals who have a serious and life-limiting illness and their families, this jumble can be as overwhelming and frightening as the illness itself. Americans facing serious and progressive illness are easily lost in a care system that does not meet their needs or even make good sense. When they need a wheelchair, they can get only surgery. When they need a home health aide, they can get only emergency room services. No policy makers have set about designing the care system that is needed for those with long-term serious illness. Instead, patients must piece together a patchwork based on services that were designed for another purpose (e.g., acute care) or developed to cope with some overwhelming public health need. Thus, heart failure patients can get pacemakers readily in a hospital service that can "do pacemakers" with alacrity. If they return to the same hospital for fatigue and shortness of breath, their needs for continuity of care, counsel, and empathy are met with pressures for rapid discharge and inattention to symptoms. Patients with dementia can easily get intravenous antibiotics and feeding tubes, but families may have to argue with health-care providers to obtain spoon feeding or guarantee a safe environment.

Clearly, the health-care system has often failed to address the physical suffering associated with the end of life. Equally troubling, to patients and families, is its failure to address the emotional and social consequences people face when dealing with chronic, disabling disease. Serious, chronic illness at the end of life is a major cause of financial disaster among Americans. Nearly one-half of all U.S. bankruptcy filings by individuals over the age of 65 were attributed to medical reasons.[1] Middle-aged family members face the emotional and financial burdens of being caregivers, an issue that will grow as baby boomers age.

Finally, as a result of demographic trends and the shortcomings of current payment mechanisms, overall health-care spending in the United States will increase over the coming decades from what are already startlingly high levels. Total U.S health expenditures reached $1.1 trillion by 1998, the last year for which these data are available.[2] Some have projected that by 2030 this number will top $16 trillion as the baby boomers reach their seventh and eighth decades.[3] The authors of one recent study estimated that "total expenditures from the age of 65 years until death increase substantially with longevity, from $31,181 (1996 dollars) for persons who die at the age of 65 years to more than $200,000 for those who die at the age of 90."[4] They estimated that between 2000 and 2015, there will be a 73% increase in combined expenditures for Medicare-covered services and nursing home care for the cohort of individuals who turn 65 in those years.

WHAT A GOOD CARE SYSTEM WOULD DO

In the last 5 years, many organizations nationwide have begun work to improve end-of-life care in thousands of hospitals, hospices, nursing homes, and private homes. Their endeavors have made a difference in the lives and deaths of hundreds of thousands of people. However, many of these groups work in isolation, sometimes in the same communities, without the benefit of coordinating programs and ideas. Their common discontent with the current state of affairs has been a critical step toward reforming the system, yet unhappiness alone will not engender lasting change. Improvement requires that several elements converge to create the energy for change: an image of what a better system would be, a will to overcome the barriers to achieving that system, the desire to learn a great deal about the care system and its society in the process, and an ability to take action to make improvement happen.

Many groups and organizations have released and endorsed statements describing the characteristics of good health care in general and end-of-life care in particular,[5-9] and these have, as one would expect, substantial areas of overlap. One particularly powerful idea is that the care system should be reliable and safe. In short, very sick people should not have to be afraid of their care system. What is it that people should be able to count on having? A patient who is seriously ill with an eventually fatal illness should be able to count on the care system that can make the promises described below. These are promises to be made to both patients and their families.[10]

MAKING PROMISES: A VISION OF A BETTER SYSTEM

There are a number of ways to construct a vision of a better care system. One way is to imagine a single health-care provider talking with a single sick and frightened patient. Imagine what that provider could promise in a care system that really worked the way it should. For patients with advanced stages of serious illness, it is just not possible to promise cure or restoration of health. What would matter to this patient? Here are seven promises that really seem to make a difference. In each case, we define the promise and its core statement and list a few examples of what it might mean for providers to put practices in place to deliver on that promise.

1. *Good medical treatment:* You will have the best of medical treatment, aiming to prevent exacerbation, improve function and survival, and ensure comfort.
   - Patients will be offered proven diagnosis and treatment strategies to prevent exacerbations and enhance quality of life as well as to delay disease progression and death.
   - Medical interventions will be in accord with the best available standards of medical practice and evidence-based when possible.

2. *Never overwhelmed by symptoms:* You will never have to endure overwhelming pain, shortness of breath, or other symptoms.
   - Symptoms will be anticipated and prevented when possible, evaluated and addressed promptly, and controlled effectively.
   - Severe symptoms, such as shortness of breath, will be treated as emergencies.
   - Sedation will be used when necessary to relieve intractable symptoms near the end of life.

3. *Continuity, coordination, and comprehensiveness:* Your care will be continuous, comprehensive, and coordinated.
   - Patients and families can count on certain professionals at all times.
   - Patients and families can count on an appropriate and timely response to their needs.
   - Transitions between services, settings, and personnel will be minimized in number and made to work smoothly.

4. *Well-prepared, no surprises:* You and your family will be prepared for everything that is likely to happen in the course of your illness.
   - Patients and families come to know what to expect as the illness worsens and what is expected of them.
   - Patients and families receive the supplies and training needed to handle predictable events.

5. *Customized care, reflecting your preferences:* Your wishes will be sought and respected and followed whenever possible.
   - Patients and families come to know the alternatives for services and expect to make choices that matter.
   - Patients never receive treatments they refuse.
   - Patients who want to live out the end of life at home usually can.

6. *Consideration for patient and family resources* (financial, emotional, and practical): We will help the patient and family to consider their personal and financial resources, and we will respect their choices about the use of their resources.
   - Patients and families will be aware of services available in their community and the costs of those services.
   - Family caregivers' concerns will be discussed. Respite, volunteer, and home aide care will be part of the care plan when appropriate.

7. *Make the best of every day:* We will do all we can to see that you and your family will have the opportunity to make the best of every day.
   - The patient is treated as a person, not a disease, and what is important to the patient is important to the care team.
   - The care team responds to the physical, psychological, social, and spiritual needs of the patient and family.
   - Families are supported before, during, and after the patient's death.

Beyond giving patients a "Good Housekeeping" guarantee, what else would a good care system require? The following attributes, related to system function, may be essential:

- Built-in learning about the system function through improvement activities and monitoring

- Formal research on important questions of diagnosis, treatment, and service delivery
- Adaptation to cultural meanings for the cultures being served
- Ways to develop and support professional caregivers, especially those providing the most direct services
- Ways to develop and support nonprofessional caregivers, including community people who are neither relatives nor previously friends
- Social patterns and mechanisms that limit the use of high-cost, low-yield interventions
- Innovations, evaluation, and implementation of efficient, sustainable, and high-value strategies for care; re-engineering the care system
- A strong grounding in data, including a meaningful epidemiology of suffering in the population of interest

WHY DO WE NOT HAVE TRUSTWORTHY CARE AT THE END OF LIFE?

Undoubtedly, many factors affect the patterns of care that are now in place; many of these factors are barriers to rapid adaptation of essential reforms. Outlined below are some key factors that appear to sustain the system's current problems.

Absence of a Consensus on Clinical Policy

Although diverse groups have set forth guidelines for pain management,[11] disease management of various chronic illnesses,[12,13] and decision making, these guidelines are widely disregarded. In addition, important aspects of good end-of-life care have no articulated standards or policies. No authoritative body has declared that patients should always lie in a clean bed, that the dying should have company if they find human presence comforting, or that whenever a crisis or question occurs families should have ready access to a professional caregiver who knows their loved one's health situation. A major professional journal published stories in which a patient's serious pain at the end of life was tolerated and explained in a way intended to be sympathetic to the physician as well as a story that described a family providing care for a severely demented person who received neither help nor continuity of care.[14] This latter situation was considered to be an example of just ordinary care, rather than "a routinized, systematic failure to serve patients and families."[15] Those working in the field need to learn to take the time to label errors and shortcomings and to find ways to correct them.

Lack of Continuity and Coordination of Care

Patients at the end of life often become quickly caught up in a care system that is almost foreign to the one that they experienced as healthy people. They may no longer see their usual primary-care physician, and his or her replacement may not have the support needed to coordinate patient care that entails an array of specialists and agencies. The patient may be referred from one health-care provider to another, without the benefit of a common and accessible medical record. The fragmentation increases the possibility of medical errors, including failure to make or implement patients' advance planning decisions. Additionally, few health-care providers have the time, financial incentive, or education to create useful, ongoing, customized care plans for these patients. Therefore, the care they provide may be reactive and piecemeal, rather than part of a long-term, well-planned strategy to control symptoms, reduce hospitalizations, and improve quality of life.

An Inadequate Payment and Coverage System for Those with Serious, Eventually Fatal Illness

Currently, most public and private payers do not cover or pay well for appropriate care provided during the chronic phases of illness that many people at the end of life experience. Health insurance generally has no provision to encourage continuity of care, self-care education, family respite, multidisciplinary care, or quality improvement. Costly prescription medications and rehabilitation geared toward maintaining function are not covered. It is almost an exact mismatch of priorities: payers generally aim to ensure ready access to surgery, diagnostic procedures, and physician services, while the patients desperately need help with understanding prescriptions, getting medical equipment, and finding personal care services. They also need continuity, reliability, symptom control, human interaction and relationship, and family support.

A Lack of Focus on Palliative Care

Many dying patients experience pain,[16,17] depression,[18] and/or underutilization of pain medications and substandard detection or management of other symptoms,[17] despite the fact most health-care providers now know how to treat or manage many of the symptoms experienced by dying patients. The practices and procedures that might ensure the appropriate use of proven treatments are not often aggressively pursued. Where good palliative care is available, it is often provided only after a patient is labeled *terminally ill* and all curative measures are discontinued. However, some recent initiatives have aimed at moving palliative care "upstream," bringing good symptom relief to patients who are still undergoing treatment for what may or may not prove to be a fatal illness.[19] Perhaps most pervasively, we simply do not see dying as a long-term process.

A Lack of Focus on Advance Planning

American society is very willing to invest time and resources in heroic efforts at treatment and extending life. Too often, we do not plan for, or acknowledge, the fact that patients are seriously ill and are never again going to be well. Advance planning services[20] are still not widely or consistently available across large systems and communities. As a result, many patients miss a valuable opportunity to plan for the kind of life and death that they would prefer.

Given the opportunity, people could make the various other arrangements that would make it more likely to live how they wish in the relatively short amount of time that they have left. Because most people with chronic diseases have a course that is very difficult to predict, failure to begin advance planning early in the course of the disease can lead to hasty decisions under distress or treatment by routine. For example, physicians may misunderstand patient's preferences for the type of measures that they would like,[21] possibly leading to the use of unwanted treatments and procedures or the failure to make these measures available.

Without a common medical record or a standardized way to make patient decisions known to all providers, many patients will not be able to have their wishes honored by emergency room staff or other new health-care providers who care for them when they are unable to communicate.

Inadequate Provider Education

Far too little attention is given to training physicians and other health-care providers about end-of-life care before they enter practice.[9,22] The inclusion of relevant content within medical school curricula and medical and other health-care textbooks has been woefully inadequate.[23–26] Although several groundbreaking programs, such as the Education for Physicians on End-of-Life Care Project[27] and the End of Life Physician Education Resource Center,[28] are working to remedy this lack of training, much opportunity for improvement remains.

Inadequate Public Education and Engagement

Patients and their families have inadequate opportunity to learn what they need to know in order to demand the kind of end-of-life care they need and to expect no less. Although the relationship between physicians and other health-care providers and their patients has slowly become less paternalistic and more collegial, patients are still learning how to demand higher-quality information and care from their health-care providers. In addition, although numerous high-quality patient education materials related to health promotion and disease prevention are available, there is much less public information widely available related to living with serious, eventually fatal illness, including the physical and socioeconomic practicalities of dying.

THE DEMAND FOR A SINGLE CAUSE OF DEATH

Another barrier to crafting an improved care system is the widespread and over-simplified tendency to insist that there is exactly one cause of death for each patient. If someone has lived with heart disease for a very long time, the eventual death is likely to be labeled as a death from heart disease even if the actual event was precipitated by a combination of factors, as is often the case with older patients with complex health conditions. In reality, the death of many patients, especially frail elders who have had a chronic, eventually fatal illness, often follows a chain of events that includes complications and co-morbidities. The events that actually precipitated a death may not be listed as the actual cause, especially when the timing of death involved a decision to stop a life-sustaining treatment or a medical error. No standardized system allows us to describe the complex chain of circumstances leading to their death. Lacking this, it is difficult to make the health-care system optimally responsive to the complex needs of these patients.

Inexperience with Serious Illness and Death

American culture has kept serious long-term illness hidden away and has viewed death as something to be surmounted, rather than a normal, expected part of life.[25] As a result, many people first encounter these situations head-on when caring for aging parents and then have no real-life experience or models to use in dealing with them. Compounding this, our popular media generally fails to include stories of people living with serious and progressive disabilities and illnesses, instead focusing on more unlikely, sensationalistic stories of sudden death or of heroic cures for acute illness or injuries. This is unfortunate because Americans are paying close attention to the medical situations that they witness on television and may be misled about the typical outcomes of heroic procedures such as cardiopulmonary resuscitation in dying patients.[29]

Strong Political and Professional Forces Aim to Protect Status and Income

Although true, it is hard to voice concerns that those who are making money on the current system may oppose its reform. Hospice and home-care aides, as well as family caregivers, generally have low status and receive inadequate support and payment. Those who act on behalf of the status quo (including some hospitals, members of certain provider specialty groups, and others) tend to have higher status and substantial assets. Often, these people are trying to provide services in the current care system and are diligently doing the best they can. Therefore, it can be difficult for them to be open to change, especially when that change might greatly alter the conditions under which they work.

ENGINEERING REAL REFORMS

How will we achieve the monumental task of changing our ways of thinking about the end of life and of better organizing and financing the care provided to individuals with serious and complex illness? Some insights will still come from basic science research, e.g., through better medications and diagnostic tools. However, more pressing now is the need is to use what we already know about relieving suffering. Most people in pain today do not have to wait for a better drug to be developed; they just need someone to prescribe correctly what we already have. Persons who want to die at home need no new device; they just need the community to figure out how to get supportive services to them at home.

The change in the epidemiology of dying has not been sudden, but the health-care and social systems that care for the dying remain ill-prepared to address the challenges that it presents. Evidence from other areas of health care suggests that sweeping change is possible if high enough priority is given to the problem being addressed. For example, up to just a few decades ago, childbirth was a risky proposition for both mothers and babies. Now, childbirth has become routinely safer and more rewarding; deaths and morbidity associated with childbirth have become newsworthy, and people feel that they can count on coming out of the experience without serious error.

Just as new mothers used to be "lucky" if their experience with childbirth was relatively comfortable and free of complications, Americans feel lucky today if a loved one has a well-supported, relatively comfortable experience with death following a serious chronic disease. Although we have seen successful attempts at improving care for some dying patients during the past several decades, most notably through hospice, widespread reform remains elusive.

Despite barriers, improvements are happening. Almost all cancer patients with pain now receive opioids, most patients die without resuscitation, and hospices serve 15%[30] of those who die in Medicare.

The Center to Improve Care of the Dying and the Institute for Healthcare Improvement have shown that rapid-cycle quality improvement is remarkably effective in this arena.[31,32] Implementation of guidelines,[16] standardization of procedures,[33] and returning control to the team that is closest to the patient have been effective at improving patient care, and, in some cases, reducing costs to health care organizations.

To push ahead, we need broad innovation by the several different stakeholder groups involved as well as some careful evaluation of these efforts. The following section describes the role of each group or stakeholder and the part they can play in improving care.

Federal Policy Makers

Legislators, federal agency leaders, and others working in government should act upon the importance of gathering data that will help us understand the changing epidemiology of dying. While we have much anecdotal evidence suggesting that the end of life is anything but ideal for the majority of patients, anecdotal evidence alone does not justify budgetary and programmatic decisions. Studies aimed at gathering good data that describe and evaluate the experience of patients in different parts of the United States and from different socioeconomic backgrounds will provide a better understanding of those parts of the system most in need of reform and will illustrate the relative merits of current attributes of different ways of providing care. Such data would also teach us much about the financial, emotional, and other impacts of the dying process on patients' families and the opportunities for providing them with appropriate support throughout the process.

Policy makers are also in a unique position to take the lead in making change happen. They need to create and test reforms within Medicare and other federal health-care delivery systems and to disseminate information about programs that have already shown some success in federal agencies such as the Veterans Administration.

Federal Agencies

A new social contract for reforming end-of-life care will require a wider acknowledgment of more appropriate categories of "persons at the end of life," more reliable promises of effective care, and more efficient and sustainable arrangements for delivering and financing this care. Federal government entities will play a leading role in developing and carrying out this social contract. The Health Resources and Services Administration (HRSA), the Agency for Health Care Research and Quality (AHRQ), the Health Care Finance Administration (HCFA), the Medicare Payment Advisory Commission (MedPAC), and the National Institutes of Health (NIH) should pursue research and demonstrations aimed at learning how to engineer an effective, efficient care system for every patient who lives with serious, eventually fatal illness. Building on the kind of success that they showed in managing the Ryan White initiative to provide care for acquired immunodeficiency syndrome (AIDS), it is especially appealing to look to the HRSA to work on end-of-life care. In HRSA's hands, we could quickly learn to implement better care strategies and to build the power and skills that will be needed. Increased development and dissemination of public information from federal health agencies, including HRSA and the Centers for Disease Control and Prevention (CDC), could begin to raise public awareness of issues surrounding the end of life. The CDC, which includes among its pledges to "base all public health decisions on the highest quality scientific data, openly and objectively derived,"[34] is a logical leader in the funding and development of studies that explore the epidemiology of dying.

State Policy Makers

Much of end-of-life care depends on Medicaid, which is funded and administered at the state level. In addition, state regulations and arrangements can make good care more possible or more difficult. State policy akers thus have an important role to play in the innovation, evaluation, and implementation of practices that encourage good care.

Provider Organizations

Provider organizations and networks need to constantly improve the reliability and scope of their services, including relieving pain, making plans to avoid emergency responses to complications, and supporting family caregivers.[31] The most effective techniques are likely to be quality improvement (www.medicaring.org)[31,35,36] and increased acceptance of accountability.

Individual Providers

Individual providers serving those with eventually fatal illness must take the initiative to improve personal practices, such as learning how best to communicate with and support seriously ill patients and families over time,[37–39] how to make symptoms manageable,[40] and how to help patients live fully within the constraints imposed by dis-

ease.[41] They should do so not only because it is the right thing to do but also because purchasers of health care, their professional associations, and consumers will be monitoring their actions carefully when making decisions about receiving or paying for the care that they provide. Indeed, there is an excellent opportunity for positive change because many professional organizations have begun to develop standards related to the care provided at the end of life, and providers therefore have evolving new yardsticks by which to measure their technical competence, and compassion, in this area.

Public and Private Health-Care Purchasers

As a result of the demographic changes detailed above, over the next two decades, the number of persons eligible for Medicare who are also very sick will grow substantially. Their needs will severely strain our political and health-care systems. To avert a national health-care crisis, we must identify, design, build support for, and implement programs that insure appropriate care for persons with serious chronic illness. Medicare is a logical place to start. Medicare is a national program that can make appropriate care for most persons with serious chronic illness widely available by developing systems that can serve as models for programs offered by private and other federal buyers of health care. This year, approximately 40 million individuals are enrolled in Medicare,[42] and 83% of all Americans die while covered by Medicare,[30] with nearly 2 million beneficiaries dying each year.[43] Of that population group, 89% will die with at least one of five chronic diseases: heart disease, stroke, dementia, cancer, or lung disease.[30] The cost of care delivered during the last year of life comprises 28% of all Medicare costs.[4]

Both the Medicare program and private purchasers of health care must demand results from providers, including the availability of coordinated, comprehensive care for dying patients. They need to use their purchasing power to help improve the value and quality of care. They also need to advocate for improvements in the payment levels and job satisfaction of professional caregivers, of whom there are not nearly enough to meet the needs of the growing numbers of individuals nearing the end of life. Additionally, the Medicare program's existing efforts to improve beneficiary information could be expanded to address the issues surrounding serious chronic illness and end-of-life issues, such as advance care planning. Private purchasers should also hold providers accountable for making sure that their patients have adequate information about their choices for care at the end of life. In addition, employers, many of whom are also purchasers of health care, need to place a higher value on informal caregiving, including granting appropriate leave benefits to employees who must take time off to care for a dying family member.

Advocacy Groups

Advocacy groups that represent the issues most important to individuals at the end of life must take the lead in educating policy makers about the needs of patients and the type of care to which they are entitled, improving our understanding of the epidemiology of dying, and urging funding of studies that will further illuminate the experiences of patients near the end of life. It will be vital for these groups to work together in this effort, rather than tackling smaller aspects of the problem in a counterproductive fashion. The poor and disenfranchised are not politically powerful, and this is the situation in which many of the chronically ill find themselves. Advocacy groups need to fill this vacuum, while ensuring that they solicit the input of those whose interests they represent. Several different types of advocacy organization have a role to play as each has a unique focus and unique perspectives to bring to bear. These groups include those with a single disease focus that work on issues ranging from research funding to patient rights (e.g., the American Cancer Society), those representing particular types of health-care provider (e.g., the National Association for

Home Care), general senior citizen advocacy organizations (AARP and the National Senior Citizens Law Center), and others.

Media

The media (and those who influence the content that it produces) must become better aware of the new epidemiology of dying and its societal implications as it makes decisions about the way that it portrays death and dying patients. America as a nation is hungry for news and entertainment, and this is borne out in the amount of time the nation spends watching television and reading newspapers. Unfortunately, Americans' view of death and dying is largely shaped by their standard portrayals in the media. It is far more often that one witnesses cardiopulmonary resuscitation (which is successful far more often than it is in real life) on television than one does in reality. The swift, expected deaths of cancer patients, accident victims, and those who fall prey to "super-viruses" are given air time at the expense of more realistic portrayals of those suffering for a long time from organ system failures or dementia.

Clearly, consumer demand plays a vital role in shaping what the media choose to highlight. It may be time for those working in end-of-life care to turn their attention to studying the consumer–media interface, to identify the most appropriate targets for education and advocacy in this area.

Patients

We know that increased public involvement is possible. A promising new level of consumerism is evident in the health-care arena,[44] along with an increase in advocacy efforts directed at a number of diseases and conditions. Celebrities and other visible individuals whose lives have been touched by them have taken on the cause of many diseases that formerly received little publicity. Even the most rare diseases have their own advocacy groups and visible supporters demanding attention on Capitol Hill. Patients also need to begin to treat inadequate medical care with the same level of suspicion that they treat more obvious medical errors.

The disorganized care system that is available for those at the end of life is rife with the potential for errors, and the patients it serves are often preoccupied with the business of dying and unable to act as watchdogs for their own care.[36]

Finally, there are also several important steps that must be taken across this broad list of stakeholders. Any effort to improve chronic illness should start with innovation, investments in creative pilot programs that test new means of delivering care. Among other improvements, such programs would introduce substantial engagement of community resources, mobilization of patient/family self-care, enhancement of home-care services, deference to the authority of patient/family choice, and more effective coordination of Medicare and Medicaid.

Legislative action is essential. At the federal level, policy changes could focus on a coordinated, national effort to improve care for people with chronic illness. This program could include pilot projects that demonstrate innovative, effective means of delivering such care. Patients and families should have access to any and all necessary services at a cost they can afford and society is willing to pay. Federal entities have a role in meeting these needs. Congress could authorize funding in several areas:

- *Hospice.* Authorize the use of a severity criterion rather than prognosis, the 6-month rule that has contributed to decreased lengths of stay, encourage the Centers for Medicare and Medicaid Services (CMS) (formerly Health Care Financing Administration) to set more appropriate reimbursement rates
- *Centers of excellence.* Contract for one or two excellent providers (in an urban area) who guarantee continuity of care for patients with fatal chronic illness; track minimum performance criteria on patient education, follow-up, continuity, utilization, comfort, advance planning, and satisfaction
- *CMS and/or CMS/HRSA demonstrations.* Fund demonstrations to learn how to effectively and efficiently deliver good care to the chronically ill, how to pro-

vide and maintain continuity for this population, and at what payment rates and strategies; ultimately, a successful CMS demonstration could become a permanent Medicare program
- *Agency for Health Research & Quality demonstration/evaluation.* Develop methods of measurement, translation of findings into usual practice, and guidelines on care of this population
- *Quality improvement and regional initiatives.* Authorize a resource center to support widespread quality improvement in the coordination of care across programs, when patients need multiple programs over time.

The time has come to consider the merits of establishing a new category of illness, namely one that represents the type of "serious and complex" illness that is not well understood in the nation's largely black-and-white view of acute versus chronic illness. Without wider acknowledgment of the particular challenges of this type of illness that would accompany formalization of the terminology used to describe it, we will continue to be less than precise in our reform efforts.

Change is already seriously overdue. We have only a few decades before our problems become significantly more pronounced. Within the next decade, the first of the baby boomers will reach Medicare-eligible age, and the numbers of people who are very sick will continue to rise, with the 65-plus age group doubling over the next three decades.[45] If we continue to do no better than we do now, the suffering will be overwhelming and the costs crippling. If we learn to do better and to deploy our knowledge effectively, we could instead have an end of life that is comfortable and meaningful in a care system that is sustainable and cost-effective. These problems are not unique to the United States,[46] so we have an opportunity to set an example for other nation struggling with meeting the needs of their aging populations.

Significant and enduring improvement in care for persons with serious chronic illness requires leadership, analysis, and much hard work. Individuals and organizations must initiate substantial efforts to learn how to serve those coming to the end of life and to translate those lessons into policy. All of us have a stake in this, and all of us will reap the benefits of learning to do it right.

The number of individuals suffering from eventually fatal chronic illness is increasing rapidly, and the current piecemeal health-care system is not arranged or financed in a way that can adequately meet their needs. We have heard much about the strains that the baby boomer generation will place on different aspects of America's social and economic landscape, but in few areas will this be as apparent as the health-care system, especially those segments of the system most likely to be relied on to provide care for individuals and populations nearing the end of life.

We are now just beginning to learn how to arrange care to serve those with serious and eventually fatal conditions. Overwhelming discrepancies remain between the characteristics of the system that can deliver reliable care at the end of life (and that many Americans say they want) and the care system that we have today. More vigorous, and even risk-taking, efforts are needed to persuade individuals, organizations, and leaders from various sectors to translate these discrepancies into actions that will lead to sustainable changes within the health-care system.

ACKNOWLEDGMENTS

This chapter is adapted from a forthcoming report, by Dr. Joanne Lynn, to be copublished by Americans for Better Care of the Dying (ABCD) and the Milbank Memorial Fund. The entire report can be downloaded (www.milbank.org). Print copies may be ordered, free of charge, from ABCD at 202-895-2660 or via e-mail (info@abcd-caring.org) and from the fund at 212-355-8400 (mmf@milbank.org).

REFERENCES

1. Warren E, Sullivan T, Jacoby M. Medical problems and bankruptcy filings. Norton's Bankruptcy Advisor May 2000.

2. Health Care Financing Administration. Highlights—National health expenditures, 1998 (2000). Available at http://www.hcfa.gov/stats/nhe-oact/hilites.htm/

3. Burner ST, Waldo DR, McKusick DR. National health expenditures projections through 2030. Health Care Financ Rev 14:1–29, 1992.

4. Spillman BC, Lubitz, J. The effect of longevity on spending for acute and long-term care. N Engl J Med 342:1409–1415, 2000.

5. Agency for Healthcare Research and Quality. Clinical practice guidelines online. (2001) Available at http://www.ahrq.gov/clinic/cpgonline.htm

6. Last Acts Task Force. Precepts of Palliative Care. Princeton, NJ, Robert Wood Johnson Foundation. 1997.

7. Cassel CK, Foley KM. Principles for Care of Patients at the End of Life: An Emerging Consensus Among the Specialties of Medicine. New York, Milbank Memorial Fund, 1999.

8. Measuring quality of care at the end of life: a statement of principles. J Am Geriatr Soc 45:526–527, 1997.

9. Cassel CK, Field MJ (Eds.). Approaching Death: Improving Care at the End of Life. Washington DC, Institute of Medicine, 1997.

10. National Coalition for Health Care and The Institute for Healthcare Improvement. Promises to keep: changing the way we provide care at the end of life (2000). Available at http://www.nchc.org/EOL101200.pdf

11. Joint Commission on Accreditation of Healthcare Organizations. Joint Commission of Accreditation of Healthcare Organizations Pain standards for 2001 (2001). Available at http://www.jcaho.org/standards_frm.html

12. Robert Wood Johnson Foundation. Overview of the Chronic Care Model (2000). Available at http://www.improvingchronic-care.org/change/model/components.html

13. Sloss EM, Solomon DH, Shekelle PG, et al. Selecting target conditions for quality of care improvement in vulnerable older adults. J Am Geriatr Soc 48:363–369, 2000.

14. Loxterkamp D. Hearing voices. How should doctors respond to their calling? N Engl J Med 335:1991–1993, 1996.

15. Lynn J. Handling conflict in end of life care. JAMA 283:3199–3200, 2000.

16. Du Pen SL, Du Pen AR, Polissar N, Hansberry J, Kraybill BM, Stillman M, Panke J, Everly R, Syrjala K. Implementing guidelines for cancer pain management: results of a randomized controlled clinical trial. J Clin Oncol 17:361–370, 1999.

17. Portenoy RK, Lesage P. Management of cancer pain. Lancet 353:1695–1700, 1999.

18. Block SD. Assessing and managing depression in the terminally ill patient. ACP-ASIM

End-of-Life Care Consensus Panel. American College of Physicians, American Society of Internal Medicine. Ann Intern Med 132:209–218, 2000.

19. United Hospital Fund. Community oriented palliative care initiative (2000). Available at http://www.uhfnyc.org/

20. Hammes BJ, Rooney BL. Death and end of life planning in one midwestern community. Arch Intern Med 158:383–390, 1998.

21. Wenger NS, Phillips RS, Teno JM, et al. Physician understanding of patient resuscitation preferences: insights and clinical implications. J Am Geriatr Soc 48:S44–S51, 2000.

22. Billings JA, Block S. Palliative care in undergraduate medical education. Status report and future directions. JAMA 278:733–738, 1997.

23. Rabow MW, Hardie GE, Fair JM, McPhee SJ. End-of-life care content in 50 textbooks from multiple specialties. JAMA 283:771–778, 2000.

24. Carron AT, Lynn J, Keaney P. End-of-life care in medical textbooks. Ann Intern Med 130:82–86, 1999.

25. Callahan, D. Frustrated mastery: the cultural context of death in America. West J Med 163:226–230, 1995.

26. Ferrell B, Virani R, Grant M, Juarez G. Analysis of palliative care content in nursing textbooks. J Palliat Care 16:39–47, 2000.

27. Skolnick A. End-of-life care movement growing. JAMA 278:967–969, 1997.

28. End of Life Physician Education Resource Center (2001). Available at http://www.eperc.mcw.edu/about/start.cfm.

29. Diem SJ, Lantos JD, Tulsky JA. Cardiopulmonary resuscitation on television. Miracles and misinformation. N Engl J Med 334:1578–1582, 1996.

30. Hogan C, Lynn J, Gabel J, et al. Medicare Beneficiaries' Costs and Use of Care in the Last Year of Life. Final Report to the Medicare Payment Advisory Commission 2000. Washington DC, MedPAC, 2000.

31. Lynn J, Schall M, Milne C, et al. Quality improvements in end of life care: insights from two collaboratives. Jt Comm J Qual Improv 26:254–267, 2000.

32. Lynn J, Schuster JL, Center to Improve Care of the Dying, Institute for Healthcare Improvement. Improving Care for the End of Life: A Sourcebook for Clinicians and Managers. New York, Oxford University Press, 2000.

33. Rocker G, Dunbar S. Withholding or withdrawal of life support: the Canadian Critical Care Society position paper. J Palliat Care 16:S53–S62, 2000.

34. Centers for Disease Control and Prevention. About CDC (2000). Available at http://www.cdc.gov/aboutcdc.htm

35. Lynn J, Lynch J. Promises to Keep: Changing the Way We Provide Care at the End of Life. Washington DC, National Coalition on Health Care, 2000.

36. Lynn J, Myers S. Errors affecting patients with eventually fatal chronic illness: disproportionate burden and exceptional opportunities for improvement. Testimony before the National Summit on Medical Errors and Patient Safety Research, September 11, 2000, Washington DC. Available at http://www.quic.gov/summit/wlynn.htm

37. EPEC Project. Education for Physicians on End-of-life Care. Available at http://www.EPEC.net

38. Buckman R. How to Break Bad News: A Guide for Health Care Professionals. Toronto, University of Toronto Press, 1993.

39. Lo B, Quill T, Tulsky J. Discussing palliative care with patients. ACP-ASIM End-of-Life Care Consensus Panel. American College of Physicians, American Society of Internal Medicine. Ann Intern Med 130:744–749, 1999.

40. Doyle D, Hanks GWC, MacDonald N (Eds.). Oxford Textbook of Palliative Medicine, 2nd ed. New York, Oxford University Press, 1998.

41. Lynn J, Harrold J. Handbook for Mortals: Guidance for People Facing Serious Illness. New York, Oxford University Press, 1999.

42. Health Care Financing Administration. Brief summaries of Medicare and Medicaid (2000). Available at http://www.hcfa.gov/pubforms/actuary/ormedmed/

43. Medicare Payment Advisory Commission. Report to the Congress: selected Medicare issues. June 1999. Available at http://www.medpac.gov/

44. Institute for the Future. Health and health care 2010. The forecast. The challenge (2000). Available at http://www.rwjf.org/iftf/intro.htm

45. Federal Interagency Forum on Aging Related Statistics. Older Americans: key indicators of well being 2000. Available at http://www.agingstats.gov/chartbook2000/default.htm

46. Chochinov HM, Janson LK. Dying to pay: the cost of end-of-life care. J Palliat Care 14:5–15, 1998.

25

Palliative Care in the Nursing Home

JOHN M. CARTER AND EILEEN CHICHIN

Nursing homes are an optimum site for palliative care. Nearly every nursing home resident suffers from at least one chronic condition where cure will not be an outcome, and a significant number of those who enter a nursing home die there. While recent statistics reveal that approximately 20% of all deaths occur in the nursing home, estimates suggest that this number will climb to about 40% by 2020.[1] Accordingly, it follows that the regular use of palliative care principles should be the norm in long-term care facilities.

Increasingly, nursing homes are integrating palliative care principles into their care. However, they are doing so in an environment that, although ideal for palliative care, is fraught with challenges that make implementation difficult. Travis and colleagues[2] reported that their review of 225 journal articles and book chapters revealed more evidence of barriers than of success to implementing palliative care in nursing homes.

Included among the barriers are issues such as the philosophical views of the clinical staff and misperceptions about the use of life-sustaining treatments, two areas that may also influence the use of palliative care in the acute-care setting. Unique to the nursing home, however, are the intimate and longstanding relationships that develop between staff and residents, resulting in staff feeling like "family" to the resident. Wanting their "family member" to live forever, it is often difficult for staff to see goals of care as other than life-extending, even in cases where what they are doing is often death-prolonging. This also brings up issues of grief and bereavement affecting staff as well as family survivors.

The uncertainties of prognostication in very frail, elderly individuals, especially those with noncancer diagnoses,[3] also affect the implementation of palliative care in the nursing home. Nursing home residents' high prevalence of cognitive impairment makes pain and symptom management an even greater challenge than in acute care. Additionally, there are challenges with respect to advance care planning. These begin with completing advance directives to making timely decisions about the four sentinel decisions that most often need addressing in the long-term care setting: cardiopulmonary resuscitation/do not resuscitate (CPR/DNR), transfer to hospital, tube feeding, and the use of intravenous fluids and antibiotics.

Finally, reimbursement issues, misperceptions, and fears about regulatory oversight also come into play.

This chapter focuses on the provision of palliative care in the nursing home, with particular emphasis on areas that are unique to long-term care.

THE NURSING HOME

Although long-term care may be provided in the community as well as in inpatient facilities, institutional long-term care, i.e., nursing homes, are the foundation of our long-term care system. These facilities provide care for many of the oldest, frailest members of our society. The nursing home industry is highly regulated by both federal and state governments. Additionally, many nursing homes seek voluntary accreditation by the Joint Commission on Accreditation of Healthcare Organizations (JCAHO). This accreditation supports palliative care since it sets standards for palliative care and pain management.[4]

Nursing homes vary in size and auspices. Around the country, there are a number of facilities with fewer than 50 beds, and many with several hundred. The majority of facilities in the United States are proprietary, with a smaller number having not-for-profit status. While nursing home residents vary in age and disability, the typical nursing home resident is a woman in her late 80s suffering from a number of comorbid conditions, one of which is likely to be dementia.[5]

With respect to the physical premises, nursing homes vary widely. Many are quite institutional in appearance, although there is a trend toward creating a "home-like" environment in nearly all long-term care institutions. In the majority of nursing homes, semiprivate rooms predominate, although some private rooms are available. Clearly, the latter are preferable when patients are actively dying.

Most facilities have common dining areas, although residents who are unable to eat in this setting may take meals in their rooms. There are generally also common rooms for recreational activities, which are mandated in nursing homes.

Staffing in nursing homes is generally "pyramid-like" in structure, with the base of the pyramid consisting of para-professional staff. These individuals, known as certified nursing assistants, provide the bulk of hands-on care to nursing home residents. Nursing homes are required to have a registered nurse as director of nursing as well as other nursing and social work staff. Generally, the nursing department is the largest clinical department in long-term care facilities.

Medical coverage varies, with the most typical nursing homes having a part-time medical director and community-based physicians following patients. Some larger facilities have a full-time medical director and at least part-time on-site physicians.[6] Increasingly, nursing homes are using nurse practitioners or physician assistants to provide primary care. Depending on the size of the facility, there may be more varied professionals. Smaller facilities, for example, may have a consulting speech and language pathologist, while larger facilities will have an entire speech–language department.

Family interactions and relationships with residents and staff are a major component of nursing home life. Although a minority of nursing home residents may have outlived all of their family members and friends, the majority remain entrenched in family networks. Members of these networks visit with regularity and retain much of a "case manager" role in which they advocate for their institutionalized relative. Integral to care planning for the nursing home resident is when the family assumes an even more prominent role when the resident loses the ability to make his or her own decisions and choices about particular treatments.

Reimbursement issues in nursing homes influence the overall functioning of the facility. Much of the emphasis for payment is on "medical need," often creating difficulties when psychosocial values and preferences are in conflict.[5] Additionally, much of what is done in nursing homes is mandated by legislation. The Omnibus Budget Reconciliation Act of 1987 includes requirements about resident assessment and care planning, as well as resident rights, quality of care, and the use of physical restraints and drug therapies.[7]

HOSPICE IN THE NURSING HOME

In recent decades, there has been a trend toward the use of hospice in the nursing home. While previously most hospice services in the United States were delivered in private homes, the impetus for providing hospice to nursing home residents was the introduction of the Medicare Hospice Benefit in 1982.[8] By the late 1990s, approximately 30% of nursing homes had at least one resident on hospice, and nursing home residents became the most rapidly growing component of Medicare hospice beneficiaries.[9]

The more traditional approach to the use of hospice in the nursing home is through the establishment of a contract between the nursing home and a local hospice provider. Far less typical in nursing homes is the establishment of dedicated beds for hospice use.[9]

Contracts between hospices and nursing homes generally allow for two different levels of care under the Medicare Hospice Benefit. The first is routine home care, which can also be provided in an assisted-living facility or a person's home. The second, general inpatient care, is that level of care provided to individuals who meet hospice acute-care criteria. Residents who require the acute level of care generally are suffering from conditions that require complex pain or symptom management or more intense attention to psychosocial issues than is required for routine care.[10]

Hospice has traditionally been utilized in the community for patients with cancer diagnoses,[11] although this is changing. While cancer patients in nursing homes also are most appropriate for hospice, there are many individuals in long-term care institutions with illnesses other than cancer for whom hospice care is effective and appropriate. Recent data suggest that approximately 20% of Medicare hospice enrollees suffer from conditions such as congestive heart failure, chronic obstructive pulmonary disease, stroke, or dementia.[9]

Patients who opt for the Medicare Hospice Benefit must be eligible for Medicare Part A and have a physician-determined prognosis of 6 months or less if the disease follows its usual course. To receive the Medicare Hospice Benefit, patients must agree to waive standard Medicare coverage and to forgo curative treatment. The hospice benefit covers pain and symptom management, bereavement, nursing assistant and volunteer visits, interdisciplinary team care, drugs and durable medical equipment, and wound care.[10]

One difficulty with the use of this benefit in the long-term care setting is that it does not cover the cost of room and board. If a nursing home resident is eligible for both Medicare and Medicaid, the cost of room and board in the nursing home is covered by Medicaid. If the patient is not Medicaid-eligible, paying for room and board becomes the responsibility of the family or the patient.[9,11] If the patient's nursing home stay posthospitalization is covered under the Medicare Part A benefit, simultaneous hospice coverage is not permitted under current regulations. When the patient opts for the Medicare Hospice Benefit, he or she must drop Medicare Part A coverage, then pay privately for the room and board if not eligible for Medicaid.

In most states, Medicaid payments for hospice patients occur through direct reimbursement to the hospice provider, who then reimburses the nursing home. Rules concerning this vary from state to state, but in general payments to the nursing home are limited to 95% of the non-hospice Medicaid rate. As a result of this 5% differential, some nursing homes have opted against hospice contracts.[10]

In addition to complexities associated with payment, another major challenge to the most appropriate use of hospice in the nursing home is prognostication in patients with noncancer diagnoses. Keay and Schonwetter[11] noted that recent concerns about regulatory enforcement of the 6-month prognostic standard in patients who have "failed to die" on time have caused a number of nursing homes to enroll only individuals who are clearly certain to die within a 6-month period. Guidelines developed by the National Hospice and Palliative Care Organization (NHPCO) can be helpful in estimating prognoses in nursing home residents with noncancer diagnoses,[12] although they have not been shown to accurately predict prognosis in prospective studies. General guidelines for determining prognosis are listed in Table 25–1. In addition, the NHCPO has developed more specific guidelines for other noncancer conditions, including pulmonary disease, human immunodeficiency virus disease, liver disease, renal disease, stroke, coma, and amyotrophic lateral sclerosis.

Another challenge that must be addressed when introducing hospice into nursing homes is one of turf. To whom does such a hospice patient in the nursing home belong, the nursing home or the hospice? Nursing home and hospice experts suggest that nursing home staff should view hospices as consultants to nursing home staff. This can help in developing a collaborative working relationship. Additionally, hospice professionals can serve as educators in nursing homes, particularly with respect to pain and symptom management programs.[8] Despite these barriers to the use of the Medicare Hospice Benefit in nursing homes, it can maximize the quality of care for nursing home residents with advanced illness.

WHO NEEDS PALLIATIVE CARE IN THE NURSING HOME?

As noted earlier, most nursing home residents can benefit from the application of palliative care principles. Because many clinicians believe erroneously that palliative care is appropriate only when an individual is actively dying, many residents who could benefit from palliative care fail to receive it. In addition, the fact that Alzheimer's disease is an ultimately terminal illness[13] is also not recognized by many nursing home staff members.

The following represent some "typical" patients who would benefit from palliative care.

> *Ms. A: one pneumonia too many.* Ms. A is a 90-year-old woman who entered the nursing home about 3 years ago after suffering a stroke that rendered her unable to both walk and speak. With attentive medical and nursing care, she has remained relatively "healthy" through much of her nursing home stay. However, in the last few months, she has had three episodes of pneumonia, all of which have been treated with intravenous an-

Table 25–1. General Guidelines for Determining Prognosis in Noncancer Conditions Patient/ Family Criteria

Patient must have life-limiting condition
Patient and/or family must be informed of prognosis
Patient and/or family must opt for maximal symptom control rather than curative interventions
Patient has *either* documented progression of disease* or documented recent impaired nutritional status† associated with terminal illness

*May include primary disease progression as documented by serial physician assessment; lab, X-ray, or other studies; multiple emergency room visits or hospitalizations in 6 months; nursing assessment if homebound; documented decline in recent functional status measured either by Karnofsky Performance Status of 50% or less or dependence in at least three activities of daily living.
†Unintentional progressive weight loss greater than 10% in 6 months or serum albumin less than 2.5 g/dl in combination with presence of life-limiting condition.
Source: Standards and Accreditation Committee, Medical Guidelines Task Force.[12]

tibiotics. Now, she has noisy respirations and is breathing about 40 times per minute. She is generally unresponsive and clearly declining. The nurses feel she is slowly dying and question why her primary-care physician is continuing to order frequent finger sticks to check her glucose levels.

Ms. B: the reluctant "transfusee." Ms. B entered the nursing home about 1 year ago. She had lived at home with live-in help for several years, but her overall condition seemed to be worsening. She came to the home with a diagnosis of Alzhiemer's disease and chronic lymphocytic leukemia. Since admission, her cognitive status declined, as did her overall physical condition. She has a health-care proxy, her cousin, and a living will outlining her treatment preferences. The living will clearly states that she would not want any treatment to keep her alive should she suffer from a terminal condition or any disorder that would render her unable to recognize her family and friends. To control the anemia secondary to her leukemia, Ms. B's primary-care physician orders a blood transfusion, generally about once a month. Ms. B is so distressed by the transfusions that she requires sedation in order for them to be administered. The staff have to hold her down while the venipuncture is being performed.

Ms. C: "well, she isn't constipated!" Ms. C is an 88-year-old woman who lives in the nursing home on a unit devoted to the care of people with advanced dementia. Several months ago, she had an above-the-knee amputation, but the stump has not healed. A few weeks ago, she stopped eating and was started on intravenous nutrition and hydration. When she is seen, she screams in response to even a gentle touch. When the nurse is asked about pain management, she responds that Ms. C is on acetaminophen around the clock; she had been on oxycodone with acetaminophen but she became constipated, so it was discontinued.

At a minimum, as Keay and colleagues[14] state, attention to a patient's previously stated wishes and management of pain and other symptoms are basic indicators of quality care for the terminally ill in nursing homes. The situations described above are not atypical in the nursing home and illustrate where good palliative care could en-

hance patient autonomy, comfort, dignity, and overall quality of life. As palliative care becomes the norm in nursing homes and as long-term care facilities begin to utilize palliative care principles, these scenarios should become the exception rather than the rule.

PALLIATIVE CARE IN THE NURSING HOME: WHO IS REFERRED? WHAT ARE THE CHALLENGES?

The typical nursing home resident is frail and dependent on staff for moderate to full assistance in some, if not all, activities of daily living (e.g., bathing, eating, dressing, and toileting). A decline in function triggers an interdisciplinary team investigation and intervention when reversibility is possible. The Minimum Data Set, a document in which staff indicate a resident's function and health, is often used as a tool to identify risk factors for decline. Frequent reassessment of goals of care in the face of irreversible illness becomes the most challenging responsibility for staff and can trigger a palliative care approach as an important, and often the primary, focus of care.

A barrier in identifying palliative care needs is the misconception that only advanced cancer patients may benefit. In fact, the very frail nursing home resident will likely suffer from more than one chronic noncancer illness and become increasingly dependent over months to years.[15,16] Degenerative diseases such as Alzheimer's disease and osteoarthritis, along with accompanying functional debility, may not always be identified as progressive disorders necessitating planning for future decline. Thus, there is a lost opportunity to employ palliative care principles early in the course of illness. The complexity of caring for the very old and the fact that predicting prognosis for noncancer illness is often inexact at best indicate that it may not be appropriate to use the model of dying developed for people with cancer for those living with different chronic disease trajectories.

Another challenge often encountered in nursing homes is inadequate awareness of the prevalence of chronic pain and other distressing symptoms in the very old.[17] Acceptance of physical discomfort as a normal aspect of aging is common, especially when routine pain assessment and management are neither expected nor required by staff. Lack of education about pain may prevent identification of residents who would benefit by a palliative care focus. Communication among the interdisciplinary team members is essential in providing a dynamic, ongoing series of discussions regarding the changing symptoms in the very ill. Demands for and expectations of restoration and improvement of function despite clear indicators of irreversible functional and health decline often create confusion in terms of goals of care and missed opportunities to emphasize palliative care.[18] Education and encouragement to step back and redefine realistic goals, ideally with consensus of the team members, enable staff to reassess the goals of care and formulate the most appropriate plan of action.

Insufficient resources and lack of training in palliative care may point to the need for a palliative care specialist who can develop a practical education program in the nursing home. The enthusiastic support of administration is invaluable in creating "buy-in" and ensuring that educational initiatives are highlighted in the required in-service training schedules. A practical approach may be to present an administrator with clear guidelines and data such as statistics regarding undertreated pain in nursing home residents with advanced cancer,[19] which justify the need for integration of palliative care in nursing home practice. Often cited concerns made by residents and their loved ones may highlight the demand for palliative care skills, such as improved pain and symptom control and enhanced communication. An increase in palliative care referrals may be expected when staff clearly understand frail residents' needs in the face of irreversible decline, and needs for staff support and education are identified by one or more primary team members.

SPECIAL ISSUES IN THE NURSING HOME

Advance Care Planning and Making Sentinel Decisions

While respect for patient autonomy is thought to be a given in our health-care setting, this does not always translate into practice. In the case of a patient or resident who can still make his or her own treatment decisions, anecdotal evidence suggests that very often nursing home staff discuss treatment options only with the family. Additionally, the extent to which potential treatments are presented in an informed manner is questionable. It is common for a physician to say to a family "Your mother cannot swallow well and is losing weight. She needs a feeding tube." Only rarely do we hear health-care providers saying "Your mother cannot swallow well and is losing weight. What do you think she would want in this situation? These are our options, and these are the pros and cons of each."

In the nursing home, when it comes to planning about health care in advance of incapacity, there are pros and cons. Like their acute-care and home-care counterparts, nursing homes that receive federal funding are mandated to review treatment preferences with patients and residents. Patient (or family) wishes with respect to DNR or CPR must be determined and documented; and where possible, health-care proxies, durable powers of attorney, or living wills should be completed. Since many people who enter a nursing home will die there, it is helpful to obtain these documents if they have been completed prior to admission or to complete them soon after. It may be difficult to complete a living will if cognitive decline precludes the patient's ability to understand particular treatments and the consequences of choosing or refusing certain treatments. However, most states now have durable powers of attorney or health-care proxies, where an individual may choose another person to make decisions for him or her in case of future loss of capacity, based on an understanding of the overall goals of care, rather than on specific treatment modalities.

Many nursing homes have policies stating that a staff member (generally a social worker or a nurse) must ask a new resident or family shortly after admission about the existence of an advance directive. If such a form exists, families are asked to bring it to the nursing home. However, very often there is little sense of urgency, with both staff and family assuming the newly admitted individual is likely to live for a prolonged period of time. Therefore, in the period of adjustment to the nursing home, the documents may be forgotten and sometimes lost.

In the case of those who do not already have advance directives, a staff member may initiate discussion, but follow-up does not always occur. In the interim, a resident may become ill and lose the ability to communicate treatment preferences or indicate who should make decisions in his or her stead. Failure to complete advance directives in a timely fashion results in increased difficulties when treatment decisions must be made for a frail individual who is unable to make his or her own preferences known. This should be an impetus for nursing homes to seek advance directives in a consistent and timely manner. In addition, a systematic program to increase the use of advance directives has been shown to minimize health-service utilization without affecting mortality or patient or family satisfaction.[20]

Yet another common situation is the lack of understanding on the part of the staff about the decision-specific nature of decision-making capacity. A patient may not be able to understand the consequences of specific treatment choices but still can easily indicate the choice of a trusted decision maker. Many nursing home residents have varying degrees of cognitive decline, but often even those with diagnoses of dementia can choose a proxy decision maker.

Many health-care professionals experience the sense that "the work is done" when a patient has completed a living will, durable power of attorney for health care, or health-care proxy. On the contrary, in the nursing home setting, it is most impor-

tant that the goals of care be reviewed periodically and decisions made in advance of a crisis. One decision that should be discussed early in the nursing home stay is hospitalization. If the resident became sicker, would he or she want to be transferred to the hospital? Or rather, would he or she prefer to remain in the nursing home and be kept comfortable, surrounded by familiar faces?

Nursing home staff are repeatedly faced with decision making regarding a long list of potential diagnostic and therapeutic interventions for each resident. Since all of the chronically ill will eventually face irreversible decline, a myriad of issues arise regarding what procedures are appropriate for each individual. The emphasis on restoration of function remains an ongoing theme, yet it often is unclear to individual staff members when to reassess the appropriateness or efficacy of each intervention. Traditions specific to a long-term care institution and cultural expectations exclusively focused on restorative care may be barriers to re-evaluating the goals of care and tailoring interventions to the specific needs of the individual. Staff may feel extraordinary discomfort when "normal procedure" is not followed. The role of the palliative care advocate is to encourage dialogue between the resident, or resident's surrogate decision maker, and staff to clearly delineate goals of care, as well as the benefits and burdens of each particular intervention. As noted earlier, there are four common sentinel decisions which patients, surrogates, and staff face in the chronically ill nursing home resident. Each is described in detail below.

Appropriateness of CPR is often the first issue to be clarified soon after nursing home admission (along with existence or clarification of health-care proxy designation). A resident, or the surrogate decision maker in the face of incapacity, should be informed about the facility's policy about provision of CPR and discuss the resuscitation procedure itself. Of utmost importance in ensuring an informed decision is clear discussion about the probable outcome of CPR in the frail nursing home resident. Multiple studies point to the poor survival rate in nursing home residents who undergo CPR, yet many residents and loved ones may never have been told these details.[21] The recommendation of a DNR order does not preclude the use of other interventions, and staff need to be clear that a DNR order pertains only to withholding CPR. All residents, regardless of the presence or absence of a DNR order, should receive continued pain and symptom management, and family and staff should be reassured that quality of care will not be compromised. Explanation of a resident's primary disease and functional status, along with the fact that CPR is ineffective and will not result in meaningful recovery, is essential to clearly delineate the likely futility of the procedure and to clarify misconceptions and unrealistic expectations. The discussion of benefits and risks of CPR and DNR orders may assist residents and loved ones in articulating other treatment goals, with support and education by staff.

The decision to transfer an ill resident to the acute-care hospital is often difficult. Without clear guidance regarding the goals of care, staff may feel obligated to recommend hospital transfer despite fears of the possible adverse consequences (increased risk of delirium, physical discomfort of transfer and removal from familiar surroundings and staff.)[2] The presence of advance directives may help to guide staff at the time of crisis, although pressure to find a quick solution may result in hospitalization when uncertainty and discomfort exist about caring for a critically ill, and maybe dying, resident. Communication with resident, surrogate decision makers, and staff is vital in preventing unwanted transfer and of particular need is a clear indicator of this goal of care in the chart documentation. A common complaint by staff is that clear guidelines regarding hospitalization directives are not highlighted in the resident's chart. An easy-to-use system of indicating resident/surrogate preferences regarding hospitalization may need to be devised by administration and the medical records staff, followed by education of

floor staff to prevent confusion at time of crisis.

The Physician Orders for Life-Sustaining Treatment (POLST) (Fig. 25–1) is an example of a successful change intervention developed to convey preferences for life-sustaining treatments during transfer from one institution to another.[22,23] The POLST form is standardized, is printed on distinctive pink paper to ensure easy recognition, and includes physician orders about specific medical treatments. Nursing home residents with a POLST indicating a desire for transfer to hospital only if comfort measures failed experienced significantly lower rates of transfer to the hospital, in keeping with their wishes.[22] Using a goal-centered advance directive may ensure that nursing home patients receive the type and intensity of medical care they prefer even if they are unable to participate in decision making at the time of an acute illness.[24]

Residents and loved ones need reassurance that a "do not hospitalize" status does not preclude solid medical and nursing care, including pain and symptom management. Along with the question of hospitalization, the use of specific diagnostic interventions should be explored for benefits and burdens in each resident. Phlebotomy, radiographic studies, fingerstick glucose monitoring, and electrocardiography are potentially helpful tools in diagnosis and may help to guide proper care. In the advanced stages of an illness or at the request of a resident at an earlier stage, some or all diagnostic testing may no longer provide benefit and, indeed, may become the source of discomfort. Open discussion with appropriate decision makers, often coupled with a reasonable recommendation by a caregiver cognizant of the patient's goals, is necessary. In addition, any directive regarding the use of diagnostic tests needs to be clearly marked on the resident's chart, where staff are expected to check such instructions. The POLST document specifies whether or not the resident is to undergo painful diagnostic procedures.

Provision of artificial hydration and nutrition poses one of the most difficult decisions encountered in the nursing home. The

SEND FORM WITH PATIENT/RESIDENT WHENEVER TRANSFERRED OR DISCHARGED

Physician Orders
for Life-Sustaining Treatment (POLST)

This is a Physician Order Sheet. It is based on patient/resident medical condition and wishes. It summarizes any Advance Directive. Any section not completed indicates full treatment for that section. When the need occurs, <u>first</u> follow these orders, <u>then</u> contact physician.

Last Name of Patient/Resident

First Name/Middle Initial of Patient/Resident

Patient/Resident Date of Birth

Section A Check One Box Only	**RESUSCITATION. Patient/resident has no pulse <u>and</u> is not breathing.** ☐ <u>R</u>esuscitate ☐ <u>D</u>o <u>N</u>ot <u>R</u>esuscitate (DNR) When not in cardiopulmonary arrest, follow orders in Sections B, C and D.

Section B Check One Box Only	**MEDICAL INTERVENTIONS. Patient/resident has pulse and/<u>or</u> is breathing.** ☐ **Comfort Measures Only.** The patient/resident is treated with dignity, respect and kept clean, warm and dry. Reasonable measures are made to offer food and fluids by mouth, and attention is paid to hygiene. Medication, positioning, wound care and other measures are used to relieve pain and suffering. Oxygen, suction and manual treatment of airway obstruction may be used as needed for comfort. These measures are to be used where the patient/resident lives. The patient/resident is not to be hospitalized unless comfort measures fail. ☐ **Limited Additional Interventions.** Includes care above. May include cardiac monitor and oral/IV medications. Transfer to hospital if indicated, but no endotracheal intubation or long term life support measures. Usually no intensive care. ☐ **Full Treatment.** Includes care above plus endotracheal intubation and cardioversion. *Other Instructions:* _____

Section C Check One Box Only	**ANTIBIOTICS. Comfort measures are always provided.** ☐ **No antibiotics** ☐ **Antibiotics** *Other Instructions:* _____

Section D Check One Box Only	**ARTIFICIALLY ADMINISTERED FLUIDS AND NUTRITION. Comfort measures are always provided.** ☐ **No feeding tube/IV fluids** ☐ **Defined trial period of feeding tube/IV fluids** ☐ **Long term feeding tube/IV fluids** *Other Instructions:* _____

Section E	Discussed with: ☐ Patient/Resident ☐ Parent of Minor ☐ Health Care Representative ☐ Court-Appointed Guardian ☐ Spouse ☐ Other:	Summarize Medical Condition

Physician/ Nurse Practitioner Name (print)	Physician/ NP Phone Number DAY: EVE:	Office Use Only
Physician/ NP Signature (mandatory)	Date	

SEND FORM WITH PATIENT/RESIDENT WHENEVER TRANSFERRED OR DISCHARGED

Figure 25–1a. The Physician Orders for Life-Sustaining Treatment (POLST) Form.

frail patient with functional decline coupled with severe cognitive loss is at significant risk of developing an irreversible feeding disorder. A clear understanding of the underlying disease process is needed for decision makers to deliberate on the benefits and burdens of artificial nutrition and hydration[25–27] and to be able to communicate

SEND FORM WITH PATIENT/RESIDENT WHENEVER TRANSFERRED OR DISCHARGED

When This Form Should Be Reviewed

This form (POLST) should be reviewed periodically and if:
- ◆ The patient/resident is transferred from one care setting or care level to another, or
- ◆ There is a substantial change in patient/resident health status, or
- ◆ The patient/resident treatment preferences change.

How to Complete the Form Review

1. Review **Sections A through F**.
2. Complete **Section G**.
   If this form is to be voided, write "VOID" in large letters on the front of the form.
   After voiding form, a new form may be completed.
   If no new form is completed, full treatment and resuscitation may be provided.

Section F	Patient/Resident (Parent of Minor Child) Preferences as a Guide for this POLST Form

I have given significant thought to life-sustaining treatment. I expressed my preferences to my physician and/or health care provider(s). This document reflects my treatment preferences. The following have further information regarding my preferences:

    Advance Directive   ☐ NO   ☐ YES
    Court-Appointed Guardian   ☐ NO   ☐ YES

Please review these orders if there is substantial change in my health status such as:

    Close to death   Improved condition   Advanced progressive illness
    Extraordinary suffering   Permanent unconsciousness

Signature of Patient/Resident, Parent of Minor, or Guardian/Health Care Representative (optional)

Signature of Person Preparing Form	Preparer Name (print)	Date Prepared

Section G	Review of this POLST Form			
	Date	Reviewer	Location of Review	Outcome of Review
				☐ No change ☐ FORM VOIDED, new form completed ☐ FORM VOIDED, *no* new form
				☐ No change ☐ FORM VOIDED, new form completed ☐ FORM VOIDED, *no* new form
				☐ No change ☐ FORM VOIDED, new form completed ☐ FORM VOIDED, *no* new form

E-MAIL: ethics@ohsu.edu

WEB SITE: www.ohsu.edu/ethics

SEND FORM WITH PATIENT/RESIDENT WHENEVER TRANSFERRED OR DISCHARGED

© CENTER FOR ETHICS IN HEALTH CARE, OHSU • Form developed in conformance with Oregon Revised Statute 127.505 et seq • July 2001

Figure 25–1b. The Physician Orders for Life-Sustaining Treatment (POLST) Form.

these facts to loved ones faced with decision making. The Alzheimer Association recommends that comfort be the primary goal of care for a person with severe irreversible dementia. In keeping with this goal, there is no medical or ethical obligation to provide artificial hydration and nutrition; rather, spoon-feeding, mouth care, artificial saliva, and ice chips are recommended for ensuring comfort. Short-term trials of intravenous fluids used to combat a potentially reversible and acute illness may be reasonable to offer a mildly demented but otherwise highly functional resident who is able to ambulate and enjoy daily social activities. The common dilemma in the nursing home is the severely cognitively and functionally impaired patient who will likely never have full restoration of eating and drinking in the last weeks of life. Staff are obligated to explore the individual's wishes regarding the use of feeding tubes and intravenous therapies in the face of irreversible decline. Discomfort with the topic coupled with easy access to these technologies may present barriers to fully exploring realistic goals of care in residents at the terminal phase of their illnesses.[28] Educating staff on the nature and progression of common illnesses, such as Alzheimer's disease or advanced heart disease, is important in creating consensus about prognosis with and without this intervention. Knowledge of and respect for advance directives and their application by a staff comfortable with end-of life care are imperative when artificial nutrition is appropriately withheld in accordance with an individual's wishes. Discomfort with "not feeding" by artificial means is a common theme, and administration and supervisory staff must be equipped to intervene and support staff who have personal objections. Spoon-feeding and meticulous mouth care should be continued in the interest of patient and family comfort.

Use of antibiotics also is an important topic to discuss for residents suffering from debilitating and rapidly deteriorating conditions. The declining resident typically experiences frequent febrile illnesses, which confront staff with the repetitive use of antibiotics to combat bacterial infections. Issues of adverse side effects, futility of specific treatment, and burden of provision may play a role in reconsidering the benefit of continued antibiotic use. The resident or surrogate may question the benefit of repeated antibiotic trials in the face of irreversible decline in baseline function. Staff need to be clear about the potential benefits of antibiotic use when viewed in the context of the total framework of the resident and the stage of illness.[29] Studies indicate that antibiotic treatment of febrile illnesses in patients with advanced Alzheimer's disease does not alter survival outcome.[30,31] Indeed, the higher severity of impairment in these patients has been associated with death within 6 months of the onset of fever.[30] In addition, staff should be educated that maximizing physical comfort in the face of febrile illness or potential infection is always an important goal, independent of antibiotic use. Frequent review of the resident's condition and disease trajectory should stimulate review and modifications of the plan of care.

Pain and Symptom Management in the Nursing Home

Symptoms encountered in the chronically ill nursing home resident are similar to those encountered in home or hospital settings. The challenge for staff, however, is to provide adequate assessment and management in those with a baseline of severe cognitive impairment. Advanced dementia coupled with delirium and a rapidly deteriorating course presents great difficulties to staff, who often have not been provided with specific training in these skills during their formal education. Multiple studies demonstrate the high prevalence of daily pain in nursing home patients with cancer who are capable of self-report.[19,32,33] The cognitively impaired are unable to clearly verbalize their concerns and are dependent on staff and loved ones to assess for signs of discomfort. Moaning and grimacing during repositioning, for example, are often clear signs of distress, yet some staff may not perceive such signs as abnormal and deserving of communication to the remainder of the team. Other signs of untreated pain include withdrawal, rigidity, unresponse to attempted care, fetal position, refusal of food and water, and change in sleep habits. Lost opportunities to assess and adequately treat acute and chronic pain may therefore result. Pain assessment scales using illustrations of objective signs, such as a series of faces from happy and content at one extreme to tearful and distressed at the other, are one type of tool to encourage staff to focus clinical assessment on nonverbal cues.[34] Regulations and institutional policies requiring pain assessments on nursing home admission and at periodic intervals also may stimulate staff to identify clues to unaddressed pain and spark a team assessment and plan of intervention. Further triggers for mandatory pain assessments may include any change in a resident's function (a change in more than one activity of daily living), change in medical status such as a new agitation, vocalizations, febrile illness, or recurrent falls. Educating staff that the nursing home resident is at high risk for chronic or recurrent pain should be given high priority in the mandatory inservice education schedule. Nursing and medical staff should take the lead in such education and share responsibility for appointing key staff as educators and role models. Facts concerning the proper use of analgesics should be clearly outlined, emphasizing the use of a standing analgesic regimen for chronic pain plus additional "rescue" medication for breakthrough discomfort. Common misconceptions regarding opioids need to be addressed, with honest analysis of potential barriers to opioid use (e.g., the frequent unavailability of opioids in nursing homes due to regulatory restrictions on storing emergency supplies). Counseling on anticipated side effects of opioids plus routine strategies to manage such side effects is essential in ensuring the success of a pain-education initiative.

Dyspnea and tachypnea are symptoms related to the subjective feeling of breathlessness and the objective finding of rapid breathing. They are commonly encountered in the nursing home during both acute and chronic illnesses, as well as in the actively dying. Education of staff in assessment and management of common case-based scenarios is essential, including reinforcement that such symptoms can be successfully palliated with both pharmacological and nonpharmacological strategies.[35,36] In addition to the liberal use of fans, bronchodilators, and steroids, the use of opioids must be reinforced as a safe and effective means to treat both dyspnea and tachypnea. Educating staff about appropriate initiation and escalation of opioids may become a particular challenge to staff who commonly express fears about eliminating respiratory drive. References to the palliative care literature regarding the safety and benefit of opioids in dyspnea and tachypnea may help allay fears of hastening respiratory failure and death.[37–39] As with education about pain, good role modeling on resident floors with respect to the treatment of tachypnea and dyspnea is invaluable.

Anorexia and dysphagia are also common problems encountered in the nursing home. Degenerative dementias, such as Alzheimer's disease, as well as cerebrovascular disease, end-stage heart/lung/kidney disease, and a myriad of other progressive illnesses put residents at risk for poor oral intake of food and fluids. Such decline causes great discomfort to staff and loved ones, who are faced with decision making and treatment options. Education about the usual and normal progression of a specific disorder and what is typically expected during decline will enable family and staff to decipher the best goals of care for that resident. Discussing the fact that hunger and thirst are not common in most terminally ill patients[40] is enormously comforting, and outlining that artificial hydration and nutrition carry significant burdens helps both staff and loved ones to refocus energies on human comfort and care rather than futile attempts at cure in the late stages of disease. Discussing interventions to provide comfort, such as mouth care and frequent assessment of symptoms common at the end of life, should empower staff to concentrate efforts on maximizing comfort and security. Involving the nursing assistant and dietitian in care planning when the resident is still eating small quantities of food will enable frequent reassessment of diet and encouragement to use favorite foods, regardless of nutritional value. Reinforcing the fact that not eating and drinking is an expression of the body slowing down during the dying process is an important intervention when staff exhibit discomfort over a resident's decline. The withholding of artificial hydration and nutrition is in the best interest of the severely demented resident who would not wish his or her life to be artificially prolonged in this circumstance, and comfort can be maintained with frequent assessment of symptoms. Reminding staff and family who fear that the patient is dying because he or she is not eating that the patient is not eating because he or she is dying is often necessary.

Gastrointestinal symptoms are common and require education about prevalence and management techniques,[41] including the treatment and prevention of nausea and vomiting. Antiemetics and anticholinergics should be included in the nursing formulary. Education on potential etiologies of gastrointestinal symptoms, including side effects of medications, is essential when counseling on treatment interventions. This is of particular note when the ill resident continues to receive enteral nutrition despite recurrent nausea or vomiting. Management of enteral feeds and reconsideration of goals of artificial nutrition should be assessed for reversible causes of distress.

Assessment and management of constipation in the nursing home patient are always a priority. Inactivity, poor oral fluid intake, and the adverse effects of medications (including opioids) contribute to constipation and increasing discomfort. Knowledge of pharmacological and nonpharmacological interventions to prevent and treat opioid-induced constipation is vital to maximizing comfort in the palliative care patient and to avoid patient and staff dissatisfaction with opioid use and efficacy in pain and dyspnea management. Involvement of the pharmacist as well as nutritionist is also advantageous to help the nurse and physician develop and monitor an effective bowel assessment and treatment program for each patient.

Depression and anxiety are symptoms which require active and ongoing palliation in the face of chronic illness. Frequent assessment for common symptoms and, in particular, atypical signs in the cognitively impaired is necessary to identify potentially treatable symptoms. Education about the prevalence of depression and anxiety and successful pharmacological and nonpharmacological interventions is essential.[42] Delirium and terminal restlessness are particularly distressing to staff and loved ones, and proficiency in assessment and management is vital to good end-of-life care.[43] Availability and the confident use of proper antipsychotic medications greatly diminish staff and family anxiety. In this clinical scenario, terminal agitated delirium is best treated with a sedating antipsychotic agent such as chlorpromazine. The ability of staff to more closely monitor the restless or agitated resident is a challenge, and supervisory staff need to prioritize staffing ratios when there is a very restless or agitated dying resident on a particular floor. Assigning a nursing assistant solely to a delirious and restless resident is an ideal plan to ensure safety, comfort, and careful monitoring, although staff shortages common in many facilities often preclude this.

Communication Issues

Care in the nursing home is traditionally provided by teams, and integral to good team functioning is regular communication among team members.[44] Thus, all members of the caregiving team, professional and paraprofessional alike, as well as the resident and family should be involved in and familiar with the resident's plan of care. This is even more important when the goals of care change from what had been a curative, restorative approach to one that integrates palliation. Inclusion of all team members is necessary to ensure that the resident's treatment preferences are respected and comfort is maximized.

While each team member plays an important role on the team, a key player on the nursing home team is the certified nursing assistant (CNA). It is vital that nursing assistants be involved in the care-planning process since they provide the bulk of hands-on and personal care. The CNA often develops a close, family-like, emotional relationship with the resident and is distressed by the resident's physical and cognitive decline.[45] Engaging the CNA in all aspects of the care-planning process, including the resident's diagnosis, prognosis, and treatment preferences, is key to his or her understanding of what is being done and why. It also enhances his or her ability to provide care to someone to whom he or she is emotionally attached while that individual's condition continues to decline.

Other members of the caregiving team need to be aware of changes in the goals of care and how these goals will be addressed. Because of the size and complexity of the teams in many long-term care facilities, several individuals beyond the core team of nurse, doctor, and social worker must be notified. For example, the recreational therapist may tailor an activity to the needs of someone who may be actively dying, e.g., choosing as one possibility to play soft music at the bedside. A physical therapist may modify an intervention to maximize comfort rather than restore function. A dietitian may, in collaboration with the physician, opt for food that might not be therapeutically optimal when cure or control of an illness is the goal but might provide the greatest degree of satisfaction to the resident when palliation is a priority.

Intrateam communication can be a source of emotional support to caregiving professionals and para-professionals who are observing the decline and eventual death of a resident who they may have known and cared for over an extended period of time. In addition to verbal communication among team members, information written in the medical record is of great benefit. It is useful for the specifics of the care plan, particularly with respect to the sentinel events mentioned earlier (CPR, hospitalization, artificial nutrition and hydration, and antibiotics), to be noted succinctly and legibly in a prominent place in the medical record so any member of the caregiving staff can have easy access to it. The POLST form, described earlier (Fig. 25–1), is an excellent mechanism to communicate this key information.[22,23]

Communication with the resident (whenever possible) and the family is equally important in palliative care. Early in the process, the family must be intimately involved in determining the goals of care, particularly with respect to the four sentinel events of CPR, hospitalization, artificial nutrition, and antibiotic use. Discussion of issues that may influence comfort should also be held. When the resident is clearly declining, for example, should painful diagnostic testing such as venipuncture be continued if no action will be taken with the results? The family's communication needs are particularly great when a resident is actively dying. This is when the support of the family is as important as the support of the dying resident. Families need to know what to expect, to the greatest degree possible, as the resident continues to fail. How long do we anticipate that the resident will live? What will the end be like? What can we do to minimize distressing symptoms and maximize comfort? Does the family wish to be present at the time of death? Are there other family members who should be called? Families should also be informed of their role as advocate for the dying resident, particularly in the case of residents who are cognitively impaired or otherwise unable to report their discomfort. Families should be encouraged to talk to their dying loved one, expressing love and gratitude and saying good-bye. They may also need encouragement to touch and hold the resident. If a family member feels the resident is in pain or experiencing other distressing symptoms, the family should report this information.

While providing information to families about dying residents' condition, the palliative care team can also inquire as to the physical and emotional well-being of the family members. Are they getting enough to eat? Are they getting sufficient rest? Most helpful to families is the 24-hour-per-day, seven-day-per-week availability of a member of a palliative care team or a knowledgeable unit team member who is well versed in palliative care. The role of this individual is to provide information and emotional support. Availability of skilled staff by telephone or beeper can be most comforting to family members overwhelmed by the dying process of a loved one. A follow-up bereavement call to the family shortly after the death of the resident provides the twofold effect of providing some closure to the caregiving staff and comforting the surviving family members. Such communication opens the door for family members to contact the staff in the future if necessary. A strong emphasis on communication in palliative care helps to create a caring, supportive environment. This has been shown to have a positive effect on the family members of residents who die in a long-term care setting.[46]

Grief and Bereavement

Loss is an everyday occurrence in the nursing home.[47] Upon admission, residents lose their previous home and whatever independence they may have had there. Over time, most residents experience declines in sensory, functional, and cognitive status. They lose roommates and other residents to death or transfer. Upon the death of a resident, the family loses someone they love and staff lose someone to whom they may have become emotionally attached. How nursing homes address these issues can have a profound effect on those who survive.

With respect to residents' reactions to their respective sensory, functional, and cognitive losses, adaptive devices that can maximize functioning are useful. Educating staff and families to allow open and honest verbalization of concerns and grief about these losses is also a positive intervention. The physical and cognitive decline of residents in nursing homes and their subsequent deaths are clearly difficult for their families, who often struggle with conflicting feelings of guilt, doubt, and relief when a many-year struggle with dementia has ended. Families need continuous emotional support through an often prolonged period of anticipatory as well as post-death bereavement, as well as the ongoing loss of the person their loved one had been.

Staff also experience loss, grief, and bereavement as residents decline and die. As noted elsewhere, relationships between staff and residents in nursing homes are quite different from those in hospitals. Many nursing home residents live in a particular long-term care facility for many months to years. Generally, their care is provided by an interdisciplinary team, and often the same team members are involved for the duration of the resident's nursing home stay. Team members develop close relationships with the residents for whom they care and are distressed by their decline and subsequent death. A particular concern here are CNAs. These individuals provide hands-on care to residents, performing for them the most intimate aspects of personal care, as well as providing emotional support. Of all staff, CNAs are most significantly affected by the decline and death of the residents for whom they care. They often liken the death of a resident to the death of a family member or close friend.[48] However, since this is perceived to be "just part of the job," CNAs do not receive the emotional support that one would receive after the death of a relative. When several deaths occur in rapid succession on the same nursing unit, the intensity of grief is clearly magnified. The high annual turnover of CNAs in the long-term care setting may be related in part to the unresolved grief and bereavement these individuals experience. Another related issue that compounds the grief is the nursing home's financial need to fill beds as soon as they become available. Staff often interpret this as an indication that the life of the individual who died was relatively meaningless and that keeping beds filled is all that matters to the home's administration. There is no time for grief because with a new admission the routine begins again. Some CNAs say they try not to become emotionally close to residents simply to avoid this repeated cycle of emotional attachment and subsequent loss.[45]

Many nursing homes have developed mechanisms to address grief and bereavement for residents, families, and staff when a resident dies. Some facilities hold a brief ceremony at the bedside immediately after a death, with available staff on the unit joining together to remember the life of the resident. We know of one facility where after a person dies and the bed is cleaned and remade, it is left empty for 24 hours and a rose placed upon it. In some facilities, a bell is rung each time a resident dies. Various types of memorial services are useful to bring closure to those who were close to a resident who has died. Many facilities hold a unit-based ceremony some time after a resident's death, inviting other residents, family members, and staff. In some, a service is held every several months, memorializing the lives of all residents who died in the period since the last service.

Some facilities permit staff to attend funerals, although this may present budgetary issues since a staff member's time away from the facility must be covered by another staff member. One relatively simple method that permits staff members to express their feelings and connect with the family is to provide all nursing units in the facility with notepaper and stamps, along with a few minutes' free time, to write condolence letters. This inexpensive mechanism can provide some closure to staff, while it lets families know that the life of their loved one affected many people.

Attitudes toward End-of-Life Care in the Nursing Home: Cultural and Philosophical Issues

Like their acute-care counterparts, nursing homes draw their staff from a wide variety of cultural backgrounds. Frequently, when it comes to end-of-life care, culture plays a dominant role. Individuals from various cultures may view the use of life-sustaining treatments differently or may have disparate views on pain management. Members of some cultures are traditionally stoic and believe others should be as well. Others feel there is meaning in suffering and in the struggle for life, so they may be reluctant to use interventions to relieve it. Some cultures shy away from patient autonomy and truth-telling. All of these views influence professionals' practice and have profound implications for the delivery of palliative care.

In addition, one's professional discipline[49,50] and when and how one learned its subject matter will influence thinking and practice. For example, patient autonomy is the dominant principle in biomedical ethics and has long been the foundation of social work practice. However, it is a new concept, relatively speaking, in medicine and nursing.[51,52] Thus, older physicians and older nurses could have greater difficulty than some of their younger counterparts in following a resident's treatment preferences to limit life-sustaining care. With respect to pain management, in the 1950s and 1960s, opioids were believed to be addictive in all cases and were underused. Thus, it is not surprising that older clinicians may be slow to use opioids in managing severe pain. Even clinicians educated in the latter part of the twentieth century had minimal, if any, education in pain management. This affects the quality of pain and symptom management.

DEVELOPING A PALLIATIVE CARE PROGRAM IN THE NURSING HOME

Increasingly, and with varying degrees of success, nursing homes across the United States are integrating palliative care principles into their daily care. Some nursing home initiatives have received foundation support (e.g., the Practice Improvement Clusters overseen by the John A. Hartford Institute for Geriatric Nursing at New York University, the Performance Improvement Collaborative in Palliative Care being developed in New York City by Rand/Institute for Healthcare Improvement with support from the United Hospital Fund, and the development of a certification examination in palliative care for CNAs by the National Board of Certification of Hospice and Palliative Nurses, funded by the Fan Fox and Leslie R. Samuels Foundation). Other nursing homes are simply quietly attempting to integrate palliative care whenever possible.

Integrating palliative care into nursing homes is a win–win situation. It optimizes patient comfort, dignity, and preference. It can potentially minimize expense by limiting the number of costly diagnostic procedures and futile treatments performed on individuals who, if they could make a choice, very often would opt not to have them. It humanizes and demedicalizes an environment that is home to many of the frailest, most vulnerable members of our society. For those who lack knowledge of palliative care and fail to see its benefits, good role modeling and the resulting improvements in quality of care and resident and family satisfaction will ultimately lead to change.

To integrate palliative care into a nursing home, there are a number of concrete steps. Key among these is obtaining administrative buy-in. Many administrators see palliative care as a positive service that maximizes quality of life and responds to the needs of residents and family members while minimizing the need for unwanted painful and unnecessary interventions

Developing a palliative care team is another major advance toward integrating palliative care into a nursing home. An interdisciplinary group consisting of individuals who are excellent role models is a good way to start. Providing this team with basic (and subsequently more advanced) palliative care education is the next step. Two effective educational programs, one for physicians and one for nurses, have been developed with support from the Robert Wood Johnson Foundation. The Education for Physicians in End-of-Life Care is designed to educate physicians on the key clinical competencies needed to provide quality end-of-life care. Information about this program can be accessed through the web (http://www.EPEC.net). The End-of-Life Nursing Education Consortium is an initiative of the American Association of Colleges of Nursing. Further information about this project can be found on the web (http://www.aacn.nche.edu).

If a local hospital has a palliative care program, forging a link with them can benefit both institutions. It allows for the sharing of educational programs as well as clinical expertise. Most importantly, it allows for the seamless transition of care when a palliative care patient is transferred from one site to the other.

To effectively integrate palliative care into a nursing home, a change in the conception of goals of care institutionwide is needed. Most nursing homes have a strong rehabilitative and restorative focus. It is difficult for staff in long-term care facilities to recognize that this is not the best approach for every resident. It is especially difficult when the resident has been in the facility for many years, suffering from a number of chronic disabilities. When is the right time to refocus the goals of care in these instances? Making this judgment requires not only clinical skill but an understanding of the end-stage nature of many of the noncancer conditions (e.g., Alzheimer's disease, advanced heart disease) that are so prevalent in nursing homes.

Another helpful step toward integrating palliative care into a nursing home is to find allies wherever and whenever possible. As a palliative care program begins in an institution, it quickly becomes apparent who supports the effort. Work with these individuals, and slowly more will join their ranks. Front-line staff buy-in is important; these are the professionals and paraprofessionals who actually do the work of patient care. In developing our program, one of our most positive experiences was a conversation with a head nurse who told us that she tells her staff that palliative care is appropriate for everyone on their unit because no one will be cured of their chronic, disabling conditions. Other allies can be found in the families of residents who have died while receiving palliative care. These individuals become the strongest advocates, having seen what a positive impact a palliative approach had on the quality of living and the quality of dying of their loved ones. Additionally, many nursing homes have organizations for relatives and friends. Aligning with these groups is also helpful to the palliative care movement, for relatives of their members are also "users" of palliative care services.

The trend toward nursing homes seeking JCAHO accreditation is a positive for palliative care. The JCAHO guidelines mandate attention to both pain and symptom management in the care of the dying.[4] These accreditation requirements can be met through the development of an institutionwide palliative care program, and this can serve as an additional institutional impetus. Simply developing these policies and procedures is an important step toward integrating good palliative care principles into nursing home care. Finally, the use of hospice contracts in nursing homes is another impetus for integrating palliative care in these facilities. Increasing numbers of long-term care facilities are opting for this approach, whereby hospice professionals work side-by-side with and support nursing home staff in their care of this highly frail and vulnerable population. This creates an environment that allows more aid to enable staff to provide humane care to residents who are dying. In addition, the presence of hospice personnel and the hospice ideology can help in the rethinking of goals of care throughout the facility.

REFERENCES

1. Brock DB, Foley DJ. Demography and epidemiology of dying in the U.S. with emphasis on the deaths of older persons. Hosp J 13:49–60, 1998.
2. Travis SS, Loving G, McClanahan L, Bernard M. Hospitalization patterns and palliation in the last year of life among residents in long-term care. Gerontologist 41:153–160, 2001.
3. Fox E, Landrum-McNiff K, Zhong Z, Dawson NV, Wu AW, Lynn J, for the SUPPORT Investigators. Evaluation of prognostic criteria for determining hospice eligibility in patients with advanced lung, heart, or liver disease. JAMA 282:1638–1645, 1999.
4. Joint Commission on Accreditation of Healthcare Organizations. 2000–2001 Standards for Long Term Care, 2000. (www.jcaho.org)
5. Wilson NL. Long-term care in the United States: an overview of the current system. In: McCullough LB, Wilson NL (Eds.). Long-Term Care Decisions: Ethical and Conceptual Dimensions. Baltimore, Johns Hopkins University Press, pp. 34–59, 1995.
6. Allen JE. Nursing Home Administration. New York, Springer, 1992.
7. Elon R. Medical practice in nursing facilities: assessing the impact of OBRA. In: Katz PR, Kane RL, Mezey MD (Eds.). Quality Care in Geriatric Settings. New York, Springer, pp. 18–36, 1995.
8. English D, Gong J. Why hospices belong in nursing homes, part 1. Nurs Homes 50,4 46–50, 2001.
9. Petrisek AC, Mor V. Hospice in nursing homes: a facility-level analysis of the distribution of hospice beneficiaries. Gerontologist 39:279–290, 1999.
10. English D, Gong J. Why hospices belong in nursing homes, part 2. Nurs Homes 50.5 44–48, 2001.
11. Keay TJ, Schonwetter RS. Hospice care in the nursing home. Am Fam Physician 57: 491–494, 1998.
12. Standards and Accreditation Committee, Medical Guidelines Task Force. Medical Guidelines for Determining Prognosis in Selected Non-cancer Diseases, 2nd ed. Arlington, VA, National Hospice Organization, 1996.
13. Post SG, Whitehouse PJ. Fairhill guidelines on ethics of the care of people with Alzheimer's disease: a clinical summary. J Am Geriatr Soc 43:1423–1429, 1995.
14. Keay TJ, Fredman L, Taler GA, Datta S, Levenson SA. Indicators of quality medical care for the terminally ill in nursing homes. J Am Geriatr Soc 42:853–860, 1994.
15. Flacker JM, Won A, Kiely DK, Ikechukwu I. Differing perceptions of end-of-life care in long-term care. J Palliat Med 4:9–13, 2001.
16. Froggatt KA. Palliative care and nursing homes: where next? Palliat Med 15:42–48, 2001.
17. AGS Panel on Chronic Pain in Older Persons. Clinical practice guidelines: the management of chronic pain in older persons. J Am Geriatr Soc 46:635–651, 1998.
18. Morrison RS, Meier DE, Cassel CK. When too much is too little. N Engl J Med 335:1755–1759, 1996.
19. Bernabei R, Gambassi G, Lapane KL, et al. Management of pain in patients with cancer. JAMA 279:1877–1882, 1998.
20. Molloy DW, Guyatt GH, Russo R, Goeree R, O'Brien BJ, Willan A, Watson J, Patterson C, Harrison C, Standish T, Strang D, Darzins PJ, Smith S, Dubois S. Systematic implementation of an advance directive program in nursing homes: a randomized controlled trial. JAMA 283:1437–1444, 2000.
21. Kane RS, Burns, EA. Cardiopulmonary resuscitation policies in long-term care facilities. J Am Geriatr Soc 45:154–157, 1997.
22. Tolle SW, Tilden VP, Nelson CA, et al. A prospective study of the efficacy of the physician order form for life-sustaining

treatment. J Am Geriatr Soc 46:1097–1102, 1998.

23. Field MJ, Cassel CK. Approaching Death: Improving Care at the End of Life. Washington DC, Institute of Medicine, Committee on Care at the End of Life, National Academy Press, pp. 120–121, 1997.

24. Gillick M, Berkman S, Cullen L. A patient-centered approach to advance medical planning in the nursing home. J Am Geriatr Soc 47:227–230, 1999.

25. Ahronheim JC. Nutrition and hydration in the terminal patient. Clin Geriatr Med 12:379–391, 1996.

26. Finucane TE, Christmas C, Travis K. Tube feeding in patients with advanced dementia: a review of the evidence. JAMA 282:1365–1370, 1999.

27. Gillick MR. Rethinking the role of tube feeding in patients with advanced dementia. N Engl J Med 342:206–210, 2000.

28. Winter SM. Terminal nutrition: framing the debate for the withdrawal of nutritional support in terminally ill patients. Am J Med 109:723–726, 2000.

29. Morrison RS, Siu AL. Survival in end-stage dementia following acute illness. JAMA 284:47–52, 2000.

30. Volicer BJ, Hurley A, Fabiszewski KJ, Montgomery P, Volicer L. Predicting short-term survival for patients with advanced Alzheimer's disease. J Am Geriatr Soc 41:535–540, 1993.

31. Fabiszewski KJ, Volicer B, Volicer L. Effect of antibiotic treatment on outcome of fevers in institutionalized Alzheimer patients. JAMA 263:3168–3172, 1990.

32. Sengstaken EA, King SA. The problems of pain and its detection among geriatric nursing home residents. J Am Geriatr Soc 41:541–544, 1993.

33. Stein WM, Ferrell BA. Pain in the nursing home. Clin Geriatr Med 12:601–613, 1996.

34. Ferrell BA, Ferrell BR, Rivera L. Pain in cognitively impaired nursing home patients. J Pain Symptom Manage 10:591–598, 1995.

35. Luce JM, Luce JA. Management of dyspnea in patients with far-advanced lung disease. JAMA 285:1331–1337, 2001.

36. Ajemian I. Palliative management of dyspnea. J Palliat Care 7:44–45, 1991.

37. Dudgeon DJ, Rosenthal S. Management of dyspnea and cough in patients with cancer. Hematol Oncol Clin North Am 10:157–171, 1996.

38. Zeppetella G. The palliation of dyspnea in terminal disease. Am J Hosp Palliat Care 6:322–330, 1998.

39. Boyd KJ, Kelly M. Oral morphine as symptomatic treatment of dyspnea in patients with advanced cancer. Palliat Med 11:277–281, 1997.

40. McCann RM, Hall WJ, Groth-Juncker A. Comfort care for terminally ill patients: the appropriate use of nutrition and hydration. JAMA 272:1263–1266, 1994.

41. Emanuel LL, von Guntun CF, Ferris FD. The Education for Physicians on End-of-Life Care (EPEC) Curriculum, Module 10, 1999.

42. Emanuel LL, von Guntun CF, Ferris FD. The Education for Physicians on End-of-Life Care (EPEC) curriculum, Robert Wood Johnson Foundation. Module 6, 1999.

43. Adam J. ABC of palliative care: the last 48 hours. BMJ 315:1600–1633, 1997.

44. Tsukuda R. Interdisciplinary collaboration: teamwork in geriatrics. In: Cassel CK, Reisenberg DE, Sorenson LB, Walsh JR (Eds.). Geriatric Medicine, 2nd ed. New York, Springer-Verlag, pp. 668–675, 1990.

45. Chichin ER, Burack OR, Olson E, Likourezos A. End-of-life Ethics and the Nursing Assistant, New York, Springer, 2000.

46. Wilson SA, Daley BJ. Family perspectives on dying in long-term care settings. J Gerontol Nurs 24:10 19–25, 1999.

47. Kane RA, Caplan AL. Everyday Ethics: Resolving Dilemmas in Nursing Home Life. New York, Springer, 1990.

48. Burack OR, Chichin ER. A support group for nursing assistants: caring for nursing home residents at the end of life. Geriatr Nurs 22:299–305, 2001.

49. Rempusheski VF. The role of ethnicity in elder care. Nurs Clin North Am 24:717–724, 1989.

50. Caralis PV, Davis B, Wright K, Marcial E. The influence of race and ethnicity on attitudes toward advance directive, life-prolonging treatment, and euthanasia. J Clin Ethics 4:155–165, 1992.

51. Tripp-Reimer T, Affifi LA. Cross-cultural perspectives in patient teaching. Nurs Clin North Am 24:613–619, 1989.

52. Murphy C. The changing role of nurses in making ethical decisions. Law Med Health Care 12:173–174, 1984.

26

Family Caregivers: Burdens and Opportunities

CAROL LEVINE

Thomas Wilson (not his real name), in his 80s, was hospitalized for a large gastric carcinoma. He also had advanced dementia and was in pain. The hospital palliative care team met with his wife, who was in a wheelchair, and their grandson. Each medical or surgical option, including the insertion of a feeding tube, presented clear risks as well as uncertain benefits. As they discussed the goals of care, it became clear that Mrs. Wilson's primary goal was to keep her husband "comfortable." She did not know, however, what option would best meet that goal. She was particularly concerned that if he did not get a feeding tube, he would suffer from hunger. Reassured by the palliative care geriatrician that this would not happen, Mrs. Wilson decided that she would take her husband home without further interventions and with adequate pain medication and family support. He died peacefully at home a few weeks later.

Selma Morgan (another pseudonym) was an agitated 83-year-old woman with dementia and inoperable rectal cancer who was brought to the hospital emergency department by her daughter. She was not a candidate for hospice because her life expectancy was longer than 6 months. The palliative care

team considered whether nerve blocks or a palliative colostomy would relieve her pain or whether the potential side effects would create more difficulties. At a team meeting, her daughter, Tanya Nolan, opposed the idea of "the bag" and felt she could manage her mother's care at home with daytime help from home care aides paid for by Medicaid. Despite the team's reservations about Mrs. Nolan's ability to work during the day and care for her agitated mother at night, Mrs. Morgan was discharged with increased pain medication and followed by the palliative care team. Over the next several months, Mrs. Morgan was hospitalized and discharged repeatedly, with the precipitating event often occurring on weekends. The team felt that Mrs. Nolan failed to understand the realities of her mother's condition and was probably not following the medication regimen exactly. They also felt that she did not manage her own health very well (she was overweight). Mrs. Nolan resisted placing her mother in a long-term care facility, but she could not manage at home. Finally, Ms. Morgan was brought to a public hospital by ambulance after her daughter called 911. She died intubated in the intensive care unit. Even though the team had tried hard, they had not been able to develop a palliative care plan that addressed Mrs. Nolan's ambivalence about her mother's care.*

As these two cases indicate, palliative care is family care. This statement can be interpreted in two equally appropriate ways. First, especially when the patient is at home, family members provide much of the direct care that is included in the broad category of palliative care. Second, family members need care themselves to sustain them through the process of their loved one's dying and its aftermath. There are certainly some elderly people who are bereft of family and friends, either because of estrangement, geographic distance, or simply longevity. This chapter, however, concerns the majority of elderly people, whose family members are shared participants in their lives and trusted caregivers in their illness and death. As these two cases also suggest, family care adds a layer of complexity to palliative care, already a multidimensional system.

While family members have always provided care to seriously ill relatives, the care that family members are expected to provide in today's health-care environment is vastly more complex than it was even a decade ago. McCorkle and Pasacreta[1] asserted that "families are increasingly replacing skilled health care workers in the delivery of unfamiliar complex care to their ill family members despite the other obligations and responsibilities that characterize their lives." These authors' review of the literature on family caregivers and the palliative phase of cancer treatment highlights "(1) the increasing number of patients who are being treated in ambulatory clinics with ongoing complex care needs, (2) the increasing number of complex tasks assumed by family caregivers, (3) the high propor-

tion of unmet needs, (4) the subjective nature of the caregiving experience that encompasses both positive and negative elements, and (5) the conceptualization of caregiver burden as positively linked to negative reactions to caregiving." This daunting context makes it imperative that palliative care teams involve family members at all stages of their relative's care and in many different ways.

WHO COUNTS AS FAMILY?

In the palliative care context, as in health care more broadly, "family" should be interpreted broadly. Spouses and adult children are the most likely relatives to take on the responsibilities of caregiving for elderly people, but others (grandchildren, nieces and nephews, cousins) may also be involved. In the nontraditional relationships that exist today, family members may not be related by blood or marriage but *fictive kin* or *families of choice*. These terms describe people whose deep attachments give them the same emotional investment, if not the same legal authority, as more traditionally recognized relationships. Robert Lipsyte's[2] moving account of his own cancer treatment and his ex-wife's death from cancer shows that even broken relationships can be important at the end of life.

This chapter uses a broad definition of *family*: "family members are individuals who by birth, adoption, marriage, or declared commitment share deep, personal connections and are mutually entitled to receive and obligated to provide support of various kinds to the extent possible, especially in times of need."[3] My more colloquial version would be "family is anyone who shows up when illness strikes . . . and stays on to help."

As early as possible, the palliative care team should find out who the patient considers family and who has been providing care of what kind. These arrangements may be the basis for continued care, or they may need revision in light of the patient's needs or the family's capacities. The palliative care team comes to a case with fresh ideas

---

*These cases are adapted from cases observed and described by Better Wolder Levin, Ph.D., a medical anthropologist, as part of the United Hospital Fund Hospital Palliative Care Initiative, 1997–98. A full report on the initiative is available in Hopper S. Building Hospital Palliative Care Initiatives: Lessons from the Field. New York, United Hospital Fund, 2001.

and skills; but the family has its own, often long, history of dealing with the disease, which should be explored and acknowledged. Sometimes that history
includes instances of conflict or dissatisfaction with previous health-care providers.
The palliative care team members need to
be aware of this history, to provide good
patient and family-centered care.

Similarly, *caregiving* should be interpreted broadly. Depending on the setting,
palliative care provided by family members
may involve medication management,
symptom control, operation of medical
equipment, record keeping, personal care,
financial and legal management, coordination of services, ordering supplies, nutrition, mobility, communication with health-
care professionals, and all of the myriad
details of running a household. Where there
are many family members willing to help,
these tasks can be assigned so that no one
person bears all of the responsibilities.
However, often, one person, the primary
caregiver, takes on most of the burden; getting others to help out then becomes yet another task to accomplish.

WHO ARE FAMILY CAREGIVERS?

Approximately 25 million American adults,
or one in four, provide some level of care
for a relative or friend who is unable to
manage alone because of illness, disability,
or frailty. The economic value of their unpaid labor is approximately $257 billion
annually, more than the cost of formal
home care and nursing home care combined.[4] Most of the care recipients are elderly; in a national random telephone survey of family caregivers conducted by the
Harvard School of Public Health, the
United Hospital Fund (UHF), and the Visiting Nurse Service (VNS) of New York,
35% of the people they cared for were
women and 27% were 80 or older ($n =$
1002).[29] The majority of care recipients
suffered from one or more chronic diseases,
such as cancer, arthritis, diabetes, or dementia. They were at the end of life, al-

though they probably had been ill for many
years. In the same survey, half the caregivers who had cared for someone in the
past year were no longer doing so. The
main reason was that the person had died.

More women than men are caregivers,
although the number of men has increased
in the past several years. Nevertheless, high-
intensity personal care is still largely a
woman's role. In a survey of 1100 terminally ill patients and their caregivers,
Emanuel et al.[5] found that 96% of the primary caregivers were family members and
72.1% of these were women; one-third of
the caregivers were over 65, and one-third
were in poor health. In a separate analysis
of the Harvard–UHF–VNS survey, Navaie-
Waliser et al.[6] found that 36% of the family caregivers were *vulnerable,* defined as
having poor to fair health or a serious
health condition. Vulnerable caregivers
were more likely than nonvulnerable caregivers to be at least 65 years old, female,
married, and a primary caregiver and to
have less than a high school education.
They were more likely than nonvulnerable
caregivers to provide more than 20 hours
of care a week. (In the survey overall, caregivers provided an average of 20.5 hours
of care a week, slightly more than the 17.9
hours reported in 1997 by the National Alliance for Caregiving/(AARP) survey.[7])

For a caregiver, being vulnerable is not
just a theoretical risk. Numerous studies
have shown that caregivers are at higher
risk than their peers for major mental
health problems such as depression, which
is itself associated with other poor health
outcomes. Caregiving stress has been
shown to alter the immune system, leaving
the caregiver at risk for immune system diseases at worst and poor immunization results at best. Less dramatic but still worri-
some are back and muscle problems related
to lifting and turning a patient. Perhaps
most pervasive is sleep deprivation, the impact on health of which is only beginning
to be understood. Most seriously, caregivers are at risk of dying. In a study of elderly caregivers who experienced strain compared to non-caregiving peers or caregivers

who did not experience strain, Schulz and Beach[8] found that the overstressed caregivers were 63% more likely to die than the other groups.

Caregivers are also at risk financially; worrying about medical bills can only add to a caregiver's other sources of stress. Perhaps because it seems selfish or crass, caregivers are often reluctant to acknowledge the financial strain, yet the drain on resources that accompanies chronic illness has long-term consequences.[9] The Study to Understand Prognoses and Preferences for Outcomes and Risks of Treatment (SUPPORT) found that families of terminally ill patients experienced serious financial problems. Almost a third (31%) lost almost all of their family savings; 29% lost their major source of income; and 55% experienced either these problems or another major life change or family illness.[10] In the Emanuel et al.[11] study, patients and families who had substantial care needs were more likely to report that they had a subjective sense of economic burden (44.9%) compared to those with lesser needs (35.3%). In objective measures, these patients and families also were more likely to report that 10% of their income was spent on health care (28.0% compared to 17%) and that they had to take out a loan or mortgage, spend their savings, or take on a second job (16.3% compared to 10.2%). The authors concluded that the families of terminally ill patients with high care needs are likely to experience economic hardship, especially if they are low-income to begin with. If any additional evidence is needed, it is only necessary to look at bankruptcy data. About 40% of the personal bankruptcies declared in the United States in 1999 were related to medical bills or illness.[12]

WHAT DO FAMILIES NEED?
WHAT DO THEY WANT?

Research on family caregivers and palliative care is quite recent and has mostly involved cancer diagnoses. Nevertheless, the results are quite consistent and applicable in most ways to other cases. Regardless of the setting and the particular medical condition, families want information and communication, education and training, and emotional support and advocacy. These of course are very broad categories, and moving them from abstractions into practical interventions requires skill and insight.

Turning first to the concrete needs for assistance, the Harvard–UHF –VNS survey of family caregivers identified two major categories of unmet needs. Of the 17.9% (n = 1063) who reported unmet needs, 55.5% said that they had a medical need (nurse, doctor, other) and 71.2% said that they had a nonmedical need (home care aide, other nonprofessional service). The Emanuel et al.[11] study of family caregivers of terminally ill patients reported that 87% of families needed more help: 62% with transportation, 55% with homemaking, 28% with nursing, and 26% with personal care. The needs of cancer patients and their families were better addressed than were the needs of those with other conditions. Of the cancer patients, 28.9% had substantial needs for care compared to 40.9% of patients with other diseases. About 15% of the cancer patients and their families reported unmet needs compared to 22.9% of patients with other diseases. While the percentage of unmet needs for cancer patients was substantial, the authors concluded that these patients probably had better access than other patients to services because the terminal nature of their disease was more predictable and because their physicians may have been more skilled at organizing assistance.

PAIN AND
SYMPTOM MANAGEMENT

Pain is a common symptom in diseases affecting elderly people. Family members are extremely sensitive to, and upset by, what they perceive to be inadequate pain control for their relative. Pain control was reported to be a key factor important at the end of life by seriously ill patients, recently bereaved family, physicians, and other care providers such as nurses, social workers, chaplains, and hospice volunteers.[13] Despite the recent attention to pain control, a 1997 study in Oregon found that for the first time in 10 years family reports of moderate or severe pain in their relative's last week of life increased, from 33% to 57%. This increase occurred during the highly charged discussion of physician-assisted suicide legislation in the state. Nearly all (96%) health-care professionals surveyed to understand the reasons for this increase believed that family members had increased expectations about pain management: 66% believed that physicians had decreased their prescribing, largely because of fears of prosecution; and 59% believed that nurses were decreasing the administration of pain medication.[14]

Some studies report discrepancies between the level of pain reported by patients and family members and between the assessments of family members and health-care professionals. Health-care professionals sometimes slight family members' concerns because family members are not objective about the situation. On the contrary, these reports should always be taken seriously. However professionals assess the patient's pain, family members who report their relative's pain are themselves suffering, and their psychic pain must be addressed. Moreover, family members may recognize verbal or nonverbal cues from the patient that others do not.

An African-American woman describes one such situation when her sister was dying in a hospital but never asked for pain medication.

The doctor said to me "Your sister is not in any pain." I replied "Yes, she is." The doctor questioned "How do you know that? You just got here." I answered "By her moans, groans, and 'oh me's.'" I explained to the doctor that we grew up in a family of 12 and that in order to be heard, you had to make a lot of noise to get attention, whether you were sick or well. Those moans, groans, and 'oh me's' meant 'get and give me what I need.' It was not required that you ask for anything. It was understood that you would get what you needed for your ailment or your pain.[15]

In many cases when the patient is at home, family members are responsible for pain management. With varying degrees of information and support from professionals, they assess pain, make decisions regarding dosage and type of medication, keep accurate records, and communicate with physicians or others about side effects or inadequate pain control.[16] If it is difficult to communicate with the health-care team, the local pharmacist becomes the primary source of information and advice. While the pharmacist can be an invaluable resource, he or she may not have all of the relevant medical information about the specific case. Family members often give medications during the night, leading to severe sleep deprivation and the possibility of error. They must often absorb the costs of medications and devices that are not covered by insurance.

Placed in this situation of heavy responsibility, untrained family members must struggle with their natural desire to keep their ill relative comfortable and free of pain with a widely held anti-drug or, more specifically, anti-opioid stance. They are afraid of giving too much pain medicine and distressed by the idea of giving too little. Some families, however, are reluctant to intervene. The family may have religious convictions that depict suffering as redemptive. African Americans who hold traditional Christian beliefs or whose cultural history includes the integration of pain into their lives may resist pain medications.[17]

Palliative care team members can make a major contribution to family caregivers by educating and reassuring them that high levels of medication for severe pain will not cause addiction. Teaching them or providing tapes about alternative methods of pain control, such as massage or relaxation techniques, can also be helpful. These methods can also be useful for family members themselves when they experience severe stress. The emotional impact of dealing with a loved one's pain can be profoundly debilitating for the caregiver.

Adequate pain and symptom control are necessary but not sufficient for family members. All three groups (patients, families, and providers) who participated in the survey cited earlier identified other valuable attributes: "clear decision making, preparation for death, completion, contributing to others, and affirmation of the whole person."[13] Of all nine major attributes, freedom from pain was ranked highest and dying at home lowest. Of the three groups that participated in the survey, physicians were more often concerned about the biomedical aspects of care, while patients and families considered psychosocial and spiritual issues to be as important as physiological ones. Patients, for example, placed a high importance on being mentally aware, being able to plan funeral arrangements, not being a burden, helping others, and coming to peace with God. Physicians, however, did not value these attributes as highly. Families ranked pain control and coming to peace with God as equally important.

In Oregon, the research team Overcoming Barriers developed a "wish list for changes to improve care of the dying," based on interviews with 475 family members.[18] In this list, families want the following:

- To have their loved ones' wishes honored regarding life-sustaining treatment
- To be respected in their role as surrogate decision maker
- To receive assistance in honoring their loved ones' wishes for location of death
- To have their loved ones' comfort be a priority
- To work with providers who aggressively manage pain and other distressing symptoms
- To receive timely responses to requests for additional pain medication
- To receive practical help with transportation and transfers between settings
- To have providers who communicate with each other and function as a team
- To receive honest information from health-care providers who are available, responsive, and caring

- To have an opportunity to speak with providers after their loved ones' death
- To be provided with emotional and spiritual support
- To have a comfortable, private room where they can say goodbye to their dying loved ones.

WHAT THE PALLIATIVE CARE TEAM CAN DO FOR FAMILY CAREGIVERS

While this wish list presents an ideal, which is probably not achievable in most situations, certainly some aspects can be implemented. In their literature review, McCorkle and Pasacreta[1] found a limited number of intervention studies. Informational or educational interventions try to meet the needs of family caregivers for information about the patient's condition and physical care, as well as about caregivers' emotional reactions. Caregivers need different kinds of information at different points in the trajectory of illness: at diagnosis, during hospitalization (especially if surgery is involved), at the start of new treatments, when there is a recurrence or destabilizing event, and during the dying phase. Caregivers can be overwhelmed by too much information as well as anxiety-ridden by too little. It is important that information be presented in terms the family will understand (which may be very simple or very technical) and that different team members present consistent information. The same information may need to be repeated because it is too emotion-laden to be absorbed all at once. Family caregivers need a number to call when they have questions, and they should be encouraged to make those calls.

von Gunten et al.[19] suggested a seven-step approach to structuring the communication of important information. The first three steps prepare the patient, caregivers, and physician for the discussion by creating a hospitable environment for the conversation, ascertaining what the patient and family already know, and determining how the information is to be shared and with whom. After the discussion (which is the fourth step in the process), the physician should respond to the emotions raised by the information, reach consensus about the goals of care and treatment priorities, and establish a plan for achieving these goals.

Support interventions are more directly aimed at assisting the caregiver to articulate and deal with the emotional turmoil that accompanies a relative's serious illness. Davies[20] provides a useful scheme for assessing family functioning, including being prepared to collect information over time and from different family members. She recommends listening to the family's story and using clinical judgment to determine where intervention is required. Her suggestions for problem solving are practical: "Be aware of the limitations of family conferences and be prepared to follow up." Family conferences, she warns, work well for cohesive families but not so well for families where more disparity of opinion exists. Some family members may not openly disagree with what appears to be a consensus but may undermine the plan anyway.[20]

While informational and educational interventions are most often implemented by nurses or other direct care providers, many different professionals, such as social workers, chaplains, and psychologists, can provide emotional support through counseling. These interventions may also be peer-led, through support groups, or through family-to-family discussions. Most of these interventions have not been rigorously evaluated, although those caregivers who participate seem to find them useful. Most caregivers, however, either do not have access to support of this kind or choose not to take part. There may be many reasons: concerns about privacy, cultural traditions, language difficulties, the press of more immediate economic survival demands.

Apart from formal interventions, everyone connected with a palliative care team can provide one extremely beneficial support: active listening. Often, family caregivers do not want anything more than a kind and compassionate listener, one who will, for those few moments, pay attention to what the caregiver is experiencing. These conversations may bring out caregivers' concerns about, for example, redefining their expectations about cure, accepting the patient's diminished capacities, struggling with ambivalence, searching for meaning, and ultimately preparing for death.

THE FINAL DAYS

Dying at home has become the gold standard of a "good death." Certainly, many, if not most, patients want to be at home, surrounded by their loved ones. A good hospice or palliative care team can usually make this possible, but there are limits to what even the most loving families can endure and provide, especially if symptoms are difficult to control. Keeping the patient at home may require considerable financial resources, for extra help, equipment, and medications that are not reimbursed. The home environment may not be one that can easily be adapted to the requirements of home death. If it becomes necessary to transfer the patient to a hospital, the family should not be made to feel that they have failed.[21]

A good death does not depend on the site (although certainly home is preferred). It can occur in a hospital (as in Lipsyte's[2] ex-wife's death) or in a nursing home. Young[22] describes her mother's last 5 days of life in a nursing home:

[S]he became confined to her bed and was given a special mattress to discourage bedsores. The nurses placed padding around her feet, gave her blankets, propped her up with pillows, and gave her oxygen to keep her comfortable and warm. Her doctor, social worker, and members of the nursing staff regularly came into her room to offer comfort. Her primary nurse's aide had grown to love Mother, so we consoled each other. Several nurses' aides shared their stories with me about the good times they had had with her. They told me how she had recently surprised them with words she had long ago lost the ability to say, an outburst of song, and displays of affectionate gratitude for their service. I had noticed that she was strangely joyful in the last few months. She died in October. I was grateful that

I had been in the light of her joy through the struggle of her dying.

When death is near, or as near as can be predicted, family members need explicit guidance about what to expect. Taylor[23] describes her dismay when she was not told that her mother was imminently dying. There were two reasons, she found out.

First, each nurse thought another nurse had told me. Second, there had been a miscommunication with the doctor during his rounds in the morning. The nurses expected him to tell me that she was dying. . . . In fact, it appears that he had missed the signs of approaching death and what he told me was that she would 'bounce back' once the antibiotics took hold.

Most people have never been present at a death and are influenced by what they have seen on television or have been told by others. They may have unrealistic expectations or fears. The palliative care team should do whatever is possible medically to make these last moments peaceful and calm. If there is a last-minute decision to transfer the patient, the relevant advance directives should be readily available and entered into the medical chart. If it is important to the patient or to the family that others be present, they should be summoned as soon as it appears that death is likely to occur. Some private moments after death allow the family to touch the body, pray, comfort each other, or simply accept the reality.

BEREAVEMENT

If American culture is uncomfortable with death, it is positively hostile to bereavement that lasts past the funeral and a period of mourning that is sanctioned by a religious authority. While most organized bereavement programs follow families for a year, one palliative medicine consultant believes that the second year is even harder than the first. The bereaved person's feelings of grief are just as strong, but he or she gets a societal message that cuts off expression of these feelings.[24] Frequently isolated from friends and colleagues during the terminal phase of the illness, the caregiver is surrounded by sympathetic well-wishers immediately after the death, only to be neglected once again if he or she does not quickly "move on with life." The medical professionals who were so closely involved in the patient's final weeks and days now disappear, often even without a condolence note or phone call. Holidays, anniversaries, even critical dates in the illness now reinforce the depth of the loss. Caregivers who had become totally invested in their relative's care may find it difficult to re-engage in social or work activities, which by contrast seem inconsequential.

Spouses in particular appear to be at increased risk of morbidity and mortality during this period. Even though they may have been under extreme stress during the illness, death is only a fleeting relief. The weight of the strains they have accumulated brings a new kind of sadness, as well as new financial and legal responsibilities to organize.[25] A caregiver dealing with a seemingly endless flow of unpaid medical bills with a reduced income is not irrational to be depressed. Supporting the caregiver through the bereavement process may be one of palliative care's most important challenges.

Interviews with caregivers after the patient's death are generally received well, despite many practitioners' fears that they would be considered intrusive. In a series of focus groups conducted by the UHF's Families and Health Care project, bereaved caregivers expressed their gratitude for the opportunity to discuss their relative's dying. For some, it was difficult at first. One young man could not even say his name during the introductions but later described his father's death and his own feelings in detail. Another participant followed the facilitator out of the room after the session ended, seeking to continue the conversation. It was clear to observers that these caregivers had not had any opportunity to discuss this momentous experience with others.[26]

A British study found that over 80% of a group of recently bereaved family members showed only mild or no distress when interviewed. Many caregivers were grateful for the chance to talk about the death and to help others in the future. Others were glad to have a chance to express their anger at their relative's care; the hope is that a good palliative care experience would eliminate this need.[27]

Still, no matter how superb the care and how compassionate the interactions with family members, someone they love has died.[28] Palliative care cannot change that awful finality, but it can help to create meaningful memories of the person's dying and death. To family caregivers, this will be a treasured gift, to be passed on as part of the family's unique history.

REFERENCES

1. McCorkle R, Pasacreta JV. Enhancing caregiver outcomes in palliative care. Cancer Control 8:36–45, 2001.
2. Lipsyte R. In the Country of Illness: Comfort and Advice for the Journey. New York, Alfred A Knopf, 1998.
3. Levine L. AIDS and changing concepts of family. In: Nelkin D, Willis DP, Paris SV (Eds.). A Disease of Society: Cultural and Institutional Responses to AIDS. New York, Cambridge University Press, p. 48, 45–70, 1991.
4. Arno PS, Levine C, Memmott MM. The economic value of informal caregiving. Health Affairs 18:182–188, 1999; updated data from 2001.
5. Emanuel EJ, Fairclough DL, Slutsman J, Alpert H, Baldwin D, Emanuel LJ. Assistance from family members, friends, paid care givers, and volunteers in the care of terminally ill patients. N Engl J Med 341:956–963, 1999.
6. Navaie-Waliser M, Gould DA, Levine C, Kuerbis AN, Donelan K. When the caregiver needs care: the plight of vulnerable caregivers. Am J Public Health 2002, in press. Vol. 92(3) March: 404–413.
7. National Alliance for Caregiving and the American Association of Retired Persons (AARP). Family Caregiving in the U.S.: Findings from a National Survey. Washington DC, NAC/AARP 1997. Available at http://www.caregiving.org
8. Schulz R, Beach SR. Caregiving as a risk factor for mortality. JAMA 282:2215–2219, 1999.
9. Rigoglioso RL. Your money or your life: the financial burden of caregiving. In:

10. Levine C (Ed.). Always On Call: When Illness Turns Family Members into Caregivers. New York, United Hospital Fund, pp. 113–130, 2000.
11. Covinsky KE, Goldman L, Cook EF, et al. The impact of serious illness on patient's families. JAMA 272:1839–1844, 1989.
12. Emanuel EJ, Fairclough DL, Slutsman J, Emanuel LL. Understanding economic and other burdens of terminal illness: the experience of patients and their caregivers. Am J Intern Med 132:451–459, 2000.
13. Jacoby MS, Sullivan TA, Warren E. Medical problems and bankruptcy filings. Norton Bankruptcy Law Advisor pp. 1–12, 2000.
14. Steinhauser KE, Christakis NA, Clipp EC, McNeilly M, McIntyre L, Tulsky JA. Factors considered important at the end of life by patients, family, physicians, and other care providers. JAMA 284:2746–2482, 2000.
15. Hickman SE, Tolle SW, Tilden VP. Physicians' and nurses' perspectives on increased family reports of pain in dying hospitalized patients: J Palliat Med 3:413–418, 2000.
16. Harper BC, Lartigue M, Doka KJ. Cultural differences: sensitivities required for effective caring. In: Doka KJ, Davidson JD (Eds.). Caregiving and Loss: Family Needs, Professional Responsibilities. Washington DC, Hospice Foundation of America, p. 148, 2001.
17. Juarez G, Ferrell BR. Family and caregiver involvement in pain management. Clin Geriatr Med 12:531–547, 1996.
18. Crawley L, Payne R, Bolden J, Payne T, Washington P, Williams S. Palliative and end-of-life care in the African American community. JAMA 284:2518–2521, 2000.
19. Center for Ethics in Health Care. The Oregon Report Card: Improving Care of the Dying. Accessed May 1, 2001. Available at http://www.ohsu/edu/ethics
20. von Gunten CF, Ferris FD, Emanuel LL. Ensuring competency in end-of-life care. JAMA 284:3051–3057, 2000.
21. Davies B. Supporting families in palliative care. In: Ferrell B (Ed.). Textbook of Palliative Nursing. New York, Oxford University Press, pp. 363–373, 2001.
22. Stajduhar KI, Davies B. Death at home: challenges for families and directions for the future. J Palliat Care 14:8–14, 1998.
23. Young CA. First my mother, then my aunt. In: Levine C (Ed.). Always On Call: When Illness Turns Families into Caregivers. New York, United Hospital Fund, p. 31, 21–32, 2000.
24. Taylor D. On dying: why was I not told? J Palliat Care 13(4):53–54, 1997.
25. Davis GF. Loss and the duration of grief. JAMA 285:1152–1153, 2001.

25. Wyatt GK, Friedman L, Given CW, Given BA. A profile of bereaved caregivers following provision of terminal care. J Palliat Care 15:13–25, 1999.

26. Levine C. Rough Crossings: Family Members' Odysseys through the Health Care System. New York, United Hospital Fund, 1999.

27. Seamark DA, Gilbert J, Lawrence CJ, Williams S. Are postbereavement research interviews distressing to carers? Lessons learned from palliative care research. Palliat Med 14:55–56, 2000.

28. Sachs GA. Sometimes dying still stings. JAMA 284:2423, 2000.

29. Donelan K, Hill CA, Hoffman C, Scoles K, Feldman PH, Levine C, Gould D. Challenged to care: Informal caregivers in a changing health system. Health Affairs 21:222–231, 2002.

27

Home Care for Frail, Older Adults

KNIGHT STEEL AND CAROLINE VITALE

Without question, the site of care preferred by almost all older persons in need of palliative care is the home. There are few who would not remain at home if needed technology and support staff could be provided in an appropriately coordinated fashion.[1-3] In contrast to the paucity of available services and the difficulty in obtaining durable medical equipment just 20 years ago in the United States, comprehensive home-care services, including hospice care, are now widespread. Home services are desired not only by those who have palliative care needs but, to the extent they can reduce the cost of more expensive services,[4] also by third-party payers.

Reimbursement mechanisms, predominantly under governmental control, have determined to a great extent the type and intensity of home-care services available to elders, be they for palliative concerns or not. In the United States many not-for-profit home-care agencies, once the predominant suppliers of home-care and palliative care services, have been replaced to a great extent by for-profit corporations.

The majority of companies providing equipment and supplies are similarly structured. These corporations, for-profit or not-for-profit, are usually financially independent of acute or long-term institutional settings and generally have incentives to provide more services or supplies if the rate of reimbursement allows for income in excess of expenses and fewer services if not. In other countries, such as Canada and the United Kingdom, access to home palliative care has been unequally distributed and is dependent on factors such as socioeconomic status, age, and rural versus urban areas.[5-9] Given the dearth of health-services research in this area, the difficulty of obtaining outcome measures, and demographic and hospital reimbursement changes, prescribing appropriate yet not excessive palliative care services in the home setting is both difficult for the practitioner and likely to be carefully monitored by the third party.[10]

In addition, most home-care services, especially those directed to long-term palliative care needs, depend on the availability and the participation of one or more informal caregivers. These persons, usually spouses or female adult children, often provide services at all hours of the day and night. Such essential caregivers often require extensive education; attention to their competing needs for employment, child care, and marital life; and respite from what may be exhausting work carried out over weeks, months, or years.[11] Regrettably, outside resources are infrequently available to address these issues. Studies have repeatedly found a strong relationship between dying at home and the presence of a primary carer.[7,12,13] The probability of dying at home is "highly dependent on the carers' ability to stay the course," whether or not professional home care is added.[7] Another recent survey related a higher likelihood of dying at home with patients who clearly stated a preference for having the place of death be at home.[14] In fact, a rising percentage of deaths in the home setting has been recently documented.[15] This is expected to increase as the population ages and as access to home palliative care improves. Lastly, the coordination of formal and informal services and the availability of immediate back-up services in the home setting are central considerations when providing home-care services. Unlike institutional settings where staff usually can fill in where necessary, the sudden unavailability of an informal caregiver, for example, may result in serious failures in patient care.

ASSESSMENT

If an older person has a palliative care need, initially that individual must be assessed to determine the cause of the problem. Thus, the provider of palliative care should never fail to attempt to determine the etiology of the symptom, although the vigor and extent to which this should be done are determined by the individual set of circumstances. Thus, abdominal pain in an individual with widespread metastatic cancer of the colon is likely due to the cancer (although not necessarily so) and therefore requires only a limited evaluation. Such patients warrant treatment directed specifically to the relief of that symptom. However, low back pain in an older man with known osteoarthritis is not necessarily secondary to that degenerative condition. He may have metastatic prostate cancer, disc disease with nerve impairment, multiple myeloma, or a host of other illnesses.

There is no substitute for a detailed evaluation including a targeted history, physical examination, and appropriate laboratory studies as sculpted by an individual's life expectancy and the potential impact on that person's quality of life should a treatable condition be discovered and addressed therapeutically. It must always be born in mind that individuals accumulate chronic diseases as they age, thus often making it more difficult to determine the etiology of a given symptom than might be true in a younger person. Also, disease may present less dramatically in older adults, and geriatric patients may attribute symptoms inappropriately to the aging process, often for long periods of time. It can be said that from a medical viewpoint individuals become increasingly unique as they age.

Perhaps for these reasons, geriatric medicine has been in the forefront of the design and utilization of standardized assessments. Domains that may require assessment in more or less detail, depending on the specific palliative care issue, include (1) physiological measures such as blood pressure, pulse, respiratory rate, forced expiratory volume in 1 second (FEV_1), and the frequency of bowel movements; (2) functional measures, including activities of daily living such as the ability to feed oneself, transfer, and toilet and instrumental activities of daily living such as the ability to shop, bank and drive a car; (3) subjective symptom distress measures, such as pain, nausea, dyspnea, weakness, fatigue, and depression; and (4) measures of family caregiver needs, including those related to stress reduction, depression, grieving, and even risk factors for elder abuse. Lastly, in the home setting, there is the need to assess the physical environment of the patient to determine what risks, such as throw rugs and diminished lighting, can be corrected. Comprehensive yet targeted care requires consideration of all of these domains.

Many symptoms, for example, nausea, depression, and pain, require first that they be recognized by the professional caregiver. In the home setting, information is typically gathered from an informal caregiver and, often, the physician or nurse may do so over the phone. Therefore, the professional may need to appreciate how a third party, the informal caregiver, may interpret a patient's symptoms due to fear, ignorance, or fatigue. To avoid missing them, the professional should ask about symptoms which may be present, even if the information is not volunteered. Recording the character of symptoms, their intensity, their precipitants, what makes them better or worse, and their change over time is essential if the efficacy of interventions is to be determined.

Circumstances will dictate whether an emphasis on one or another parameter is indicated. Palliative care often requires a detailed evaluation of one or more distressing symptoms to determine what is likely to be effective. Sometimes simple interventions may be used. Thus, if sitting upright relieves dyspnea, advising the homebound person to use couch cushions underneath a pillow for sleeping may be helpful. Similarly, providing stairs over the side of a bathtub may not only diminish the risk of falling but may markedly decrease the pain associated with hip flexion when bathing is desired. Appropriate bracing and splinting of painful joints or pathological lesions similarly may diminish pain and may prevent sudden movements, either passive or active, from being so feared that a person chooses to lie motionless.

Information obtained from a targeted history and physical examination may need to be supplemented with laboratory data. It is axiomatic that tests should be obtained only when the results will likely influence outcomes. At least two circumstances bear special consideration. The first, of course, is when a symptom is being initially evaluated. The decision as to which tests are warranted is driven by the ease and potential burden of obtaining them, the value to the clinician of a positive or negative result, the likelihood of a false-positive or false-negative result, and on occasion costs to the patient and family. The second is when a person's symptoms are likely to be aggravated by an easily remedied condition. Thus, for example, fatigue may well be made worse by a low hemoglobin level. Similarly, dyspnea may be markedly improved in a person with chronic obstructive pulmonary disease if there is an element of congestive heart failure as well which is amenable to therapy. Thus, in such a circumstance, measurement of the ejection fraction may be warranted even if this requires a trip to an ambulatory setting.

Social and economic circumstances also may require thoughtful consideration, and the caregivers themselves may require monitoring to be sure they are adequately educated. It is not always appreciated how difficult it is for a lay caregiver to recall and follow directions about a new procedure in the home setting. Thus, if an individual is going home from a hospital with a feeding tube for the first time, detailed instructions may need to be provided legibly in writing on more than one occasion and the caregiver assessed as to his or her ability to carry out the instructions shortly after discharge.[16]

One system for a comprehensive assessment of older adults' palliative care needs was developed by a research organization, InterRAI, Inc.[17] (www.interrai.org) This not-for-profit group of scientists and clinicians bases its series of assessment tools on the Resident Assessment Instrument, mandated for use in all nursing homes in the United States. Modified to address more specifically palliative care needs, the Resident Assessment Instrument for Palliative Care (RAI-PC) has been field-tested recently and found to be reliable. It includes questions directed to the following domains: mental state, symptom presence and management, caregiver stress, continence, skin care, functional state, cognition, ability to communicate, and patients' wishes, among others. This assessment tool is designed to be used in all settings but especially the home. It will provide an overview of an individual's needs and allow data to be grouped so that settings for the provision of palliative care can be compared and groups of individuals risk-adjusted so that outcomes of interventions can be more accurately measured.

In considering how best to provide comprehensive palliative care in the home setting, professionals and informal caregivers alike must prioritize according to which needs are most troublesome to the patient. At times, individuals may prefer having pain to being sedated or dyspnea to delirium. No matter the wishes of the patient, the provider is still well advised to follow the Hippocratic treatises of the fifth and fourth centuries B.C. The author of *On Diseases*, Book I (Chapter 6), wrote "it is right in treating patients to cure curable ('feasible') conditions fully but in the case of incurable ('infeasible') ones to know why they cannot be treated and, in treating those who have such (untreatable) diseases, to help them as much as is feasible on the basis of one's treatment" (reference kindly supplied by Professor Heinrich von Staden, Institute for Advanced Study, Princeton, NJ).

PROFESSIONAL ORGANIZATION AND STAFF

The Physician

The decision to provide palliative care in the home setting presupposes that an appropriate mix of professionals is available. Although in the United Kingdom and some other nations, home visiting by physicians remains at least a recognized option, in the United States, housecalls by a doctor continue to be the exception rather than the rule.[18] This situation may improve in the future with the introduction of a better reimbursement schedule for home visits by physicians and the introduction of an examination in home care in the year 2000 under the aegis of the American Academy of Home Care Physicians.[19] Still, at this time, few physicians make home visits, and

of these only a modest number are knowledgeable about palliative care.[20]

In part to overcome this deficit, most palliative care services when provided in the home setting in the United States are coordinated by hospices. Modeled after St. Christopher's and other such facilities in the United Kingdom, they have significant advantages in that they generally take a comprehensive multidisciplinary approach to managing symptoms and are usually staffed by knowledgeable professionals.[21,22] Furthermore, funding, although often inadequate given the costs of modern palliative therapies, allows for the delivery of care of a reasonable quality to most older recipients. Unfortunately, in general only persons at or very near the end of life are eligible for hospice care under Medicare. This falsely dichotomous relationship between palliation and life prolonging care effectively guarantees that persons will receive palliative care services at home under the hospice benefit for only a short time (often a few weeks or less), due to the desire of most individuals to employ life-prolonging treatments until death is imminent. Also, once patients are enrolled in hospice, more often than not primary-care physicians participate little, if at all, in their care beyond the perfunctory signing of forms.[23] Some argue that palliative care services organized under hospice programs should therefore be more collaborative in character, helping the primary-care provider assume a leadership position in a multidisciplinary team and facilitating communication among professionals, family members, and patients.[24,25] The importance of the primary physician's role in home palliative care is underscored by a recent study showing that terminally ill patients who are most compliant with taking their medications viewed their general practitioner as their main prescriber and not the hospice or home-care nurse.[26]

Still, experience with hospice services in the home setting in the United States, the United Kingdom, and other nations such as Sweden, demonstrates that comprehensive care directed to palliation can be delivered effectively over a considerable period of time.[27] The availability of both equipment and services is driven to a great extent by the reimbursement system. It is apparent that palliative care services under hospice will increase in quantity and variety if targeted for sufficient funding and likely will become less available if they are capitated or the budget process forces them to compete with other services for resources.[28] How incentives might be formulated to facilitate the best palliative care system for the home setting in the United States, for example, is not clear at this time. As noted, higher reimbursement rates for physician visits have been introduced too recently to determine their effect.

Physicians are poorly trained in palliative care.[29–31] In both undergraduate and postgraduate education, the emphasis has been on cure rather than comprehensive symptom management and support for families.[32–34]

The Social Worker

The social worker who works as a member of the hospice team has traditionally concerned him- or herself with the needs of both patients and their caregivers. This professional may well also take a lead role in managing the grieving process after the death of the patient. With respect to a geriatric individual who is near the end of life, this professional must be familiar with community resources such as meals-on-wheels programs or church-organized support services. In addition, since the range and degree of sophistication of volunteer agencies vary from location to location, the social worker may need to be especially adept at finding a way to "make do" with existing resources.

Financial concerns may be paramount to both patients and families, especially if palliative care needs are protracted in time and if the older adult has a fixed income. In some countries, for example the United States, reverse mortgages permit an older couple to access the assets in their home. In countries where drugs need to be purchased by the consumer, knowledge of prescription-support programs may be helpful. Transportation requirements are central for older persons who may need assistance with ambulation or who do not have a spouse or relative who drives.

It is often the social worker who encourages the older adult in need of palliative care to continue to participate in enjoyable activities where still possible (e.g., card games can be moved to the bedside) and to order those services at home that may be perceived by the patient as essential for social intercourse, such as manicures or hair styling. Social workers may well need to foster a life review and facilitate a positive reframing of life's events. This professional must encourage the patient to use coping skills that worked in the past, especially if palliative care needs can only be partially fulfilled by pharmacological or other interventions.

Patients and their families may simply need time to vent. Palliative care needs are often the triggers for the surfacing of long-standing difficulties between patient and caregiver. It is unrealistic to expect these issues, which may extend back for decades, to be easily resolved. Rather, the social worker may suggest formal counseling for the caregiver so that some aspects of these long-time problems can be recognized as less important than other more positive aspects of a relationship that may have been extant for even a half-century. Caregivers may also benefit substantially from respite services, be they for a few hours or a few days. In the words of more than one social worker "You can't pour from an empty pitcher." Younger children in the household may need special attention, with opportunities both to participate in care and to be sheltered from situations which are especially threatening or sorrowful.

Although not exclusively an issue for social workers, these professionals may highlight and find it necessary to address the fears, both spoken and unspoken, of patient and caregiver surrounding palliative care needs.[35,36] Does the symptom suggest progression of an illness? Will a functional decline ever be reversed? Will the stress on a family member of caring for a needy person be harmful to the caregiver? Will the palliative care needs result in economic hardship? Palliative care in the home encompasses more than the strictly medical aspects of palliative care needs. Assessment and ongoing monitoring of the social and psychological well-being of each patient as well as that of caregivers should be more than perfunctory in nature if the care is to be exemplary.[37,38]

In addition, if the patient has palliative care needs at the end of life, appropriate long-term planning is necessary. Once the patient dies, the family may need considerable attention for some time. The natural grieving process may require monitoring, and persons who have sustained a loss should have access to support groups and, when necessary, professional intervention. In fact, a recent analysis suggests that carers of patients who die at home versus those who die elsewhere are likely to experience higher and longer-lasting levels of psychological distress in bereavement, necessitating close follow-up by a social worker or other appropriate professional. If there is no formal chaplaincy service available to the patient and family or if they do not wish to see a chaplain, the social worker may need to facilitate access to other supportive resources in the community. In addition, arrangement for funeral services may be required.

The Nurse

When palliative care is envisioned, it is the nurse who is likely viewed as the principal professional. This is with good reason, given the scope of the nurse's responsibility for both primary care and administration of services. To a great extent, nurses have come to replace physicians as principal providers in the home-care setting, especially when hospice services in the home are offered. It is usually the nurse who both recognizes and attempts to alleviate the distressing symptoms associated with the dying process, often acting to palliate symptoms within pre-

scribed boundaries established in advance of their appearance.

The nurse's primary-care responsibilities may be grouped into three categories. First, this individual usually establishes and maintains the bridges between family members, the patient, the professionals, and the required durable equipment agencies. Second, it is the nurse who must recognize and evaluate the intensity of palliative care needs, arrange for therapy, and determine the efficacy of interventions. Third, it is the nurse who must anticipate needs when possible and prevent symptoms and the whole array of negative consequences of the disease or medications from occurring.

With respect to the first role, nurses traditionally encourage both patients and their families to express their concerns and to address them with the social worker should one be available. Thus, the nurse usually must be an "ear" for the entire professional community and farm out concerns to the professional or service agency most likely to be helpful. The nurse likely works closely with a physician, who may rely to an exceptional degree on this professional in the home setting.

The second and third roles, the traditional ones, may be most time-consuming. A series of domains may need to be addressed either continuously or sequentially: (1) nutrition and hydration, (2) the urinary tract, (3) skin care, (4) dyspnea, (5) bowel functioning including nausea and vomiting, (6) spirituality and mental health, (7) safety, (8) pain and other symptoms in need of pharmaceuticals, as well as (9) other less frequent symptoms and needs. After assessing the symptoms and needs of a palliative care patient in the home, the nurse may occasionally conclude that home palliative care is not feasible, due either to lack of caregiver/social support or to a failure to control symptoms at home, necessitating an inpatient admission. Readmissions to the hospital are usually due to lack of symptom control, caregiver stress, or lack of communication and coordination between the different professionals.[3,40–42] The nurse plays a pivotal role in assessing, treating, and preventing symptoms; coordinating care by facilitating communication; and supporting the caregiver, thereby preventing potential hospitalization or institutionalization as much as possible.

Nutrition and hydration

Families caring for persons with palliative care needs not infrequently place considerable emphasis on nutrition, perhaps because providing food is associated with affection and caring. Also, family members may equate food intake with helping to increase their loved one's strength and well-being. While family members may feel helpless as they watch the relentless progression of a devastating illness, they may view nutrition as something which has intrinsic value and which they can provide to the patient to help the situation. In addition, eating is something the family can do together. Therefore, families may need to be educated about the patient's illness and its effect on both the ability and the desire to eat. Families may need to be advised that forcing an individual to eat is not likely to be beneficial and may actually provoke bloating and vomiting.[43]

It is possible to make a rough estimate of the individual's daily caloric needs so as to maintain his weight. As a general rule, the total caloric requirement is obtained by multiplying the nonedematous weight in kilograms by about 30. Thus, an individual weighing about 130 lb (about 60 kg) who does not have significant amounts of edema will require about 1800 calories per day. This assumes that there are no exceptional factors, such as high fever, severe chronic obstructive pulmonary disease, (COPD) or malabsorbtion secondary to abnormal bowel function. Furthermore, it assumes that the individual's activity is minimal.

The olfactory sense is diminished with age, affecting both the taste and enjoyment of food. This may necessitate stronger flavors that are especially pleasing to the patient. Furthermore, swallowing may be impaired especially for thin liquids. Some-

times this may be ameliorated by thickening the fluid with commercially available products or mixing it with thicker foods, such as puddings or applesauce. The patient may also decrease the risk of aspiration by "chin-tucking" when swallowing.

More food may be consumed when it is offered in small quantities more frequently than the traditional three times daily and when supplements are especially to the liking of the patient. Carbohydrate supplements tend to be better received than supplements high in lipids, although they usually have fewer calories per unit volume. Even with attention to such details, many near the end of life may continue to lose weight. It should always be appreciated that persons who are dying are rarely symptomatic from malnutrition or even dehydration.[43] Thus, the use of parenteral means, nasogastric tubes, or percutaneous tubes is discouraged in that circumstance.

When a percutaneous esophageal-gastric (PEG) tube is required, for example, in persons with severe swallowing difficulties following a cerebrovascular accident, most families can be taught to manage the feeding routine. Usually, it is recommended that they install one can (about 240 cc) of feeding, followed by about 60 cc of water five or six times daily. A bolus of air should not be instilled to "clear" the tube as it may cause gas pains. Initially and periodically thereafter, the stomach should be aspirated about an hour after feeding, to be sure it has emptied satisfactorily. In addition, the patient's bed should be maintained at a thirty-degree angle at all times, to minimize the risk of aspiration. Nonetheless, aspiration of oral secretions may still occur, as may aspiration of stomach contents on occasion. The family should be advised of this, to prevent a feeling of guilt should aspiration occur. It is not at all clear that PEG tubes diminish the risk of aspiration.[44]

The urinary tract

Use of Foley catheters is associated with multiple problems. They may be uncomfortable, are associated with both local and systemic infections, and often are difficult for families to manage properly. Thus, for example, the Foley should never be raised above the level of the patient, thereby allowing urine to flow backward; but keeping the bag below the patient when changing the bedsheets may be very difficult for informal caregivers, especially when the patient is in a double bed or one that is larger. Nonetheless, toward the end of life, a Foley catheter may serve the needs of both patient and family by obviating the need to change the sheets frequently and allowing the patient to remain dry. Families must be instructed to empty the bag at least daily, and arrangements should be made to change the Foley about every 4–6 weeks.

Skin care

Attention to the integrity of the skin is critical in palliative care. Much skin care in the home setting, however, has to be provided by family members. Thus, all persons who provide personal care to the patient will require considerable instruction in how to prevent pressure ulcers and how to manage any areas of breakdown that have occurred, to diminish the likelihood of their further enlargement. Turning a patient who has significant impairment of mobility about every 2 hours throughout a 24-hour period may be especially time-consuming, anxiety-producing, and exhausting for the caregiver. If air pressure mattresses cannot be obtained because of unavailability or cost, the primary caregiver must almost certainly arrange for assistance, either professional or nonprofessional, to minimize the risk of skin breakdown.

Once redness or incipient skin breakdown occurs, the foremost consideration is to diminish or, much preferred, eliminate any further pressure on that site. This is often easier said than done, and positioning multiple pillows so that a patient's sacrum, for example, is raised off the bed is often especially difficult for a single caregiver. In addition, if the patient is defecating in bed, preventing fecal matter from contaminating the site is a very substantial undertaking and may not be possible even in the best of circumstances. Also, in the home setting,

a single family member may find it very difficult to pull the patient up in bed without applying considerable sheer force to the back. The patient should almost always be pulled up in the horizontal position unless there is some contraindication such as COPD. A draw sheet is helpful but requires two individuals who must have sufficient strength to lift the patient.

In certain situations, such as patients in the terminal stages of dying or who experience significant pain with turning, it may be advisable to avoid repositioning the patient frequently and to do so for hygiene purposes only, thereby keeping the patient as comfortable as possible.

Dyspnea

Of all symptoms, dyspnea ranks at or near the top of any list ordered according to the most likely to trouble both patient and family caregiver.[45] A sense of "air hunger," whether or not oxygen is in use, can at times be alleviated by fans blowing directly on the patient or by opening the windows widely. The use of home oxygen is common and certainly should be considered. Family members as well as the patient should be warned not to smoke around oxygen containers; and, of course, if they are essential for patient welfare, a back-up source of electricity (a generator) is required if oxygen is being supplied from a concentrator or a motorized apparatus. In the terminally ill patient, small amounts of morphine may result in a marked improvement in dyspnea and may be given while monitoring the respiratory rate.[46] For patients with increased respiratory secretions or "death rattle" who are in the terminal stages of dying, anticholinergic medications, such as hyoscine, are helpful to alleviate this symptom, which can be very distressing to family members.[47]

Spirituality and mental health

Many persons near the end of life express concerns that may be grouped under the heading of spirituality. Such persons may have been fervent and orthodox in their religious beliefs, agnostic, or atheist prior to a life-ending illness. They may ask very personal questions of both nurse and caregiver: "Why me?" or "What did I do wrong to deserve this?" However, they may be concerned more with theological matters, such as "What follows death?" or with the very process of death.[48] Sometimes the local pastor, especially if the patient was active in the church, will make a home visit. Hospice services in the United States require the inclusion of both pastoral care and social worker support. For persons who are homebound but not at the end of life, such questions are often very difficult to address. Few psychiatrists or consulting social workers make home visits on a regular basis. Thus, nurses often must be as helpful as possible and try to arrange for in-home support when available or, in some locations, consultation by telephone.

Depression in both the older individual with palliative care needs and the person's caregiver is common. Those with long-standing depressive symptoms may be especially vulnerable; chronic physical illness and chronic pain are known risk factors for depression. Recently, it has been shown that depressive symptomatology and hopelessness are strong predictors of desiring a hastened death in terminally ill patients.[49] Therefore, it is important to look for these symptoms in patients receiving palliative care. When contact with a professional may be quite limited, as is true in the home setting, it is important for the nurse to have a high degree of suspicion that the patient and perhaps the family caregiver are depressed if this symptom is to be addressed adequately. Sometimes the family member is in desperate need of a respite period, be it for an evening or a few days. Just recognizing the need and giving the family member permission, so to speak, to have time off may preclude the collapse of the informal care system altogether. Furthermore, providing the caregiver with a respite period may allow the older adult to remain home for a longer period of time. If in spite of respite care and whatever professional support can be provided, significant amounts of depres-

sion persist, the nurse may determine that home care is no longer feasible.

Sometimes the nurse may be faced with an especially difficult problem when a patient displays a serious psychiatric disturbance, such as suicidal ideation, and no formal psychiatric support is available. Under these circumstances, it is necessary for the professional to advise the responsible physician of the signs and symptoms of the disorder, especially if newly present. Under such circumstances, it may be judged that acute hospitalization is required, even if it is carried out against the patient's will. These occurrences are rare but not unheard of in the home setting and may be more frequent when services are first introduced and patient, family, and the professional team do not know each other well.

Safety

Few, if any, homes were designed with an eye toward lowering the risk of accidents. Lighting may be poor, especially for the elderly patient with poor eyesight, and stairs may lack banisters on both sides or may not be designed for those who experience pain when ambulatory. Bathrooms rarely have well-placed grab bars or even easy access to a bathing place, and toilets may be too low and not fitted with bars to allow ease of getting on or off with safety. Access to many rooms may be impossible if an ambulatory aid or wheelchair is required. In addition, each person has "individualized" the home, be it with scatter rugs or lengthy extension cords that must be stepped over. Nurses usually must assume some responsibility for pointing out particularly hazardous situations and offering families the names and telephone numbers of appropriate durable medical equipment providers to address other safety issues.

In addition, nurses should give consideration to the general overarching aspects of safety, such as the ability of the older adult to exit the home in a fire or to be protected from undue risk of burglary or violence when doors cannot be locked. Alert systems that are easily transportable by the patient may provide considerable comfort to the geriatric patient and the caregivers who may need to leave the patient alone for short periods, to go shopping, for example.

Pain and other symptoms in need of pharmaceuticals

Likely the most common palliative care need is pain management. Although the drugs utilized in the home setting may be identical to those used in the hospital, the route of administration may be different. Some families find pumps and intravenous arrangements difficult to manage even when professional competency is readily available. Some hospice services report that families find rectal suppositories difficult, perhaps because of the degree of intimacy involved. Oral or sublingual medications are almost always best and may be used in conjunction with patches when available. For optimal pain control, pain medications are best used when prescribed around the clock and not on an as-needed basis.[21]

Sometimes nurses must work with the patient and more frequently the family to alleviate the fear of producing harm when drugs are required to provide adequate pain relief. Because of cultural reasons, widespread ignorance, and misinformation, families may even be concerned that they are hastening death if pain is adequately controlled. In addition, some side effects may have to be tolerated to achieve pain control, especially when a new medication or higher doses are initiated. Some of these negative effects may become less of a problem over time.

Under any circumstances, a total drug list detailing all drugs being administered, their doses, and the routes of administration should be kept up to date and immediately accessible to both professional and caregiver. This will allow the family member to provide appropriate information to the nurse by telephone should a new distressing symptom or sign be noted.

In addition, for patients near the end of life, a group of drugs that might be required should be kept in the patient's home. Then,

after appropriate consultation with the professional team, they can be drawn upon for use in the middle of the night or at odd hours should a symptom occur. In addition to oral morphine, consideration should be given to including an antiemetic, a drying anticholinergic agent for secretions, an anxiolytic agent, a drug for seizures, and an antipsychotic.[40] The exact contents of this medicine package must be individualized to reflect the likely needs of the patient.

Less frequent symptoms and needs

Restlessness, a sign of delirium, is both frequent in occurrence in the terminally ill and usually very concerning to families. The nurse may be especially helpful by educating family members in advance about what to expect as death approaches and by explaining that restlessness may be ameliorated by a host of ancillary measures. Sometimes success can be achieved with music, massage, or leaving the television or radio playing at a low level. Lighting should be adjusted to the most helpful level, recognizing that bright, intense lighting is usually particularly unpleasant. Extraneous or sudden noise should be eliminated to the extent possible. Warm drinks, such as warm milk with honey or warm water with rum and butter, may be very soothing to the patient and often are easily prepared by the caregiver.

Note should also be taken of odors that may be offensive not only to close friends who may be discouraged from visiting but to caregivers and patients as well. They often act as a constant reminder of illness. An old home remedy is to cut up onions and place them under the bed. Some odors are difficult to mask, but with the wide range of flavored aerosol products and the use of perfumes applied directly to the patient, most offensive odors can be concealed.

Persons with striking degrees of disfigurement, such as those resulting from oral tumors, may not wish outside visitors. Family members may not be as disconcerted by the sight of these deformities, in part due to their seeing the patient daily, thereby allowing them to accommodate slowly to a progressive disfiguring lesion. For individuals with tracheostomies because of end-stage neurological disease, a home visit by a speech therapist may be especially helpful, although nurses are usually the ones to teach the families how to care for the ostomy and to arrange for the emergency back-up availability of an ambu bag should that be indicated. Computer-generated sound may allow communication when none was possible previously, although such devices are rarely used in an end-of-life setting.

HOME MEDICAL EQUIPMENT AND MEDICAL SUPPLIES

To provide in-home care, a number of medical supplies as well as medical equipment (durable medical equipment) may be needed. These supplies and equipment can usually be either purchased or rented from medical/surgical supply stores, pharmacies, or medical supply catalogs. It is important to know first what types of equipment and supply are recommended by the physician, visiting nurse and perhaps physical therapist or occupational therapist before actually purchasing them. With proper documentation of need from the physician or nurse, part or all of the expense of certain types of durable medical equipment may be covered by Medicare or private insurance in the United States. In addition, some home modifications may be necessary to improve the safety and feasibility of caring for a loved one at home. In this regard, forward planning is important to individualize the care to the patient's specific needs.[40]

General supplies that are often useful to have readily available when taking care of a loved one at home include but are not limited to, the following:

- Bandages, gauze pads, paper (nonstick) tape
- Extra bed linens, including sheets, pillows, easily washed blankets
- Disposable rubber gloves (nonpowdered)
- Adult diapers and/or large absorbent pads

- A mechanism to allow the patient to signal for help if alone in the room (e.g., a bell) or in the home (e.g., an emergency response system)
- Soft, disposable cleaning rags
- Lotion
- Baby shampoo
- Basins
- Antibiotic ointment (always check for patient allergy)

Certain types of durable medical equipment are often necessary to successfully deliver palliative care to the terminal ill patient or ongoing care to the chronically ill person in the home setting. As a person becomes more frail and unable to perform various activities of daily living, the use of durable medical equipment can help to compensate for any decrease in function, ease the physical burden often placed on family members, and provide a measure of safety. Some of the more common and useful types of equipment can be categorized as follows.[50]

Devices to Aid in Mobility and Function

Assistive devices are used to help improve mobility, including ambulation and transferring from bed and chair. Examples include slide boards and partial bedside rails for transfer, canes (which provide only minimal support with gait and balance), walkers (which offer much increased support), wheelchairs of varying types, and even electric scooters. Walkers may be standard, that is, without wheels but with rubber caps, or adapted for persons who have a tendency to fall backward (e.g., Parkinson's patients) by placing wheels on the front posts, thereby obviating the need to lift it between steps. Other walkers or canes have armrests, which allow persons who have painful deformities of the hands or wrists (e.g., persons with rheumatoid arthritis) to use them. Some walkers have a seat to allow the user to sit and rest. If appropriate, the home-care patient should be assessed by either the physician or physical therapist to determine the safest and most appropriate assistive device.

An array of smaller devices can enable an older person or anyone with some degree of restricted mobility to continue to perform everyday tasks. Examples include Velcro closures for shoes instead of shoestrings and for clothing instead of buttons, long-handled shoehorns to assist in putting on shoes, and large rubber grip tubes placed on handles of toothbrushes, hairbrushes, etc. for easier gripping. Other examples include rocker wall switches, which do not require the dexterity that traditional toggle light switches do to turn on the light, and telephones with large push buttons. For reaching items in high or low places, a long-handled "reacher" is very useful and lightweight. This can be used to grab items such as sweaters from closet shelves or canned foods from top pantry shelves.

Depending on the mobility of the patient, one or more of the following types of equipment for the bathroom should be considered. A raised toilet seat enables someone who has generalized weakness to rise up from the toilet more easily. The same is true for a toilet frame, which is a unit that fits over the toilet and provides support on both sides. Grab bars in the tub and shower sufficiently well attached to hold a person's weight are important and may require the assistance of an outside contractor to install. A bath transfer bench, another useful piece of equipment, aids a person who has difficulty with rising from sitting on the bottom of the bathtub. This type of bench straddles the tub and allows the patient to sit at the side of the tub and slide over, rather than step over the side when getting in and out. This may also enable a patient to take a much-desired shower without the fear of falling due to loss of balance or fatigue. Also, a hand-held shower is for many more comfortable to use than the regular shower while sitting on a tub bench. The hand-held shower can usually be easily attached to the existing shower apparatus.

Equipment Useful in Caring for the Bed-Bound Patient

If the home-care patient is essentially bed-bound, as with many patients in the terminal stages of dying, the focus shifts from mobility and ambulation to keeping the patient as comfortable as possible in bed. In this scenario, patients will become more dependent in their activities of daily living such as transferring and toileting. Various types of durable medical equipment can help the patient and caregiver compensate for the loss in function. For example, an electric hospital bed allows the patient to assume a seated position without exertion and to elevate the foot of the bed if there is significant lower extremity edema. The hospital bed may well improve comfort by allowing frequent repositioning and better respiration for those with pulmonary disease. It may also facilitate the transfer in and out of bed by allowing the height to be adjusted.

If a hospital bed is not needed, a handrail can be attached to the bedframe or supported by projections under the mattress, which will allow the patient to sit up without personal assistance or with less strenuous effort on the part of the caregiver. In this same way, a trapeze apparatus may be of benefit to help the patient's mobility in bed. This usually consists of a triangular handle suspended over the bed that the patient can hold on to for support when rising to sit or to shift positions in bed. For some caregivers tending to a loved one who is now bed-bound, a Hoyer lift can help to transfer such a patient from bed to chair, easing the physical strain on the caregiver. This apparatus consists of strong canvas-type material that is slid under the patient's back and pelvis and attached to a strong steel support from above. The patient is then hoisted from the bed and moved over to a chair. With a small amount of training by the home visiting nurse or physical therapist, a caregiver can learn to use this apparatus, thereby enabling a frail or weak patient to spend some time out of bed if so desired. Various mattresses, such as a low-air-loss mattress, are also available to help reduce pressure on skin tissue, thereby reducing the risk of developing a pressure ulcer.

In addition, the use of a bedside commode, urinal, or bedpan especially at night can help prevent physical strain on the caregiver, as well as diminish the discomfort of the patient when he or she is no longer able to ambulate easily to the bathroom even with assistance.

Specialized Medical Equipment

Depending on the patient's medical conditions and symptoms, there are a variety of specialized medical devices that may be of considerable value when deemed necessary by the physician. These include pieces of equipment that allow for therapies usually given in a hospital setting to be brought into the home. In addition, some types of equipment play an especially important role in allowing palliative care to be rendered at home. For example, a patient with advanced COPD or end-stage lung cancer will likely benefit from home oxygen therapy to help with any symptoms of dyspnea. This requires the use of either oxygen tanks or an oxygen concentrator.

An oxygen concentrator is a device using the existing room air as the source of oxygen. The device concentrates the oxygen from the room air up to approximately 5 liters per minute via nasal cannula. The use of an oxygen concentrator obviates the need for continued oxygen tank replacement as there is a continuous, unlimited supply of oxygen through the concentrator. These devices also come with a humidifier; the patient or caregiver is usually taught how to fill the humidifier with distilled water. For patients using an oxygen concentrator, it is also standard to be given a spare oxygen tank to be used in case of a power outage as the concentrator runs on electricity. The spare tank usually supplies enough oxygen for about 6 hours, depending on its size. It is important to clarify this in advance with the company supplying the home oxygen so that one is prepared in the case of a power outage. One drawback to most oxygen concentrators is the level of noise they typically produce. Some patients may find it better to have a concentrator in the living area for use during the daytime and to switch to an oxygen tank in the bed-

room at night to allow for a more quiet night's rest.

The oxygen tubing should be long enough to allow some ambulation around the room for the ambulatory patient. However, the tubing should not be longer than 35 feet so as to guarantee that the patient is still getting the necessary level of oxygen. Beyond approximately 35 feet of tubing, the concentration of oxygen getting to the patient is likely less than the prescribed amount. Also, although longer tubing allows more freedom for the patient, the tubing may get tangled and presents a fall risk to the patient.

There are several other mechanical devices used in the home setting to address palliative care needs. With each device, the caregiver is usually taught by the home visiting nurse how to use it and the appropriate situation in which it should be used. For example, some patients with COPD may benefit from using a home nebulizer for delivering medications such as bronchodilators to help ease dyspnea. For patients with continued production of oral secretions, a home oral suction device may be appropriate to gently clear secretions from the patient's mouth. It is not uncommon for patients receiving palliative care at home to have, for one reason or another, a pre-existing percutaneous gastrostomy tube through which he or she is fed the appropriate nutritional supplements. Sometimes the patient tolerates the feeding better when it is given slowly over a long period of time with the use of a pump. This device can be easily worked by a family member, once instructed by the nurse. Other pumps, such as those used for home intravenous therapy (for antibiotics or pain medications), are much less commonly used for patients receiving palliative care. Families of palliative care patients often are easily overwhelmed when required to administer highly technical therapies in the home. In addition, there are some patients who are maintained in the long term on home ventilators (e.g., patients with amyotrophic lateral sclerosis) who may not be in the terminal stages of dying but whose care is palliative in nature. For these persons, ongoing communication among the physician and home support service personnel, such as the respiratory therapist, home heath aide, and visiting nurse, and most importantly the family members is crucial for optimal palliative care in the home.

ADAPTATION OF THE HOME

When planning to care for a chronically ill or terminal patient at home, it is important to adapt the home environment to accommodate the patient and to anticipate any potential safety hazards.[51] For example, when arranging the patient's bedroom and choosing the location of the bed, it is important to take into consideration both the patient's wishes if possible and the view from the bed both when lying flat and when upright. Items important to the patient, such as photographs and perhaps reading material, should be in view and within reach if practical. The use of a mobile hospital table is helpful because it rolls directly over the bed. It may also be helpful to move the patient's bed to the center of the room, to be able to tend to the patient from either side.

When adapting the home for rendering medical care to a loved one, it is important to make sure that there is sufficient electricity to support the necessary medical equipment. The advice of an electrician may be needed prior to installing the equipment. Also, if high-tech equipment, such as a home ventilator, is being used, the utility company should be notified so that a generator can be supplied during a power outage.

Emergency response systems may be very simple or rather complex. They usually consist of a small radio transmitter worn as a pendant or necklace and activated by a push of a button. A 24-hour emergency monitoring center is then contacted. The emergency staff will try to contact the patient through a small two-way remote box placed in the home. If there is no response, then emergency assistance is automatically called. Other systems require a response from the patient about every 12 hours or a response team is activated. This prevents an older adult living alone from lying on the floor after a fall for a considerable period of time.

It is very important to take into consideration the lighting, especially in the rooms where the patient will be living. A sensor device can be installed without new wiring that detects motion and automatically turns on lights as one enters the room. This may be useful for bathrooms or hallways, to prevent an older person from walking through a dark hallway on the way to the bathroom during the night. Lighting should also be bright at both the top and bottom of stairways, allowing the entire stairwell to be well lit as many falls occur on stairs. It is important to make sure that there is adequate lighting in the areas traversed by any ambulatory person, especially in those with any visual impairment. Also in some cases, too much light can be bothersome to the home-care patient. Bright sunlight, streetlights, or headlight glare coming in through a window can be alleviated with curtains or blinds.

For older persons who may be somewhat frail yet are ambulatory with a walker, it is important to have chairs with firm seats and solid arms for use when rising. Also useful are recliners that are made with an electric or pneumatic rising device that can assist people to rise from the sitting to the standing position. This may be particularly valuable to people with arthritis or conditions in which there is reduced lower extremity muscle strength.

It is likely that many older persons being cared for in the home setting, even those receiving palliative or terminal care, may have some days in which they are able to ambulate with or without an assistive device such as a walker and some days that may be spent entirely in bed. To help prevent a fall, all area rugs should either be removed or securely taped in place and nonslip treads should be used on stairs. Also, it is important to install handrails on both sides of stairs if they are used by the patient and sometimes in hallways. If possible, living should be consolidated on one floor, to avoid stairs altogether. All hallways and pathways to the bed and bathroom should be free of clutter with enough space for a walker or wheelchair.

ACKNOWLEDGMENTS

We offer our most sincere gratitude to Elizabeth Steel, M.S.W., for her detailed review of the section on social work and her insights and advice, to Patricia Puchalik, R.N., M.S.N., and Ana Cernadas, R.N., C.H.P.N., for their most thoughtful comments on the section on hospice and nursing.

REFERENCES

1. Thorpe G. Enabling more dying people to remain at home. BMJ 307:915–918, 1993.
2. Grands GE, Todd CJ, Barclay SIG, Farquhar MC. Does hospital at home for palliative care facilitate death at home? Randomized controlled trial. BMJ 319:1472–1475, 1999.
3. Brown P, Davies B, Martens N. Families in supportive care. Part II: Palliative care at home: a viable care setting. J Palliat Care 6:21–27, 1990.
4. Ferris FD, Wodinsky HB, Kerr IG, Sone M, Hume S, Coons C. A cost-minimization study of cancer patients requiring a narcotic infusion in hospital and at home. J Clin Epidemiol 44:313–327, 1991.
5. Holstein BE, Due P, Almind G, Holst E. The home-help service in Denmark. In: Home Care for Older People in Europe: A Comparison of Policies and Practices. New York, Oxford University Press, pp. 38–62, 1991.
6. Roe DJ. Palliative care 2000—home care. J Palliat Care 8:28–32, 1992.
7. Grande GE, Addington-Hall JM, Todd CJ. Place of death and access to home care services: are certain patient groups at a disadvantage? Soc Sci Med 47:565–579, 1998.
8. Fainsinger RL, Demoissac D, Cole J, Mead-Wood K, Lee E. Home versus hospice inpatient care: discharge characteristics of palliative care patients in an acute care hospital. J Palliat Care 16:29–34, 2000.
9. Wilkinson EK, Salisbury C, Bosanquet N, et al. Patient and career preference for and satisfaction with specialist models of palliative care: a systematic literature review. Palliat Med 13:197–216, 1999.
10. Peruselli C, Marinari M, Brivio B, et al. Evaluating a home palliative care service: development of indicators for a continuous quality improvement program. J Palliat Care 13:34–42, 1997.
11. Ramirez A, Addington-Hall J, Richards M. The careers. BMJ 316:208–211, 1998.
12. Bradshaw P. Characteristics of clients referred to home, hospice and hospital palliative care services in western Australia. Palliat Med 7:101–107, 1993.
13. DeConno F, Caraceni A, Groff L, et al. Effect of home care on the place of death of advanced cancer patients. Eur J Cancer 32A:1142–1147, 1996.
14. Karlsen S, Addington-Hall J. How do cancer patients who die at home differ from those who die elsewhere? Palliat Med 12:279–286, 1998.
15. Higginson IJ, Astin P, Dolan S. Where do cancer patients die? Ten-year trends in the place of death of cancer patients in England. Palliat Med 12:353–363. 1998.
16. Vitale CA, Benoff M, Steel K. Role of a transition nurse when discharging frail elderly from hospital to home. Abstract presented at The Annual Meeting of American Geriatrics Society, May 2001.
17. Steel K, Ljunggren G, Topinková E, et al. Tha RAI-PC, an assessment instrument for palliative care in all settings. J Hospice Pall Care (in press).
18. Meyer GS, Gibbons RV. House calls to the elderly—a vanishing practice among physicians. N Engl J Med 337:1815–1820, 1997.
19. Ratner ER. Show what you know: a credentialing examination in home care. Home Health Care Consult 7:31–39, 2000.
20. Meier DE, Morrison RS, Cassel CK. Improving palliative care. Ann Intern Med 127:225–230, 1997.
21. Rhymes JA. Home hospice care. Clin Geriatr Med 7:803–817, 1991.
22. Bonneh DY, Shvartzman P. Profile of a home hospice care unit in Israel. Isr J Med Sci 33:17–81, 1997.
23. McWhinney IR, Stewart MA. Home care of dying patients: family physicians' experience with a palliative care support team. Can Fam Physician 40:240–246, 1994.
24. Charlton RC. Palliative care: home or hospice? J R Coll Gen Pract 347, 1989.
25. Kedziera P, Harris D. End-of-life care: hospice or home? Cancer Pract 6:188–190, 1998.
26. Zeppetella G. How do terminally ill patients at home take their medication? Palliat Med 13:469–475, 1999.
27. Beck-Fries B, Strang P. The organization of hospital based homecare for terminally ill cancer patients: the motala model. Palliat Med 7:93–100, 1993.

28. Maltoni M, Nanni O, Naldoni M, Serra P, Amadori D. Evaluation of cost of home therapy for patients' with terminal diseases. Curr Opin Oncol 10:302–309, 1998.

29. Carron AT, Lynn J, Keaney P. End-of-life care in medical textbooks. Ann Intern Med 130:82–86, 1999.

30. Billings JA, Block S. Palliative care in undergraduate medical education. JAMA 278:733–738, 1997.

31. Doyle D. Domiciliary palliative care. In: Doyle D, Hanks GWC, MacDonald N (Eds.). Oxford Textbook of Palliative Medicine, 2nd ed. New York, Oxford University Press, pp. 957–973, 1998.

32. Schvartzman P, Singer Y. Community education in palliative medicine. J Palliat Care 14:75–78, 1998.

33. Cassel CK. Overview on attitudes of physicians toward caring for the dying patient. In: Caring for the Dying: Identification and Promotion of Physician Competency Educational Resource Document. Philadelphia, American Board of Internal Medicine pp. 1–4, 1995.

34. Field MJ, Cassel CK (Eds.). Approaching Death: Improving Care at the End of Life. Washington DC, National Academy Press, 1997.

35. Hileman JW, Lackey NR, Hassanein R. Identifying the needs of home caregivers of patients with cancer. Oncol Nurs Forum 19:771–777, 1992.

36. Levine C. Rough Crossings: Family Caregivers' Odysseys through the Health Care System. New York, United Hospital Fund, 1998.

37. Axelsson B, Sjoden P. Quality of life of cancer patients and their spouses in palliative home care. Palliat Med 12:29–39, 1998.

38. Hinton J. Can home care maintain an acceptable quality of life for patients with terminal cancer and their relatives? Palliat Med 8:183–196, 1994.

39. Addington-Hall J, Karlsen S. Do home deaths increase distress in bereavement? Palliat Med 14:161–162, 2000.

40. O'Neill B, Rodway A. Care in the community. BMJ 316:373–377, 1998.

41. Jones RVH, Hansford J, Fiske J. Death from cancer at home: the carers' perspective. BMJ 306:249–251, 1993.

42. Hinton J. Which patients with terminal cancer are admitted from home care? Palliat Med 8:197–210, 1994.

43. McCann RM, Hall WJ, Groth-Juncker A. Comfort care for terminally ill patients: the appropriate use of nutrition and hydration. JAMA 272:1263–1266, 1994.

44. Finucane TE, Christmas C, Travis K. Tube feeding in patients with advanced dementia: a review of the evidence. JAMA 282:1365–1370, 1999.

45. Mercadante S, Casuccio A, Fulfaro F. The course of symptom frequency and intensity in advanced cancer patients followed at home. J Pain Symptom Manage 20:104–112, 2000.

46. Luce JM, Luce JA. Management of dyspnea in patients with far-advanced lung disease: "Once I lose it, it's kind of hard to catch it . . ." JAMA 285:1331–1337, 2001.

47. Bausewein C. Comparative cost of hyoscine injections. Palliat Med 9:256–258, 1995.

48. Lynn J, Schuster JL, Kabcenell A. Improving Care for the End of Life: A Sourcebook for Health Care Managers and Clinicians. New York, Oxford University Press, 2000.

49. Breitbart W, Rosenfeld B, Pessin H, et al. Depression, hopelessness and desire for hastened death in terminally ill patients with cancer. JAMA 284:2907–2911, 2000.

50. Meyer MM, Derr P. The Comfort of Home: An Illustrated Step-by-Step Guide for Caregivers. Portland, OR, Care Trust, 1998.

51. Bakker R. Elderdesign: Designing and Furnishing a Home for Your Later Years. New York, Penguin, 1997.

28

Hospital-Based Palliative Care

DANIEL FISCHBERG AND DIANE E. MEIER

Palliative care is interdisciplinary care that aims to improve quality of life and function and relieve suffering for patients and their families. It is a kind of care that should be available to all patients with chronic, severe, or life-limiting illness independent of their diagnosis or prognosis. It should be provided from the time of diagnosis, along with curative efforts, for any serious illness. This definition has evolved from the narrower one used by the World Health Organization: "the active total care of persons whose disease is no longer responsive to curative treatments."[1] While largely pioneered in the United States in the home setting through hospice programs, palliative care is rapidly advancing as a hospital-based form of care. In this chapter, we examine why these hospital-based palliative care programs have proliferated, how they function, and what data exist as to their effectiveness.

THE EPIDEMIOLOGY OF DEATH IN THE UNITED STATES: A CENTURY OF CHANGE

In essentially every manner conceivable, death in the United States has changed dramatically over the last 100 years. Advances in sanitation and hygiene early in the century and the advent of the antibiotic era at mid-century were responsible for the marked changes in the demographics of death. In 1900, the median age at death was 50 years and infectious diseases were leading causes of death. By century's end, the median age at death was 76 years and heart disease, cancer, and stroke accounted for the majority of all deaths in the United States.[2] As a consequence of these changes in longevity and leading causes of death, the usual death is no longer a sudden or unexpected event as it was in the past. Modern death more typically follows a period of chronic illness and progressive disability, which may last for years, if not decades.

In the early 1900s, the role of medicine was also significantly different from today. There were precious few medical therapies that significantly altered the natural history of a disease. People recovered from or succumbed to their illness almost entirely independent of medical interventions. The role of the medical and nursing professions was to provide prognostication and comfort whenever possible. Indeed, the few pharmaceuticals available at the time that continue in use in some form today (e.g., opiates, salicylates, cardiac glycosides, atropinergics, and sympathomimetics) were what we would now consider wholly palliative in that their role is to ameliorate symptoms and not to cure or otherwise modify disease progression.

At the beginning of the twenty-first century, both the general public and the medical profession have accepted disease-modifying therapies, specifically cure or control of disease, as the norm. Patients are encouraged to fight for life prolongation at all costs, and death is often considered not the natural and inevitable end of all living things but a failure of modern medical care. This is despite the fact that, for all of its remarkable advances, modern medicine offers a relatively small number of cures. Most advances in medicine result not in cure of illness but in prolongation of the lives of those with chronic illness.

The site of death has also changed significantly. Early in the twentieth century, most people in the United States died where they were born, at home. As medical therapies advanced, people with serious illness began to receive more of their care in hospitals; and at the present time, half of Americans die in a hospital and another quarter die in nursing homes. Only the remaining quarter of Americans die at home, despite the fact that home is the preferred site of care for nearly 90% of Americans according to data from two Gallup polls.[2]

These statistics on site of death hide tremendous regional variation. Different areas of the country, even those within close proximity, have marked differences in location of death. These variations are not based, as one might hope, on regional variations in preferences regarding the site of death. Instead in-hospital death is increased in regions with high numbers of available hospital beds and reduced in areas with fewer available hospital beds and proportionately higher nursing home bed and hospice availability. These health-system factors, and not patient-specific factors and preferences, account for 80% of the regional variation in rates of in-hospital death.[3]

DYING IN THE HOSPITAL: A CRISIS OF CARE

If most of us are dying in hospitals despite our preferences, what then is the experience like? Certainly, the most comprehensive data we have on the experience of the dying in our hospitals come from the Study to Understand Prognoses for and Preferences for Outcomes and Risks of Treatments (SUPPORT).[4] This ambitious, multimillion dollar project funded by the Robert Wood Johnson Foundation, enrolled 4301 seriously ill patients over 2 years at five high-quality academic medical centers in its first, descriptive, phase. Multiple assessments were made to describe the quality of the care of these patients at the time of their deaths. Several disturbing findings were highly publicized at the time of the study's publication in 1995.

- Among patients preferring to avoid resuscitation, their physicians were unaware of their preference more than 50% of the time.
- Thirty-eight percent of patients who died spent more than 10 days in an intensive care unit (ICU) and a median of 8 days unconscious, on mechanical ventilation, or in an ICU.
- Even in the final 3 days of life, pain control was so poor that family members of 50% of conscious patients who died reported that their loved one was in moderate or severe pain at least half of the time.
- Nearly one-third of the families, all of whom had medical insurance, reported the loss of most or all of their savings during the serious illness.

The disturbing findings of SUPPORT stand in stark contrast to what we know about the preferences of people with serious or chronic illness. When asked what they want from the health-care system, such patients ask for adequate pain and symptom management, avoiding inappropriate prolongation of dying, achieving a sense of control, and strengthening relationships with and not burdening loved ones as important elements of quality medical care.[5]

It is this discordance between the care that those with serious illness desire and that which they receive that has driven the development of the hospice and palliative care movement. Beginning in the 1970s, some of those caring for the seriously ill and dying in hospitals began to pioneer a new type of care, one that was modeled on the basic precepts of the hospice movement to provide comprehensive, compassionate, and competent care focused on the relief of suffering and the promotion of quality of life for patients facing a life-threatening illness. Like hospice, this new type of care was often delivered by interdisciplinary teams of nurses, physicians, social workers, and other allied professionals working toward the implementation of a treatment plan concordant with the values and preferences of the patient and family. While these teams have used different names at different institutions, including *terminal care support team*, *symptom control team*, *support care team*, and *comfort care team*, *palliative care team* seems to have become the favored term.[6] Hospitals with early palliative care services included St. Luke's Hospital in New York, McGill's Royal Victoria Hospital in Montreal, and St. Thomas's Hospital in London.[7–9]

ROLE OF THE HOSPITAL-BASED PALLIATIVE CARE TEAM

Dunlop and Hockley[6] described multiple roles for hospital-based palliative care teams:

- Advise the ward team on symptom control and psychosocial/existential issues
- Provide additional support and counseling to families
- Provide support and advice to staff
- Participate in education of hospital staff
- Act as liaison between hospital and hospice/home-care services or other institutions
- Lead research efforts in the study of relief of symptoms and other sources of distress in patients and families with life-threatening illness

In practice, of course, different hospital-based palliative care teams will emphasize different roles. Some will focus on providing advice, support, and education to the primary team in a purely consultative model. At other institutions, the palliative care team may assume primary responsibility for many patients, aspiring to the comprehensive palliative care associated with traditional hospice care. The culture of each institution will often dictate the model. Failure to adopt a role compatible with the needs of the primary providers at the institution can be disastrous for a palliative care team.

A common source of confusion is the distinction between hospice and palliative care. Both may be delivered in inpatient as well as community settings, and both focus on the relief of suffering and the provision of care to patients and their families that is concordant with their values and beliefs. However, in the United States, hospice is regulated as a Medicare benefit. The Medicare Hospice Benefit regulations stipulate that only patients with an expected prognosis of 6 months or less are eligible. Patients receiving the hospice benefit must agree to forsake curative therapies. In return, they receive comprehensive nursing, physician, and allied services; durable medical equipment; and medications related to the relief of symptoms due to their terminal illness.

Palliative care has no such requirements and is paid for like standard medical services. Palliative care may be offered at any time during the course of a chronic, serious, or potentially life-limiting illness concurrently with curative and disease-modifying treatments. It is appropriate independent of diagnosis and prognosis.

TEAM STRUCTURE AND FUNCTION

The hospital-based palliative care team, following the model of hospice, is typically an interdisciplinary team. From early on, clinical nurse specialists led or were key personnel on these teams.[7] At some smaller programs or at programs early in development, a clinical nurse specialist may be the sole member of the team. Larger hospital-based palliative care teams commonly include physician and social worker members.[10] Hospital-based palliative care teams at tertiary-care hospitals may find that the culture of their institution requires strong physician and nursing leadership on the team. Allied professionals who may be members of the core team or may be consulted regularly include pharmacists, nutritionists, chaplains, bereavement counselors, therapists, and others.[10]

The team may function exclusively on a consultation model. Alternatively, it may assume primary responsibility for all referred patients, providing care on a dedicated inpatient palliative care unit or throughout the hospital using scattered beds. Many teams offer both types of service.[10]

Patients and families with severe distress may benefit from transfer to a dedicated palliative care unit, where maximal palliative therapies may be administered under the direct supervision of the palliative care team. Palliative care units may serve as models for excellence in clinical care as well as educational centers for the teaching of palliative care to nurses and physicians. Balanced against these benefits may be the loss of the opportunity for ongoing involvement with the referring or primary team as a result of transfer to a dedicated palliative care unit. This not only translates into lost educational opportunities but may deliver subtle and undesirable messages regarding the primary physician's obligation to care for patients throughout the course of a serious illness. In addition, this pattern of transferring dying patients to the palliative care unit may also unintentionally communicate that expert care of the dying is the province of a handful of skilled professionals and not the expected standard of care for all physicians and nurses. Finally, clustering deaths on one unit of a hospital may unintentionally promote the belief that death is a shameful failure of medical care that needs to be hidden, or at least segregated, and not the natural and inevitable outcome of all things living. Each team will

weigh the relative merits of both models of care, often on a patient-by-patient basis, before choosing the model that best serves the needs of the patient and family and the broader needs of the team and institution.

The model that a palliative care team adopts will often guide how the team is used as a resource by colleagues at the hospital. Teams that predominantly accept primary care responsibility for patients will largely focus on the treatment of distressing physical, emotional, social, or spiritual issues and, when possible, the development of a safe and supportive discharge plan. Teams that serve in a consultive role will also often spend a great deal of time fostering communication between the patient and family and the primary team regarding prognosis, goals, and plan of care.

THE EDUCATIONAL IMPERATIVE

Beyond the epidemiological and clinical imperatives described above, a universal role for the hospital-based palliative care team must be to participate in the education of nursing and physician colleagues, especially at teaching hospitals. Medical and nursing school curricula as well as textbooks contain scant material regarding the provision of quality palliative care,[11-17] and clinicians, as a consequence, are often poorly prepared to care for the dying.[18-20]

Teaching hospitals are the major site of training for both physicians and nurses, yet data from SUPPORT clearly demonstrate that an unsatisfactory standard of end-of-life care is the norm at many of these institutions. Palliative care teams based at teaching hospitals are in an ideal position to correct these traditional educational deficits by actively teaching and promoting the practice of optimal care for the seriously ill and dying.

Multiple hospital-based palliative care teams have attempted to document their educational impact. Von Gunten and colleagues[21] initiated a rotation in hospice and palliative medicine for hematology/oncology fellows and found increases in confidence in pain and symptom management, communication skills, and knowledge regarding hospice and palliative care approaches to end-of-life care. At another institution, the establishment of a hospital-based palliative care service led to improved analgesic-prescribing patterns.[22] At our own institution, we have documented improvements in knowledge among residents and geriatrics and hematology/oncology fellows following a rotation with the palliative care service.[23,24]

PREVALENCE AND IMPACT OF HOSPITAL-BASED PALLIATIVE CARE PROGRAMS

Billings and Pantilat[10] surveyed a random sample of 100 teaching hospitals and found that 26% had either a palliative care consultation service or inpatient unit and 7% had both. The average daily census on the consultation services was six, and the inpatient units had an average of 12 beds.

Of 4797 hospitals responding to the American Hospital Association (AHA) 1998 Annual Survey, 1751 (36%) reported having a pain service and 719 (15%) reported having an end-of-life service. Further survey of the programs with at least one of these services yielded 1120 responses, of which 337 (30%) reported having a palliative care program. Of the hospitals without a palliative care program, 228 (20%) reported plans to establish one.[25] More than half of these programs were in community hospitals.

The top five reasons cited for consultation of the palliative care service in the survey by Pan et al.[25] were pain management, goals of care, other symptom management, discharge plans and options, and terminal diagnosis.

Virik and Glare[26] prospectively evaluated 50 cases referred to a palliative care service at a tertiary teaching hospital in Sydney. Consistent with the AHA survey data, pain management was the most common reason for consultation. The median number of recommendations per patient was three. Advice regarding discharge planning was given in 62% of cases, and recommendations in this area were rated as most helpful by the referring team. Abrahm et al.[27] studied the impact of a hospice consultation team on the care of veterans with advanced cancer. In the first year of service, they resolved 85% of the medical/nursing problems identified. Ninety percent of the patients referred to the team with unacceptable pain achieved acceptable pain control.

PALLIATIVE CARE AT MOUNT SINAI HOSPITAL: A CASE STUDY

Mount Sinai Hospital (MSH) in New York is a private, urban, tertiary-care teaching hospital with 1171 beds. The hospital is the main teaching site for the Mount Sinai School of Medicine of New York University, at which the authors are full-time faculty in the Departments of Geriatrics and Medicine.

The Palliative Care Service (PCS) at MSH was initiated in 1997 following a 2-year faculty development program. This program was composed of a series of monthly seminars on palliative care topics. The seminars were open to all members of the hospital community. Beginning in April 1997, a clinical nurse specialist and physician began to see patients referred for palliative care consultation. Three attending physicians from the Department of Geriatrics, including one of the authors (D.E.M.), shared the physician duties at that time. The number of consultations grew steadily to the present level of approximately 50 new referrals per month (Fig. 28–1).

In 1998, leadership in the Department of Medicine designated four float beds on one of the medical teaching floors of the hospital as the Palliative Care Unit (PCU). Patients admitted to this unit were managed by residents of the Department of Medicine under the direct supervision of the physician and nurse of the PCS. In 2000, a formal curriculum of palliative care education was implemented for the residents rotating on the PCU. At the present time, 12 part-time physicians and three full-time advanced practice nurses oversee the clinical

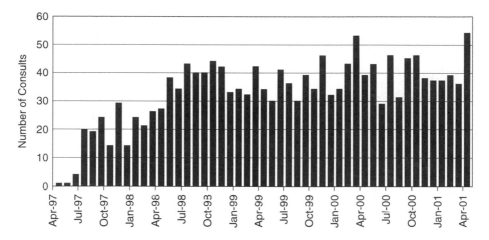

Figure 28–1. New consults per month, Mount Sinai Hospital Palliative Care Service, April 1997–April 2001.

care of patients referred to the PCS and PCU. A full-time bereavement coordinator joined the team in 2001. A team of part-time and volunteer licensed massage therapists works with the PCS, employing non-pharmacological interventions, such as relaxation and massage, to reduce distress. The PCS consults regularly with social work, chaplaincy, pharmacy, and therapist colleagues in the hospital.

Approximately 50% of the patients referred to the MSH PCS have a primary cancer diagnosis. The remaining 50% of patients are evenly divided among other common noncancer diagnoses including advanced heart, lung, and liver disease; dementia; stroke; and acquired immunodeficiency syndrome (AIDS) (Fig. 28–2). Patients referred to the PCS have a median age of 71 years, 52% are female, 49% are white, 25% are African American, and 20% are Latino. In 2001, 55% of the patients referred to the PCS died at MSH. Analysis of the disposition of patients who were discharged alive after referral to the PCS revealed the following:

- 36% went home with nonhospice home care
- 26% were transferred to a skilled nursing facility (including nursing homes with palliative care)

- 20% were discharged home with hospice care
- 16% were transferred to an inpatient hospice setting
- 2% had another disposition

To assess their clinical impact, the PCS at MSH prospectively studied 325 consecutive referred patients and assessed the number of recommendations per patient and the rate at which recommendations were implemented by the primary team.[28] An average of 4.2 recommendations were made per patient, with an overall implementation rate of 91%.

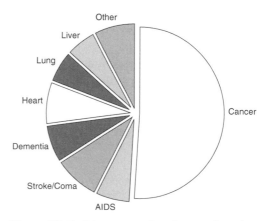

Figure 28–2. Diagnoses of patients referred to the Mount Sinai Palliative Care Service, April 1997–April 2001.

Since the goal of palliative care is the relief of distress, all palliative care services must document the degree to which they succeed in this mission. The clinicians of the MSH PCS measure symptom distress daily and document their measurements at initial consultation, at discharge, and every 72 hours in between using a four-point numeric rating scaled based on a modification of the Edmonton Symptom Assessment System.[29] A comparison of the level of symptom distress at the time of consultation and at death or discharge is shown in Figure 28–3 for the prevalent symptoms of pain, dyspnea, and nausea. For all three of these burdensome symptoms, clinically and statistically significant reductions were seen for patients with mild, moderate, or severe initial symptoms. Subgroup analysis between patients discharged alive versus those who died showed that the symptoms of both groups improved comparably.

FISCAL IMPACT OF HOSPITAL-BASED PALLIATIVE CARE SERVICES

In the current medical economic environment, the fiscal impact of each intervention must be studied so that informed decisions may be made regarding its cost-effectiveness. Hospital-based palliative care programs have been shown to improve the symptoms of patients with serious and life-threatening illness as well as to have a positive impact on the education of clinicians,

but at what cost? Palliative care services spend considerable time counseling patients and families regarding treatment options and alternatives in the face of serious illness. There are currently no mechanisms for clinician reimbursement that adequately account for the time-intensive nature of these interventions. For this reason, many palliative care services cannot fund themselves exclusively through clinical income and often rely on varying amounts of philanthropic and institutional support. Several authors have attempted to quantitate the fiscal impact of communication interventions regarding goals of care upon their institution.[30–33] All of these studies have demonstrated a reduction in hospital and ICU length of stay, more appropriate utilization of high-technology therapies, and no increase in risk-adjusted mortality associated with ethics, palliative care, and intensive communication interventions applied to critically and seriously ill patient populations. When medically realistic goals of care and prognoses are communicated to patients and families, they often elect to avoid high-technology, death-prolonging therapies in favor of the palliative goals of comfort. Length-of-stay analysis at MSH has shown similar benefits in terms of documented reductions in ICU and hospital lengths of stay for patients who die in the hospital following a palliative care consult versus patients who die without such a consult.

Palliative care services provide additional fiscal benefits that are more difficult to measure: often, palliative care communica-

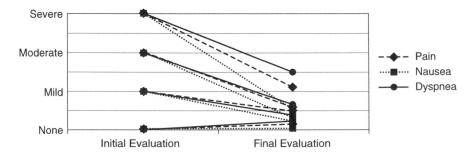

Figure 28–3. Impact of palliative care service consultation on the symptoms of pain ($n = 884$), nausea ($n = 843$), and dyspnea ($n = 844$) at Mount Sinai Hospital, September 1998–April 2001.

tion interventions will clarify the goals of care sufficiently that a patient and his or her family may choose to leave the hospital for either hospice or certified home health agency care at home, in a skilled nursing facility, or an inpatient hospice unit. Without clarification of the goals of care, no rational discharge plan can be agreed upon, resulting in long ICU and hospital stays and a high rate of in-hospital deaths.

BARRIERS TO OPTIMAL UTILIZATION OF HOSPITAL-BASED PALLIATIVE CARE

Multiple factors prevent full utilization of hospital-based palliative care. These include fiscal limitations, gaps in palliative care expertise and leadership, and cultural issues that prevent timely referral for palliative care services.

Frequent, repeated counseling of patients and families and education of clinical colleagues can be extremely time-consuming. The inadequacy of current strategies for compensation for clinical services of this nature has been mentioned. Improved and more consistent financial support for institutional palliative care initiatives will be required to develop the number and quality of programs needed to care for the aging population.

Palliative medicine, as a specialty, is a new field. The field currently lacks the American Board of Medical Subspecialty certification required for government support of graduate medical education, and as a result, there are very few academic training programs in palliative care.[34] The limited number of academic training programs translates into a limited number of academic leaders in the field, which in turn inhibits the training of future physicians so necessary to good care of the seriously ill. To place a specialist in palliative medicine in every hospital or community will require exponential growth in the number of trainees and training programs. A far more achievable goal is the education of every physician in the basics of palliative care. This has been the goal of the Educating

Physicians in End-of-life Care project sponsored by the American Medical Association and the Robert Wood Johnson Foundation, which educated over 1200 physicians and other health-care professionals as of April 2002.[35] A comparable program for nurses, The End-of-Life Nursing Education Consortium Project is also available.[36]

Cultural attitudes toward disease and death are more pervasive issues that serve as barriers to optimal employment of hospital-based palliative care services. Our culture celebrates activity, accomplishment, and youth and denies death. The consumer society seems to consider itself entitled not just to health but also to immortality. Advances in public health and the technologies of medicine feed this death-denying culture, and patients, families, and physicians may pursue questionably effective, burdensome therapies rather than confront the simple truth that a life may be coming to its natural end. For these reasons, palliative care consultation is often deferred until the final days or hours of life. At MSH 77% of patients referred to palliative care are already severely disabled or moribund at the time of consultation.

A more rational model is to begin palliative care interventions to some degree at the time of diagnosis of any serious, chronic, or life-limiting illness, regardless of prognosis and whether or not curative treatments are likely to be beneficial. At this time, disease-modifying therapies will likely comprise the bulk of interventions. However, as disease progresses, disease-modifying therapies may become more burdensome and limited in terms of their benefits; and correspondingly, palliative care interventions may come to comprise the greater share of care. The concurrent delivery of disease-modifying and palliative types of care allows for smoother transitions in care as disease progresses and the goals of care shift.

THE FUTURE: HOSPICE–HOSPITAL RELATIONS

Since only a fraction of our hospitals currently have a palliative care service, alternative means are necessary to ensure that the continuum of care is uninterrupted. An effective solution for both hospitals with palliative care services as well as those without them is to collaborate with community hospices. Partnering hospitals with hospices has advantages for all parties involved. A number of the nation's hospice programs have already forged strong, mutually beneficial partnerships with hospitals in their communities.[37] These partnerships have benefited a range of communities, types of hospice program, and forms of partnership.

Most importantly, these collaborations benefit patients and their families. Partnering with hospice can give hospitalized patients access to an untapped repository of palliative care expertise. Hospices bring interdisciplinary palliative care expertise and the ability to case-manage the care of very complex and seriously ill patients across multiple settings, spiritual services, volunteer supports for both patient and family caregivers, and bereavement programming and support for family members for at least 1 year after the patient has died. For patients in hospice, hospitals may provide acute-care expertise and secondary- and tertiary-care specialty services. Together these institutions can meet most, if not all, of the needs of the seriously ill for a range of illnesses, disease stages, and clinical settings.

Collaboration benefits hospices and hospitals as well, from both a patient care and a business perspective. From the hospice perspective, since many terminally ill patients are cared for in hospitals, a hospital partnership allows hospices to reach and care for a much larger group of patients and families earlier in the course of their illness. The MSH PCS substantially increased hospice referrals in the first year of its existence. Other programs have reported similar trends (M. Twaddle, personal communication, 2002).

While an increased number of referrals earlier in the disease course has obvious potential fiscal benefits for hospice, most importantly, it increases access to palliative care services for patients in greatest need of these specialized services. A strong link between hospitals and community hospices can also help to overcome one of the main barriers to hospice referral: the implication of abandonment by the hospital's primary medical team and the resultant patient and family feeling of a forced transfer out of the hospital that inhibits many referrals. If hospice professionals and hospital staff work together and see themselves and are seen by patients as part of the same team, the discontinuities inherent in the experience of the transfer are minimized. Collaboration also improves hospice access for a much broader segment of the patient and provider community, including cardiologists, intensivists, transplant teams, nephrologists, and their patients, groups of patients and providers who seldom access hospice care, at least in part due to unfamiliarity with hospice and its benefits.

From the hospital perspective, hospice collaboration creates instant capacity to meet the clinical palliative care needs of the sickest and most complex patients. Linkage with hospice professionals can provide clinical expertise not only to patients in the hospital but also to their families, both during and after the hospital stay. Hospices can create the bridge between the hospital and home that is so often lacking in the acute-care setting, leading to long hospital stays and frequent readmissions. The hospice partnership markedly enhances discharge options for seriously ill persons with high professional care needs upon return to the home. Hospice professionals are familiar with and feel secure about caring for the predictable crises that are a routine part of care at home for persons with serious and complex illness.

Finally, the financial incentives for hospitals favor hospice partnerships. Under capitation arrangements, hospices help prevent frequent and costly hospital readmissions for the sickest 5% who utilize more than 30% of the health-care dollar.[38] Under case rate and per diem models, hospice partnerships and their associated discharge options can help reduce length of stay for some of the longest-stay, sickest, and most costly patients in the hospital, thus increasing bed capacity for new admissions. Even if a hospitalized patient cannot be discharged to another care setting, hospice involvement can lead to marked reductions in cost per day, largely because of the impact on pharmacy costs, number of diagnostic procedures, and use of intensive care. For hospitals that participate in contracts for inpatient hospice beds, some long-stay but hospice-eligible patients can choose to be "paper-transferred" to hospice care while remaining in the hospital setting. In such circumstances, the hospital recovers approximately $500 in per diem income from the hospice, as opposed to zero dollars from the typical long-stay Medicare patient whose diagnosis-related group payment has long been exhausted.

Clearly hospice–hospital collaborations provide earlier and increased access to palliative care for persons with serious illness. These collaborations permit a broader array of clinical services to both hospitalized patients as well as those already in hospice. Financial benefits for both hospices and hospitals make these collaborations mutually feasible.

SUMMARY

Hospital-based palliative care teams have evolved as a natural outgrowth of the modern hospice movement. Too often, people with chronic, serious, or life-limiting illness experience extraordinary levels of physical, emotional, social, and spiritual distress. The ability of hospital-based palliative care teams to address the suffering of these patients, independent of their prognosis and diagnosis, allows wider and earlier access to these critical services to people in need. While palliative care is clearly needed for people with serious but curable disease, hospital-based palliative care services will also play a critical role as doctors and their patients and families struggle with the transition from caring and curing to caring. Partnerships between hospitals and hospices are a mutually beneficial way to maintain high-quality and continuous care throughout this transition at the beginning of the end of life.

REFERENCES

1. World Health Organization. Cancer Pain Relief and Palliative Care. Geneva, WHO, 1990.
2. Field MJ, Cassel CK (Eds.). Approaching Death: Improving Care at the End of Life. Washington DC, National Academy Press, 1997.
3. Pritchard RS, Fisher ES, Teno JM, et al. Influence of patient preferences and local health system characteristics on the place of death. SUPPORT Investigators. Study to Understand Prognoses and Preferences for Risks and Outcomes of Treatment [see comments]. J Am Geriatr Soc 46:1242–1250, 1998.
4. SUPPORT Principal Investigators. A controlled trial to improve care for seriously ill hospitalized patients. The Study to Understand Prognoses and Preferences for Outcomes and Risks of Treatments (SUPPORT). JAMA 274:1591–1598, 1995.
5. Singer PA, Martin D, Kelner M. Quality of end of life care: patients' perspectives. JAMA 281:163–168, 1999.
6. Dunlop RJ, Hockley JM. Hospital-based Palliative Care Teams: The Hospital–Hospice Interface, 2nd ed. Oxford, Oxford University Press, 1998.
7. O'Neill WM, O'Connor P, Latimer EJ. Hospital palliative care services: three models in three countries. J Pain Symptom Manage 7:406–413, 1992.
8. Mount BM. The problem of caring for the dying in a general hospital; the palliative care unit as a possible solution. Can Med Assoc J 115:119–121, 1976.
9. Bates T, Hoy AM, Clarke DG, et al. The St Thomas' Hospital terminal care support team. A new concept of hospice care. Lancet 1:1201–1203, 1981.
10. Billings J, Pantilat S. Survey of palliative care programs in United States teaching hospitals. J Palliat Med 4:309–314, 2001.
11. Oneschuk D, Hanson J, Bruera E. An international survey of undergraduate medical education in palliative medicine. J Pain Symptom Manage 20:174–179, 2000.
12. Billings JA, Block S. Palliative care in undergraduate medical education. Status report and future directions. JAMA 278:733–738, 1997.
13. Rabow MW, Herdle GE, Fair JM, et al. End-of-life care content in 50 textbooks

from multiple specialties. JAMA 283:771–778, 2000.

14. Ferrell B, Virani R, Grant M. Analysis of symptom assessment and management content in nursing textbooks. J Palliat Med 2:161–173, 1999.

15. Hill TP. Treating the dying patient. The challenge for medical education. Arch Intern Med 155:1265–1269, 1995.

16. Merman A, Gunn D, Dickinson G. Learning to care for the dying: a survey of medical schools and a model course. Acad Med 66:35–38, 1991.

17. Plumb JD, Segraves M. Terminal care in primary care postgraduate medical education programs: a national survey. Am J Hosp Palliat Care 9:32–35, 1992.

18. Buss MK, Marx ES, Sulmasy DP. The preparedness of students to discuss end-of-life issues with patients. Acad Med 73:418–422, 1998.

19. Ogle KS, Mavis B, Rohrer J. Graduating medical students' competencies and educational experiences in palliative care. J Pain Symptom Manage 14:280–285, 1997.

20. Ferrell BR, McCaffery M. Nurses' knowledge about equianalgesia and opioid dosing. Cancer Nurs 20:201–212, 1997.

21. Von Gunten CF, Von Roenn JH, Gradishar W, et al. A hospice/palliative medicine rotation for fellows training in hematology-oncology. J Cancer Educ 10:200–202, 1995.

22. McQuillan R, Finlay I, Branch C, et al. Improving analgesic prescribing in a general teaching hospital. J Pain Symptom Manage 11:172–180, 1996.

23. Fischberg DJ, Pan CX. Design and evaluation of a palliative care curriculum for internal medicine residents on an inpatient palliative care unit. J Palliat Med 4:277, 2001.

24. Pan CX, Fischberg D, Morris J, et al. Through the looking glass: looking at a palliative care consult service from an educational perspective. J Palliat Med 5:203, 2002.

25. Pan CX, Morrison RS, Meier DE, et al. How prevalent are hospital-based palliative care programs? Status report and future directions. J Palliat Med 4:315–324, 2001.

26. Virik K, Glare PG. Profile and evaluation of a palliative medicine consultation service within a tertiary teaching hospital in Sydney. J Pain Symptom Manage 23:17–25, 2002.

27. Abrahm JL, Callahan J, Rosetti K, et al. The impact of a hospice consultation team on the care of veterans with advanced cancer. J Pain Symptom Manage 12:23–31, 1996.

28. Manfredi PL, Morrison RS, Morris J, et al. Palliative care consultations: how do they impact on the care of hospitalized patients? J Pain Symptom Manage 20:166–173, 2000.

29. Bruera E, Kuehn N, Miller MJ, et al. The Edmonton Symptom Assessment System (ESAS): a simple method for the assessment of palliative care patients. J Palliat Care 7:6–9, 1991.

30. Lilly C, De Meo DL, Sonne LA, et al. An intensive communication intervention for the critically ill. Am J Med 109:469–475, 2000.

31. Dowdy MD, Robertson C, Bander JA. A study of proactive ethics consultation for critically and terminally ill patients with extended lengths of stay [see comments]. Crit Care Med 26:252–259, 1998.

32. Carlson R, Devich L, Frank RR. Development of a comprehensive supportive care team for the hopelessly ill on a university hospital medical service. JAMA 259:378–383, 1988.

33. Campbell ML. Program assessment through outcomes analysis: efficacy of a comprehensive supportive care team for end-of-life care. AACN Clin Issues 7:159–167, 1996.

34. Billings J. Palliative medicine fellowship programs in the United States: Year 2000 survey. J Palliat Med 3:391–396, 2000.

35. EPEC. The EPEC Project: Education for Physicians on End of Life Care. Chicago, 2001.

36. American Association of Colleges of Nursing. The End-of-Life Nursing Education Consortium (ELNEC) Project. Washington, DC, 2001.

37. National Hospice and Palliative Care Organization and the Center to Advance Palliative Care. Hospital–Hospice Partnerships in Palliative Care: Creating a Continuum of Service. 2001.

38. Lubitz JD, Riley FF. Trends in Medicare payments in the last year of life. N Engl J Med 328:1092–1096, 1993.

Index

Page numbers followed by f and t indicate figures and tables, respectively.

Abandonment, 74–75
Abuse, elder, 74–75
Access to care
  medical professionalism and, 57
  racial differences, 84–85
Accountability, 56–57, 76
Accreditation, nursing home, 358, 373–74
Acetaminophen, for pain management, 214, 216t
Active listening, 382
Activities of daily living, 143t
Acupuncture
  for dyspnea, 247
  for pain management, 224t
Acute care of the elderly (ACE) units, for
      hospitalized frail elder, 105
Acute stroke unit, 137–38, 137t
Addiction, to opioids, 218
Advance care planning, 307–13
  communication issues, 322–24
  in dementia, 170
  disease progression and, 308–9
  in dying patient, 311–13
  early in disease trajectory, 309–11
  ethical issues, 66
  goals, 308
  lack of focus on, 349
  in nursing home patient, 362–67, 365f–366f

possible issues and actions, 311t
sentinel time periods for, 309
vs. advance directives, 308, 308t
Advance directives, 308, 324, 334, 362–63
Advanced lung disease, 173–85
  dyspnea in, 174–81, 231. *See also* Dyspnea
    burden, 174–75
    complementary/alternative therapies, 247
    nonpharmacological approaches, 180–81,
      242–44
    pharmacological approaches, 175–80, 235–42
    psychological burden, 184–85, 247–48
    surgical approaches, 181–83, 244–47
Advocacy
  end-of-life care reform, 352–53
  ethical issues, 76–77
Aesthetic well-being, in dementia, 33
Affect, in communication, 318
African Americans
  attitudes toward end-of-life care, 82–83
  experience and treatment of aging and dying, 84–85
  life expectancy, 84
Ageism, 72–73
Agency for Health Care Research and Quality
      (AHRQ), in end-of-life care reform, 351,
      354
Aggrenox, for stroke prevention, 139

Aging. *See also* Elderly person
  attitudes toward
    bias, 72–73
    ethnic differences, 80–81
  experience and treatment of, diversity in, 84–85
  and quality of life, 73–74
Agitation
  in dementia, 165–66
  in dialysis withdrawal, 199
  in end-stage dementia, 296–97, 297t
  in nursing home patient, 369
  tube feeding–induced, 40
Air humidification, for dyspnea, 244
Air movement, for dyspnea, 244
Airway obstruction, in lung cancer, 183, 246
ALD. *See* Advanced lung disease
Alprazolam, for dyspnea, 241
Alternative medicine
  for dyspnea, 247
  for pain management, 225
Altruism, forced, in research for elders with terminal
    illness, 70
Altruistic love, 30–31
Alzheimer's disease
  dementia in, 160. *See also* Dementia
  depression in, 167
  hallucinations in, 166
  incapacity in, 332, 333t. *See also* Incapacitated
    patient
  intracerebral hemorrhage and, 135
  pain assessment in, 164
  palliative care in, love's place in, 30–35
Amitriptyline
  in advanced lung disease, 185, 248
  for pain management, 220, 221t
Amphetamine, for stroke patient, 148, 149–50
Amyloid angiopathy, hemorrhage from, 135
Analgesia
  epidural, 223t
  intrathecal, 223t
Analgesics, for pain management
  epidemiology, 206
  overview, 213–19, 216t–217t
  route of administration, 213–14
  timing, 214
Anesthesia, for pain management, 222, 223t
Anesthetics, local, for pain management, 220, 221t
Aneurysm, saccular, subarachnoid hemorrhage from,
    134, 135
Angiopathy, amyloid, hemorrhage from, 135
Angiotensin-converting enzyme (ACE) inhibitors
  for heart failure, 111
  for stroke prevention, 138
Anorexia
  management, 259–60
  in nursing home patient, 368–69
Anti-inflammatory interventions, in frail elder, 104
Antiarrhythmics, for pain management, 221t
Antibiotics
  in advanced dementia, 168
  ethical issues, 69
  in nursing home patient, 367

Anticholinergic drugs, delirium from, 289
Anticoagulation
  for stroke prevention, 139, 140t
  for stroke therapy, 137
Anticonvulsants, for pain management, 220, 221t
Antidepressants
  in advanced lung disease, 180, 184–85, 241–42,
    248
  in dementia, 167
  for depression, 295–96
  for dyspnea, 180, 241–42
  for fatigue, 281, 282t
  in heart failure, 114–15
  for post-stroke depression, 147–48
  tricyclic
    in advanced lung disease, 185, 248
    for fatigue, 282t
    in heart failure, 114
    for pain management, 220, 221t
    for post-stroke depression, 148
Antiemetics
  for intestinal obstruction, 264
  for nausea and vomiting, 261–63, 262f, 262t
Antihistamines, in end-stage renal disease, 198–99
Antihypertensive agents, for stroke prevention, 138,
    140t
Antiplatelet therapy, for stroke prevention, 139–40,
    140t
Antipsychotics
  for delirium, 290
  for dyspnea, 180, 241–42
Anxiety
  in advanced lung disease, 184–85, 247–48
  assessment and treatment, 291–92
  clinical features, 291
  diagnosis, 291
  epidemiology, 291
  nausea and vomiting from, 261
  in nursing home patient, 369
  screening for, in pain assessment, 209
Anxiolytics, for dyspnea, 180, 241–42
Appetite, stimulation, 259–60
Aspiration risk
  in home palliative care, 392
  tube feeding and, 38–39
Aspirin
  for pain management, 216t
  for stroke prevention, 139
  for stroke therapy, 137, 137t
Assisted suicide, 20, 69–70
Assistive devices, in home palliative care, 396–97
Asthenia
  cachexia-related, 273
  fatigue and, 272
Atherothrombotic stroke, large vessel, 136–37
Atrial fibrillation, and stroke, 136, 139
Autonomy, in death, 20

Baclofen, for post-stroke spasticity, 147
Bacterial infection, oral, 257
Bad news, delivering, 319–22, 320t

Bankruptcy, medical reasons for, 346, 379
Barriers to palliative care, 49–50
  hospital-based, 409
  in nursing home, 357–58
Bathroom equipment, in home palliative care, 397
Bed-bound patient, home equipment, 397–98
Bedside rails, 396, 397
Behavioral therapy, for pain management, 225
Bend, Oregon
  end-of-life care, 14
  Medicare spending, 6, 7–8, 7f
Benzodiazepines
  in advanced lung disease, 180, 185, 241–42, 248
  for anxiety, 292
  in dementia, 166
Benzydamine, for mucositis, 257
Bereavement
  communication issues, 327
  cultural differences, 86
  in nursing home, 371–72
  support
    in dialysis withdrawal, 199–200
    to family caregivers, 371, 383–84
"Best interests," in decision-making hierarchy, 334
Beta$_2$-agonists, for dyspnea, 175, 235
Beta blockers, for heart failure, 111
Bisacodyl, for constipation, 266
Bowel obstruction. See Intestinal obstruction
Bran, for constipation, 267
Breakthrough pain, 214
Breast cancer, 123, 124f, 125, 125f, 128, 129
Breathlessness. See Dyspnea
Bronchodilators, for dyspnea, 175, 235
Bullectomy, for dyspnea, 181, 244
Buspirone
  in advanced lung disease, 180, 185, 241, 242, 248
  for anxiety, 292
Butorphanol, adverse effects, 219

Cachexia
  asthenia and, 273
  fraility and, 99
  nutrition and, 41–43
Calciphylaxis pain, in end-stage renal disease, 196–97
Calcitonin, for pain management, 220, 221t, 222
Caloric requirement, estimation, 392
Cancer, 123–31. See also site of cancer, e.g., Breast cancer
  cachexia-related asthenia in, 273
  caregiver's role, 130–31
  chemotherapy, 127–29
  delirium in, 289
  fatigue in, 273, 274–75
  incidence, 124, 124f
  intestinal obstruction in, 263
  management algorithm, 126
  radiation therapy, 129–30
  research on, 124–25
  scope of problem, 123–25, 124f, 125f
  surgical management, 130

taste alterations in, 257–58
  tumor behavior, 125
Candidiasis, oral, 257
Cannabinoids, for nausea and vomiting, 263
Capacity. See also Incapacitated patient
  assessment, 65
  communication issues, 326–27
  decision-specific nature, 363
  definition, 333
  full mental, frail patient with, 64
  prior to death, 332, 333t
Capsaicin, for pain management, 221t
Carbamazepine, for pain management, 220, 221t
Cardiac cachexia, fraility and, 99
Cardioembolic stroke, 136
Cardiologist visits, supply of cardiologists and, 9, 9f
Cardiopulmonary resuscitation (CPR)
  in nursing home patient, 363–64
  in Oregon, 12–13
Caregivers
  informal. See Family caregivers
  stress in, 378–79
Carotid body resection, for dyspnea, 182–83, 245
Carotid endarterectomy, for stroke prevention, 140, 140t
Cause of death
  changes in, 402
  demand for single, 350
Celecoxib, for pain management, 215, 216t
Celiac plexus blockade, for pain management, 223t
Centers for Disease Control and Prevention (CDC), in end-of-life care reform, 351
Centers of excellence, 354
Cerebrovascular disease, end-stage renal disease in, 192
Certified nursing assistant (CNA)
  bereavement support, 371
  communication with, 369–70
  palliative care certification, 372
Chemotherapy
  for breast cancer, 128–29
  for colon cancer, 128–29
  in elderly person, 127–29
  fatigue from, 275
  for lung cancer, 183–84, 246–47
Chinese culture, dementia in, 32
Chiropractic medicine, for pain management, 224t
Chlorpromazine
  for delirium, 290
  in dementia, 166
  for dyspnea, 180, 241, 242
  for nausea and vomiting, 262t
Cholesterol, stroke risk and, 138, 140t
Cholestyramine, for diarrhea, 268
Chronic obstructive pulmonary disease
  bullectomy for, 181, 244
  dyspnea in, 174. See also Dyspnea
  fatigue in, 274
  and hypoxemia, oxygen therapy, 177, 238–39
  incidence, 173
  prognosis, 174t
  psychological burden, 184–85, 247–48

Cigarette smoking, stroke risk and, 139
Cimetidine, in end-stage renal disease, adverse effects, 198
Cisapride, for nausea and vomiting, 263
Clinical nurse specialist, in hospital-based palliative care team, 404–5
Clopidogrel, for stroke prevention, 139
Clorazepate, for dyspnea, 241
Codeine
  for diarrhea, 268
  for dyspnea, 179, 240
  for pain management, 217t
Cognitive-behavioral therapy
  in advanced lung disease, 185, 248
  for pain management, 224t, 225
Cognitive impairment
  communication issues, 326–27
  decision-making issues, 332–40. See also Incapacitated patient
  and depression, 293–94
  from opioids, 215, 218
  pain assessment in, 211–12
Cognitive interventions
  for fatigue, 278, 279f
  for pain management, 225
Colic, in intestinal obstruction, 264
Colon cancer
  chemotherapy, 128–29
  in elderly person, 123, 124f, 125f, 128–29
Communication, 314–27
  about advance care planning, 322–24
  about transition to palliative care, 324–25, 325t
  in advanced illness
    effective, 317–19
    present state, 314–15
  affect in, 318
  of bad news, 319–22, 320t
  with bereaved patient, 327
  with cognitively impaired patient, 326–27
  dreaded questions in, 325–26
  emotion-handling skills in, 318–19, 319t
  empathy in, 318
  ethical issues, 61–63
  with family caregivers, 370–71, 381–82
  with heart failure patient, 115–16
  of hope in context of palliative care, 319
  information transmittal, 61–62
  informed consent, 62–63
  in nursing home, 369–71
  poor, etiology, 315–16
  principles, 316–17, 316t
  responding to illness meaning, 62
  value differences and, 63
Community, professional obligations to, 59
Competence, definition, 333
Complementary therapies
  for dyspnea, 247
  for pain management, 225
Conflict of interest, ethical issues, 71–72
Congestive heart failure (CHF). See Heart failure
Congressional funding, for health care system reform, 354

Conservation withdrawal system, 274
Constipation
  assessment, 265
  background, 265
  in end-stage renal disease, 197–98
  management, 266–67
  in nursing home patient, 369
  opioid-induced, 165, 215, 218
Constraint-induced movement therapy, for stroke patient, 146
Coping strategies, for fatigue, 278–79
Cordotomy, for pain management, 223t
Coronary artery disease
  depression in, 114
  end-stage renal disease in, 192
Corticosteroids
  for anorexia, 259–60
  for dyspnea, 176–77, 236–37
  for fatigue, 281, 282t
  for pain management, 221t
Cortisol, in frail elder, 97
Cost effectiveness, in palliative care, 50
Cough suppressants, for dyspnea, 242
Creatinine, serum, in elderly person, 193
Cultural competence, ethical imperative, 63–64
Culture. See also Diversity
  and approach to death, 81
  definition, 80
  and ethical approaches, 63–64, 81
  and grieving experience, 86
  and pain management, 86
Cyclizine
  for intestinal obstruction, 264
  for nausea and vomiting, 261, 262t
Cyproheptadine, for diarrhea, 268

Daily living, activities of, 143t
Danthron, for constipation, 266
Dartmouth Atlas of Health Care, 3–6, 4f–5f, 4t
Death and dying. See also End-of-life care; Terminally ill patient
  attitudes toward, ethnic differences, 80–81
  capacity prior to, 332, 333t
  cause of
    changes in, 402
    demand for single, 350
  conversations about, communication skills, 324–25, 325t, 326
  cultural inexperience with, 350
  with dignity, 20–21
  experience of, 19–20
    communicating, 17–18
    diversity in, 84–85
  family caregiver support prior to, 382–83
  at home
    factors associated with, 10
    patient preference for
      and place of death, 10, 10f
      reasons for, 20
    and presence of primary carer, 387

in hospital, experience of, 403–4
physician and, 21–22
physician anxiety regarding, 316
process, in older adult, *xxiii*
quality of, measurement, 26–27
site of
    changes in, 403
    and patient preference, 10, 10f
    regional variation, 403
time dimension, 18–19
in United States, epidemiology, 402–3
"Death rattle," 169, 393
Deathbed vigil, dialysis withdrawal and, 196
Decision-making capacity. *See* Capacity;
    Incapacitated patient
Deliberative model, in patient–physician
    relationship, 60
Delirium, 286–91
    assessment and treatment, 289–91
    clinical features, 287–88
    definition, 160, 286–87, 287t
    in dementia, 165–66
    diagnosis, 288
    in dialysis withdrawal, 199
    epidemiology, 288–89
    in nursing home patient, 369
    outcome, 289
    risk factors, 288
Delirium Rating Scale, 288
Delusions
    in delirium, 288
    in dementia, 166–67
Dementia, 160–70
    advance care planning, 170
    aesthetic well-being in, 33
    in Alzheimer's disease, 160
    caregiver issues, 297–98
    causes, 160–61
    deaths associated with, impairments related to,
        161
    emotional and relational well-being in, 33
    end-stage
        love's place in, 30–35
        psychiatric disturbances in, 296–97, 297t
        tube feeding in, 37–40, 169
    family issues, 169–70
    with Lewy bodies, 160–61
    nutritional issues, 169
    prognosis, 161–64, 162t, 163t
    spiritual well-being in, 33–34
    stages, 161
    stigma associated with, 32
    symptom management, 164–69
        agitation and delirium, 165–66
        "death rattle," 169
        delusions and hallucinations, 166–67
        depression, 167, 297
        dry mouth, 168–69
        dyspnea, 169
        fever and infection, 167–68
        incontinence, 168
        insomnia, 167

pain, 164–65
skin care, 168
vascular, 160
Dependence, on opioids, 218
Depression, 292–96
    in advanced lung disease, 184–85, 247–48
    assessment, 294–95
    caregiver issues, 297–98
    cognitive impairment and, 293–94
    in dementia, 167, 297
    dialysis withdrawal and, 195–96
    in elderly person, 113–14
    epidemiology, 292–93
    in family caregivers, 394
    fatigue and, 275
    in home palliative care, 394
    hopelessness and, 294
    in nursing home patient, 369
    physical illness symptoms and, overlap, 292
    post-stroke, 147–48
    risk factors and complications, 293–94
    screening for, in pain assessment, 209
    treatment, 295–96, 295t
    underdetection and undertreatment, 293
Deschutes County, Oregon, end-of-life care, 14
Desipramine, for pain management, 220, 221t
Developmental challenges, end-of-life, 17–22
Dexamethasone
    for anorexia, 259–60
    for dyspnea, 237
    for fatigue, 281, 282t
    taste alterations from, 258
Dextroamphetamine
    for fatigue, 281, 282t
    for stroke patient, 148, 149
Diabetes mellitus, end-stage renal disease in, 192
Diagnostic tests, in nursing home patient, 364
Dialysis
    in elderly person, 193
    methods, 193
    mortality rate, 193
    peritoneal, 193
    symptoms related to, 193
    "washout" after, 193
    withdrawal, 194–200
        agitation during, 199
        bereavement after death, 199–200
        delirium during, 199
        family involvement in decision making, 195
        gastrointestinal symptoms, 197–98
        mouth care, 198
        myoclonus during, 199
        pain management, 196–97
        pruritus during, 198–99
        psychosocial issues, 195–96
        skin care, 198
        symptoms during last 24 hours, 195, 195t
Diarrhea, 267–68
Diaschisis, 149
Diazepam, for dyspnea, 241, 242
Diet. *See also* Nutrition
    in cachectic patient, 42

Diflunisal, for pain management, 216t
Digoxin, for heart failure, 111
Dihydrocodeine, for dyspnea, 179, 240
Dilation, of malignant esophageal stricture, 259
Diphenhydramine, for intestinal obstruction, 264
Diphenoxylate, for diarrhea, 268
Disclosure
    of concerns, communication skills, 316–17, 316t
    of conflict of interest, 71–72
Discomfort Scale for Dementia of the Alzheimer's
        Type, 164
Disease. *See* Illness
Disfigurement, in home palliative care, 395–96
Disillusion, at end-of-life, 19
Diuretics, in heart failure, 111
Diversity, 79–88
    in attitudes toward aging and dying, 80–81
    in attitudes toward end-of-life care, 81–84
    in experience and treatment of aging and dying,
        84–85
    strategies of caring, 85–88
        disagreements about informing patient, 87–88
        guiding questions, 87t
        LEARN acronym, 86–87
        for severely ill and dying patient, 87, 87t
        spiritual assessment, 87t
Do-not-resuscitate orders
    in nursing home patient, 363–64
    in Oregon, 12–13
Docusate sodium, for constipation, 267
Domperidone, for nausea and vomiting, 262–63,
        262t
Dopaminergic agonists, for stroke-related
        impairments, 150–51
Drowsiness, from opioids, 215, 218
Dry mouth
    in dementia, 168–69
    in end-stage renal disease, 198
Dulcolax suppositories, in dementia, 165
Durable power of attorney, in nursing home patient,
        362
Dying. *See* Death and dying; End-of-life care;
        Terminally ill patient
Dyspepsia, in end-stage renal disease, 197–98
Dysphagia
    assessment, 258
    investigation, 258
    management, 258–59
    in nursing home patient, 368–69
Dyspnea, 230–49
    in advanced lung disease, 174–81, 231
    assessment, 232–33, 232t
    burden, 174–75
    causes, 232, 233
    complementary/alternative therapies, 247
    definition, 174–75, 230
    in dementia, 169
    differential diagnosis, 233, 233t
    exercise tests, 234
    in heart failure, 111
    in home palliative care, 393

    in lung cancer, 174, 183–84, 183t
    management, 234–48
    measurement, 233–34
    multidimensional aspects, 230–31
    nonpharmacological approaches, 180–81, 242–44
        exercise training, 243
        humidified air, 244
        increased air movement, 244
        inspiratory muscle training, 243
        noninvasive positive pressure ventilation, 181,
            243–44
        positioning, 244
        progressive muscle relaxation, 243
        pulmonary rehabilitation, 180–81, 242–43
    in nursing home patient, 368
    in older adult, 231–32
    pharmacological approaches, 175–80, 235–42
        antidepressants, 180, 241–42
        anxiolytics, 180, 241–42
        bronchodilators, 175, 235
        corticosteroids, 176–77, 236–37
        cough suppressants, 242
        local anesthetics, 242
        neuroleptics, 180, 241–42
        opioids, 179–80, 239–41
        oxygen therapy, 177–79, 178t, 238–39
        progesterone compounds, 237–38
        theophylline, 176, 235–36
    prevalence, 231
    psychological burden, 184–85, 247–48
    quality of life and, 233
    surgical approaches, 181–83
        carotid body resection, 182–83, 245
        lung transplantation, 182, 245
        lung volume reduction, 182, 244–45
        vagotomy, 182–83, 245
    terminal, ethical considerations, 247

Eastern Cooperative Oncology Group Performance
        Status score, in elderly person, 125–26
Eating problems. *See also specific disorder, e.g.*
        Anorexia
    as marker of advanced disease, 38
    reversible causes, 42
Education
    on end-of-life care, 373, 409
        inadequacy, 349–50
    on fatigue management, 278, 279f
    on pain management, 221, 224t, 225
    on palliative care, 50, 75, 409
        hospital-based, 405–6
        in nursing home, 362, 373
    as support to family caregivers, 381–82
Education for Physicians in End-of-Life Care, 373,
        409
Elderly person. *See also* Aging
    abuse of, 74–75
    advance care planning of, 308–9. *See also*
        Advance care planning
    bias against, 72–73

cancer in. *See* Cancer
chemotherapy in, 127–29
comprehensive assessment. *See* Geriatric
    assessment, comprehensive
death and dying. *See* Death and dying
demographics, *xxi*
depression in, 113–14
dialysis in, 193
dyspnea in, 231–32
end-of-life care. *See* End-of-life care
fatigue in, 272
frail. *See* Fraility
goals of medicine for, 48–49
medical illness in. *See* Illness
pain in. *See also* Pain
    assessment, 208–12
    causes, 206
    chronic, 362
    epidemiology, 206
    management, 205–6
palliative care claims of, 51–53. *See also* Palliative
    care
professional obligations to, 57–58
terminally ill. *See* Terminally ill patient
vulnerability, 57–58
Eldernapping, 74
Electrical stimulation
    for stroke patient, 146
    transcutaneous, for pain management, 224t
Electricity, in home palliative care, 399
Emergency care decisions, ethical issues, 65–66
Emergency response systems, in home palliative
    care, 399
Emetic pattern generator, 261, 262f
Emotion-focused coping strategies, for fatigue, 279
Emotion-handling skills, in communication, 318–19,
    319t
Emotional incontinence, in stroke patient, 147
Emotional support, for family caregivers, 382
Emotional symptoms, in delirium, 288
Emotional well-being, in dementia, 33
Empathy, in communication, 318
Emphysema, lung volume reduction surgery for,
    182, 244–45
End-of-life care, 3–15. *See also* Death and dying;
    Terminally ill patient
    attitudes toward
        diversity in, 81–84
        in nursing home, 372
    balance of palliative care and disease-directed care
        in, 337, 337f
    culturally diverse strategies, 87, 87t
    educational programs, 373
    evidence-based medicine, 10
    geographic variability, 4–6, 4f, 5f
    good
        characteristics, 346–47
        system attributes, 347–48
    health care system for, 345–55. *See also* Health
        care system
    medical culture and, 21

Medicare spending and, 6–8, 6f, 7f
    more is better assumption
        influence, 10–11
        validity, 11–12
    in Oregon, 12–15, 12f–13f
    patient preference and, 10, 10f
    physician discussion of, indications, 22
    problems
        insurance coverage, 348–49
        lack of consensus on clinical policy, 348
        lack of continuity and coordination, 348
        lack of focus on advance planning, 349
        lack of focus on palliative care, 349
        provider education, 349
        public education and engagement, 349–50
    sources of variation, 8–11, 8f–10f
    stakeholder roles in reforming
        advocacy groups, 352–53
        federal agencies, 351–52
        federal policy makers, 351
        individual providers, 352
        media, 353
        patient, 353–54
        provider organizations, 352
        public and private health care purchasers,
            352–53
        state policy makers, 352
End-of-Life Nursing Education Consortium, 373,
    409
End-stage dementia. *See also* Dementia
    love's place in, 30–35
    psychiatric disturbances in, 296–97, 297t
    tube feeding in, 37–40, 169
End-stage renal disease
    comorbid disorders, 192
    dialysis for, 193. *See also* Dialysis
        withdrawal, 194–200
    epidemiology, 192
    quality of life in, 193
Endarterectomy, 140, 140t
Endobronchial stents, 183, 246
Endocrine changes, in frail elder, 96–97
Enema, 267
Energy balance and conservation, 279–80
Epidural analgesia, 223t
Error reduction, research on, 76
Erythropoietin
    in end-stage renal disease, 199
    for fatigue, 281, 282t
Esophageal stricture, malignant, dysphagia in, 258,
    259
Estrogen, in frail elder, 96
Ethical issues, 55–77
    advocacy, 76–77
    communication, 61–63
        illness meaning, 62
        information transmittal, 61–62
        informed consent, 62–63
        value differences, 63
    conflict of interest, 71–72
    culture and, 63–64, 81

Ethical issues (*continued*)
  incapacity, 64–66
    emergency care decisions, 65–66
    frail patient with full mental capacity, 64
    global, 65
    partial, 64–65
  informed consent, 62–63
  life-support decisions, 66–70
    advance care planning, 66
    antibiotics, 69
    artificial nutrition and hydration, 68–69
    assisted suicide or euthanasia, 69–70
    futility, 66–67
    mechanical respiration, 68
    withdrawing and withholding interventions, 67–69
  medical professionalism, 55–60
  patient–physician relationship, 60–61
  research for elders with terminal illness, 70–71
  social context, 72–75
  social policy, 75–77
  therapeutic decisions, 60–66
  value differences, 63
Ethics
  medical, sources, 55–57
  professional, 55–56
Ethnicity. *See also* Diversity
  and attitudes toward end-of-life care, 81, 82t
  definition, 80
  and hospice services, 88
  and pain management, 88
Euthanasia, assisted, ethical issues, 69–70
Evidence-based medicine, in end-of-life care, 10
Exercise
  for dyspnea, 243
  for fatigue, 280
  in frail elder, 102–3
  for pain management, 224t, 225
Exercise tests, for dyspnea, 234
Exhaustion, in frail elder, 99t
External beam radiotherapy, for dysphagia, 259

Families of choice, 377
Family caregivers, 376–84
  assignment of responsibilities, 378
  bereavement support, 371, 383–84
  communication with, 370–71, 381–82
  definition, 377–78
  depression in, 394
  epidemiology, 378
  evaluation, in pain assessment, 209
  fatigue in, 282–83
  financial problems, 346, 379
  impact of serious illness on, *xxiii–xxiv*
  issues
    cancer patient, 130–31
    dementia patient, 169–70
    depressed and/or demented medically ill elder, 297–98
    dialysis withdrawal, 195
  frail elder, 106
  nursing home patient, 370–71
  participation, in home palliative care, 386–87
  professional obligations to, 59
  support
    emotional, 382
    during final days, 382–83
    informational/educational, 381–82
    in pain and symptom management, 379–81
    in whole-person care, 59
  unmet needs, 379
  vulnerability, 378–79
  "wish list" of, 381
Fatigue, 271–83
  acute, 274
  assessment, 276–77, 277t
  in cancer patient, 273, 274–75
  causes, 274–75
  central, 273
  chronic, 274
  in chronic obstructive pulmonary disease, 274
  concept, 272–73
  correlates, 275
  definition, 272
  depression and, 275
  in family caregivers, 282–83
  in heart failure, 111, 275
  management, 278–81
    coping strategies, 278–79
    education/cognitive interventions, 278, 279f
    energy balance and conservation, 279–80
    exercise, 280
    nutritional considerations, 280
    pharmacological, 281, 282t
  measurement, 277–78
  multidimensional aspects, 273–74
  in older adult, 272
  peripheral, 273
  prevalence, 271–72
  and quality of life, 275–76
  in stroke patient, 275
Fatigue journal, 278, 279f
Federal agencies, in end-of-life care reform, 351–52
Federal policy makers, in end-of-life care reform, 351
Feeding
  hand, 42
  tube. *See* Tube feeding
Fentanyl, for pain management, 217t
Fever, in dementia, 167–68
Fexofenadine, in end-stage renal disease, 198–99
Fiber, dietary, for constipation, 266
Fibromyalgia, fatigue in, 275
Fictive kin, 377
Field of Dreams effect, 8–9
Financial problems, family caregivers, 346, 379
Fluconazole, for oral candidiasis, 257
Fluids, for constipation, 266
5-Fluorouracil, for colon cancer, 128, 129
Fluoxetine
  for fatigue, 281, 282t
  for pain management, 220, 221t

Fluticasone, for dyspnea, 177, 237
Foley catheter, in home palliative care, 392–93
Folstein Mini-Mental State Examination (MMSE),
        288
Fraility, 93–106
    biologic basis, 95–99, 96f
        disease-induced physiologic changes, 98–99
        endocrine changes, 96–97
        inflammatory changes, 97–98
        molecular changes, 98
        sarcopenia, 96
    clinical presentation, 94–95
    comprehensive geriatric assessment, 100–101
    conceptualization, 94, 94f
    consequences, 94–95, 95t
    cycle, 95, 96f
    definition, 94
    end-stage, 100
    ethical issues, 58, 64
    home care, 386–400. See also Home palliative
            care
    identification
        in hospital setting, 105
        for targeted treatment and prevention, 99–100,
            99t
    as indication for palliative care, xxiii
    palliative care
        alternative models, 105–6
        family involvement, 106
        hospital-based, 105
    primary, 96, 97f, 98
    secondary, 96, 97f, 98–99
    spectrum, 101f
    treatment, 100–106, 101f
        ambulatory, 100–104
        anti-inflammatory interventions, 104
        comprehensive geriatric interdisciplinary
                treatment plans, 101–2
        exercise interventions, 102–3
        geriatric evaluation and management units, 102
        hormonal interventions, 104
        hospitalized, 104–6
        nutritional interventions, 103
        pain interventions, 103–4
        palliative care, 104–6
        physiologic system-targeted interventions, 102
Functional Assessment Rating Scale (FAST), in
        dementia, 162–64, 162t, 163t, 296
Functional Independence Measure (FIM), stroke
        outcome and, 151, 152
Functional status
    definition, 24
    in pain assessment, 208–9
    tube feeding effects on, 39–40
Futility, ethical issues, 66–67

Gabapentin, for pain management, 220, 221t
Gastrointestinal symptoms, 256–68
    anorexia, 259–60
    constipation, 265–67

    in dialysis withdrawal, 197–98
    diarrhea, 267–68
    dysphagia, 258–59
    intestinal obstruction, 263–65
    mouth problems, 256–58
    nausea and vomiting, 260–63
    in nursing home patient, 369
Gastrostomy, percutaneous venting, for intestinal
        obstruction, 264–65
Gastrostomy tubes
    infections and, 39
    informed consent for, 37
Gemcytabine, for prostate cancer, 128
Generosity, just, 34–35
Geriatric assessment, comprehensive
    in cancer, 125–26, 127t
    of frail elder, 100–101
    for home palliative care, 387–89
Geriatric Depression Scale, 295
Geriatric evaluation and management units, for frail
        elder, 102
Geriatric interdisciplinary treatment plans,
        comprehensive, for frail elder, 101–2
Geriatric Pain Measure, 103–4
Glomerular filtration rate, in elderly person, 193
Grief. See Bereavement
Grip strength, in frail elder, 99t
Growth hormone
    in frail elder, 97
    replacement, 104
Growth opportunities, end-of-life, 17–22
Guardian, court-appointed, in decision-making
        hierarchy, 334–35

Hallucinations
    in delirium, 288, 290
    in dementia, 166–67
Haloperidol
    for delirium, 290
    in dementia, 166
    in end-stage renal disease, 198, 199
    for intestinal obstruction, 264
    for nausea and vomiting, 262t
Hand feeding, 42
Head trauma, subarachnoid hemorrhage from, 135
Health Care Finance Administration (HCFA), in
        end-of-life care reform, 351
Health care proxy, 65, 324, 334, 362. See also
        Advance care planning
Health care purchasers, in end-of-life care reform,
        352–53
Health care reimbursement. See Reimbursement
Health care resources
    allocation. See Rationing of palliative care
    and end-of-life care, 8–10, 8f, 9f
    and mortality rates, 11–12
Health care system
    current problems, 348–50
    reforms
        Congressional funding requirements, 354

Health care system (*continued*)
  engineering, 350–55
    implemented, 351
    requirements, 346, 354–55
  vision of better, 346–48
Health expenditures, 346
Health insurance, for end-of-life care, 348–49
Health outcomes, patient-assessed, 23
Health promotion, as goal of medicine, 48
Health-related quality of life (HrQoL), definition, 24
Health Resources and Services Administration (HRSA)
  demonstration funds, 354
  in end-of-life care reform, 351, 352
Health status, and quality of life, distinctions and
      overlap, 23–24, 24f
Heart disease
  death from, symptoms associated with, 112–13
  pain in, 113
Heart failure, 110–19
  clinical features, 111
  definition, 110
  depression in, 113–15
  end-stage renal disease in, 192
  epidemiology, 111–12
  etiology, 110
  fatigue in, 275
  fraility and, 99
  information and communication in
    about prognosis, 115–16
    about treatment regimes, 115
  "Medicaring" in, 118
  pain in, 113
  palliative care, 116–19
  pharmacological management, 111
  prognosis, 112, 115–16
  supportive care, 118
  symptom control, 112–13
Hemiplegia, post-stroke, 145
Hemispatial neglect, dopamine and, 150
Hemodialysis, 193. *See also* Dialysis
Hemorrhage
  intracerebral, 135–36
  subarachnoid, 134–35
Heparin, for stroke therapy, 137
Herpes infection, oral, 257
Home
  death at
    factors associated with, 10
    patient preference for
      and place of death, 10, 10f
      reasons for, 20
  oxygen therapy in, 393, 398
    Medicare reimbursement for, 178, 178t, 239
Home palliative care, 386–400
  adaptation of home, 399–400
  assessment, 387–89
  equipment, 396–99
    for bed-bound patient, 397–98
    for mobility and function, 396–97
    specialized, 398–99
  family caregiver participation, 386–87

general supplies, 396
hospice services, 389–90
nurse's responsibilities, 391–96
  dyspnea, 393
  medications, 395
  mental health, 394
  miscellaneous symptoms and needs, 395–96
  nutrition and hydration, 392
  pain management, 395
  safety, 394–95
  skin care, 393
  spirituality, 393–94
  urinary tract, 392–93
physician's responsibilities, 389–90
reimbursement system, 386, 390
social worker's responsibilities, 390–91
Homocysteine, elevated, stroke risk and, 139
Hopefulness
  in context of bad news, 321
  in context of palliative care, 319
  in dementia, 33
  at end-of-life, 19
Hopelessness, and depression, 294
Hormonal interventions, in frail elder, 104
Hospice services
  collaboration with hospitals, 409–11
  for dementia, 164
  ethnicity and, 88
  funding needs, 354
  in home palliative care, 389–90
  for incapacitated patient, 338–40
  Medicare reimbursement for, 359, 404, *xxii*
  in noncancer conditions, prognostic guidelines,
      360, 360t
  in nursing home, 359–60, 360t
Hospital, dying in, experience of, 403–4
Hospital Anxiety and Depression Scale (HADS), 295
Hospital-based palliative care, 402–11
  barriers to optimal utilization, 409
  collaboration with hospices, 409–11
  educational imperative, 405–6
  fiscal impact, 408–9
  impact, 406
  at Mount Sinai Hospital, case study, 406–8, 407f,
      408f
  prevalence, 406
  role of, 404
  team structure and function, 404–5
Hospital beds
  electric, 397
  and hospitalization rate, 8–9, 8f
  and mortality rates, 11–12
Hospitalization
  at end-of-life
    death in hospital and, 10, 10f
    geographic variability, 4, 4f–5f
  of incapacitated patient, 338
  of nursing home patient, 363, 364
Hoyer lift, 397
Human subject concerns, in research for elders with
      terminal illness, 70–71

Humidified air, for dyspnea, 244
Hunger, in terminally ill patient, 40, 368–69
Hurley Discomfort Scale, 211–12
Hydration
    artificial, 36–43. *See also* Tube feeding
        in dementia, 169
        ethical issues, 68–69
        in incapacitated patient, 337–38
        in nursing home patient, 364–67
    in home palliative care, 392
    by hypodermoclysis, for delirium, 290
Hydrocodone, for pain management, 217t
Hydromorphone
    for dyspnea, 179, 240
    for pain management, 217t
Hyoscine, for nausea and vomiting, 262t
Hypercalcemia, nausea and vomiting in, 260, 261
Hyperhomocysteinemia, stroke risk and, 139
Hyperpnea, definition, 230
Hypertension
    intracerebral hemorrhage and, 135
    stroke risk and, 138
Hyperventilation, definition, 230
Hypoxemia, chronic obstructive pulmonary disease
        and, oxygen therapy, 177, 238–39

Ibuprofen, for pain management, 216t
Illness
    advanced
        communication in
            effective, 317–19
            present state, 314–15
        eating problems as marker of, 38
        in older adult, experience of, *xxii–xxiii*
    chronic, staging of palliative care during, *xxv,
        xxvi(t)–xxvii(t)*
    personal meaning of, 62
        nationality and, 83
    physiologic changes due to, in frail elder, 98–99
    prevention, as goal of medicine, 48
    serious
        cultural inexperience with, 350
        culturally diverse strategies of caring for, 87,
            87t
        demography of, *xxi–xxii*
        impact on patient and families, *xxiii–xxiv*
        "serious and complex," establishing category of,
            354
    trajectory, advance care planning and, 308–9
Immobility, post-stroke, 145–46
Implantable pumps, for pain management, 223t
Incapacitated patient, 64–66
    communication issues, 326–27
    emergency care decisions, 65–66
    global, 65
    palliative care and hospice for, 338–40
    partial, 64–65
    in research for elders with terminal illness, 70
    surrogate decision making for
        challenges, 335–36

        consensus-based approach, 336–38, 337f
        hierarchy, 334, 334t
        legal involvement, 334–35
Incontinence
    emotional, in stroke patient, 147
    urinary, in dementia, 168
Individual providers, in end-of-life care reform, 352
Infection
    in dementia, 167–68
    oral, 257
    tube feeding and, 39
Inflammatory mediators, in frail elder, 97–98
Information transmittal
    disagreements about, 87–88
    ethical issues, 61–62
    in heart failure, 115–16
Informational model, in patient–physician
        relationship, 60
Informational support, to family caregivers, 381–82
Informed consent
    ethical issues, 62–63
    for tube feeding, 37
Insomnia, in dementia, 167
Inspiratory muscle training, for dyspnea, 243
Instructional model, in patient–physician
        relationship, 60
Insulin-like growth factor, in frail elder, 97
Intensive care
    and mortality rates, 11
    during terminal hospitalization
        geographic variability, 4, 4f–5f
        in Oregon, 12, 12f, 13f
Interleukin-6, in frail elder, 97–98
Interstitial lung disease
    dyspnea in. *See* Dyspnea
    idiopathic pulmonary fibrosis in, 177, 237
    prednisone-responsive, 177, 237
Interstitial pneumonitis, usual, 177, 237
Intestinal obstruction, 263–65
    causes, 263
    clinical assessment, 263
    management, 263–65
Intracerebral hemorrhage, 135–36
Intrathecal analgesia, 223t
Ipratropium bromide, for dyspnea, 175, 235
Irinotecan (CPT-11), for colon cancer, 129
Ischemic stroke, 136–37
Ispaghula, for constipation, 267
Itraconazole, for oral candidiasis, 257

Japanese culture, dementia in, 32
Joint mobilization, for stroke rehabilitation, 141
Judgment, substituted, in global incapacity, 65
Just generosity, 34–35

Karnovsky score, in elderly person, 126
Ketoconazole, for oral candidiasis, 257
Ketorolac, for pain management, 216t
Kin, fictive, 377

Lactulose, for constipation, 267
Lacunar stroke, 136
Large vessel atherothrombotic stroke, 136–37
Laxatives
    lubricant, 267
    oral, 266–67
    rectal, 267
    softening/osmotic, 266–67
    stimulant, 266
    surfactant, 267
LEARN acronym, 86–87
Leukemia, 123, 125f
Levodopa, for stroke-related impairments, 150
Levomepromazine
    for intestinal obstruction, 264
    for nausea and vomiting, 261, 262t
Lewy bodies
    dementia with, 160–61
    in Parkinson's disease, 161
Lidocaine, for pain management, 220, 221t
Life expectancy
    African Americans, 84
    changes in, 402, xxi
Life-prolonging care, palliative care and,
        simultaneous, xxvii–xxviii, xxviii(f)
Life review, 21, 22
Life-support decisions, 66–70
    advance care planning, 66
    antibiotics, 69
    artificial nutrition and hydration, 68–69
    assisted suicide or euthanasia, 69–70
    futility, 66–67
    mechanical respiration, 68
    withdrawing and withholding interventions,
        67–69
Life-sustaining treatment
    in incapacitated patient, 337–38
    racial differences, 84–85
Lighting, in home palliative care, 399
Listening, to family caregivers, 382
Living will, 324, 334, 362. See also Advance care
        planning
Local anesthetics
    for dyspnea, 242
    for pain management, 220, 221t
Loperamide, for diarrhea, 268
Lorazepam
    for delirium, 166
    for dyspnea, 169, 242
Love
    in palliative care, 30–31
    and personhood, 31–32
    quality of, as love's creation, 32–34
    vulnerability and, 34–35
Lumbar sympathetic blockade, for pain
        management, 223t
Lung cancer
    dyspnea in, 174, 183–84, 183t, 240, 245–47
    in elderly person, 123, 124, 124f, 125f
    incidence, 173
    psychological burden, 184–85

Lung transplantation, for dyspnea, 182, 245
Lung volume reduction surgery, for dyspnea, 182

Magnesium, for constipation, 267
Malnutrition. See also Nutrition
    in dementia, tube feeding effects, 37–40
    nutrition and, 37
McGill Pain Questionnaire, 209
Mechanical respiration, ethical issues, 68
Media, in end-of-life care reform, 353
Medicaid
    in end-of-life care reform, 352
    nursing home care under, hospice benefit and, 359
Medical culture, and end-of-life care, 21
Medical ethics, sources, 55–57. See also Ethical issues
Medical professionalism, 55–60. See also
        Professionalism
Medical specialist visits
    geographic variability, 5
    supply of specialists and, 9, 9f
Medicare
    in end-of-life care reform, 352–53
    reimbursement
        for home oxygen therapy, 178, 178t, 239
        for hospice services, 359, 404, xxii
    spending, and end-of-life care, 6–8, 6f, 7f
Medicare Payment Advisory Commission
        (MedPAC), in end-of-life care reform, 351
"Medicaring," in heart failure, 118
Medications, in home palliative care, 395
Medicine
    evidence-based, in end-of-life care, 10
    goals of
        description, 47–48
        for elderly person, 48–49
        ethics and, 56, 58–59
Medroxyprogesterone
    for anorexia, 260
    for dyspnea, 238
Megestrol acetate, for anorexia, 260
Memorial Delirium Assessment Scale, 288
Memorial services
    at dialysis units, 199–200
    in nursing home, 372
Mental capacity. See Capacity; Incapacitated patient
Mental health, in home palliative care, 394
Mental status examination, 288
Meperidine, adverse effects, 197, 219
Mesalazine, for diarrhea, 268
Mesothelioma, malignant, chemotherapy, 128
Methadone, for pain management, 219
Methylcellulose, for constipation, 267
Methylphenidate
    in dementia, 167
    for fatigue, 281, 282t
    for stroke patient, 148, 149
Metoclopramide
    in end-stage renal disease, 198
    for intestinal obstruction, 264
    for nausea and vomiting, 262–63, 262t

Metronidazole, for diarrhea, 268
Mexiletine, for pain management, 220, 221t
Miami, Florida, Medicare spending, 6, 7–8, 7f
Minimum Data Set, 361
Minneapolis, Minnesota, Medicare spending, 6, 7–8, 7f
Mixed pain syndromes, 207
Mobility, constipation and, 266
Mobility devices, in home palliative care, 396–97
Molecular changes, in frail elder, 98
Morality, in patient–physician relationship, 61
Morphine
    for dyspnea, 169, 179, 239, 240, 241
    in end-stage renal disease, 197
    for pain management
        continuous infusions, 222, 223t
        in dementia, 165
        overview, 217t
Mortality
    dialysis and, 193
    health care resources and, 11–12
    socioeconomic status and, 84
    tube feeding and, 38
Mount Sinai Hospital, hospital-based palliative care, 406–8, 407f, 408f
Mouth, dry, management, 256–57
Mouth care, in dialysis withdrawal, 198
Movement therapy, constraint-induced, for stroke patient, 146
Mucositis, 257
Muscle relaxants, for pain management
    continuous infusions, 222, 223t
    overview, 221t
Musculoskeletal examination, in pain assessment, 208
Myocardial infarction, depression after, 114
Myoclonus, in dialysis withdrawal, 199
Myofascial pain, 222

Nabilone, 238
Nabumetone, 216t
Naproxen, 216t
Nasogastric tubes, infections and, 39
National Comprehensive Cancer Network guidelines, for older cancer patient, 126, 127t
National Hospice and Palliative Organization
    dementia guidelines, 163–64, 163t
    prognostic guidelines in noncancer conditions, 360, 360t
National Institutes of Health (NIH), in end-of-life care reform, 351
Nationality
    and attitudes toward end-of-life care, 83
    and experience and treatment of aging and dying, 84
Nausea and vomiting
    anticipatory, 261–62
    causes, 261–62
    clinical assessment, 260–61

    in end-stage renal disease, 197–98
    management, 261–63, 262f, 262t
    from opioids, 218
Navajos, use of language, 86
Nebulizer, home, 398
Nefazodone, 185, 248
Neglect, 74
Nerve block
    for pain management, 223t
    for post-stroke spasticity, 146–47
Neuralgia, trigeminal, carbamazepine for, 220
Neuroablation, for pain management, 223t
Neuroleptics
    for delirium, 290
    for dyspnea, 180, 241–42
Neurological examination, in pain assessment, 208
Neuropathic pain, 207, 220
Neurostimulation, for pain management, 223t
Neurosurgical pain management, 222, 223t
NMDA inhibitors, for pain management, 221t
Nociceptive pain, 207
Noncompliance, in heart failure patient, 115
Noninvasive positive pressure ventilation, for dyspnea, 180–81, 243–44
Nonsteroidal antiinflammatory drugs
    in end-stage renal disease, 197
    for pain management, 214–15, 216t
Noradrenergic system, in stroke-related impairments, 149–50
Nortriptyline
    for fatigue, 282t
    for post-stroke depression, 148
Nurse, role
    in home palliative care, 391–96
    in stroke rehabilitation, 144
Nursing home(s)
    accreditation, 358, 373–74
    attitudes toward end-of-life care, 372
    characteristics, 358–59
    communication issues, 369–71
    grief and bereavement, 371–72
    palliative care
        barriers, 357–58, 361–62
        current referrals, 361
        education program, 362, 373
        potential patients, 360–61, 360t
        program development, 372–74
        special issues, 361–72
    reimbursement issues, 359
Nursing home patient
    advance care planning, 362–67, 365f–366f
    care levels for, 338t
    hospice services, 359–60, 360t
    pain management, 206, 367–68
    sentinel decisions, 363–67
        antibiotics, 367
        artificial hydration and nutrition, 364–67
        cardiopulmonary resuscitation, 363–64
        diagnostic tests, 364
        hospitalization, 363, 364
    symptom management, 367–69

Nutrition. *See also* Malnutrition
  artificial, 36–43. *See also* Tube feeding
    in dementia, 169
      ethical issues, 68–69
      in nursing home patient, 364–67
    in cachectic patient, 41–43
    fatigue and, 280
    in frail elder, 103
    in home palliative care, 392
    malnutrition and, 37
Nystatin, for oral candidiasis, 257

Obsessive-compulsive disorder, anxiety in, 291, 292
Obstructive pulmonary disease, chronic. *See* Chronic
    obstructive pulmonary disease
Occupational therapist, role in stroke rehabilitation,
    143–44
Occupational therapy
  for pain management, 224t
  for stroke rehabilitation, 142
Octreotide
  for diarrhea, 268
  for intestinal obstruction, 264
Odor control, in home palliative care, 395
Olanzapine, in dementia, 166
Ondansetron
  in end-stage renal disease, 198
  for nausea and vomiting, 262, 262t
Opioids
  addiction to, 218
  for anxiety, 292
  cognitive impairment from, 215, 218
  constipation from, 165, 215, 218, 265
  delirium from, 165–66, 289
  in dementia, 165–66
  dependence on, 218
  for diarrhea, 268
  drowsiness from, 215, 218
  for dyspnea, 179–80, 239–41, 368
  iatrogenic pseudoaddiction to, 219
  nausea from, 218
  in nursing home patient, 368
  for pain management
    continuous infusions, 222, 223t
    overview, 215, 217t, 218–19
  respiratory depression from, 215, 218
  rotation, for delirium, 290
  side effects, 180
  for tachypnea, 368
  tolerance to, 215
  withdrawal reactions, 218
OPQRST assessment, of dyspnea, 232, 232t
Oral infections, 257
Oral suction device, in home palliative care, 398
Orange County, California, Medicare spending,
    7–8, 7f
Oregon, end-of-life care practices, 12–15, 12f–13f
Orthostasis, post-stroke, 145
Orthotic devices, for stroke patient, 146
Orthotist, role in stroke rehabilitation, 145

Outcome measures
  development, 76
  on quality of death and dying, 26–27
Oxycodone, 217t
Oxygen concentrator, 398
Oxygen therapy
  for dyspnea, 177–79, 178t, 238–39
  home, 393, 398
    Medicare reimbursement for, 178, 178t, 239

Paclitaxel, for breast cancer, 128
Pain, 205–25
  assessment
    in cognitively impaired patient, 211–12
    in elderly person, 208–12
    in frail elder, 103–4
    history, 208
    in nursing home patient, 367–68
    physical examination, 208–9
    scales, 210–11, 210t
  breakthrough, 214
  chronic, 208, 362
  in dementia, 164–65
  in elderly person
    causes, 206
    epidemiology, 206
  in heart failure, 113
  mixed, 207
  myofascial, 222
  neuropathic, 207
  nociceptive, 207
  perception, age-related changes, 207–8
  physiology, 206–7
  psychological, 207
  unrelieved, negative outcomes associated with,
    206
Pain management, 212–25
  analgesics for, 213–19
    acetaminophen, 214, 216t
    nonsteroidal antiinflammatory drugs, 214–15,
      216t
    opioids, 215, 217t, 218–19
    route of administration, 213–14
    timing, 214
  anesthetic and neurosurgical approaches, 222, 223t
  barriers, 205
  cultural differences, 86
  in dialysis withdrawal, 196–97
  economic issues, 213
  in elderly person, 205–6, *xxiii*
  ethnic differences, 88
  family caregiver support, 379–81
  in frail elder, 103–4
  as goal of medicine, 48
  in home palliative care, 395
  nondrug strategies, 222, 224t, 225
  nonopioid medications for, 219–22, 221t
  in nursing home, 367–68
  placebos in, 214
  WHO approach, 212–13, 212f

Palliative care. *See also* End-of-life care
  barriers to, 49–50, 357–58, 409
  cost effectiveness, 50
  definition, 402
  education on, 50, 75, 409. *See also* Education
    hospital-based, 405–6
    in nursing home, 362, 373
  ethical aspects. *See* Ethical issues
  family involvement. *See* Family caregivers
  fraility as indication for, *xxiii*
  geriatric
    markers for initiation, *xxiv–xxv, xxv(t)*
    staging, *xxv, xxvi(t)–xxvii(t)*
  in heart failure, 116–19
  in home, 386–400. *See also* Home palliative care
  hope in context of, 319
  hospital-based, 402–11. *See also* Hospital-based
    palliative care
  for hospitalized frail elder, 104–6
  for incapacitated patient, 338–40
  lack of focus on, 349
  and life-prolonging care, simultaneous,
    xxvii–xxviii, xxviii(f)
  love in, 30–31
  in nursing home, 357–74. *See also* Nursing home,
    palliative care
  rationing, 46–53. *See also* Rationing of palliative
    care
  reimbursement issues, 359, 386, 390
  transition to, communication about, 324–25,
    325t
Palliative care team
  family caregiver interventions, 381–82
  hospital-based, 404–5
  in nursing home, 369–70
  in whole-person care, 59–60
Pancreatic enzyme replacement, for diarrhea, 268
Panic disorder, anxiety in, 292
Panic sensations, in advanced lung disease, 185, 248
Paraffin, for constipation, 267
Paralysis, post-stroke, 145–46
Parkinson's disease
  dementia in, 161. *See also* Dementia
  hallucinations in, 166
  sleep disorders in, 167
Paroxetine
  in advanced lung disease, 185, 248
  for fatigue, 281, 282t
Paternalistic model, in patient–physician
    relationship, 60
Patient(s)
  education
    on end-of-life care, 349–50
    on pain management, 221, 224t, 225
  end-of-life care preference of, place of death and,
    10, 10f
  in end-of-life care reform, 353–54
Patient-centered social policy, professional advocacy
    for, 76–77
Patient–physician relationship, 60–61
Pemoline, for fatigue, 281, 282t

Pentazocine, adverse effects, 219
Perceptual disturbances, in delirium, 288
Percutaneous esophageal-gastric (PEG) tube, in
    home palliative care, 392
Percutaneous gastrostomy tube, in home palliative
    care, 398
Peripheral vascular disease, end-stage renal disease
    in, 192
Peritoneal dialysis, 193. *See also* Dialysis
Personhood, love and, 31–32
Phenothiazines, for nausea and vomiting, 261
Physiatrist, role in stroke rehabilitation, 141, 143
Physical activity. *See also* Exercise
  fraility and, 99–100, 99t
Physical modalities, for pain management, 224t
Physical therapist, role in stroke rehabilitation, 143
Physical therapy
  for pain management, 224t
  for stroke rehabilitation, 141
Physician
  care intensity at end-of-life, geographic variability,
    4–6, 5f
  death anxiety, 316
  home visits, 389
  role in home palliative care, 389–90
  visits to dying patient, geographic variability, 4–5,
    5f
Physician-assisted suicide, 20, 69–70
Physician Orders for Life-Sustaining Treatment
    (POLST), 68
  in nursing home, 364, 365f–366f, 370
  in Oregon, 13–14
Physician-patient relationship, 60–61
Pick's disease, dementia in, 161
Pilocarpine, for dry mouth, 257
Placebo, in pain management, 214
Pleural effusion, malignant, 183–84, 245–46
Pleurodesis, for malignant pleural effusions, 183,
    246
Pneumonia
  aspiration, tube feeding and, 38–39
  in dementia, 168
Pneumonitis
  aspiration, tube feeding and, 38–39
  interstitial, usual, 177, 237
Polyethylene glycol, for constipation, 267
Positioning, for dyspnea, 244
Post-traumatic stress disorder, anxiety in, 291, 292
Practice norms and standards
  adherence to, 56–57
  development, 76
Prayer, in dementia, 33–34
Prednisolone, for dyspnea, 237
Prednisone
  for dyspnea, 176, 177, 236, 237
  for fatigue, 281, 282t
Pressure sores
  in dementia, 168
  in end-stage renal disease, 198
  in home palliative care, 393
  tube feeding and, 39

Priority setting
in palliative care for elderly person, 52–53
in rationing of palliative care, 49–51
Problem-focused coping strategies, for fatigue, 279
Prochlorperazine, for dyspnea, 242
Professional ethics, 55–56. *See also* Ethical issues
Professionalism
goals of care, 58–59
obligations to elders and terminally ill, 57–58
obligations to family and community, 59
respectful therapeutic relationship, 59
sources, 55–56
team orientation, 59–60
whole-person care, 59
Progesterone compounds
for anorexia, 260
for dyspnea, 237–38
Prognostic guidelines, in noncancer conditions, 360, 360t
Program for All-Inclusive Care of the Elderly, 105–6
Progressive muscle relaxation, for dyspnea, 243
Progressive resistance exercise, in frail elder, 102–3
Promethazine, for dyspnea, 180, 241, 242
Propensity to refer index, geographic variability, 5–6
Propoxyphene, in end-stage renal disease, adverse effects, 197
Prostate cancer, in elderly person, 123, 124f, 125f
Provider organizations, in end-of-life care reform, 352
Proxy, health care, 65, 324, 334, 362. *See also* Advance care planning
Pruritus, in dialysis withdrawal, 198–99
Psychological evaluation, in pain assessment, 209
Psychological pain, 207
Psychologist, role in stroke rehabilitation, 144
Psychosocial issues, in dialysis withdrawal, 195–96
Psychotherapy
for depressed heart failure patient, 115
for depression, 295, 295t
Public, in end-of-life care reform, 353–54
Pulmonary disease
advanced. *See* Advanced lung disease
chronic obstructive. *See* Chronic obstructive pulmonary disease
Pulmonary fibrosis, idiopathic, 177, 237
Pulmonary rehabilitation, for dyspnea, 180–81, 242–43
Pulmonology, interventional, for lung cancer, 183, 246

Quality
of death and dying, 26–27
of end-of-life care, 26
of life
aging and, 73–74
definition, 24
dyspnea and, 233
at end of life
implications for clinical practice, 27
measurement, 26
patient treatment preference and, 24–26
physician prediction of patient treatment preference and, 26

in end-stage renal disease, 193
fatigue and, 275–76
health status and, distinctions and overlap, 23–24, 24f
of love, 32–34
Quality improvement, funding needs, 354
Questions, dreaded, 325–26

Race. *See also* Diversity
and attitudes toward end-of-life care, 82–83
definition, 79–80
and experience and treatment of aging and dying, 84–85
Radiation therapy
for dysphagia, 259
in elderly person, 129–30
fatigue from, 275
for lung cancer, 184, 247
Ramipril, taste alterations from, 258
Range of motion (ROM) exercises, for stroke rehabilitation, 141, 146
Rationing of palliative care, 46–53
for elderly person, 51–53
goals of medicine in, 47–48
age and, 48–49
priority setting, 49–51
Recreational therapist, role in stroke rehabilitation, 144–45
Rectal laxatives, 267
Referral propensity, geographic variability, 5–6
Refocoxib, for pain management, 215, 216t
Rehabilitation nurse, role in stroke rehabilitation, 144
Rehabilitation psychologist, role in stroke rehabilitation, 144
Reimbursement issues, 50
home palliative care, 386, 390
mismatch with needs of older adult, *xxiv*
nursing home palliative care, 359
Relational well-being, in dementia, 33
Relaxation and distraction techniques, for pain management, 224t
Religion, and attitudes toward end-of-life care, 83–84
Renal failure. *See* End-stage renal disease
Research
for elders with terminal illness, ethical issues, 70–71
needs, 76
Resident Assessment Instrument for Palliative Care, 388–89
Resistance exercise, in frail elder, 102–3
Resource allocation. *See* Rationing of palliative care
Respect, in whole-person care, 59–60
Respiratory depression, from opioids, 215, 218
Respite period, for family caregivers, 394
Restlessness
in home palliative care, 395
terminal, in nursing home patient, 369
Risperidone, for delirium, 166
Roemer's law, 8–9
Role morality, in patient–physician relationship, 61

Saccular aneurysm, subarachnoid hemorrhage from, 134, 135
Safety, in home palliative care, 394–95
Saliva, artificial, 257
Salivary flow, stimulation, 257
Salsalate, for pain management, 215, 216t
Sarcopenia, in frail elder, 96
Scopolamine
    for colic, 264
    for nausea and vomiting, 261
Sedation, for delirium, 290–91
Senna, for constipation, 266
Serotonin reuptake inhibitors, selective
    in advanced lung disease, 184–85, 248
    for anxiety, 292
    in dementia, 167
    for depression, 295
    for fatigue, 281, 282t
    for post-stroke depression, 148
Sertraline
    in advanced lung disease, 185, 248
    for fatigue, 282t
    in heart failure patient, 114
Service capacity, development, 75–76
Sex steroids, in frail elder, 96–97
Situational model, in patient–physician relationship, 60
Skeletal muscle, loss, in frail elder, 96
Skin care
    in dementia, 168
    in dialysis withdrawal, 198
    in home palliative care, 393
Sleep disorders, in dementia, 167
Sleep/rest patterns, assessment, 277, 277t
Slide boards, in home palliative care, 396
Sloan Kettering Pain Card, 210t
Smoking, stroke risk and, 139
Social evaluation, in pain assessment, 209
Social issues, ethical aspects, 72–75
Social policy, ethical issues, 75–77
Social worker, role
    in home palliative care, 390–91
    in stroke rehabilitation, 145
Socioeconomic status
    and attitudes toward end-of-life care, 83
    and experience and treatment of aging and dying, 84–85
Sodium picosulfate, for constipation, 266
Spasticity, post-stroke, 146–47
Speech-language pathologist, role in stroke rehabilitation, 144
Spinal cord compression, radiation therapy, 129
Spiritual well-being, in dementia, 33–34
Spirituality
    in Alzheimer's disease caregivers, 33
    assessment, 87t
    and attitudes toward end-of-life care, 83–84
    in home palliative care, 393–94
Spironolactone, for heart failure, 111
Standards of care
    adherence to, 56–57
    development, 76

State policy makers, in end-of-life care reform, 352
Statins, for stroke prevention, 138
Stellate ganglia blockade, for pain management, 223t
Steroids. See also Corticosteroids
    for intestinal obstruction, 264
    sex, in frail elder, 96–97
Stimulants
    for depression, 296
    for fatigue, 281, 282t
    for post-stroke depression, 148
Stool samples, in diarrhea, 268
Stool softeners, for intestinal obstruction, 264
Stress
    caregiving, 378–79
    post-traumatic, 291, 292
Stroke, 134–52
    acute therapy, 137–38, 137t
    atrial fibrillation and, 136, 139
    fatigue after, 275
    from intracerebral hemorrhage, 135–36
    ischemic, 136–37
    outcomes, 151–52
    prevention, 138–40, 140t
    rehabilitation, 141–48
        for depression, 147–48
        inpatient, 142–43
        for paralysis and immobility, 145–46
        pharmacological interventions to improve recovery, 148–51
        prescription, 142
        process, 141–43
        for spasticity, 146–47
        team, 141t, 143–45
    from subarachnoid hemorrhage, 134–35
Subarachnoid hemorrhage, 134–35
Substance P inhibitors, for pain management, 221t
Substituted judgment
    in decision-making hierarchy, 334
    in global incapacity, 65
Sucralfate, for mucositis, 257
Suffering, relief of, as goal of medicine, 48
Suicide
    assisted, 20, 69–70
    dialysis withdrawal and, 196
Supportive care, in heart failure, 118
Suppositories, rectal, for constipation, 267
Surgery, fatigue from, 275
Surrogate decision making. See also Advance care planning
    challenges, 335–36
    communication issues, 324
    consensus-based approach, 336–38, 337f
    hierarchy, 334, 334t
    legal involvement, 334–35
Survival, tube feeding and, 38
Symptom management
    in dementia, 164–69
    family caregiver support, 379–81
    in nursing home, 367–69

Tachypnea
  definition, 230
  in nursing home patient, 368
Tai-chi balance intervention, in frail elder, 102–3
Tamoxifen, for breast cancer, 129
Taste alterations, 257–58
Team. See Palliative care team
Terminally ill patient. See also Death and dying;
      End-of-life care
  advance care planning in, 311–13
  family caregivers of
      financial problems, 379
      unmet needs, 379
      vulnerability, 378–79
  hunger and thirst in, 40, 368–69
  professional obligations to, 57–58
  tube feeding in
      alternatives to, 41–43
      effectiveness, 37–40
      symptoms due to, 40–41
Testosterone, in frail elder, 96
Theophylline, for dyspnea, 176, 236–37
Therapeutic decisions, ethical issues, 60–66
Therapeutic relationship, respectful, 59
Thirst, in terminally ill patient, 40, 368–69
Thoracentesis, for malignant pleural effusions, 183,
      246
Thoracoscopy, medical, for malignant pleural
      effusions, 183, 246
Thrombolysis, for stroke, 137, 137t
Thyroid cancer, in elderly person, 125
Ticlopidine, for stroke prevention, 139
Tissue plasminogen activator, for stroke, 137
Tolerance, to opioids, 215
Tracheostomy, in home palliative care, 396
Tramadol, for pain management, 217t
Transcutaneous electrical nerve stimulation, for pain
      management, 224t
Trazodone
  in advanced lung disease, 185, 248
  in dementia, 167
  for fatigue, 281, 282t
  for post-stroke depression, 148
Triamcinolone, for dyspnea, 176–77, 236
Tricyclic antidepressants
  in advanced lung disease, 185, 248
  for fatigue, 282t
  in heart failure patient, 114
  for pain management, 220, 221t
  for post-stroke depression, 148
Trigeminal neuralgia, carbamazepine for, 220
Trigger point injections, for myofascial pain, 222
Triglycerides, stroke risk and, 138–39
Trustworthiness, 56
Tube feeding, 37–43
  alternatives to, helping families think about,
      41–43
  decision making about, 36–37
  in dementia, 37–40, 169
  effects
      aspiration, 38–39
      functional abilities, 39–40

infections, 39
pressure sores, 39
survival, 38
  ethical issues, 68–69
  in home palliative care, 392
  in incapacitated patient, 337–38
  informed consent for, 37
  in nursing home patient, 364–67
  symptoms due to, 40–41

Universal vulnerability, 34–35
Uremia
  in end-stage renal disease, 198
  itching in, 198
  nausea and vomiting from, 261
Urinary incontinence, in dementia, 168
Urinary tract, in home palliative care, 392–93
Usual interstitial pneumonitis, in idiopathic
      pulmonary fibrosis, 177, 237

Vagotomy, for advanced lung disease, 182–83,
      245
Values
  differences, 63, 85. See also Diversity
  patient, exploring, 323–24
  vulnerable, protection of, 63
Vancomycin, for diarrhea, 268
Vascular dementia, 160
Ventilation
  mechanical, ethical issues, 68
  positive pressure, noninvasive, for dyspnea,
      180–81, 243–44
Ventilator, home, 398–99
Ventilatory capacity, drugs that increase, 175–77,
      235–38
Ventilatory demand, drugs that decrease, 177–79,
      238–39
Visual analogue pain scale, 210t
Vocational counselor, role in stroke rehabilitation,
      145
Vomiting. See Nausea and vomiting
Vomiting center, 261, 262f
Vulnerability
  of elders and terminally ill, 57–58
  medical professionalism and, 57
  universal, 34–35

Walkers, in home palliative care, 396
Walking speed, in frail elder, 99t
Warfarin, for stroke prevention, 139
Wasting syndrome, in frail elder, 98–99
Weight loss, in frail elder, 99–100, 99t
Wheelchairs, in home palliative care, 396
Whole-person care, 59–60
Withdrawing and withholding interventions, ethical
      issues, 67–69
Women, as caregivers, 378
World Health Organization, pain management
      approach, 212–13, 212f